9 KEYS TO OPTIMAL HEALTH

CRACKING THE METABOLIC CODE

JAMES B. LaVALLE, R.Ph., C.C.N., N.D.
with STACY LUNDIN YALE, R.N., B.S.N.

To Paris! A wish of Vibrant Health to you + your family!

Basic Health
PUBLICATIONS, INC.

The information contained in this book is based upon the research and personal and professional experiences of the author. It is not intended as a substitute for consulting with your physician or other healthcare provider. Any attempt to diagnose and treat an illness should be done under the direction of a healthcare professional.

The publisher does not advocate the use of any particular healthcare protocol but believes the information in this book should be available to the public. The publisher and author are not responsible for any adverse effects or consequences resulting from the use of the suggestions, preparations, or procedures discussed in this book. Should the reader have any questions concerning the appropriateness of any procedures or preparation mentioned, the author and the publisher strongly suggest consulting a professional healthcare advisor.

Basic Health Publications, Inc.
8200 Boulevard East
North Bergen, NJ 07047
1-201-868-8336

Library of Congress Cataloging-in-Publication Data

LaValle, James B.
    Cracking the metabolic code : 9 keys to optimal health / by James
LaValle with Stacy Yale.
        p. cm.
Includes bibliographical references and index.
    ISBN 1-59120-011-3
    1. Health. 2. Medicine, Popular. 3. Metabolism. I. Yale, Stacy.
II. Title.

    RA776.L418   2004
    613—dc22

                                    2003024686

Editor: Cheryl Hirsch
Typesetting/Book design: Gary A. Rosenberg
Cover design: Mike Stromberg

Printed in the United States of America

10   9   8   7   6   5   4   3   2

Contents

Dedication

When I considered the list of people this book should be dedicated to, I first had to realize that when you have traveled a long journey there are so many people to mention. Both the journey of the creation of this book and the journey of my professional lifetime seem long, sometimes complex, and yet very rewarding. In fact, I have written several other books in the process of putting this book together. While some of the people noted here I met along my way, others have happily accompanied me for a portion of my journey.

And so, to the following, this book is dedicated: First, to David Polen, D.C., who passed away a little over a year ago. He gave unselfishly to his friends, family, and patients. Then, to my mentor and dear friend Alexander Wood, D.C., N.D., from whom I have learned so much over the years. To my family—my brother Lou, you have always been my pillar of strength, especially in those tough and confusing teenage years; to my mom and dad who just love me and I need say no more; to my wife, Laura, who has brought a real sense of peace and perspective into my life; to my son Christian, who at age four teaches me so much about the joy of living.

This book is also dedicated to my partners at the Living Longer Institute: Steve Pomeranz, M.D., and John Zerbe, M.D., thank you for the opportunity to build such a dynamic and integrative facility. And special thanks to my staff at Living Longer: Pam Cordes, R.N., M.S., N.D., and Linda Solitz, Annette Hyde, and Maureen Pelletier, M.D., who are the real backbone to my work.

Acknowledgments

I must acknowledge those who have helped me write this book. This book is a synthesis of a lot of great work and research that has come before it. There are too many authors to mention by name, but to all the professionals out there who are dedicated to the teaching and mentoring process in integrative medicine, I commend your tireless efforts.

And I, myself, have the best colleagues that anyone could ask for. Without the help of Ernie Hawkins, Stacy Yale, and Ross Pelton, this book would not have happened—my thanks and appreciation to you for your work. This book has been a three-year project and a complex one that likely would never have been completed without your help. I must also make a special note of thanks to my wife, Laura, who is not only a supportive and very patient spouse, but also a talented professional in nutrition and dietetics, who contributed endless hours of editorial help.

I would like to thank Cheryl Hirsch, a very skilled and patient editor, who took my thoughts, ideas, and ramblings, and worked magic. Thank you so much.

Lastly, I would like to thank my publisher Norman Goldfind for giving me the opportunity to write this book—a book I have wanted to write for a very long time—and for sticking with it when deadlines came and went, and for seeing through this tough project. I do not underestimate the commitment you showed. Thank you.

Foreword

At some point in life, each of us begins to slowly turn an invisible corner. It is often so subtle and so gradual that we have no awareness of its effect on our lives. We look in the mirror and something about us looks a little different. We climb a flight of stairs and we feel winded, we move up another size in our clothes, and so on. We might tend to shrug these things off as "ordinary" age-related changes. But if we peered deep inside the body, we would realize that a slow, steady shift in our body chemistry has been happening and it affects virtually all of our systems. Our nervous system begins to send signals that begin to alter hormonal and endocrine function, and this gives rise to changes in blood chemistry.

A visit to the doctor confirms this. Cholesterol is slightly up, triglycerides are high, blood pressure has nudged itself out of the comfort zone, and blood sugar levels look a little suspicious. The doctor may also note the obvious. You are overweight and the excess weight will affect your health. The doctor's earnest advice to you is to eat differently, watch your sugar intake, and get some regular exercise.

Recent studies now reveal that roughly 150 million Americans are overweight and that this will lead to an already growing epidemic of diabetes, cardiovascular disease, and other life-threatening health problems. For most of us, though, these are just statistics. Some startling new evidence may make this a bit more personal and . . . a bit more urgent. Those extra pounds that you've been accumulating are not just uncomfortable baggage. A growing number of studies conducted over the past five years have revealed that fat cells are virtual *inflammation factories.* This is especially true of the fat that accumulates around the belly.

As fat cells grow, they produce larger and large amounts of chemicals known as *cytokines.* These cytokines have cumbersome names such as *tumor necrosis factor alpha* (TNF alpha) and *interleukin-6* (IL-6). These messengers activate a whole host of systems throughout the body associated with inflammation. In fact, they can even activate the same pain and inflammation—headache, body aches, and the like—that pain-relieving drugs such as aspirin (Bayer), ibuprofen (Motrin, Advil, Nuprin), and acetaminophen (Tylenol) are used to treat. Moreover, these same inflammation messengers being churned out by fat cells have a negative effect on insulin and blood sugar.

Some recent studies have shown us how true it is that excess belly fat can be a virtual engine of inflammation. In one study, obese women had much higher levels of the inflammatory chemical TNF alpha (*Eur J Endocrinol,* 2001). Obese children also had higher levels of TNF alpha (*J Pediatr Endocrinol,* 2001). Another dangerous inflammatory compound IL-6 was found to be higher in overweight people. This was especially true if the weight was carried in the belly (*Circulation,* 2002). These and many other studies show that increased belly fat is associated with the release of inflammatory chemicals.

We've heard it from our mothers since we were young: "Too much sugar is bad for you." As we got older, we heard the same refrain from our doctors and the medical press. Most people probably think there is a sliver of truth to this, but I'll bet most shrug it off.

Recent studies tell us that we should put new faith in this old adage. It turns out that sugar intake can trigger oxidative stress. Put simply, that means that increased sugar intake can initiate free-radical activity in the body and lead to damaged cell membranes.

The sugar story gets even more interesting. In one study, healthy middle-aged women were asked to eat diets with a high-glycemic load. This means they were given foods that tend to rapidly spike blood sugar levels, much like feeding sugar. The women were then tested for another inflammatory compound called *C-reactive protein* (CRP). Women fed high-glycemic diets had higher levels of CRP. This was even more the case in women who were overweight (*Am J Clin Nutr,* 2002).

The findings of these and related studies are quite extraordinary. In short, they suggest that the intake of too much sugar and high-glycemic foods may fuel the inflammation pathways in the body and that sugar is a possible engine of this inflammation.

What is also compelling about this research is the discovery that simple interventions can have a profound effect. In the studies cited above, exercise lowered the levels of the inflammatory compounds TNF alpha and IL-6. Imagine, using a simple activity to lower the levels of inflammatory chemicals in one's body! This is akin to going on a walk to achieve the effect of taking a drug.

It gets even more fascinating. Studies have also shown that consuming simple nutrients such as those found in fish oil (found in high levels in omega-3 essential fatty acids) also lowers the inflammation chemicals associated with increased body fat (IL-6, TNF alpha, CRP, and others).

This is only the most basic introduction to the story presented in *Cracking the Metabolic Code: Nine Keys to Optimal Health.* But it illustrates a principle: Our lifestyle significantly affects our body chemistry—all the way down to the level of our genes.

Most people are unaware of the extent to which our lifestyle and choices affect the most basic elements of heredity—our genes. We tend to think of genes as fixed, unchangeable elements that confer things like blue eyes, red hair, or diseases like cystic fibrosis. While this is true to a strong degree, genes are quite pliable. They are a little like Silly Putty in some respects. Genes can become more active or more passive based on what we do.

In this regard, how our genes express themselves is strongly dependent upon how we live. Studies in which subjects exercised one leg while leaving the other leg untrained revealed a startling 65 percent difference in the amount of an enzyme that affects fat burning called *lipoprotein lipase.* The change occurred because exercise "switched on" the gene for lipoprotein lipase. Studies have also shown that ingestion of eicosapentaenoic acid (EPA), a form of omega-3 essential fatty acid, leads to an activation of genes that burn fat and a slowing of the genes that make fat.

In a remarkable way, eating, sleeping, exercising, conflict, love, and virtually all the activities of life are involved in managing the ways in which our genes express themselves. This, in turn, affects the metabolic code that orchestrates the complex array of activity that guides our bodies toward health or disease.

Dr. LaValle has taken on the arduous task of making simple what is an unusually complex subject. The basic message is that there are sets of events that begin to change our body chemistry as we mature. Many of these are within our control, but if we do not seize this control, the whole of our bodies' adaptive responses will become activated. In other words, if we take certain actions, our bodies will oblige with a certain set of responses.

We know what many of these are. With others, we have a great deal to learn. *Cracking the Metabolic Code: Nine Keys to Optimal Health* weaves together the pieces with the goal that, in the end, you will be able to take precise steps to hasten your path to optimal health.

Cracking the Metabolic Code also comes with a warning: Failure to recognize the trends and to take action can predictably lead to changes that begin with a condition called *metabolic syndrome* or Syndrome X. Metabolic syndrome is a name given to a set of factors that signal troublesome changes are occurring to your metabolism. The typical definition of metabolic syndrome includes elevated triglycerides, elevated cholesterol, elevated blood pressure, above ideal body weight, and elevated blood glucose.

On the surface, these changes may not seem like much. However, if you were able to look inside your cells, you would witness an intense amount of activity normally aimed at correcting body chemistry beginning to shift dangerously in the wrong direction. You would also observe that the inflammatory system had become almost silently engaged, harming systems that you didn't even know you had.

In *Cracking the Metabolic Code,* Dr. LaValle makes practical sense of these changes. As you read this book, you may want to keep in mind this basic introduction to the "code." In order to bring your biochemistry more favorably within your control, there are four basic points to consider:

1. Blood Sugar and Insulin. Sugar (glucose) is the basic fuel of all cells and insulin is the agent that gets this fuel into the cell. The effectiveness with which insulin does its job of getting sugar into the cell begins to change in many people as they mature. It also changes dramatically by simply being overweight. If your insulin and glucose response are not functioning properly, it can lead to a cascade of events that begin to have dramatic, if not subtle, effects on your health initially. With time, the effects are loud and damaging.

2. Inflammation, Oxidative Stress, and Glycation. As noted above, changes in weight, body fat, and blood sugar control activate a host of messenger systems and responses that take on a life of their own. Fat cells and white blood cells become engines of inflammation that can affect everything from the heart to the brain to the joints. Free-radical changes begin to tax the antioxidant defense mechanisms.

   Glycation is a troublesome, slowly occurring process in which sugar binds tightly to one of your body proteins. This can be a protein that circulates throughout the body, such as insulin. It can also be a longer-lived protein, such as the tissues that hold your ligaments together or the lens of your eye. The sugar-protein reaction (glycation) causes wrinkling, browning (a characteristic associated with oxidation), and stiffening of the proteins, which ages them more quickly and changes their function. In fact, the glycation reaction may be one of the principal factors of accelerated aging. Various nutrients and dietary factors affect inflammation, oxidative stress, and glycation. Attention to all of these is part of cracking the metabolic code.

3. Neuropsychological. Mood and stress have an immense bearing on our overall biochemistry. Cortisol is a key stress hormone. As chronic stress infiltrates our senses, cortisol begins to shift hormonal response, leading to a change in other hormones being produced. For example, as cortisol rises in response to stress, a set of biochemical changes are set in motion that contribute to all of the physical changes described thus far. In addition, various mood states such as depression and anxiety are associated with increased food cravings, which, if acted upon, further aggravate the biochemical changes taking place. In one study, depressed males who exercised experienced none of the expected rise in growth hormone that usually occurs with exercise. Since growth hormone is one of the key repair

hormones in the body, it makes us aware that stabilizing mood is crucial if we wish to correct adverse shifts in body chemistry (*Psychoneuroendocrinology,* 1999).

4. Optimum Nutrition. All processes critical to optimum health are only possible in the presence of fundamental nutrients. Precursors, or building blocks, are needed to manufacture neurotransmitters, hormones, and the active substances that make the body work. Cofactor vitamins and minerals, the substances that help the body transform nutrients, are vital to all metabolic function. Fatty acids form the very structure of cells, much like bricks form the foundation of a building. Accessory nutrients such as flavonoids from fruits and carotenoids from vegetables form the protective matrix that allows the body to function in the most strenuous environments. A deficiency of almost any combination of nutrients can dramatically alter the body's metabolic efficiency.

In reading this book, I hope you will come to understand its core message that so much of our ability to live inspired, fruitful, and healthy lives is within our control. So many people desire the richness and possibility that life has to offer, but are frustrated by the demands of life and effort needed to make simple changes.

In this book, Dr. LaValle offers his insights based on emerging science, his experience as a health professional, and a sincere desire to help others. I invite you to digest this book in however small or large bites you desire. Consider that all of the positive changes you make will benefit your life and will build upon those made before.

Also, please consider that while this book strongly advocates the means to improve your body chemistry, there is no substitute for the richness of loving, intimate relationships. Nurture these fully as you journey on the road to wholeness.

—Michael A. Schmidt, Ph.D.
Author of *Brain-Building Nutrition,*
Bio-Age, and *Nutritional Pharmacology*
and Clinical Neuroscience

Looking Deeper Than the Eye Can See

This book is about looking—about looking in the mirror at yourself and honestly deciding whether or not you are satisfied with what is looking back at you. It is about looking at your whole body and assessing it honestly. Are you satisfied with your state of health?

Today, a state of ill health is a reality for many millions of Americans. Despite the many miracles in modern medicine and our scientific advances, we seem to be faced with significant health challenges—challenges that, in part, are arising from our lifestyles. It is not uncommon for me to see patients who suffer from several conditions or diseases simultaneously, and many or most of these patients do not realize the extent that their lifestyles have influenced those diseases. This book is, of course, for those people. It is for the millions of Americans who are just plain sick and tired of feeling sick and tired.

If you're one of the lucky few who, so far, is enjoying good health, you should still read on. Why? Because this book will help you to get in tune with your body; it will help you to recognize problems before they start to pull you down. It will help you to look deeper than the eye can see to help you maintain your health throughout the aging process.

Whether this book finds you in a state of illness or a state of health, these challenges and these forces that you have faced during your lifetime have created changes within your metabolism. And one day, even if it has not happened yet, these forces will gain enough momentum that you begin to notice a change in your health. That change may be subtle, or it may be harsh, but it will signal the beginning of the breakdown of your health.

The ideas central to this book have become more and more important to me over my years of practice as I have seen and treated many thousands of people with the same challenges and the same complaints. The idea of putting these unifying concepts of my practice into book form has been a passion of mine for ten years.

Now, I want to teach my readers as I have already taught my patients and fellow healthcare professionals. I want to teach you about how your body works so that you can become proactive with your health and become as healthy as you can be.

Typically, books like this are written with the premise that they will give you the absolute answers to all your problems. Unfortunately, I don't have all the answers. But this book represents an evolution of more than twenty years in my own growth both as a healthcare practitioner and as a human being. Perhaps more important, this book represents many thousands of successful outcomes with patients who have problems just like yours.

I was fortunate to have been exposed to natural medicine at an early stage in my career. While I was in pharmacy school in the late 1970s, I had a cousin who was importing natural medicines from Germany. Of course, at first I scoffed at my cousin; I doubted his medicines and their effectiveness. But a personal life crisis turned me around. While I was still a supposedly healthy student in my twenties, I began getting light-headed after eating. Sometimes I would even pass out. This was, of course, alarming to me since both my grandmother and my father were diabetic. I feared that I was going to follow their genetic footprints! After searching for some answers through traditional methods without success, I decided to search for other options.

That search lead me to David Polen, D.C., whose explanation of my health challenge changed my perspective on medicine forever. He explained to me that although it was obvious that I was having blood sugar regulation issues, my health history most likely had a great deal to do with why my chemistry was misbehaving. Moreover, it didn't seem to surprise him that, although I had just won a bodybuilding championship, I felt old, that my energy was low, that I was achy, and that I would break out in welts and bumps when stressed. In addition, I had developed Raynaud's syndrome, a circulatory disorder, and the skin on my fingers would crack and ulcerate especially during the winter months.

Dr. Polen then did something that no other doctor had ever done before. He asked me about my life. I told him that I had had double pneumonia at four months old and had almost died, and that the next sixteen years of my life were basically made up of memories of going to the pharmacy and getting the "pink and the purple stuff to take." I was on antibiotics and decongestants so often that I thought they were part of my meal plan. I also had severe allergies. They were so bad that when we went on family vacations, there was no doubt I would end up getting sick from the new environment. At sixteen, I came down with a severe case of mononucleosis and lost thirty-five pounds and six weeks out of my life. Along with all of my physical complaints, I had trouble concentrating at school, which got progressively worse as the years passed.

There were emotional challenges, as well. A neck injury in an all-star game ended my days of playing football. I didn't know which was worse—the neck injury or the fact that, in a single instant, I had gone from being a star to being a "nobody," a failure.

I wish I could say that I met these challenges head-on, but, in reality, my head proved harder than my neck. Over the next several years, my health continued to decline. After high school, I enrolled in the pharmacy program at the University of Cincinnati, and those first few years were an intense emotional and physical struggle.

I remember one day when I was quite literally in the depth of despair. Physically, I felt as if I were eighty although I was only twenty-one. Emotionally, I felt that my life was over instead of just beginning. I found myself at the most critical crossroad of my life. I could continue to spiral downward or I could map out a new path for my life. With determination, a decision rose from deep within me. In that moment of decision, I made a conscious choice to begin the journey of re-creating my life and my health on a physical and emotional level.

After that, I opened my mind and my heart to the "new view" of health that Dr. David Polen and another naturopath, Alexander Wood, D.C., N.D., provided me. I found that it was a view that made sense, both from what my training as a pharmacist had taught me, and what I was learning about natural medicine. What I learned is that good health is, to a great degree, a question of balance. The effects of the environment, the foods we eat, the stress we're under, our genetics, and even our jobs can all act as forces to disturb our natural metabolic balance. And what truly influences our health is our ability to cope with these various stressors and maintain our balance.

Since then, I have dedicated my life to studying health and all that promotes good health. I have noticed again and again what works and what doesn't. And I have seen such wonderful changes in people's lives. I have studied various disciplines of healing and I have been fortunate to have been guided by some great physicians along the way. After all this, I can honestly say that the most profound process I have discovered is the ability, inborn in all of us, to change and grow.

That's what led to this book. While I am the author of eight other books and hundreds of articles, I can honestly say that no other work has come as much from my heart as has this one. It is not only the product of my years of study, but also the product of my life's journey.

Presently, I am in clinical practice at the Living Longer Institute located in Cincinnati, Ohio. At Living Longer, we combine state-of-the-art medical science with the best of natural medicine to create an integrative approach to health. We have the leading medical imaging services (MRIs, CT scans, DEXA scans, and spectroscopy) and do research combining medical imaging and the use of nutraceuticals. In addition to practicing internal medicine and women's health, we offer physical therapy, massage therapy, functional fitness training, and exercise along with a host of other services, including performance enhancement and preventative programs for people who are interested in staying as healthy as they can.

The goal of all this work is to truly help our patients—whether they are suffering from cancer, fibromyalgia, multiple sclerosis, obesity, autism, or irritable bowel syndrome—live longer and better lives by helping them to choose the safest options when dealing with their health challenges. After our patients have come through the program, they tend to be amazed by how they feel as the symptoms they have lived with for so long begin to slip away into memory.

I feel truly blessed to have the honor of working with my patients as they move toward reclaiming their metabolism and their health. For those I cannot work with personally, with whom I cannot personally share all that I have learned over these past twenty years, I wanted to create a guide from which they still could learn how to regain control of their health. This is that book. I offer it to all of you who feel as though your health is spiraling downward.

I hope this book serves to help you get back on the path toward good health. If you have had your own moment of clarity and want to take charge of your health, if you want to lift that fatigue and indifference in your life and manage your metabolism so that you can live a lifestyle that promotes health and weight management, then I invite you to read on. Learn how your body functions. Learn the nine keys to your metabolic code. The more you learn, the less mystery will be surrounding how and why you may be feeling the way you feel. And the more you practice what you learn, the better you will feel.

—James LaValle, R.Ph., C.C.N., N.D.
Director, Co-Founder, Living Longer Institute

A Healthy Metabolism Promises a Healthy Future

Metabolism is the term used collectively for all of the physical and chemical reactions that occur in the body. The chemical reactions of metabolism take the food we eat and transform it into fuels and building blocks for our bodies. These chemical reactions are necessary for providing energy for activities such as movement and thinking, and for organ function such as digestion and the formation of urine. These reactions are also critical for breaking down old tissue and building new tissue. All glands and body systems are either directly involved in, rely on, or influence metabolism.

Most people think of metabolism as simply the body's ability to burn calories properly and to maintain a health body weight. They understand the term to mean "the resting energy expenditure," that is, the amount of calories used by the body at rest, while it is really the sum total of all the *catabolic* (breakdown of substances in the body) and *anabolic* (tissue-building) processes in the body. When we refer to metabolism throughout this book, we will be referring to all the metabolic pathways that influence not only the rate of energy expenditure (calorie burning) but also total health. These are the metabolic pathways that make up your "metabolic code." Your metabolic code is your personal chemistry. If your metabolism is out of balance as evidenced by weight gain and/or any other health problem, there are measures that can be taken to create balance among these metabolic pathways within the body.

Many people who have difficulty losing weight suspect some metabolic culprit, but oftentimes are thwarted in their pursuit of correcting their metabolism, because typically, the traditional medical route is to test the thyroid's function. If the test result is normal, you are considered to have a "normal" metabolism. However, from an integrative viewpoint, there are many factors that can disrupt metabolism. Most people are surprised to learn of the complex web of factors that can in fact influence their metabolism. The well-balanced interplay of your liver, your thyroid gland, your gastrointestinal tract, your adrenal glands, your pancreas, the water you drink, the foods you eat, and the oxygen you breathe, as well as the environment in which you live, are all key to a healthy metabolism and the ability to maintain an ideal body weight.

BREAKING THE "CODE" AND RECLAIMING YOUR METABOLISM

Because there are so many factors that can affect metabolism, there are also many reasons you may be having difficulty either losing or controlling your weight. And you don't have to be overweight, necessarily, to be feeling the effects of disturbances in metabolism. You may, for example, just be extremely fatigued and having trouble figuring out why. This book was written to give you the information and the tools you need to "crack your metabolic code," to find out what may be influencing your metabolism, and therefore your health.

The first tool is the System Discovery Assessment questionnaire in which there is a section on each of the key influences on metabolism—for example, the thyroid, the pancreas, and the adrenals. After a great deal of thought as to the best time to complete the questionnaire, either before or after reading the rest of the book, the questionnaire was placed at the end of the book in Chapter 17. As you read through each chapter, you will be learning about each of the key components of metabolism, as well as the external and internal influences that may be affecting it and your health, and you may begin to recognize what some of your problems may be. Completing the questionnaire will then confirm for you the areas that may be affecting your metabolism. If you score high in a section, say, for example, on the adrenals, you can suspect that to be a factor that will be affecting your health and metabolism. That is why this book is called *Cracking the Metabolic Code.* We are going to help you become a detective to discover what it is that is making it so difficult for you to lose weight, overcome fatigue, solve chronic aches and pains, lower high blood pressure or cholesterol, and/or to just feel good again.

Some readers may decide to skip right to the questionnaire to get to the "bottom" of their health problem. That's alright, but I don't recommend it for several reasons. Reading through the book will educate you on exactly how it is that this particular "key" effects metabolism and how it may be manifesting in the symptoms that you are feeling. This is important because with knowledge—the second tool—comes not only power, but also conviction. As you read through each chapter, you may begin to identify with it as you hear yourself described. Then you begin to understand, "Oh, so that's how stress might be causing my cravings for sugar, midday fatigue and sleep problems!" Or "So that's how a diet high in refined sugars keeps my weight on!" Once you really understand the underlying causes, you know why you have to make the needed changes. Remember when you were a child and sometimes it seemed so much easier to follow your parent's or teacher's orders once you understood why? Not much has changed since then. When you really understand how it is your metabolism has gotten out of whack, it makes it much easier to do what you have to do to correct it—especially when you understand the long-term consequences of having your chemistry functioning out of sync.

For you to truly take command of your metabolism and your health, you will first have to learn how your body functions. Otherwise, you will be forever searching for that "magic bullet" or the nonexistent "drink-from-the-fountain-of-youth" miracle cure. One reason I wanted to write this book is because it seems as though people are continuously trying to oversimplify causes of weight gain and obesity, as well as many of the other chronic problems that seemingly come out of nowhere. I wish that it were so simple that there was one cause for weight, and likewise a simple solution. The truth is our bodies work as integrated machines—each individual system is dependent on the proper functioning of others. The sooner we, as a society, understand this fact, the sooner we can come to longer-lasting solutions for our health issues and stop looking for one-pill cures.

The third tool is contained in the summary chapters for each section of the book. Each summary chapter contains strategies and supplement protocols to address each area that may be affecting your personal chemistry. You can begin to use these strategies immediately, or ideally wait until you have read the entire book and completed the final questionnaire, which will help you develop a plan of action that addresses all body systems and factors affecting your metabolism.

The fourth tool is lab testing. If you have any doubts or just want to verify your suspicions on the health status of a particular metabolic key, you may choose to utilize lab testing and the evaluation of it from a trained health practitioner. Information on lab tests that are most likely to reveal problems is included throughout the book.

In the upcoming chapters, there is a lot of information of various body systems and related functions—from the effects of stress on your body chemistry to detoxification of the liver, the intestines role in your health, the thyroid gland and its functions, the pancreas and blood sugar control, the adrenal glands and their hormones, the enzymes in our bodies and their important roles, the water we drink, the foods we eat, and the air we breathe. Reclaiming your metabolism is the process of understanding these vital bodily functions and where your body's systems may be breaking down. Learning about your metabolism will show you how to unwind your past body chemistry, so you can create a roadmap back to health and more youthful vitality and energy.

So, the first step to reclaiming your metabolism is discovering where your metabolism is breaking down. The second step is determining what you can do to correct your metabolism and making your plan for change; this will involve your lifestyle choices.

Once you understand the changes that need to be made and you have your plan, the third step is to just do it one by one. Not only should you be able to correct any underlying problems, which may be affecting metabolism, the steps you take will also help restore better nutritional status and overall health. In other words, you should begin to feel much better, because the same problems that bog down metabolism will bog you down and deplete your energy. Understand how powerful it is for you to make health-promoting choices on a daily basis. Those choices are the foundation you will stand on as you age from decade to decade. You can either gain momentum with the right choices or lose speed, spiral downward, and decay.

USING THE THREE SETS OF KEYS

Cracking the "Metabolic Code" is about the interrelationship of everything you do in life and how it affects your health. For these reasons, I strongly recommend that you read this book from beginning to end even if a particular "key," or health concept, doesn't seem to apply to you. Understanding the interrelationship of these important health concepts is what the metabolic code is about.

The first three keys are about the endocrine hormones—one of the hottest topics in medicine today—your pancreas and blood sugar regulation, your thyroid and metabolism, and your adrenal glands and chronic stress. Gaining control and learning how to balance each of these glands are essential to reclaiming your metabolism and regaining your health.

- **Key One:** Balancing Your Blood Sugar—Fighting Insulin Resistance, Cardiovascular Disease, and Belly Fat

- **Key Two:** Balancing Your Thyroid—Overcoming Fatigue and Burning Fat

- **Key Three:** Balancing Your Adrenals—Relieving Symptoms of Chronic Stress (Cravings, Low Energy, Memory Loss, and Insomnia)

The second set of keys is dedicated to detoxification and rejuvenation of your body systems. One of the major health issues today is how to protect yourself from the harmful effects of toxins in order to enjoy optimal health and increase longevity. You can't escape toxin exposure in today's world. Certainly decreasing the amount of toxins you ingest and minimizing exposure will help, but what can you do if you're already toxic? Key Four is about how to take care of your liver, the body's primary organ of detoxification. Key Five discusses the intestines, the role they play in protecting you from toxins, and how a healthy bowel is essential for health. Key Six examines the major toxins in our environment and their repercussions on our health.

- **Key Four:** Detoxifying Your Liver—The Body's Garbage Collector and Recycler

- **Key Five:** Detoxifying Your Intestines—From Managing Toxins to Improving Immunity

- **Key Six:** Detoxifying Your External Environment—The Effects of Environmental Toxins on Your Health

The third set of keys deals with optimizing your health through what you eat, drink, and breathe. These keys will help you incorporate nutrition, drinking water, and getting adequate oxygen into ways of maintaining your peak metabolism. A healthy diet, quality water, and clean oxygen combined give the vital elements needed to keep all the metabolic pathways in the body operating unencumbered and efficiently. These are the keys that you must use on a daily basis.

- **Key Seven:** Understanding Diet and How to Get the Most from What You Eat

- **Key Eight:** Understanding Your Need for Water—The Body's Most Essential Nutrient

- **Key Nine:** Understanding the Two Sides of Oxygen—Breath of Life or Harbinger of Aging, Inflammation, and Disease?

Once you have read through the sixteen chapters and understand how the body and its metabolic functions are interconnected and must work in harmony, I encourage you to complete the questionnaire, score it, and utilize the tips given based on your scores to help you put together a plan of action for your health. Your total score from the questionnaire will give you an overall profile of your health, and your scores in different areas of the questionnaire will indicate which of the keys you need to tend to and in what order of importance (concentrating on highest scores first). Using this questionnaire, you can map out your own personalized plan of action in your journey to optimal health.

Does cracking the "Metabolic Code" work every time? There may be some people who are beyond the point of being able to rebuild their health by implementing the steps in this book. However, the majority of the people who begin to take charge of their metabolism by applying the nine keys described in this book will gain significant health rewards, increase their vitality, and reduce the symptoms of their present health crisis. If this information is not enough to help you overcome your personal health challenges, I encourage you to seek out a healthcare professional experienced in natural therapeutics who can guide you back to the path of vitality and health.

Why Do I Feel So Unhealthy?

CHAPTER 1

Losing Your Balance: How the Downward Spiral of an Unhealthy Metabolism Begins

Each of us at one point in our lives is faced with a health challenge. The challenge can be big or small, but regardless of its size, it affects our well-being. For many folks, the first wake-up call is stubborn weight gain or cholesterol levels that are slowly creeping up. Others think they are sailing along fine when suddenly their doctor tells them their blood sugar is above normal. Hopefully, you are not one of the unfortunate folks whose first wake-up call is something quite serious, such as a heart attack.

A new approach of medicine is emerging to address these health challenges. It is one that is more preventive-minded and bridges the best of modern science with our past healing traditions. The new approach encourages working with the body as a whole (wholistic medicine) and watching for early warning signs that your health may not be on track. When you examine systems of medicine such as traditional Chinese medicine (TCM) or Ayurveda (the traditional medical system of India) that have successfully developed over thousands of years, you will find they all have a common theme. Simply stated, the theme tells us that all of the body works together at any given moment to create our current state of health. One faltering or overworked system impacts on another organ or system, which can then translate into a symptom or even a disease. Even seemingly minor health problems can cascade into large ones if left unaddressed.

Your liver, intestines, and kidneys act as filters and recyclers of your body fluids, extracting what you have taken in from your diet and what you have been exposed to in your environment. All the while, communication is going on with your brain. This harmony of function between the organs dictates the balance in the body's systems, which include the nervous, immune, gastrointestinal, and endocrine (hormonal) systems, among others.

The process of organs and systems working in harmony or disharmony is not difficult to grasp. It is just the same with the engine of a car. The engine has multiple parts that all need to be working properly in order to be safely driven. A problem may even go undetected for years before the car one day breaks down. And even small problems can cause a total breakdown in function. An oil leak for instance, if undetected, can cause the whole motor to break down. Similarly, in the human body, correcting the integral components that lay the foundation for your metabolism can make sweeping changes in how well your body functions, how well you feel, and whether or not you will progress to a disease or diseases.

HOW DISEASE BEGINS

How does disease (or *dis*-ease) come about? Disease can be caused by exposure to a pathogen (anything that makes us sick, like a bacteria or virus), or by anything that causes a disruption in the normal functioning of the body, including missing or damaged genes. Lifestyle has a tremendous effect on whether or not you become ill, because many lifestyle factors affect whether or not you have a strong immune system to fight the pathogens and whether or not your normal functions will be maintained. In many countries of the world, people are well aware of the huge importance of lifestyle, including diet, exercise, smoking, drinking or drug habits, and proper attention to stress and emotional health. Yet, here in the United States, we tend to believe that whether or not you get certain diseases depends almost entirely upon your genes.

Health is determined by what our genes tell our cells to do. Our lifestyle, however, has a tremendous impact on our genes. So while your genes may make you somewhat more susceptible to certain diseases, your lifestyle can be the difference as to whether they actually develop.

Some diseases are *predisposed,* meaning we obtained the genes for them when we were in the womb. This genetic information had been passed on to us by our parents from their own health-related genetic information. The genes that cause diseases, over which we have very little control, are largely based on factors such as familial or inherited genetics. Some experts believe that around 25 percent of our health or disease is due to our genetic inheritance.

In most cases, genes that initiate a disease are expressed, or "turned on," during growth and maturity as a result of many lifestyle factors. These factors include environmental exposures during prenatal development (including maternal nutrition and exposure to substances such as cigarette smoke, chemical pollutants, recreational drugs, and certain pharmaceutical drugs); nutrition during the formative years and in adulthood; the environment; physical factors such as chronic stress; exercise; drugs (prescription and recreational), and emotional health. Environmental factors are a broad category and can include exposure to chemicals and solvents (such as in new carpeting or cleaning solutions), pollution, cigarette smoke, pesticides, and food preservatives, among others.

All these factors interact with our genes and have an impact on our health and susceptibility to disease. Take cancer, for example. Cancer begins with what is known as an initiator. An initiator is something that causes the first damage to the genetic material of the cell, the DNA. A person may have been exposed to an initiator in childhood or in young adult life, but initiation can happen at any stage of life, even while in the womb. Many people, for example, were exposed while in the womb to the pesticide, DDT. Babies whose mothers were exposed to DDT had a greatly increased chance of developing cancer. An initiator can be anything from a chemical in the environment, to a sunburn or cigarette smoke. The damaged cell (or cells) may be removed by a strong immune system, it can remain in that semi-damaged state for some time, or may obtain further damage by *promoters,* that is, substances or circumstances that continue to damage the genetic material of the cell. Promoters can be the same as initiators or something different, but it is known that having steady exposure to two or more potential promoters, such as cigarette smoke and excessive alcohol, greatly increases one's chances of getting cancer. Poor diet and free radicals are other promoters. Cancer occurs when sufficient damage has occurred to the genes in the cell, the immune system is unable to eliminate the aberrant cells, and they begin to multiply out of control.

So the choices made before and after birth virtually affect us on a cellular level. The bottom line is that our metabolic code, which develops during our lifetimes, must be in harmony for us to lead a healthy, productive life. Over the years, as our cells begin to change during the process of aging, the door to diseases is opened even wider. When our genetics have been disrupted (whether by familial or lifestyle/ environmental causes), we enter a world of altered biochemistry and metabolism, cellular dysfunction, and disease. If there is a family history of heart disease, diabetes, or cancer, those genetic switches will be the most likely to get turned on *when our metabolism becomes stressed.* Bear in mind that it takes many, many insults to cellular health and function to finally end up in chronic disease. That is why lifestyle choices can be so powerful in helping us to prevent disease. The body has many mechanisms to survive insult. Giving the body an extra boost with good nutrition, exercise, and stress control can make all the difference between chronic illness and health.

The Role of Metabolism in Disease

While some diseases, such as cancer, can be a result of the expression of genes, many diseases or conditions are a result of the direct disturbances in metabolism, either through interfering with the enzymes in the body, directly interfering with hormones, or by losing proper functioning of body systems as a result of lifestyle or environmental exposures.

One example of how the downward spiral of metabolic health can occur with just one lifestyle influence is the effect that stress has on the body. In fact, many people can trace when their health problems began back to a single event in their lives that created a lot of stress and forever changed their lives.

Chronic stress alters adrenal gland function. Under stress, the adrenal glands produce more stress hormones such as cortisol. Rising cortisol levels begins a disruptive chain reaction that impacts several other organs and systems. Chronic stress depletes certain neurotransmitters in the brain, which can trigger carbohydrate cravings and eating binges. If this scenario continues the lack of the neurotransmitter can lead to disturbed sleep patterns, which in turn can cause changes in the release of growth hormone, blood sugar regulation, and immune function.

Chronically elevated cortisol levels can also cause increased insulin release and lead to insulin resistance, a condition in which the body does not respond to insulin efficiently, which in turn, can result in abdominal weight gain. If the person is eating the sugar and carbohydrates to quell the stress and to try to build the neurotransmitters, the insulin resistance is fed, which in turn perpetuates the weight gain. This vicious cycle of metabolic chaos can quickly cause an increase in *body mass index* (lean to fat ratio). Excess insulin leads to a weight gain that is characterized by most of the weight being gained around the abdomen (or belly fat). Belly fat is known to contribute to inflammation in the body, resulting in even more destructive metabolic disruption.

Meanwhile, the elevation in cortisol also stimulates the production of extra cholesterol and triglycerides (a primary form of fat in the blood), which leads to increased cardiovascular risk. Cortisol also stimulates the production of *neuropeptide Y,* a chemical messenger, which turns off the body's natural killer cell activity, a critical component of a healthy immune system. In addition, cortisol lowers the production of other immune cells. And if that is not enough, cortisol itself stimulates the release of many inflammatory chemicals, which cause systemic inflammatory reactions that trigger increased free-radical damage of the cells (oxidation).

As the body continues to churn out more cortisol, dehydroepiandrosterone (DHEA), a hormone produced primarily by the adrenal glands, is used up in the process. When the available DHEA stores are depleted, the production of sex hormones slows and libido begins to decline.

Finally, with chronic cortisol elevation, changes in thyroid function begin to occur, which in turn lowers the body's metabolic rate and makes it even more difficult to utilize nutrients and to lose weight.

This is how delicate and interdependent the balance of our body systems are and how any alteration in this balance can cause a cascade of reactions that leads to a decline in health. A person in such a situation may see their weight gain as the problem. They might try to reduce calories and increase activity, and get modest or no results. Then, they might hear about a low-carbohydrate diet approach and try that. Again, the person may see only modest, if any, results. You see, these approaches alone will not correct the underlying problem of the adrenal exhaustion that has impacted thyroid function, and more.

The Effect of Lifestyle on Metabolism

In the upcoming chapters, we will be talking a lot about a condition known as *metabolic syndrome,* also called Syndrome X, because it is a condition that affects increasing numbers of Americans. It is also a perfect example of a condition that is a result of lifestyle habits that lead to an out-of-control metabolism and to other serious diseases. This condition was initially named Syndrome X because the cause of the cluster of symptoms that characterize it were unknown. Today, the causes of Syndrome X are no longer such a mystery and that is why throughout this book I will refer to it as metabolic syndrome.

Metabolic syndrome isn't a disease in itself. It is a set of simultaneously occurring symptoms that includes primarily abdominal weight gain with high blood sugar (glucose), high blood pressure, high triglycerides, and high cholesterol. You see, it is normal to have an increase in blood glucose after eating. However, once insulin (a key metabolic hormone responsible for controlling the rate at which glucose and other nutrients are taken up by cells) is secreted, it will carry glucose and other nutrients into the cells, which will in turn lower blood glucose and insulin levels. But in metabolic syndrome excess body weight and other factors cause the cells, especially the fat, muscle, and liver cells, to be unable to respond to insulin. This is known as insulin resistance. When blood sugar and insulin levels remain chronically high, eventually it will cause an increase in the blood fats, cholesterol, and triglycerides. Metabolic syndrome often results in complete resistance to insulin and the high blood sugar of type 2 diabetes, or non-insulin dependent diabetes.

The symptoms of metabolic syndrome are known to increase risk of other diseases. For instance, chronically elevated blood insulin levels are known to be associated with hypertension, and elevated cholesterol and triglycerides are associated with increased risks of cardiovascular disease, such as atherosclerosis. This is why the symptoms of metabolic syndrome, have come to be called "the deadly quartet." Not only does metabolic syndrome usually lead to type 2 diabetes and/or result in heart disease and high blood pressure, but it is also known to cause a variety of problems, including an increased risk of stroke and possible kidney failure. Metabolic syndrome can also accelerate aging and set the stage for catastrophic health problems, such as Alzheimer's disease, cancer, and other age-related diseases.

Although not all people with metabolic syndrome are overweight, rates of metabolic syndrome have skyrocketed concurrently with the growing population of overweight and obese people, and it is becoming a problem even in young age groups. In 2002, the American College of Endocrinology (ACE) and the American Association of Clinical Endocrinologists (AACE) declared metabolic syndrome as epidemic in the United States.

What are the factors most closely linked to development of metabolic syndrome? Excess body fat and a sedentary lifestyle. With excess body weight and lack of exercise, the cells of the body become insulin resistant, and the problems continue to mount from there.

Insulin resistance and metabolic syndrome are also caused in part by a diet high in refined carbohydrates and sugars, such as bread, chips, candy, and soft drinks—foods that not only raise glucose and insulin levels, but are also lacking the vitamins and minerals our bodies need to properly utilize these foods. Equally as important are the hidden or subtle contributors to metabolic syndrome, which will be discussed throughout this book, factors such as the effect that chronic stress (adrenal function), subclinical hypothyroidism and oxidative stress may play in the chemistry leading to metabolic syndrome and beyond. Later chapters discuss these factors and what we can do to intervene and help put our metabolism back on the right track.

In many cases, the body will struggle for years to restore balance against external and internal assaults before overt illness is detected. As Figure 1.1 on page 15 illustrates, although the body will try its best to restore balance among all its metabolic systems, once you have entered into the realm of imbalance or disease, it can literally be like slipping down a spiral staircase, spiraling downward ever more from year to year, from one condition to another, from one medication to another, each stage resulting in less vitality and worsening health.

Modern science validates this approach to health, which recognizes that many of our most dreaded diseases have underlying related causes. Ideally, preventive medicine can head off health problems. But if health problems have already occurred, the best approach involves looking deeper. True health comes when we begin to take the steps to correct the underlying causes of disease, which will get our metabolism back on track and reduce the factors creating the pathway toward disease.

TAKING CHARGE OF YOUR HEALTH

The practice of naturopathic medicine is based on a wholistic approach. My training as a health professional was first in pharmacy, then in nutrition, and finally in naturopathic medicine. *Cracking the Metabolic Code* is based on the knowledge I have gained over the years in all these disciplines. Like an increasing number of practitioners that have received training in Western medicine (allopathic medicine) I use an approach toward health that is based on tenants of wholistic medicine, but it is also integrative, meaning it attempts to blend the best of Western medical and scientific research with the concept of whole-body relationships in traditional medicines in order to reclaim and balance your metabolism.

This approach is beginning to take hold because for the last fifty years medicine has been dominated by research that looks for a "cure in a pill" for every ill. However, because the body's organ systems and its functions are interconnected, a single medication may be a temporary fix but not a solution to the underlying causes. This does not devalue modern pharmaceutical research—countless lives have been extended

Figure 1.1. The Downward Spiral of Health

At any given moment the various factors that influence your health can send you spiraling from metabolic wellness down a path of metabolic disruption. It can start in your mother's womb or at any point in your life.

Conception and Birth
- Genetics
- Birth trauma
- Drug therapy
- Neonatal nutrition

Poor Diet
- Skewed nutrition
- Toxic nutrition
- Increase in fat, sugar and carbohydrates

Drug Therapy
- Alters gut function
- Alters nutrition status
- Changes in immune response

Lack of Oxygen and Exercise

Weight Gain
- Increase in fat deposition
- Increase in inflammation chemistry

Fatigue
- Decrease in energy-generating capacity

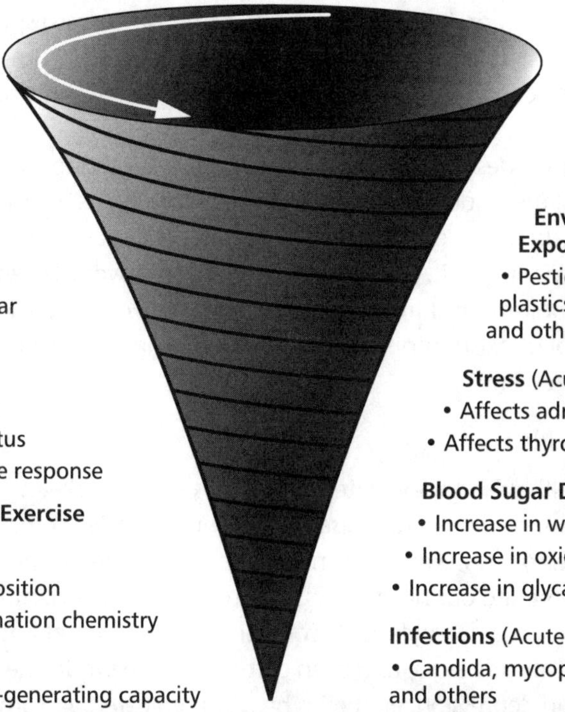

Blood Pressure and CVD

Water Quality and Quantity

Environmental Exposure
- Pesticides, solvents, plastics, heavy metals, and others

Stress (Acute and Chronic)
- Affects adrenal function
- Affects thyroid function

Blood Sugar Dysregulation
- Increase in weight gain
- Increase in oxidative stress
- Increase in glycation

Infections (Acute and Chronic)
- Candida, mycoplasm, parasites, and others

RESULT

- Increases inflammation
- Increases glycation
- Increases oxidative stress
- Increases aging rate
- Increases cellular damage
- Increases risk for diabetes, cancer, cardiovascular disease, Alzheimer's disease, Parkinson's disease, autoimmune diseases, and obesity

Your biochemistry is the sum total of your life up to today!
One event or exposure can break down your metabolic code.

and saved through modern pharmacology—but today there is renewed interest in combining the best of modern medicine with traditional healing practices.

Of utmost importance in whole-body approaches is to prevent health problems by recognizing early warning signs, such as those mentioned above. Maybe you have gained weight and are having trouble getting it off. Maybe your cholesterol has started to elevate. Maybe you are having above normal blood sugars or insulin levels. Or maybe you are just under a great deal of stress from a job or an unsatisfying relationship. As you can see from the examples above these are not situations to be taken lightly. *Cracking the Metabolic Code* will educate you as to how you can take charge and either stop yourself from entering into, or extracting yourself from, the downward spiral of health. Because once you enter it, you may be getting into more health problems than you bargained for.

It is not uncommon for people who enter this downward spiral to be diagnosed with two, three, four, and even five conditions or diseases. They are seemingly unrelated. In these circumstances, a person can be left without hope of ever feeling better.

The approach described in this book leads you to discover and then take the steps to control the underlying causes to those conditions, so that you can begin to crack your metabolic code and unravel the issues that have kept them from reclaiming health and vitality. In it, I hope I can help you discover what influences are affecting your metabolism, and in the process improve your overall health, in order to improve control of existing diseases or conditions, in order to prevent more serious future health problems.

The Time Is Now

We are in a health crisis today. Rates of diabetes are skyrocketing in the teenage and adult population; cardiovascular disease continues to take its toll in record numbers; autoimmune disorders, obesity, metabolic syndrome, depression, and cancer increasingly dominate our healthcare system. Children are getting more serious diseases at earlier and earlier ages. Girls come into my practice at age fifteen with insulin resistance, with fibromyalgia, and even chronic fatigue syndrome. Children, suffering from anxiety and depression, are being heavily medicated. At some point, we have to say enough is enough.

Every day, science is pointing at the common threads of chemistry that are intertwined in many of these conditions. Our challenge is to "turn off" the messengers that bring on disease and to stop the wave of disordered biochemistry, which envelopes and eventually incites chaos and disruption into the function of our cellular health.

Although this book is intended as a total approach to health, I know many of you will focus primarily on the weight loss aspects. An estimated 70 percent of the American population is overweight of which 30 percent are obese. Understandably, many people are looking for answers. The problem with many of the current approaches to weight loss is that they either exploit people with "miracle weight loss pills" that claim you don't have to change your diet or exercise, or they concentrate on diet and exercise only. And although many people are willing to do the work of reducing calories and increasing exercise, long-term maintenance of weight loss eludes them. Even the most reputable of weight-loss programs have very low success rates. This is because the many factors that can be working against a balanced metabolism are not being addressed. Many people are overweight or obese due to a biochemistry that has somehow become skewed. The chapters that follow will reveal many of the biochemical-related issues that result in weight gain and how to reestablish the balance of the biochemistry in our bodies. Some people have one issue; others may have multiple roadblocks to reclaiming their metabolism. With the information in the following chapters and the questionnaire in the final chapter you should be able to identify some of, if not most of, your underlying health issues.

Understanding what can go wrong in the chemistry of our bodies can help us to understand how to prevent problems before they start, or how to unravel problems after they have begun. By understanding where your systems have faltered, you can target a program of food selection, lifestyle, and supplement use that is specific to reclaiming your metabolism.

Basically, long-term health is about the choices that we make and have made in our lives. *Your health is the sum total of your life experience up to today.* That is, the health status of your mother when you were in her womb, the drug therapy you may have had, the diet you ate, the chemicals to which you were exposed, the genes you carry, environmental and work stresses, spiritual challenges, personal and family relationships, exercise, as well as influences that we may have not even uncovered, create the current status of your health equation. Some of these factors you obviously had no control over; others you did. To rebuild health, you have to get back in control of your lifestyle choices. I am no purest, but I have always tried to teach people to make responsible choices for their health. It's the choices you make six out of seven days that count.

People do not live in a test tube. They have a variety of influences that affect their health at any given moment. It is literally a "symphony of health" or "chaos of disease" that is playing out. Your challenge is to take action and actively extract yourself from the downward spiral of health that is affecting the majority of people today. You can choose to change that downward spiral to a continuum of health, longevity, and vitality; however, it will take effort, a good understanding of how your body works and what influences it, the use of appropriate nutrients and cofactors to optimize your metabolism, and striving toward emotional well-being and a connection to spirit in your life.

Now let's get started on your road to health. . . .

Hormonal Balance: The Keys to Reclaiming Your Metabolism

CHAPTER 2

The Masters of Metabolism: Why You Need to Balance Your Hormones

We don't usually think much about the glands that make up our endocrine system until something goes wrong with them. The endocrine glands, the "masters of metabolism," direct activities within the body by releasing chemical messengers, called *hormones,* into the bloodstream. More than fifty hormones regulate our mood, our metabolism, and sexual function, as well as growth and development and other functions. The endocrine system works closely with the nervous system, stimulating or inhibiting the flow of nerve impulses; these impulses, in turn, can stimulate or inhibit the release of hormones. So when hormone function is altered or becomes unbalanced, it can have far-reaching body-wide effects.

The major endocrine glands include the pituitary, the hypothalamus, the thyroid and parathyroid, the adrenals, the pancreas, and the ovaries and the testes. In addition, the stomach, the small intestine, the skin, the heart, and the placenta all contain some endocrine tissue. These glands and endocrine-containing organs secrete hormones that relay important information to *target cells,* cells that are genetically designed to respond to a certain hormone(s). Target cells each have receptor sites specifically for the hormones it needs to carry out its functions. Without hormones, cells would be unable to carry out important metabolic and regulatory functions because they would lack direction.

The hypothalamus serves as the primary link between the nervous system and the endocrine glands. The hypothalamus senses conditions from the environment such as temperature, light, and even emotional feelings, and relays this information to the pituitary. The hormones of the pituitary gland, in turn, regulate the amount of hormone production among several endocrine glands. It is for this reason that the pituitary gland is known as the "master gland" of the endocrine system.

MASTER OF THE ENDOCRINE SYSTEM

The pituitary gland is a peanut-sized gland (about 1 cm) located at the base of the brain, just below the hypothalamus. The gland is divided into two distinct lobes: the anterior and posterior pituitary glands.

The anterior pituitary gland secretes what are known as *tropic hormones,* or hormones that control the levels of other hormones. The tropic hormones exert their effect on the thyroid gland, the adrenal glands, the ovaries, and the testes. The pituitary releases *thyroid-stimulating hormone* (TSH, which turns on thyroid hormone production), *adrenocorticotropic hormone* (ACTH, which stimulates adrenal hormone production), and *follicle-stimulating hormone* (FSH, which stimulates the production of eggs and sperm). These glands, in turn, produce their own hormones.

The anterior pituitary gland also secretes *growth hormone* (GH) and *prolactin.* Growth hormone stimulates growth and cell division. The target cells for GH are located in bone, muscle, and adipose (fat) tissue. GH encourages cells to utilize fats, conserve carbohydrates, and assist in the synthesis of proteins, making it an important metabolic regulator. Prolactin stimulates the mammary cells to produce milk in nursing mothers.

The posterior pituitary gland secretes two hormones: *antidiuretic hormone* (ADH) and *oxytocin.* Antidiuretic hormone affects the kidneys and urinary output and thereby controls water balance and blood pressure. Oxytocin causes contractions of the smooth muscle lining the uterus thereby stimulating the contractions felt during childbirth. It also initiates what is known as the "let down" reflex, the release of milk from milk ducts in response to infant suckling.

HOW HORMONES COMMUNICATE WITH TARGET CELLS

Each target cell has a receptor site with a "code" that regulates its activity. *Protein substrates* within the receptor sites contain the code for each target cell. There are two ways in which hormones cause action in cells.

The first way is by generating a chemical signal inside the target cell. To do this, the hormone changes the shape of the receptor site once it binds to it. The change in shape causes a messenger chemical such as *cyclic adenosine monophosphate* (cAMP) to activate other chemicals inside the cells to produce the target cell action. An important substance in this process of hormone activity is *adenosine triphosphate* (ATP). This molecule is known as the body's "universal energy molecule" because it provides the energy needed for the cells to do their work. In this instance, ATP is used by the protein substrate to bring about the cellular changes.

Figure 2.1 on page 23 illustrates this pathway by which hormones communicate their message to target cells.

The second way hormones bring about action in target cells is actually by passing through the cell membrane and binding with the receptor there. The hormone-receptor complex will then bind to DNA and activate genes for production of proteins (such as an egg or sperm cell and sex hormones).

The secretion of hormones is generally controlled by a *negative feedback mech-*

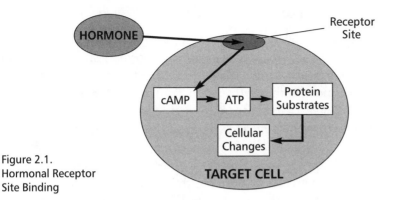

Figure 2.1.
Hormonal Receptor
Site Binding

anism. This mechanism can operate directly between target cell and gland, or indirectly, by way of the hypothalamus, which coordinates endocrine, behavioral, and nervous system functions. When hormones are secreted and cellular activity occurs, a message is sent to the endocrine gland to stop producing the hormone. When activity of the cell declines, the gland responds by increasing hormone production. Figure 2.2 below illustrates this process.

Another mechanism of controlling hormone secretion is in response to nerve impulses. For example, sympathetic nerve impulses are initiated by stimuli such as fear and anger. (The sympathetic nervous system is part of the autonomic nervous system, which controls body activities that are beyond conscious control, such as pupil dilation, intestinal motility, and heart rate.) This triggers the adrenal glands to release adrenaline. Adrenaline generates the "fight-or-flight" response: heart rate and blood pressure increase, blood flow is redirected to the major organs, and there is a sudden burst of physical energy and mental clarity. Digestion slows, the kidneys retain water, glycogen is converted to glucose for energy, and the airways of the lungs dilate. All of these activities work in biochemical harmony to protect us in times of danger or perceived threat. Each organ is activated as a result of its target cells' knowing how to respond to the influence of a given hormone.

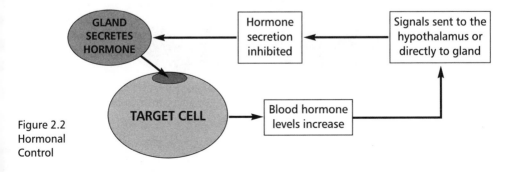

Figure 2.2
Hormonal
Control

ENDOCRINE DISORDERS

Endocrine disorders can be classified as primary or secondary. Primary disorders originate from the gland responsible for producing specific hormones. Malfunction of the endocrine system is typically a result of problems with hormone secretion. The glands may produce too much hormone (hyperfunction) or too little (hypofunction). Aging, congenital (birth) defects, infection, inflammation, autoimmune disease, and tumors can all cause endocrine malfunction, as can damage to the glands from drug therapy, poor nutrition, stress, trauma, or exposure to radioactive toxins. Sometimes, antibodies (cells that destroy foreign substances) destroy circulating hormones before they reach their target cells. In addition, the receptors on target cells can become nonfunctional either because they are blocked or otherwise interfered with.

Because the endocrine system is a network of glands and organs, a breakdown in any one gland or organ will influence equilibrium. The struggle to reestablish harmony places stress on the body, and, ultimately, affects health and well-being. Figure 2.3 below highlights the factors most influential to the integrity of the endocrine system: nutrition, drug therapy, enzyme function, bowel (intestinal) terrain, environmental exposures, and stress.

The endocrine system does not work in isolation. It is intimately linked to the immune, gastrointestinal, and nervous system functions. The next three chapters in this section will focus on three major organs and glands within the endocrine system—the pancreas, the thyroid (parathyroid), and the adrenals—and on the key roles they play in your metabolism.

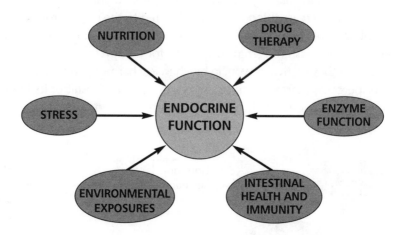

Figure 2.3 Keys Factors that Influence the Endocrine Glands

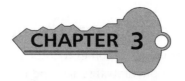

CHAPTER 3

KEY ONE:
Balancing Your Blood Sugar—
Fighting Insulin Resistance,
Cardiovascular Disease,
and Belly Fat

You hear it every day on the news—the United States is experiencing record levels of diabetes. This disease is rising rapidly in this country, with the sharpest jump being in thirty to forty year olds. More alarming, however, are the record levels of childhood and teenage diabetes, which are increasing alongside record levels of obesity (where there is one, there is usually the other).

Diabetes is a result of problems with the pancreatic hormone insulin. Insulin controls the amount of glucose (blood sugar) circulating in the blood and the rate at which it is absorbed into the cells. Glucose is the body's primary fuel. Every cell in the body is nourished by glucose. It is the principal source of energy for most organs in the body and has a critical influence on the way the body performs. Too much or too little glucose in the blood can wreak havoc on your metabolism.

Poor blood sugar regulation is the precursor to insulin resistance—one of the most severe side effects of weight gain and the primary symptom of metabolic syndrome. It is also a leading risk factor in the development of diabetes, as well as cardiovascular disease, kidney disease, obesity, nerve disorders, polycystic ovary disease (a hormonal disorder characterized by menstrual irregulatory, infertility, increased hair growth, and obesity), and a host of serious conditions that result when insulin levels are not kept at a constant level.

There are two major types of diabetes: Type 1, or insulin-dependent diabetes, and type 2, or noninsulin-dependent diabetes. Type 2 is by far the most common type, accounting for 90 to 95 percent of all cases. Until recently, this type of diabetes developed primarily in adults over the age of fifty and was often called adult-onset diabetes. Today, it is becoming commonplace in the young, occurring in children and teenagers. In this chapter, we will concern ourselves mostly with discussions of insulin resistance and type 2 diabetes and their pervasive impact throughout the body.

THE NEGATIVE IMPACT OF EXCESSIVE SUGAR INTAKE

The primary dietary concern when it comes to insulin resistance and diabetes is excessive intake of refined carbohydrates, sugar, and high-glycemic foods. The connection between sugar consumption and diabetes is indirect to date, but it does exist. We are aware that the number of Americans who are overweight or obese is steadily rising. Studies have shown that obese children and adults consume much more refined sweeteners, especially in the form of soda, compared to their normal-weight counterparts. Therefore, we see a connection between high sugar consumption and being overweight or obese. And being overweight or obese is one of the primary causes of type 2 diabetes—hence, the connection. There are also studies showing that high sugar intakes result in the wasting of some minerals. These minerals have significant roles in helping insulin to work better.

At the very least, we know that when a person consumes lots of sugary foods and drinks, they do so in place of taking in healthy nutrient-dense foods, and do not get all the nutrients they need for good health. However, many people either refuse to believe or refuse to act on the fact that excessive sugar intake has a negative impact on their health.

To illustrate, a young client of mine with attention-deficit hyperactivity disorder (ADHD) could have easily entered the downward spiral of health at a very young age. The boy's mother, also a client, had type 2 diabetes. On taking a complete health history from the boy, I found that he was underweight and that his diet consisted almost exclusively of high-sugar foods. (Don't let this confuse you: While excessive sugar intake usually leads to weight gain, I find that in some cases young people who are underweight gain weight after they give up sugar and begin to consume more nutrient-dense foods.) As a part of the boy's program, I suggested to his mother that she reduce his sugar intake drastically. (She had not taken this step previously because she felt that it was important for her underweight child to at least take in the calories, whatever the form. However, nutrient depletion can occur from excessively high-sugar intakes and can be very detrimental to the body as a whole. Given the family history of diabetes, it made sense to decrease the boy's sugar intake.) His mother willingly "put away the sugar" because she did not want to see her child suffer as she had suffered.

Within ninety days, the boy had gained weight and his mood and concentration greatly improved. He was well on the way to recovery. Yet his pediatric psychiatrist criticized our staff for altering the child's sugar intake. The psychiatrist stated emphatically that intake of sugar had nothing to do with the status of the child's health and that it had nothing to do with ADHD. From my perspective, however, had this child not changed his diet, he probably would not have gained weight or experienced an improvement of his symptoms. This nine-year-old body had already entered the downward spiral. Fortunately, his and his mother's willingness to change his diet allowed him to have much improved health. Hopefully, both he and his mother will continue on their journey to good health.

This type of thinking (that sugar has no ill effects) has contributed to the growing number of young children and adolescents with insulin resistance and obesity today—and therefore to the number of chronically ill young people whose future may contain one or more of the real-life consequences of diabetes.

The trend toward excessive sugar consumption starts when our children are young. Advertising brainwashes our children into thinking that sugary snacks and treats are good for them. Many parents do not restrict their children's sugar intake, either because they are ignorant of the possible ill effects of too much sugar or because strong cultural influences make it very difficult to limit the children's intake, especially when they are already used to eating it. Some misguided parents reward their children with sugar-laden foods in exchange for good behavior. This sets up children for a life-long pattern of wanting to reward themselves with treats. It used to be that sugary foods, snacks, and desserts were saved for special occasions and holidays. These days, candies, desserts, and especially sodas are consumed on a daily basis.

If you are like a lot of the people who come to my office, you probably crave soft drinks, sweets, and salty carbohydrates, on a daily basis. These cravings are often driven by imbalances in your biochemistry due to chronic stress and other nutritional imbalances. People have gotten used to regular sugar consumption and don't realize just how much they are consuming. Did you know that the average American eats more than 150 pounds of sugar annually? Just one can of a soft drink, on average, contains nine to eleven teaspoons of sugar. To make matters worse, in these days of the "super-sized" soft drink, one serving of soda contains between twenty-five and thirty teaspoons of sugar. And still, customers rush up for a free refill.

Our passion for sugar and packaged, processed "convenience" foods comes at a great cost to our society. It is estimated that 16 million adults in the United States have diabetes. That's 8 percent of all men and women age twenty and over. Thirty percent of the population is obese (obesity and diabetes are partners in crime). It is estimated that 42 million diabetics will be added to that number during the next five years. That's one in three people in our country who are obese and seven out of ten who are overweight. Put that all together and we have a serious problem.

HOW THE PANCREAS BALANCES INSULIN

At first, the following discussions may not seem important enough for the average person to know. However, if you understand the workings of the pancreas and insulin, you will be able to understand the metabolic changes that lead to weight gain and other undesirable effects; you will see how this one area alone can have such a far-reaching impact on your health.

The pancreas is located behind the stomach and is attached to the small intestine. The pancreas has two functions. As an *excretory gland,* it secretes digestive juices into the small intestine by way of the pancreatic duct. As an endocrine gland, the pancreas secretes hormones from a group of specialized cells known as the *islets of Langerhans.* The islets of Langerhans contain three types of hormone-secreting cells—the *alpha cells,* which secrete glucagons (hormones that increase blood sugar levels); the *beta cells,* which secrete insulin (which lowers blood sugar levels); and the *delta cells,* which secrete somatostatin (a hormone that inhibits gastric-acid release important in proper digestion). Somatostatin is also secreted in other parts of the body.

Each hormone has an important role in maintaining blood glucose concentration and supplying cells with energy. Glucose is the molecule used to produce energy for cells in the form of adenosine triphosphate (ATP), the "energy molecule" that runs body functions. The hormones work synergistically, performing a delicate balancing act in response to fluctuations in blood glucose.

Insulin acts to decrease the concentration of glucose in the blood. Insulin performs several functions that ultimately have this effect. First, it stimulates the conversion of glucose to *glycogen* by liver cells. Glycogen is a polysaccharide, which acts as a storage molecule for glucose. Glycogen synthesis causes a decrease in blood glucose. Second, insulin prevents the conversion of fat and protein molecules to glucose. It protects the glucose stores in these cells and inhibits their release into the blood. In fact, insulin promotes the synthesis of protein and the storage of fat. Insulin also transports the branched-chain amino acids *leucine, isoleucine,* and *valine* into muscle tissue. These amino acids are essential for maintaining lean muscle tissue.

Finally and most important, insulin facilitates the transport of glucose across the cell membranes of certain cells. These cells, including skeletal and cardiac muscle, as well as cells in adipose (fat) tissue, have insulin receptors. Glucose uptake by these cells results in a decrease in the blood glucose concentration. Some cells, like neurons in the central nervous system, lack insulin receptors and are dependent on a continuous supply of glucose from the blood. Because insulin facilitates storage and preserves the integrity of proteins and fats, it is considered an *anabolic* hormone. This is a significant point for understanding its role in metabolism and body-fat distribution. Anabolic hormones promote weight gain.

Glucagon has the opposite effect of insulin; it serves to increase blood glucose concentrations. Glucagon stimulates the conversion of glycogen back to glucose (a process called *glycogenolysis*) and its release into the blood. Glucagon also regulates the conversion of amino acids to glucose, in a process called *gluconeogenesis,* and the breakdown of fats into fatty acids and glycerol. The role of glucagon in the breakdown of glucose, proteins, and fats makes it a *catabolic* hormone. Insulin and glucagon are regulated by a negative feedback mechanism (a way in which the body turns off hormones after they've done their job, for example, when sugar levels drop, insulin does also). When blood sugar is high (hyperglycemia), insulin is secreted and glucagon is suppressed.

Somatostatin, secreted by delta cells in the islets of Langerhans, helps to inhibit secretion of glucagon. When blood sugar is low (hypoglycemia), insulin is suppressed and glucagon is secreted.

CONDITIONS ASSOCIATED WITH POOR BLOOD SUGAR REGULATION

Many serious, chronic conditions are associated with impaired pancreatic function and blood sugar regulation. One of the more serious is type 2 diabetes and its complicating factors. The inability to lower blood sugar in people with type 2 diabetes is linked to several predisposing conditions, including impaired insulin secretion, hyperinsulinemia, insulin resistance, impaired glucose tolerance, and increased glucose production by the liver. All these conditions occur when the pancreas is not working properly.

Hyperinsulinemia

Hyperinsulinemia is an overproduction of insulin by the pancreas. The causes of hyperinsulinemia, which creates elevated glucose levels due to an intolerance of glucose, are associated with age, obesity, and a high-carbohydrate or high-sugar diet.

Frequent spikes in blood sugar require the pancreas to release insulin, resulting in overstimulation of the beta cells and increased insulin secretion. Hyperinsulinemia promotes excessive storage of fat, increasing the risk of major cardiovascular events such as stroke and heart attack. The underlying physiology of hyperinsulinemia is linked to the phenomenon of *insulin resistance.*

Impaired Glucose Tolerance (IGT)

Glucose tolerance (borderline hyperglycemia) is measured by administering an oral glucose load (12 ounces of juice, for example) after a twelve-hour fast, and measuring the level of sugar in the blood.

Until recently, hyperglycemia was largely untreated unless it was accompanied by a fasting blood sugar level of 140 mg/dl. However, a fasting blood sugar level of 126 mg/dl is the new standard that determines type 2 diabetes, while borderline hyperglycemia (110–126 mg/dl) is recognized as *impaired glucose tolerance* (IGT).

This is considered by many experts to indicate a "prediabetic" condition, in which many cases could be controlled with diet, exercise, stress management, and nutritional supplements. It is estimated that 13.5 million individuals are affected by IGT. Some estimates are even much greater with as many as 40 million people at risk.

Abdominal obesity is considered a major risk factor for the development of IGT. That means that if you have *visceral adiposity* (a nice term for belly fat), you probably are becoming or already have impaired glucose tolerance and are one metabolic step away from becoming a person who has diabetes.

Insulin Resistance

Insulin resistance is defined as an inability of insulin to facilitate glucose uptake from the blood into the cells. It is characterized by poor insulin binding at the receptor cells, particularly skeletal muscle cells. Insulin is produced and carried to the cells, but glucose uptake is sluggish. Consequently, blood sugar remains elevated. To compensate, the pancreas initially releases more and more insulin (hyperinsulinemia). Blood glucose can be maintained within normal limits if enough insulin is produced.

Type 1 Diabetes

Type 1 diabetes (insulin-dependent diabetes) affects 5 to 10 percent of the population and is a condition in which the pancreatic beta cells fail to secrete insulin. This is known as an *absolute insulin deficiency.* Without adequate insulin, glucose cannot be transported into the cells. The result is a state of cellular "starvation" and glucose accumulation in the blood. Type 1 diabetes is characterized by *hyperglycemia* and by the breakdown of fats and protein, which are used to meet the energy demands of the body. The catabolism of fats and protein predisposes insulin-dependent diabetics to a dangerous metabolic condition known as *ketoacidosis.* Ketoacidosis is a condition in which the pH (acid-alkaline balance) of the body is too acidic and high in ketones, the waste products of partially burned (or metabolized) fat. Insulin-dependent diabetics require a continuous supply of insulin to prevent ketoacidosis and to maintain a stable blood sugar concentration.

It is thought that type 1 diabetes is a caused by a genetic predisposition for an abnormal immune response to beta cells in the islets of Langerhans. Islet cell antibodies have been detected in 60 to 95 percent of persons with type 1 diabetes. However, genetic predisposition, vaccinations, Coxsackie's virus (virus with cold and flulike symptoms, which can mutate into a strain that inflames the heart muscle, leading to cardiomyopathy and heart failure), milk antigens, and mycotoxins (poisonous substance produced by a fungus) have also been implicated as triggers for the elevated immune responses that may destroy beta cells as well.

Type 2 Diabetes

Ninety to ninety-five percent of diabetics are type 2 or non insulin-dependent diabetics. Type 2 diabetes is distinguished from type 1 in a number of ways. As I have already stated, type 2 diabetes is a progressive disease rooted in diet and lifestyle. I believe that other factors such as the cumulative effect of your daily interaction with your environment, past drug history (amounts, frequencies, specific medications, and recreational drug use), and the level of stress in your life can also influence progression toward this disease.

Type 1 diabetes typically strikes at a young age. It is due to an autoimmune reaction that can be initiated by various factors, including bacterial and viral exposure. While type 1 diabetes is generally discovered in childhood, type 2 is typically diagnosed in middle age. However, as was mentioned earlier, there is also an alarming rise in the number of teenagers and preadolescents who have developed type 2 diabetes.

While type 1 is caused by impaired insulin secretion, type 2 is caused by *insulin resistance,* an impaired ability of insulin to perform its task at the cellular level. It is characterized by poor binding of insulin to receptor cells and consequently poor uptake of glucose by the cells, resulting in *impaired glucose tolerance.*

In type 2 diabetes, insulin secretion is normal or slightly above normal, but the body cells aren't recognizing the insulin that is made. The result is the pancreas pushes harder to make more insulin because the body's blood sugar is continuing to rise. As insulin levels continue to rise in the body, the person will gain weight because insulin causes weight gain.

Hyperinsulinemia and repeated insult with highly refined carbohydrate and sugar intake can ultimately lead to underproduction of insulin by the beta cells of the pancreas. Physiology books tell us that the high blood glucose levels become toxic to the beta cells and that our high intake not only of sugary foods, but also of refined foods, in general, simply calls upon the pancreas for too much insulin production. The insulin-producing part of the pancreas is an endocrine gland. Endocrine glands can wear out over time. For instance, that the adrenal glands and the thymus glands can basically shrivel up from overuse is well known. It is theorized by some that the same thing could happen to the pancreas.

This concept should not be difficult to grasp. Think about it: How many people could work overtime for years on end without eventually wearing out? The pancreas faces the same fate. Years of overburdening from cookies, cakes, colas, and the endless "hidden sugars" in processed foods and carbohydrates eventually result in the pancreas losing its ability to function at optimal metabolic performance. This leads you down the spiral of metabolic chaos.

Table 3.1 on page 32 summarizes the difference between type 1 and type 2 diabetes.

Risk Factors for Type 2 Diabetes

Obesity and diabetes often occur together. A person who is over age forty-five and is overweight is a prime candidate for developing type 2 diabetes. America is the most obese nation in the world. It is as if we are purposefully cultivating our own population of diabetics. According to some sources, it is estimated that approximately 30 percent of the population is obese. An astounding 20 percent are considered *morbidly obese* (in excess of 20 percent of normal weight for sex, height, and build). There is a greater prevalence of obesity among teenage girls than ever before. This

Table 3.1. Differences Between Type 1 and Type 2 Diabetes

BETA CELLS	RECEPTOR CELLS	BLOOD SUGAR	RISK FACTORS	SYMPTOMS
TYPE 1				
No insulin secretion	No glucose	>140 mg/dl	autoimmune responses, fungi, genetics, high milk intake, vaccinations, viruses	cardiovascular disease, excessive thirst, fatigue, ketoacidosis, polyuria, wasting
TYPE 2				
Normal insulin secretion progresses to hyperinsulinemia	Insulin resistance, Impaired glucose tolerance	>126 mg/dl	abdominal obesity in middle age, high sugar diet, obesity, African or Hispanic descent	blurred vision, cardio-vascular diseases, constant hunger, excessive thirst, obesity, polyuria, poor wound healing

could be attributed to a variety of factors, but excessive carbohydrate intake is one of the most important. Seven in ten Americans are overweight. Look around. It does not take long to observe this trend among our population. Obesity is now a bigger risk factor for developing related health risks than smoking.

Research has shown a strong correlation between upper body obesity ("apple shapes") and the development of type 2 diabetes. In one study, apple-shaped women with waist-to-hip ratios of 0.8 or more, or waist measurements of thirty inches or more, had a greater risk of developing cardiovascular disease and diabetes than their "pear-shaped" counterparts.

Young and middle-aged adults who gain weight are at highest risk for insulin resistance and hyperinsulinemia (overproduction of insulin). One study concluded that each 5 percent increase in weight gain over the age of twenty was accompanied by an almost 20 percent greater incidence of insulin resistance. Even without dramatic weight gain, an age-associated trend toward hyperinsulinemia and insulin resistance has been identified. It is estimated that 10 to 25 percent of the adult American population may be insulin resistant. In my opinion, this number is *very* conservative.

Figure 3.1 on page 33 illustrates how insulin resistance, if untreated, can develop into a truly serious condition.

Conditions Associated with Type 2 Diabetes

To see such an increase in the incidence of diabetes is unfortunate because the secondary problems such as diabetic retinopathy, kidney failure, and cardiovascular disease that can develop from diabetes are very serious and debilitating. What makes this so sad to me as a practitioner is that many people are not even aware of these secondary health problems. All too often, I have heard people claiming that if they had known more, they would have worked harder to stay healthy.

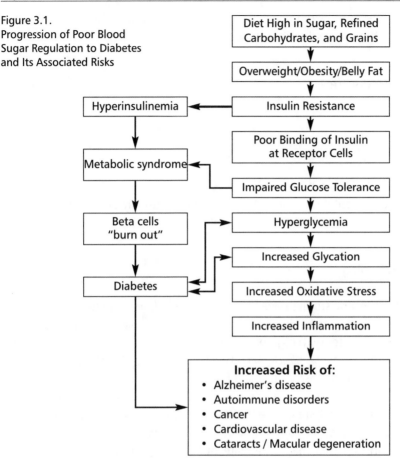

Figure 3.1.
Progression of Poor Blood Sugar Regulation to Diabetes and Its Associated Risks

Keep in mind that the progression toward insulin resistance and/or type 2 diabetes occurs over time. You don't wake up one morning and say, oh no, I can really feel that insulin resistance working on me today! This condition can go pretty much undetected into your thirties and forties as poor regulation of blood sugar. But then when you reach your fifties or sixties, it becomes official. The doctor says to you, "You have diabetes." There is no such thing as "getting over" diabetes, and the complications that can result from it not only take a devastating toll on health and well-being, they are also very expensive. The average annual medical expense for a patient with diabetes ranges from $10,000 to $12,000.

Many diabetic complications are a direct result of uncontrolled blood sugar. The accumulation of sugar in the blood generates free-radical damage to the capillaries and blood vessels, elevating *isoprostanes* (inflammatory mediators formed when arachidonic acid, a naturally occurring fatty acid, is oxidized by free radicals), resulting in destruction of the retina, peripheral vessels of the limbs, the kidneys, and the heart. Impotence is common among diabetic men.

Diabetes is the third leading cause of death when combined with complicating factors. Some of these complications include:

- Blindness

- Cardiovascular disease

- Fatigue

- Impotence

- Kidney failure

- Neuropathy (damage to the nerves)

- Non-traumatic amputation (not due to an accident), usually of extremities such as small bones in the feet or removal of ulcerated areas

- Obesity

- Poor wound healing

The results of several studies have highlighted the relationship between diabetes and incidence of heart attack. The Prospective Cardiovascular Munster Study (PRO-CAM) found that diabetes with high blood pressure increased the risk of heart attack by as much as eight times. *Dyslipidemia* (abnormal blood lipid profile) increased the risk by sixteen times, and those with high blood pressure, diabetes, and high cholesterol levels had a twenty times greater risk of heart attack. Because insulin resistance and hyperinsulinemia precipitate type 2 diabetes, they contribute to premature cardiovascular disease and other complications associated with diabetes. Insulin resistance and hyperinsulinemia may aggravate obesity, hypertension, atherosclerosis (hardening of the arteries), and dyslipidemia. The three major components of dyslipidemia associated with insulin resistance include:

- Decreased high-density lipoprotein (HDL or healthy) cholesterol

- Increased triglyceride (primary form of fat in blood) levels

- Negative changes in the composition of low-density lipoprotein (LDL or harmful) cholesterol

Since insulin resistance impairs glucose uptake by cells, blood sugar remains elevated. How does insulin resistance or diabetes cause dyslipidemia? With nowhere to go, excess glucose is converted to fat by the liver and triglyceride levels increase. Changes in LDL cholesterol, stimulated by insulin, promote plaque formation and atherosclerosis.

Insulin enhances the glycation (an enzymatic reaction of sugars) of LDL, a molecular change that ultimately stimulates macrophages (white blood cells involved in immune response) to attack the modified LDL. The arteries that house the LDL undergo free-radical damage and form fatty deposits leading to plaque. So you can see that, in addition to oxidation, glycation may well be a key risk factor for heart disease development.

Hyperinsulinemia also leads to sodium and fluid retention, which can lead to hypertension. Insulin also stimulates the autonomic nervous system (the part of the nervous system that governs involuntary actions) and the growth of smooth muscle cells (which contribute to the formation of plaque) through growth factors related to insulin. Both of these conditions cause the blood vessels to become rigid and constrict. If your blood vessels get smaller and more rigid, it is harder for your heart to pump blood through them. So, over time, your blood pressure will go up. High blood pressure (a precursor of heart disease), like insulin resistance (a precursor of diabetes), is one of the key identified problems in metabolic syndrome.

Type 2 diabetes is a highly preventable condition. Now let's look at the primary diet and lifestyle factors that affect the pancreas and blood sugar regulation.

KEY INFLUENCES ON INSULIN REGULATION

Nutrition is clearly the key most intimately connected to the health of the pancreas. The pancreas is influenced by nutrition in two major ways. First, the synthesis of insulin and glucagon (a hormone that opposes insulin and is needed for the maintenance of healthy metabolism) are dependent on enzymes and nutrients from the diet. Second, and more important, insulin secretion from the pancreas is regulated by fluctuations in blood glucose. And the rise and fall of blood sugar is a direct function of dietary choices.

Diet and Insulin Regulation

Carbohydrates are the primary source of blood glucose for the body. The most readily available forms of glucose are *simple carbohydrates* found in table sugar, honey, milk products, natural fruit sugars, molasses, and other modified sweeteners such as corn syrup. (Refined white flour products, which have been stripped of fiber, are not technically simple carbohydrates, but because of the lack of fiber, they are quickly converted to glucose.) These simple carbohydrates actually serve as empty calories, meaning that they provide little nutrition to the body in the way of fiber, vitamins, or minerals. But they add plenty of calories.

Complex carbohydrates are also made up of sugars, but the sugar molecules are lengthier with more complex structures. These strands of sugars actually form a substance called starch. Complex carbohydrates, or starches, are found in whole foods and fiber-containing foods such as legumes, grains, vegetables, and fruits. The strands of sugars in complex carbohydrates are eventually broken down by digestive enzymes into the individual sugar molecules. So complex carbohydrates are a significant source of glucose.

Even within these two carbohydrate groups, some foods are more readily converted to glucose than are others. Therefore, we need to identify carbohydrates in terms of their *glycemic index.* The glycemic index of a food measures the rate at which a carbohydrate breaks down into glucose in the bloodstream. Foods with a high glycemic index are considered to be fast acting because they release glucose into the bloodstream quickly, causing a rapid rise in blood sugar, which in turn signals the pancreas to produce insulin. Foods with a low glycemic index are considered slow acting and release glucose into the bloodstream slowly.

The formula for determining a food's glycemic index is derived by the absolute change in blood glucose after consuming a food, divided by the change in blood glucose after consuming white bread, multiplied by 100. (We'll talk about foods that are considered high glycemic foods in Chapter 13.)

A food's glycemic index does not necessarily measure its effects when part of a mixed meal. For example, green beans, which have a somewhat high glycemic index, are typically consumed with foods that contain protein and fat. This lowers the overall effect of a food with a higher index.

With the help of insulin, carbohydrates provide the fuel that feeds our cells. Carbohydrates supply us with quick bursts of energy. When we eat carbohydrates, there is a simultaneous release of insulin into the bloodstream. If these carbohydrates are low in fiber and are eaten without fat and protein, which slow the release of glucose into the blood, then insulin rapidly transports glucose into the cells. Sometimes this results in a dramatic decline in blood sugar, which is known as *reactive hypoglycemia.*

Why is this significant? Well, for one thing, a reduction in blood sugar signals us to eat more and replenish the supply. Because the drop in blood sugar is rapid and dramatic, our cravings are for quick fuel, usually more carbohydrates. When we eat carbohydrates again, we aggravate another insulin response, and so on. This eating cycle of constant carbohydrate cravings can lead to what is, in effect, a *carbohydrate addiction.* Other factors can also cause this craving to occur. For instance, stress can have an impact on cravings by depleting the neurotransmitter serotonin, the chemical messenger that delivers the sensation of fullness to the brain. Over time, this constant carbohydrate loading from cravings can lead to weight gain, impaired glucose tolerance, and hyperinsulinemia.

The Effects of High Carbohydrate Intake

In 1988, the U.S. Surgeon General issued dietary recommendations for a new food guide pyramid in hopes of ameliorating three of our nation's top health concerns: cardiovascular disease, diabetes, and obesity. The recommendations, based on the food guide pyramid from the United States Department of Agriculture (USDA), were to substantially reduce fat and increase carbohydrates. Most people were happy to comply. Carbohydrates, for one, taste good. They initially satisfy hunger by providing bulk with fewer calories than fat. They also satisfy our craving for sugar.

Removing fat from the diet seemed like a good idea. The recommendations were based on the connection between saturated fat intake and cholesterol. Elevated cholesterol had been identified as a risk factor for cardiovascular disease, and it was known that high fat intakes, in general, and saturated fat, in particular, could lead to elevated cholesterol levels. The idea was to get Americans to eat less total fat and less saturated fat from animal protein sources. It seemed to be relatively simple, as well.

However, by cutting out saturated fat from animal products like eggs and red meat, an important change took place. We eliminated excellent sources of quality protein. We also abandoned the "good" fats, the essential fatty acids. Unfortunately, most people still poorly understand the role of quality sources of fat in maintaining health, managing weight, and providing satiety. (See the inset "The Fat You Need" on page 38.)

The problem with the food guide pyramid was not so much the recommendations that were made, but the interpretation that people made of them and the health practices that people adopted as a result. Americans did lower their fat intake, but they did not lower their intake of refined carbohydrates or sugar, nor did their consumption of fruits, vegetables, and whole grains increase enough.

In the late 1980s, food manufacturers began to meet the demands for high-carbohydrate, "fat-free" products. Based on the dietary recommendations, these foods were marketed as "healthy" choices. After all, they had no fat. And they tasted good. Refined carbohydrates, sugar, salt, "fake fat," and artificial flavors were used to replace the flavor that had been lost by removing the fat. The results were disastrous!

Our "fat-free" choices of the past two decades have sped up that spiral downward to poor health. Weight gain and obesity are at an all time high. The prevalence of cardiovascular disease, diabetes, and cancer are on the rise. Today, children are getting "middle-age" diseases. As a nation, our reliance on inordinate amounts of processed foods is taking a toll.

The Effects of Low-Carbohydrate Intake

By the late 1990s, some scientists, nutritionists, physicians, and biochemists began to recognize the ill effects of low-fat, high-carbohydrate diets, primarily the now-evident contribution to the obesity rate in our country. Their research was based on empirical evidence, but the tendency for high-carbohydrate diets to cause weight gain and cardiovascular disease has been seen in ancient cultures and noted by some individuals in past centuries.

The ancient Egyptians, according to one author, exemplified the first example of the fattening effect of carbohydrates. This primarily agricultural society existed on a diet high in complex carbohydrates, with little meat. Upon examination of ancient text and the remains of mummies, it appears that there was widespread cardiovascular disease, obesity, and premature death. Later, the writings of Jean-Anthelme Brillat-Savarin, author of the legendary *The Physiology of Taste* published in 1825, described his success with a carbohydrate-restricted weight-loss diet.

The Fat You Need

The role of dietary fat is one of the most misunderstood areas of nutrition. Fat, like carbohydrates, has been given a bad name. We have been conditioned to think that reducing dietary fat will help eliminate body fat. The connection, while seemingly simple, is not. In fact, most people are deficient in essential fatty acids (EFAs) caused by an imbalanced intake of these fats, as well as the fact that there are few quality sources for them. EFA deficiency has been linked to diabetes, impaired glucose tolerance, hyperinsulinemia, and hypothyroidism, among other diseases.

EFAs are critical for the rebuilding and producing of new cells, and for the proper functioning of cellular membranes. Cellular membranes are responsible for maintaining the integrity of the cell, as well as allowing substances to bind with and permeate the cell. Without a healthy cell membrane, insulin binding at receptor cells may be impaired, triggering impaired glucose tolerance, insulin resistance, and hyperinsulinemia.

EFAs fall into two categories: omega-3 fatty acids, which come in three types—alpha-linolenic acid (ALA), docosahexaenoic acid (DHA), and eicosapentaenoic acid (EPA)—and omega-6 fatty acids, which are made up of linoleic acid (ALA) and gamma linolenic acid (GLA).

Omega-3s are found in cold-water fish (anchovies, haddock, mackerel, salmon, tuna, and trout) and in flaxseeds and flax oil. Borage and evening primrose oils are quality sources of omega-6 EFAs. Although both are good for us, the ratio of omega-3 to omega-6 from quality oils in our diet should be 1:3.

Modern diet plans found in books such as *Dr. Atkins' Diet Revolution* by Robert C. Atkins, M.D. (Bantam, 1981) and *The Scarsdale Diet: Plus Dr. Tarnower's Lifetime Keep-Slim Program* by Herman Tarnower, M.D. (Bantam, 1995) advocated high-protein, low-carbohydrate diets and became sweeping bestsellers. These diets offered weight-loss regimens that provided the weight-loss solutions many people had been seeking.

Now, twenty plus years later, books advocating high-protein and low-carbohydrate diets are once again appearing on the *New York Times* bestseller list. Books like *Protein Power: The High Protein/Low Carbohydrate Way to Lose Weight, Feel Fit, and Boost Your Health—in Just Weeks!* by Michael Eades (Bantam, 1997), *The Carbohydrate Addict's Diet: The Lifelong Solution to Yo-Yo Dieting* by Rachael Heller (New American Library, 1999), and *Dr. Atkins' New Diet Revolution* by Robert C. Atkins, M.D. (Avon, 2001) all advocate carbohydrate-restricted eating plans to control insulin and lose weight. Their programs are primarily based on the principle that carbohydrate restriction helps to balance insulin release and glucose transport to the skeletal muscle and fat cells. The body turns to fat stores to maintain blood sugar and energy for cellular metabolism, many times resulting in rapid weight loss.

The role of EFAs in health and disease is associated with their conversion to *eicosanoids,* a group of "superhormones" that act as hormonal gatekeepers of the cells known as prostaglandins. Prostaglandins are powerful hormonelike molecules that affect virtually every mechanism in the body. In the presence of specific enzymes, EFAs are converted into several types of prostaglandins, generally classified as inflammatory or inflammatory reducing in nature.

The inflammatory prostaglandins (PGE2, thromboxane A2, and leukotrienes) are made from arachidonic acid, which is produced from the oxidation of various lipids and fatty acids. These prostaglandins are overproduced for several reasons, but the primary dietary factor is not getting enough omega-3 EFAs. These prostaglandins contribute to inflammation, cardiovascular disease, allergies, an overactive immune response, and hyperlipidemia.

Omega-3-formed prostaglandins (PGE1 and PGE3) enhance the immune system, prevent platelet aggregation (and hence, blood clots, strokes, and heart attacks), dilate arteries, and fight inflammation.

Like the EFAs, both types of prostaglandins have important functions. But it is important that they be present in a healthy ratio. If pro-inflammatory prostaglandins are produced in excess of the healthy series, a variety of conditions may result. For more information on fatty acids and their importance, I highly recommend *Brain-Building Nutrition: The Healing Power of Fats and Oils* by Michael A. Schmidt, Ph.D. (North Atlantic Books, 2001), a leading authority on fatty acids and their essential role in brain function, weight management, and general health.

I want to credit all the many authors and health practitioners over the years for doing a tremendous job of making Americans aware of their excessive carbohydrate intake. However, once again, some problems can develop if low-carbohydrate diet approaches are taken to the extreme for too long. The following will explain how low-carbohydrate diets work and their potential risks.

Low-carbohydrate diets deprive the cells of glucose from carbohydrates. This forces the body to use its glycogen reserves (stored in the liver) to feed the cells. Once glycogen is depleted, the body enters a state of "metabolic emergency," where fat and protein are converted to glucose (gluconeogenesis) in order to fuel the *citric acid cycle.* The citric acid cycle is itself a biochemical process that takes place within the mitochondria (the "powerhouse") of the cells. It is the process that uses glucose to create ATP.

When fat is mobilized to provide energy, the breakdown of fatty acids release metabolic compounds known as *ketone bodies.* Ketone bodies are produced as secondary sources of fuel for the central nervous system. In small amounts, they are of use to the body. In large amounts, they can alter the acid-base balance of the blood.

In extreme situations, when ketone bodies are produced faster than they can be eliminated (through the lungs and kidneys), the blood is acidified and a condition called *ketoacidosis* can develop. This is one of the risks of a prolonged low-carbohydrate diet. Ketone production must be monitored and controlled.

The conversion of fat to glucose for energy production is inefficient. Only 5 percent of a fat molecule is made up of the three-carbon glycerol chain needed to make glucose. Of the remaining fatty acids, some are used to provide energy in the form of ketone bodies. While this satisfies the energy requirements of most cells, the brain and nerve cells require a continuous supply of glucose. The nervous system consumes about two-thirds of the glucose used every day. Since fat reserves are a poor source of glucose, in the absence of carbohydrates, protein stores are used to sustain the brain and nervous system.

Amino acids from protein can be converted to glucose when other sources of fuel are unavailable. This process, however, diverts protein from its primary functions. Protein is needed to reinforce the structural components of the body, to help stabilize insulin secretion, and to provide the building blocks for hormones, tissues, neurotransmitters (found everywhere that we excite or inhibit *target cells*), and enzymes. Protein is the substance of lean muscle throughout the body. When lean mass is used as fuel, *catabolism* (the breakdown of muscle) occurs. As lean mass is lost, so is the ability to burn calories efficiently. Thus, losing muscle mass is detrimental because it negatively affects the metabolism, making it even more difficult to lose weight in the future. This is another potential risk of low-carbohydrate diets. If not enough protein is consumed, the body will break down the proteins in muscle. This is why the low-carbohydrate diets emphasize and recommend high-protein intake. However, high-protein intake is not without its own potential problems.

Animal-protein-based diets can lead to increased cancer risks and other health risks. We know this because vegetarian diets historically have proven to have the lowest cancer, cardiovascular disease, and hypertension rates. Also, high-protein diets force the liver and kidneys to work overtime to detoxify and excrete *ammonia*. Ammonia is the byproduct of amino acid breakdown, which must be converted to *urea* and flushed out in the urine. This requires a large amount of water in order to prevent dehydration. Along with urea, valuable minerals (potassium, sodium, magnesium, and calcium) are lost in the urine. This process can lead to a variety of health problems over time including *osteoporosis*. (Recent evidence has shown, however, that if you eat enough vegetables with protein, you can avert the calcium loss from your bones.)

As I have explained, carbohydrate restriction will lead to weight loss in most cases. The reason is that it forces the body into burning fat as a fuel source. Clinically, however, I observe two problems with low-carbohydrate diets. First, carbohydrate restriction becomes difficult to maintain long term because the eventual cravings for carbohydrates, especially when dieters are under a lot of stress, push them to extremes. Carbohydrates trigger the production of a neurotransmitter called serotonin. Serotonin not only makes us feel happy and calm, but also when serotonin levels are adequate, it provides a signal to the brain that we are full and can stop eating. Adequate serotonin is also needed for restful sleep. So restriction of carbohydrate foods may contribute to low serotonin levels and, therefore, may affect mood, sleep, and the ability to feel full after eating. In addition, low serotonin levels are a cause of depression. Recent studies have revealed that people with chronically low serotonin levels (characterized by feeling depressed and trouble sleeping) have the hardest time keeping off weight.

Second, many, if not most, people regain the lost weight once they start eating carbohydrates again. Recent evidence points to the possibility that ketogenic diets (diets so low in carbohydrate intake that the body is forced to form ketones) may actually *increase* the ability of fat cells to attract and store fat once the diet is discontinued. The reason for this may be that the underlying problem of insulin resistance has not been improved, just averted through avoidance of any glucose challenge. Ketosis-based diets have been around for years, but they are not the entire solution to our obesity problems. They are simply a way to manipulate the body into burning up fat stores, and many times, they still do not go to the root of the problem.

You have to go beyond just the pancreas to understand the factors involved in blood sugar regulation. Low-carbohydrate dieting that does not include regular generous servings of vegetables is like putting a Band-Aid over a bullet hole. It covers up the problem, but many times, it does not deal with the reason for the insulin-related chemistry. It is true that people eat way too many carbohydrates, especially refined sugars. However, eliminating all carbohydrates, even healthier ones, is going to the extreme, the same kind of extreme that led to the low-fat and low-protein diets of the 1980s. It is also true that you may need to restrict carbohydrates especially from grains, pastas, and cereals when beginning a weight-management program, but to never eat these foods again is restricting valuable sources of fiber and other nutrients the body needs. I know that low-carbohydrate dieters have become extreme when they come into my office and tell me that they are off carrots. Believe me, people are not getting fat in this country due to a rabbitlike appetite for carrots!

Common sense and historical evidence tell us that dietary extremes are difficult to maintain for any length of time. The role of complex carbohydrates in our diet is to provide calories, fiber, minerals, vitamins, and *phytochemicals* (biologically active substances in plants that protect the body against illness) unavailable in meat. Without them, we are dangerously deprived of important nutrients and fiber. Carbohydrate restriction removes the component of our diets that provides satiety and a feeling of fullness. The neurotransmitter serotonin is activated by carbohydrates at mealtime to tell us when to *stop* eating. When we cut out carbohydrates from our diet, we cut down on serotonin and lose the ability to feel satisfied, to feel pleasantly full. That is why when you are craving carbohydrates and try to eat protein to quench the craving, many times it just doesn't work. Fix the serotonin depletion and the craving stops. And all the dietary changes in the world will not make this happen if you are under a great deal of stress.

A restricted-carbohydrate diet is also unappealing, a fact that some use to point out the success of these programs. After all, without carbohydrates, one simply eats less since there are fewer foods to choose from. And, based on the principles of *thermodynamics* (properties of heat and matter), eating less in some people will result in weight loss.

Some authors argue that we are not physiologically designed to eat carbohydrates. This simply is not true. Our teeth show us to be a species of omnivores, with both molars and incisors to handle a variety of foods. And we have a lengthy gastrointestinal tract, designed to extract nutrients and eliminate waste from a variety of foods. We have digestive enzymes specifically to break down carbohydrates. It seems obvious that our prehistoric ancestors ingested carbohydrates from fruits, starchy vegetables, and plants. And, from all indications, our ancestor's bodies accepted these foods readily and well.

A Well-Balanced Diet

Some advocates of carbohydrate-restricted diets take the position that the body responds to *all* carbohydrates in the same way, with an unmitigated insulin response. In truth, this approach bypasses the importance of complex carbohydrates and downplays their role in the production of energy. It also categorically condemns insulin, despite its many critical functions throughout the body.

The most important component of insulin-mediated weight loss is beginning a *drastic reduction in the intake of sugar and refined carbohydrates.* Refined carbohydrates and sugar, which have been stripped of fiber, nutrients, and enzymes, have a higher glycemic index than complex carbohydrates because they are rapidly broken down and released into the blood as glucose. Unrefined, complex carbohydrates (whole grains) are important sources of nutrients and fiber. The fiber in whole grains slows the digestion of carbohydrates, allowing for a slower release of glucose into the blood and a steady insulin response. Some nutrients that help regulate the insulin response (chromium, for example) are found in whole grains, but are destroyed in the refining process. But, once again, when people hear this message, they overindulge in whole grains—*eat them sparingly.* Carbohydrates are best eaten in the evening, because they help in the manufacture of serotonin, which, as mentioned earlier, has a calming effect and helps you sleep.

The dietary culprits of modern living are *not* whole grains, but an excessive intake of sugar, refined carbohydrates, overconsumption of carbohydrates in general, artificial flavors and colors, pesticides, processed foods, and a skewed intake and ratio of fats (omega-6 and omega-3) and trans-fatty acids (harmful byproducts from hydrogenated fats and oils, margarines, and fried foods)—all that, plus the huge amount of food that the average American eats at any given meal.

Also, people consume excessive amounts of complex carbohydrates (in the form of grains) at the expense of nutrient-dense vegetables. Although it is difficult to convince people to eat vegetables, it is essential that they become the center of a healthy food plan. I refer you to the book *What Color Is Your Diet* by David Heber, M.D., Ph.D. (Regan Books, 2002). His book can help us all understand the importance of fruits and vegetables and what their colors may mean to our health.

The ideal diet provides adequate protein to maintain anabolic activity (repair and maintenance) without stressing the liver and kidneys or depleting water and minerals. It also contains complex, unrefined carbohydrates, including a rich supply of vegetables, in amounts appropriate for individual levels of activity, to maintain stable blood sugar without inducing excessive insulin response. And it provides enough quality fat to fuel energy and supply essential fatty acids vital to the brain, immune system, and cellular membranes.

All foods—whether they are carbohydrates, fats, or proteins—contain calories. If more calories are consumed than expended, the excess calories are stored as glycogen and fat for later use. This excessive caloric intake is compounded to a point of an efficient fat-producing factory when other metabolic key factors are out of balance and contributing to lowered cellular efficiency. In other words, if too much energy is brought into the factory and the furnace is turned down, the excess is stored in reserve. In the body, the energy is food, the furnace is metabolism, and the storage units are fat cells.

Enzymes and Insulin Regulation

The pancreas produces and secretes enzymes essential for digesting food and regulates enzymes critical for the conversion of essential fatty acids to prostaglandins. (See the inset "Enzymes: What Makes Things Happen" on page 45.) The pancreas secretes protein-digesting, carbohydrate-digesting, and fat-digesting enzymes into the small intestine. These enzymes break down large food molecules so that they may be absorbed by the intestinal villi and transported into the bloodstream. So critical are pancreatic enzymes that deficiency results in acute digestive symptoms, including diarrhea and weight loss. Without them, food passes through the digestive tract undigested and unabsorbed.

Pancreatic enzyme deficiency has a number of proposed causes. One is pancreatic exhaustion from a diet high in cooked foods. A diet of mostly cooked foods—and devoid of naturally occurring enzymes—relies exclusively on the pancreas' store of enzymes to break down food. Another theory is that a highly acidic diet from sugar and refined carbohydrates, upsets the alkaline environment required for pancreatic enzymes to function. A low-fiber diet is also thought to decrease pancreatic function. Infection, particularly by intestinal microorganisms such as *Helicobacter pylori* and *Giardia lamblia,* can obstruct the flow of pancreatic enzymes.

The second most common cause of pancreatic enzyme deficiency is a scarcity of *cofactors* (nonprotein, organic molecules essential for enzyme activity). Enzymes of all types depend on nutritional cofactors to perform their functions. Magnesium is a cofactor in more than 100 enzyme-induced pathways. For example, the metabolic enzyme delta-6-desaturase is dependent on magnesium in order to convert omega-6 to gamma linolenic acid (GLA) and dihomogamma linolenic acid (DGLA), two types of omega-6 essential fatty acids (EFAs). Magnesium is also required for the synthesis of the healthy prostaglandins PGE1 and PGE3.

The conversion of dietary omega-6 EFAs to healthy prostaglandins is regulated, in part, by *delta-6-desaturase,* which is stimulated by insulin. Delta-6-desaturase is inhibited by several conditions, including age and diet, especially trans-fatty acids, byproducts of hydrogenation (a process used to make oil more solid, as is commonly done in the production of margarine). A diet high in refined carbohydrates slows delta-6-desaturase activity and decreases production of healthy prostaglandins.

Another enzyme involved in the production of prostaglandins is *delta-5-desaturase.* In the presence of delta-5-desaturase, GLA becomes arachidonic acid, which is ultimately converted to PGE2, an unhealthy or proinflammatory prostaglandin. Delta-5-desaturase is regulated, to a large degree, by endocrine hormones specifically secreted by the pancreas. Glucagon inhibits the enzyme, while insulin promotes it. A diet high in refined carbohydrates, hyperglycemia, and hyperinsulinemia stimulates delta-5-desaturase and the production of arachidonic acid and the inflammatory cascade.

The overproduction of the inflammatory prostaglandins is a major cardiovascular risk factor for those with elevated insulin. Hypertension, atherosclerosis, blood clotting, and cholesterol synthesis are all directly linked to unhealthy prostaglandins. Controlling body fat, dietary intake, and insulin levels are significant ways to limit delta-5-desaturase, and control the production of arachidonic acid.

Omega-3 fatty acids, especially eicosapentaenoic acid (EPA), also utilize delta-5-desaturase. Thus, higher intakes of EPA will competitively inhibit the amount of delta-5-desaturase that is available to convert GLA to arachidonic acid and the proinflammatory prostaglandins. This is why a balanced intake of a 1:3 ratio of omega-3 to omega-6 fatty acids is important in the diet.

Stress and Insulin Regulation

Stress is a contributing factor in almost every psychological condition and in many physical ones. While stress does not cause diabetes, it aggravates the pancreas and the adrenal glands and interferes with blood sugar regulation. The stress response, best known as "fight or flight," involves the secretion of stress hormones from the adrenal glands. These hormones, including *epinephrine, norepinephrine, glucocorticoids,* and *mineralocorticoids,* prepare the body for physical danger in a number of ways.

Nervous system activity increases, heart rate and blood pressure rise, surface

Enzymes: What Makes Things Happen

Your metabolism can do nothing without enzymes. Enzymes are catalysts required for virtually every function within the body. They are specialized proteins that act as catalysts to promote the billions of biochemical reactions that occur inside of you. A catalyst is anything that lowers the metabolic energy required for a particular reaction to take place. Without properly functioning enzymes, metabolic function is greatly inhibited, and metabolism slows down.

Thousands of different enzymes have been identified in the human body, with as many as 10,000 enzymes altogether. Each enzyme has a specific function in the body that no other enzyme can duplicate. Enzymes are often divided into three groups: *metabolic, digestive,* and *food-based.*

Those that follow play the most critical roles in the promotion of your personal metabolic code. You'll be learning more about them and just how important their function is to our health as we discuss each key in later chapters.

Metabolic Enzymes

Metabolic enzymes catalyze the reactions that enable life. Among their many functions, they activate cellular processes, break down chemical byproducts, convert food to energy, and generate chemical messengers.

Some examples of metabolic enzymes that impact your chemistry include:

• *Delta-6-desaturase.* Delta-6-desaturase is critical for the conversion of the omega-6 essential fatty acid *linoleic acid* (LA) into its metabolically active form, *gamma linolenic acid* (GLA). GLA is a key precursor for prostaglandin synthesis. Prostaglandins are regulatory chemicals that control a variety of body functions, including pain, inflammation, swelling, blood pressure, cholesterol levels, digestive processes, synthesis of sex hormones, fluid retention, blood clotting, nerve transmission, and the immune system.

• *5-alpha-reductase.* 5-alpha reductase is responsible for transforming testosterone, the male sex hormone, to 5-dihydrotestosterone (5-DHT). Excessive conversion of testosterone to 5-DHT is considered a major factor in several male-related hormone disorders, including prostate cancer, benign prostatic hyperplasia (BPH), acne, and baldness.

• *Alcohol dehydrogenase.* Also known as acetaldehyde dehydrogenase, this enzyme catalyzes the reduction of acetaldehyde, an extremely toxic breakdown product of ethanol (found in alcohol). If alcohol dehydrogenase is insufficient, acetaldehyde accumulates in the tissue, causing a host of problems such as liver damage and mental disorders. Most people who lack this enzyme cannot tolerate the effects of alcohol consumption, including some Asian groups and Native Americans.

• *Glutathione peroxidase.* A powerful antioxidant enzyme found within every cell of the body, particularly the brain and liver, which neutralizes free radicals, specifically *hydroperoxides,* which generate the highly destructive hydroxyl radicals. Low levels of glutathione peroxidase have been implicated in a wide array of diseases, including Parkinson's disease, Alzheimer's disease, and human immunodeficiency virus (HIV-1).

• *Glucose-6-phosphate dehydrogenase (G6PD).* G6PD is one of the primary enzymes needed for glucose metabolism. When your cells do not have enough glucose, cells cannot perform their intended tasks efficiently. G6PD deficiency is a common genetic abnormality. It is estimated that 100 million people suffer from a deficiency in G6PD. With G6PD deficiency, oxidative stress in the red blood cell leads to the reduction of hemoglobin, the oxygen-carrying protein in red blood cells, and structural changes within the cell.

• *Cyclooxygenase (COX).* COX is the enzyme that catalyzes the conversion of arachidonic acid (an inflammatory chemical mediator) to prostaglandins. The enzyme is found in two forms, known as COX-1 and COX-2. COX-1 is found in all tissue, where it continuously produces protective prostaglandins in response to the presence of hormones and changing conditions. The gastrointestinal lining, the kidneys, the heart, and blood platelets are major sites of COX-1 activity. COX-2, in contrast, is not active in most normal tissue, except in response to proinflammatory stimuli. The destructive prostaglandins synthesized in the presence of COX-2 increase inflammation and platelet aggregation (clotting).

• *5-Lipoxygenase (5-LOX).* 5-LOX is an enzyme that can insert oxygen into the molecule of arachidonic acid and thereby increase a type of inflammatory chemical known as leukotriene B4, which is even more destructive than proinflammatory prostaglandins. Leukotrienes are particularly dangerous to brain cells, where they may

blood vessels constrict (allowing for increased blood flow to the vital organs), and the liver releases stored glycogen to increase blood sugar. In order to fuel this intense metabolic state, the body relies on glycogen and protein stores. Fat replaces muscle mass lost in protein catabolism. The chief adrenal hormone responsible for changes in blood sugar metabolism and insulin activity is *cortisol.*

Cortisol decreases insulin sensitivity by receptor cells, decreases glucose uptake, and increases blood sugar. The rise in blood sugar is intended to serve as a reservoir for the central nervous system, which requires a continuous supply of glucose to function. Problems arise when this stress state becomes chronic. When cortisol levels (and, therefore, blood sugar levels) are chronically elevated due to the stress in our lives, the risk of insulin resistance and hyperinsulinemia increases, and you start to gain weight. So, by being chronically stressed out, you gain weight.

Stress hormones also increase urinary excretion of magnesium, which is an important cofactor in the synthesis of healthy prostaglandins. Additionally, epinephrine (also known as *adrenaline*) decreases the activity of delta-6-desaturase, interfer-

cause inflammation and degradation of cellular function. This elevation has been linked to prostate cancer, as well. The expression of the 5-LOX gene and the activity of the 5-LOX pathway are increased in the elderly subjects and in individuals taking NSAIDs. Wide-ranging disastrous effects occur to your personal metabolic code when this enzyme is elevated.

Digestive Enzymes

Digestive enzymes break down food and are grouped into several categories. *Proteases* (or proteolytic enzymes) specifically *catabolize* (or to break down) proteins, *lipases* aid in breaking down fat, and *amylases* break down carbohydrates. Without these enzymes, which are secreted by the salivary glands and the pancreas, digestion of food and absorption of nutrients would be impossible. A research study in the early 1990s concluded that more than 20 million Americans suffer from digestive disorders. Many of these disorders may be rooted in insufficient digestive enzymes.

Food-Based Enzymes

Food-based enzymes are those that occur naturally in raw foods. They support the digestive process by removing some of the burden on digestive enzymes. Examples are *papain* (from papaya) and *bromelain* (from pineapple), among others. Raw foods contain naturally occurring enzymes that are destroyed by heat and processing. Since the modern Western diet is comprised primarily of cooked foods, we lack the intake of food enzymes that nature intended. This places the burden of digestion on the digestive organs, which must produce the enzymes needed to digest the food we eat rather than the metabolic enzymes need for health and healing.

ing with the production of healthy prostaglandins. Moreover, cortisol increases the pancreatic secretion of insulin, and insulin stimulates the activity of delta-5-desaturase. Delta-5-desaturase increases the production of arachidonic acid and unhealthy prostaglandins. In other words, stress hormones have a double-negative effect. They inhibit healthy prostaglandin synthesis and enhance unhealthy prostaglandin synthesis. This is an important link between stress, cardiovascular disease, and diabetes and insulin resistance.

While most people consider stress emotional or physical in origin, diet also plays a major role. The adrenal stress hormones are stimulated by a diet high in carbohydrates and low in protein. An excessive intake of sugar, as well as hypoglycemia, triggers the release of adrenal hormones.

Other Endocrine Hormones and Insulin Regulation

Many authors, nutritionists, physicians, and biochemists have suggested that metabolic syndrome is controlled by the pancreas. Although the pancreas is the key organ in insulin regulation, it relies on other glands within the endocrine system—specifically, the thyroid and pituitary glands—to function properly. To place all of the blame on the pancreas limits your ability to regain control of your metabolism and, therefore, your health.

The hormones of the pituitary gland help regulate the amount of hormone production among several other endocrine glands, including the thyroid, adrenals, and the pancreas. The thyroid gland assists the pancreas and liver in maintaining stable blood sugar. A hormone released by the thyroid, *thyroxin,* increases insulin response. *Hypothyroidism* (low thyroid hormone output) threatens this supportive role and contributes to hyperglycemia and poor insulin response.

The exact effects of thyroid hormone on insulin secretion and action remains poorly understood. However, a recent clinical trial demonstrated that a hypothyroid state resulted in a reduction in both insulin binding and a number of insulin receptors in the livers of experimental rats. The thyroid gland also controls *thermogenesis,* or the ability of the body to convert caloric energy from carbohydrates and fat to heat and energy.

Bowel (Intestinal) Terrain and Insulin Regulation

Leaky gut is a condition characterized by increased permeability of the mucosal wall in the intestines. The "holes" in the intestinal wall may be a result of injury, infection, nutritional deficiencies, and even stress. The inflamed intestinal mucosa allows unusually large molecules to "leak" into the bloodstream. These large molecules are interpreted as foreign bodies and the immune system responds. The result is an allergic and/or inflammatory reaction, which can occur locally, producing gastrointestinal symptoms.

Leaky gut syndrome is implicated as a contributing factor in a host of conditions, including eczema, psoriasis, asthma, and arthritis. One autoimmune condition that may be linked to leaky gut is the spontaneous development of type 1, insulin-dependent diabetes from the T-lymphocyte (immune cell)-mediated destruction of pancreatic beta cells from which insulin is secreted. Many factors can influence the permeability of the gut, including food allergies, drugs, inadequate digestive enzymes, and dysbiosis.

Dysbiosis is defined as a disruption in the normal balance of microorganisms in the oral, gastrointestinal, or vaginal mucosa. Certain conditions promote the harmful overgrowth of otherwise harmless organisms, including yeast, bacteria, and protozoa. These organisms can alter the immune response of their host, deplete nutrients, and produce harmful endotoxins (those found within the body). Endotoxins are the waste products of the metabolic cycle of these organisms. *Candida albicans* is a common yeast, which, in a favorable terrain, can proliferate to dangerous levels. *C. albicans* destroys healthy intestinal bacteria, weakens the immune system, and can infect the blood and tissues. Systemic yeast infection (candidiasis) is associated with many obscure and difficult-to-treat conditions.

The most favorable condition for yeast overgrowth is hyperglycemia. A "high-sugar" environment feeds yeast, and any condition resulting in elevated blood glucose promotes yeast overgrowth. A diet high in sugar and refined carbohydrates, insulin resistance, and impaired glucose tolerance all encourage yeast proliferation.

During the *proliferative* (growing) stage of yeast growth, several endotoxins are produced: *acetaldehyde, ethanol,* and *alloxan.* These endotoxins destroy enzymes, damage cell membranes, and alter cellular response to hormones. When the yeast transforms from the bud to mycelial state, an enzyme is released, which attacks cell membranes. Free-radical damage, cell membrane rigidity, and decreased permeability of cells can result. These changes all influence the ability of the cell to carry out normal functions, including the utilization of glucose and cellular respiration.

Endotoxins can interfere with hormonal influence over cells. They do this by binding with receptor sites of target cells, and tricking the cells into believing they have bound with a hormone. While no hormone has actually reached the cell, negative feedback is initiated and the hormone production diminishes. This phenomenon, known as *hormone masking,* can affect insulin receptors and pancreatic secretion of insulin. Disrupting insulin production and glucose uptake has the effect of creating an even more favorable environment for yeast growth, thus feeding a toxic cycle. Bacteria and viruses through stimulation of T-cell-mediated autoimmunity can indirectly influence the pancreatic beta cells.

Oxygen and Insulin Regulation

Cellular metabolism is the mechanism by which food energy is converted to adenosine triphosphate (ATP), the chemical compound used by the cells to fuel metabolism. Cellular respiration is dependent on two vital components: glucose (derived from food) and oxygen.

Without oxygen, *anaerobic respiration* takes place, yielding a lower output of ATP, and therefore, less efficient energy production. Insulin influences the availability of oxygen at the cellular level. One way it does so is by promoting delta-5-desaturase and arachidonic acid production, which shifts the balance of prostaglandin synthesis in favor of the proinflammatory series (PGE2). This shift, among other things, constricts blood vessels. Constriction of blood vessels means restriction of blood flow to the cells. And blood is the oxygen transport vehicle for the body.

Oxygen increases insulin sensitivity of cells, particularly muscle cells. Since the cells need glucose to fuel cellular metabolism, it makes sense that in the presence of oxygen, cells are more receptive to insulin-mediated glucose transport.

The most important and effective method of increasing the oxygen content of blood, and oxygen availability to the cells, is exercise. Exercise has long been recommended for the prevention and treatment of diabetes. One major effect of exercise is to increase insulin sensitivity and, thus, reduce the risk of developing insulin resistance and type 2 diabetes. Research indicates that exercise may also improve existing insulin resistance, hyperinsulinemia, and impaired glucose tolerance.

In a recent study, conducted at the Washington University School of Medicine, exercise training increased glucose uptake of the cells by 56 percent in individuals with abnormal glucose tolerance. Furthermore, exercise can reduce insulin requirements of insulin-dependent diabetics. The effect of exercise on glucose uptake and insulin action does not appear to be affected by age, meaning that the benefits are realized across the life span.

Exercise plays an important role in preventing cardiovascular damage associated with poor insulin regulation. It is well known that exercise lowers triglyceride levels, reduces hypertension, and prevents atherosclerosis. Endurance exercise promotes glucagon secretion, which inhibits delta 5-desaturase. Exercise also helps control stress and obesity, two primary risk factors for developing both diabetes and cardiovascular disease. Another contributing factor of cardiovascular disease is oxidative stress. Oxidative damage occurs when free radicals, byproducts of cellular metabolism, inhibit or destroy normal chemical pathways. Free radicals damage enzymes, cell membranes, and DNA (genetic material) and are associated with many degenerative conditions, including cardiovascular disease. The body has a natural defense against normal, metabolic free-radical damage in the form of antioxidants. However, a constant barrage of external free radicals from pollution, radiation, diet, inflammatory response, and other sources can overwhelm the natural defenses of the body, leaving it highly susceptible to free-radical damage.

Those with poor insulin regulation appear to be at high risk of free-radical damage. According to an unpublished study conducted at Duke University Medical Center, the ability of type 2 diabetics to defend against free-radical damage is almost half that of nondiabetic subjects. High blood sugar triggers free-radical production and oxidative stress in the blood vessels, which contributes to some of the major complications associated with diabetes. Remember that for many of us, insulin resistance places us just a few dangerous steps away from diabetes and the cascade of health problems associated with it.

Insulin secretion may be partially regulated by intracellular production of ATP, the chemical compound used by the cells to fuel metabolism. As ATP levels increase, and the need for glucose transport into the cells diminishes, there is a reduction in pancreatic secretion of insulin. When ATP is used up, as during exercise, the pancreas is stimulated to secrete more insulin.

LAB TESTS FOR ASSESSING BLOOD SUGAR REGULATION

If you are unsure whether you have poor insulin regulation, consider requesting a *metabolic dysglycemia profile* from your healthcare provider. This is a unique test that measures a number of metabolic parameters affecting blood glucose. These include fasting and post-challenge glucose and insulin levels; glycated hemoglobin

A_1C; fructosamine; DHEA; cortisol; and IGF-1. By looking at these values, early detection of impaired glucose regulation can be detected long before signs of overt diabetes develop. A separate lipid profile is also available to measure any effects of impaired glycemic control. The test utilizes blood and saliva samples taken before a glucose challenge test, and a blood test two hours afterward.

TREATING POOR BLOOD SUGAR REGULATION

Conventional medicine has myriad drugs for regulating blood sugar despite an individual's lifestyle. Although this sounds attractive, we all know that there is a price to pay when we take multiple medications. Although this may control the problem, it rarely leads to true health. An integrative approach, which may include conventional drug therapy, focuses on a process that includes improving food selection, exercising, getting the needed nutrients that are responsible for blood sugar regulation, and taking advantage of the various nutraceuticals available to improve your health and to reduce the risks of developing metabolic syndrome and other conditions. Learning to eat well, making sure you get physically active, and supplementing your diet with chromium and magnesium (the two most important nutrients for blood sugar regulation) is a good start to managing your blood sugar. I'll be providing you with specific recommendations in Chapter 6.

Matthew's Story

Before seeing Dr. LaValle, I had a host of health problems and complaints. My primary problem was that I had become what my medical doctor called "an incipient diabetic." I had severe carbohydrate cravings and had gained a lot of weight. I had other problems such as sleep disturbances, fungal infections on my toes and feet, low energy, and blemishes on my face. I could not exercise because I would get a painful itching in my legs when I did. Within three days of taking the supplements that Dr. LaValle recommended and making some dietary changes, the carbohydrate cravings ceased and my blood sugar normalized. After several weeks, my foot fungus and skin blemishes cleared up. Over five to six months, I lost forty pounds and began sleeping better. I can exercise now without the painful itching and I have not had a sore throat or cold since starting with Dr. LaValle's recommendations.

I was excited when Matthew started taking his health into his own hands. Many people simply accept their nagging health symptoms as normal. Matthew's rejuvenation program focused on improving his blood sugar response. This, along with detoxification, helped him to overcome his fungus-related itching, sore throat, and fungal nails. In the end, he dramatically improved the quality of his life, and hopefully, his longevity.

INSULIN BALANCE IS KEY

Controlling your blood sugar will have far-reaching implications on your personal metabolic code. It is an essential component that must be regulated if you are to achieve the goal of long-term health. In Chapter 6, I'll give you information on how to balance your insulin using diet and supplements, along with important lifestyle choices. The consequences of poor blood sugar regulation are clear. Increasing your risks of developing insulin resistance and diabetes has a devastating impact on your health.

Now that we've talked about the pancreas, the battle of proper insulin levels and keeping our bodies healthy through blood sugar regulation, let's continue to seek a balance of hormones throughout the body. A normal functioning thyroid gland and a balance of its hormones are imperative in keeping our bodies healthy. Let's look further.

Now, onward for Key Two . . .

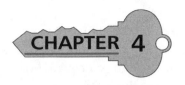

CHAPTER 4

KEY TWO:
Balancing Your Thyroid—Overcoming Fatigue and Burning Fat

I f you are puzzled by your sluggish metabolism and by your almost total lack of energy, then you need to read this chapter carefully. There are millions of people who, along with you, are wondering why their metabolism moves at a snail's pace. Are you tired of feeling tired all day long? Do you feel depressed? Do you have dry skin and cold hands and feet? Do you seem to gain weight no matter what you seem to do? These and other all-too-common symptoms can signal a larger problem. Hypothyroidism—defined as underactive thyroid, or, as the underproduction of thyroid hormones—is estimated to affect 11 million Americans, 9 million of who are women.

There are several factors that can affect thyroid function and hormone utilization in the body. Chronic stress may be getting the best of your thyroid function. Or environmental toxins, which can bind to thyroid receptors and alter thyroid hormones, may be affecting your chemistry. Food allergies may be contributing to thyroid dysfunction. Even overconsumption of soy products has been associated with thyroid dysfunction. Any and all of these factors and more could be affecting your thyroid's ability to function at optimal efficiency.

A recently published Italian study of people 100 years or older suggests that endocrine, metabolic, and immune functions are interdependent and are paramount in maintaining health as we age. Preserved functions of the thyroid and parathyroid hormones, as well as integrity of muscle mass and vitamin D, were associated with longevity and high natural killer (NK) cell immunity (a type of immune cell that destroys cancer and virus-infected cells).

Since the thyroid gland is responsible for regulating many functions in the body, it makes sense that the underproduction or underutilization of thyroid hormones leads to a host of symptoms ranging from weight gain and fatigue to high cholesterol levels and, possibly, even infertility. Furthermore, thyroid function can be reduced for years before clinical tests indicate a diagnosable problem. Despite the appearance of many of the classic symptoms of low thyroid function, vast amounts of people are untreated because their thyroid function tests are within normal clinical limits, or just slightly off. The term *subclinical hypothyroidism* has been used to describe this state, and thanks to the practitioners who recognize and treat it, many people are finally being spared unnecessary suffering.

Subclinical hypothyroidism is one of the most common complaints that I come across in my practice. Working with patients like these over the years, I have come to understand that no other single gland seems to have as wide an effect on symptoms than does the thyroid. If the thyroid is not functioning well, symptoms can range from weight gain to depression; dry skin to constipation; and cold hands and feet to brittle hair, skin, and nails. Other symptoms of low thyroid function include:

- Aching muscles
- Decreased metabolism
- Elevated cholesterol
- Fatigue, insomnia
- Heartburn
- Hoarseness
- Increased menstrual flow

- Infertility
- Intolerance to cold
- Poor appetite
- Poor concentration
- Poor coordination
- Reduced rate of breathing
- Slow heart rate

Within the endocrine system, the thyroid is the biological engine that ultimately directs hormonal function and, therefore, metabolism. The thyroid gland produces the hormones that make the body burn calories. Thyroid hormones are what drive your basal metabolic rate (the energy required for internal or cellular work when the body is at rest), in other words, your metabolism.

HOW THE THYROID GLAND REGULATES METABOLISM

The thyroid is a large, butterfly-shaped gland with two lobes connected by a body (or isthmus) over the trachea. Embedded within the thyroid gland are four masses of tissue called the parathyroid glands. The thyroid produces and secretes three major hormones: *thyroxine, triiodothyronine,* and *calcitonin.* Thyroid hormones influence almost every cell of the body. The thyroid gland has a crucial role in metabolism, fat burning, and oxygen utilization, as well as in gastrointestinal and neuromuscular function.

Thyroxine and triiodothyronine are produced when iodine combines with the amino acid tyrosine. Thyroxine, or T4, is tyrosine bound to four molecules of iodine. Triiodothyronine, or T3, is tyrosine bound to three molecules of iodine. Iodine and tyrosine must be present in adequate amounts in the diet for the synthesis of T4. When thyroid hormone was first discovered, T4 was given exclusive credit for the metabolic activity at the cellular level. Later, it was discovered that T3 was four times more active than T4 at the target cells. It is now understood that much of the circulating T4 is actually converted to T3 prior to cellular metabolic activity.

The anterior pituitary gland and the hypothalamus regulate thyroid hormone levels. Initially, the hypothalamus responds to a metabolic change such as low body temperature, stress, or sleep by releasing thyrotropin releasing factor (TRF), while simultaneously signaling the anterior pituitary gland to release thyroid stimulating hormone (TSH). TSH stimulates the thyroid, which traps iodine, synthesizes T4, and releases the thyroid hormone. As levels of T4 increase, the activities of the hypothalamus and pituitary are inhibited. (Figure 2.2 on page 23 illustrates this mechanism.)

T4 increases the metabolic rate of almost every tissue in the body. Its effects on metabolism are astonishing. For example, a person whose thyroid gland reduces the production of T4 will experience as much as a 40 percent drop in metabolism, or *basal metabolic rate* (the rate at which the body spends energy for the maintenance activities of the body). Meanwhile, overproduction of T4 can increase normal metabolic activity by 100 percent. T4 increases the basal metabolic rate by impacting the rate of ATP (energy) production in the mitochondria (the energy-producing components of cells). The thyroid uses much of this energy to convert caloric energy to heat in a process called *thermogenesis.* In other words, how your body uses food determines your metabolism.

Thyroid hormone increases the utilization of carbohydrates and fat from food, and the rate of protein synthesis. It stimulates the appetite and the movement of food through the digestive tract. In the presence of thyroid hormone, muscle catabolism increases, which increases the resting metabolic rate (muscle burns more energy than fat). Thyroid hormone also increases the sensitivity of skeletal muscle to impulses from the spinal cord. (An excess of thyroid hormone is known to cause tremors, and a deficiency results in sluggish muscle response.) Thyroid hormone increases the uptake of oxygen into the cells, which speeds aerobic respiration. Finally, thyroid hormone actually increases the number of mitochondria within the cells.

Aging, poor nutrition, stress, and exposure to environmental toxins can all damage the thyroid gland and ultimately undermine metabolic function. As we age, thyroid activity diminishes, contributing to the weight gain that many people experience as they approach middle age. By keeping the integrity of the endocrine system, and particularly thyroid function, the seemingly inevitable "middle-age spread" many times can be avoided.

When metabolism is increased, the demand for oxygen also increases to fuel the aerobic energy cycle within the cells. The cardiovascular system responds by dilating blood vessels and increasing the heart rate, blood volume, and rate of breathing. The heart works harder and faster to meet increased metabolic demands. This creates a precarious balance between oxygen availability and free-radical potential. While extra oxygen supply is needed to support increased metabolism, too much oxygen generates free radicals that can damage mitochondrial DNA (DNA within the mitochondria).

Calcitonin is the hormone released from the parathyroid tissue that influences calcium and phosphate levels of the blood and bones. Calcitonin lowers blood concentrations of these minerals by increasing their absorption into bones. Blood calcium levels regulate the release of calcitonin through the negative feedback mechanism (a way in which the body turns off hormones after they've done their job). When calcium levels are high, calcitonin is released. When calcium levels drop, calcitonin is inhibited.

Table 4.1 below summarizes the metabolic roles of the thyroid gland's three major hormones.

Table 4.1. Thyroid Hormones and Their Functions

HORMONE	SOURCE	ACTION
Thyroxine (T4)	TSH from anterior pituitary	Increases metabolism of fats, carbohydrates and proteins; promotes protein synthesis; stimulates growth and activity of the nervous system
Triiodothyronine (T3)	Converted from T4 to active T3	Same as action as thyroxine
Calcitonin	Stimulated by increases in serum calcium and digestive secretions	Stabilizes blood calcium and phosphate levels by conserving ions in the bones, and increasing excretion in the urine

The Parathyroid Gland

The parathyroid gland consists of tightly packed cells. These cells secrete *parathyroid hormone* (PTH, also known as *parathormone*), whose primary function is to increase the blood concentration of calcium and decrease the concentration of phosphate. Parathyroid hormone works with calcitonin to maintain a stable blood concentration of these minerals. This is very important for neuromuscular control, as a drop in calcium can cause the muscles to lose their ability to expand and contract properly. When calcium in the blood is too high, muscles and reflexes are weak and slow to respond.

CONDITIONS OF THE THYROID GLAND

Hypothyroidism is a condition resulting from the *underproduction* of thyroid hormone, and hyperthyroidism is a condition resulting from the *overproduction* of thyroid hormone. Hypothyroidism that can be clinically diagnosed is called overt hypothyroidism. Hypothyroidism is also sometimes referred to as *suboptimal* or *functional hypoythyroidism.* This condition has virtually the same symptom profile as hypothyroidism, but remains undiagnosed and untreated because blood tests are within normal clinical range. Many side effects and illnesses can be caused by a poorly functioning thyroid.

Hyperthyroidism

Hyperthyroidism is not as common as hypothyroidism. However, hyperthyroidism like hypothyroidism is more prevalent in women than men. Although it can occur at any age, it is most likely to occur after age fifteen and more so in those who have reached their thirties and forties. The annual incidence of hyperthyroidism in the United States is about one per a thousand women.

When the thyroid gland produces too much thyroxine, despite normal levels of TSH, the signs and symptoms of hyperthyroidism (sometimes called thyrotoxicosis) appear. Hyperthyroidism causes a high increase in basal metabolic rate, sensitivity to heat, restlessness, decreased menstrual flow, rapid heartbeat, hand tremors, weight loss, and mental alertness. These symptoms, as well as the contrary symptoms of hypothyroidism are listed in Table 4.2 on page 59.

The most common type of hyperthyroidism is Grave's disease. This disorder is accompanied by exophthalmos (bulging of the eyes) and goiter (an enlarged thyroid gland). Grave's disease, like Hashimoto's thyroiditis, which is discussed below, is an autoimmune condition. Antibodies (cells that normally destroy foreign substances) that mimic the action of thyroid-stimulating hormone (TSH) bind to receptor sites in the thyroid gland, stimulating the production of thyroid hormones.

An uncommon but serious form of hyperthyroidism is *thyroid storm.* This condition usually comes on suddenly and can result from an infection, trauma, severe emotional distress, or preeclampsia (a condition that occurs during pregnancy). High levels of thyroid hormone circulating in the system can result in high fever, muscle wasting, wild mood swings, liver enlargement, and cardiovascular and central nervous system complications.

Hypothyroidism

When your thyroid is either underactive, nonfunctioning, or has been all or in part surgically removed, you are considered *hypothyroid* (low thyroid). Millions of people worldwide are affected by hypothyroidism; it is estimated that 10 to 20 percent of women experience hypothyroidism during their lifetime.

Myxedema, or *acquired hypothyroidism* (terms for adult hypothyroidism), is a condition that appears in late childhood or in early to middle adulthood. Symptoms of myxedema develop slowly, sometimes over the course of several years. The predominant clinical symptoms are severe mental and physical fatigue: tasks that once seemed effortless can become overwhelming. Depression, intolerance to cold, weight gain, hair loss, dry skin, and constipation are other indicators of acquired hypothyroidism. There is also a marked reduction in heart rate. Women may experience heavy, extended menstrual periods. The term myxedema characterizes the collection of a mucous substance in the connective tissue throughout the body. Subsequently, there is swelling (edema) of the face, vocal cords, inner ears, and hands.

The most common type of hypothyroidism is caused by an autoimmune reaction to the thyroid gland, known *as Hashimoto's thyroiditis.* In this disorder, the body in effect becomes allergic to thyroid hormone. It then produces antibodies against its own thyroid tissue, or autoantibodies. Hashimoto's thyroiditis affects ten times as many women as men and is the primary cause of hypothyroidism in older children.

The specific origin of autoimmune thyroiditis is unknown, although several research articles have pointed to its association with other autoimmune disorders. In one study, 41.6 percent of patients with systemic lupus erythematosus (SLE, a chronic inflammatory disease that can affect many of the body's organs) also had thyroid autoantibodies in their blood samples. There is also a high correlation between the presence of thyroid autoantibodies and diseases of the adrenal glands. For example, among a group of 212 patients with *Addison's disease* (severe underactivity of the adrenal glands), 188 tested positive for antibodies against thyroglobulin (the storage form of T4 within the thyroid gland). Eighty-one had antibodies against thyroid peroxidase (an enzyme necessary for thyroid hormone activity).

A recent study found that patients treated for *Cushing's disease* (severe overactivity of the adrenal glands) have an increased prevalence of thyroid autoimmunity and autoimmune thyroiditis.

Autoimmune diseases of the pancreas, such as insulin-dependent diabetes mellitus (type 1 diabetes), are also strongly associated with autoimmune thyroid disease. It is proposed that these autoimmune diseases share a common autoantibody that cross-reacts between various organs and tissues. The endocrine system appears to be the most vulnerable to these autoimmune attacks.

Hashimoto's thyroiditis is a common cause of *simple* or *endemic goiter,* a swelling of the thyroid gland. It primarily affects those who live in areas with naturally poor sources of iodine in the soil or drinking water, and those who lack iodine in the diet. In this case, the lack of iodine needed to synthesize thyroxine T4 results in low serum T4 levels. In response, the pituitary gland secretes thyroid-stimulating hormone (TSH) in an effort to "wake up" the thyroid gland. Continuous stimulation of the thyroid causes it to swell, but it is still unable to manufacture adequate hormone levels. Consequently, symptoms of hypothyroidism accompany goiter.

There can be many causes of low thyroid that may not be easily discovered. Heavy metal intoxication, stress, adrenal exhaustion, infections, food allergies, dysbiosis, along with nutrient deficiencies, can all play a role in slowing thyroid function.

Subclinical Hypothyroidism

It is estimated that 15 to 25 percent of the population, approximately 43 to 72 million Americans, has some degree of subclinical hypothyroidism. Subclinical hypothyroidism is also sometimes referred to as *suboptimal* or *functional hypoythyroidism.* These are people who display symptoms of hypothyroidism, but whose blood tests

Table 4.2. The Differences between Hypothyroidism and Hyperthyroidism

SYMPTOMS	HYPOTHYROIDISM	HYPERTHYROIDISM
Behavior and mood	Depression, fatigue, sleepiness, poor concentration, hallucinations	Nervousness, restlessness, irritability, exhaustion, insomnia
Cardiovascular	Slow pulse rate (<70 bpm); prolonged condition may result in weakened heart muscle	Heart palpitations, rapid pulse, and atrial fibrillation, inhibited in platelet function
Cholesterol	Elevated cholesterol	Decreased cholesterol
Features	Coarse voice, stunted growth in children, enlarged thyroid	Bulging eyes, enlarged thyroid
Gastrointestinal	Slowed digestion, constipation, bloating, hard stools, heartburn, poor appetite	Diarrhea, increased appetite
Menstrual/Sexual	Heavy periods, milky discharge from breasts, infertility, loss of libido	Scant periods, infertility, loss of libido, impotence
Metabolism	Decreased basal metabolic rate: weight gain	Increased basal metabolic rate: weight loss
Muscles and reflexes	Muscle aches, cramping, poor coordination, numbness in hands and feet	Muscle weakness, tremors
Respiratory	Breathing slows, poor ventilation	Hyperventilation
Skin and hair	Dry, rough skin texture, yellow/orange skin tone, decreased sweating; hair thin and dry, loss of body hair	Silky, thickened skin, increased sweating, hives; thinning hair, hair loss
Tolerance to temperature	Intolerance to cold	Intolerance to heat

will fall within the normal range. Many clients who walk into my practice complaining of fatigue and intolerance to cold have been previously diagnosed with fibromyalgia (a disorder with no obvious physical cause characterized by chronic, achy, muscular pain; extreme fatigue; and skin sensitivities). In short, while they complain mostly of symptoms related to hypothyroidism, the results of conventional tests claim that their thyroid function is normal.

There are two possible reasons for this scenario: Either the thyroid hormones are in the bloodstream but are not binding to target tissue and creating the desired activity, or the current "normal" range of thyroid hormones and TSH on lab tests needs to be changed. This second reason, which is discussed later in this chapter, is actually a current topic of discussion in the medical community. Subclinical hypothyroidism has virtually the same symptom profile as hypothyroidism, but it remains undiagnosed and untreated because blood tests are within normal clinical range. That is, serum T3 and T4 levels are normal, or low to normal, and TSH is only slightly elevated. The problem may stem from the inability of target cells to convert T4 to T3.

The negative feedback mechanism fails because serum T4 remains within normal limits. (TSH is stimulated in response to drops in serum T4.)

Many patients who complain to their physicians of symptoms such as cold hands and feet, intolerance to cold weather, nausea, headache, fatigue, irritability, dry skin and hair, hair loss, insomnia, weight gain, and many other vague complaints are told that nothing is wrong. Although their symptoms clearly indicate that there is a problem, current lab tests are either not sensitive enough to determine that there is a problem or the results need to be redefined for treatment. Subclinical hypothyroidism can eventually lead to overt hypothyroidism.

Because thyroid function appears to decline with age, the elderly are at particular risk for subclinical hypothyroidism. A recent population-based, cross-sectional study found that subclinical hypothyroidism increases the risk of atherosclerosis and myocardial infarction among postmenopausal women. Because thyroid hormone has such a profound impact on other hormones in the body, subclinical hypothyroidism can even lead to reproductive difficulties in women of childbearing age. If a woman does conceive, but has a deficiency of thyroid hormone, the fetus can suffer because thyroid hormone is responsible for regulating tissue growth and development, particularly the growth of nerve tissue.

Conditions Associated with Thyroid Dysfunction

The thyroid gland, with the help of the pituitary, is the most important organ in the body for controlling weight and body fat. Thyroid hormones define the rate of cellular metabolism. If the thyroid gland is functioning properly, and enough thyroid hormone is getting to the cells, then energy from food is properly utilized. If there is a problem with the gland itself or if something is interfering with the thyroid hormone's ability to bind to its target cells, metabolism alters, slowing down or speeding up every process in the body, which in turn can cause many recurring problems. The following discussions cover the most common problems associated with the underproduction or overproduction of thyroid hormone, several of which are directly associated with metabolic syndrome.

Fatigue and Free-Radical Damage

Fatigue can be directly related to problems with the thyroid. The process by which energy from food is released and transferred to usable energy by the cells is a complex chain of chemical reactions known as *cellular respiration.*

Some energy is released from food in the absence of oxygen (anaerobic respiration), but most is derived in the mitochondria of the cells in the presence of oxygen (aerobic respiration). In the mitochondria, aerobic respiration produces cellular energy in the form of ATP (a large energy molecule). Triiodothyronine (T3) and thyroxine (T4) are needed to utilize oxygen during aerobic respiration. If T4 or T3 levels are low, cellular respiration and energy are depleted, excess oxygen builds up in the cells, and oxidative, or free-radical, damage occurs. When these levels are low, the number of mitochondria in our cells actually begins to decrease.

Most, if not all, diseases associated with or caused by free-radical damage (for example, cancer, cardiovascular disease, diabetes, arthritis, and premature aging) may be accelerated by insufficient thyroid hormone. Furthermore, without oxygen, the cells must rely on anaerobic respiration for energy. This metabolic pathway is insufficient for energy production and leads to lactic acid accumulation (an acid that when elevated can interfere with the biochemical interactions needed for muscle contractions), fatigue, and cellular destruction.

Since low thyroid function slows down every process in the body, including circulation, those with hypothyroidism are often mildly anemic. Iron is an essential component of hemoglobin, the protein in red blood cells that transport oxygen throughout the body. Iron deficiency anemia results from poor dietary iron intake, and subsequent inadequate production of hemoglobin. Mild anemia can be corrected by insuring sufficient dietary intake of iron. Heme iron, found in meat, is the most readily absorbable form of iron. Non-heme iron is found in whole grains, seeds, nuts, vegetables, blackstrap molasses, and nutritional yeast.

Grave's disease and Hashimoto's thyroiditis are both associated with pernicious anemia, an anemia resulting from a deficiency of vitamin B_{12} (cyanocobalamin). Under normal conditions, the epithelial cells of the gastrointestinal tract produce a substance known as intrinsic factor, which allows the body to absorb vitamin B_{12} from food. Pernicious anemia produces antibodies, which attack the intrinsic factor and prevent the body from absorbing this vitamin. Pernicious anemia can be treated with intramuscular B_{12} injections.

Both hypothyroid and hyperthyroid conditions can create fatigue and exhaustion. In hypothyroidism, the ability of the cells to produce ATP is inhibited by low thyroxine. In hyperthyroidism, excessive rates of cellular function leads to metabolic exhaustion.

Cardiovascular Disease

The metabolism of fats and absorption of essential fatty acids (EFAs) are important functions of the thyroid. Insufficient thyroxine to stimulate fat metabolism can lead to *hyperlipidemia,* or elevated cholesterol. Without the benefit of cardioprotective nutrients from essential fatty acids, you may be at an increased risk of cardiovascular disease. If you have a high cholesterol reading, be sure to have your thyroid function evaluated before beginning medication.

T3 is necessary for the utilization of oxygen by the mitochondria during cellular respiration. Inadequate T3 in the cells has a negative effect on oxygen consumption. Excess oxygen results in an increase in the oxidation of lipids (fats) and free-radical damage. Increased oxidation of the low-density lipoprotein (LDL) form of cholesterol, often referred to as "bad" cholesterol, has been identified in hyperthyroid and hypothyroid states.

Insulin Resistance

T4 also influences how quickly glucose (sugar) is absorbed from the intestines and then taken up by the cells. Thyroxine stimulates the conversion of proteins and fats to glycogen when blood sugar is high and the transformation of glycogen to glucose when blood sugar is low. The thyroid gland assists the pancreas and liver in maintaining stable blood sugar. In other words, thyroxine increases insulin response.

Hypothyroidism threatens this supportive role and contributes to poor insulin response and blood sugar regulation. The exact effects of thyroid hormone on insulin secretion and action remains poorly understood. However, a recent clinical trial demonstrated that a hypothyroid state resulted in a reduction in both insulin binding and number of insulin receptors in the livers of experimental rats. These alterations help to explain the indirect effect of thyroid function on a wide spectrum of metabolic functions.

Malabsorption

Poor absorption of dietary nutrients in the intestines is associated with hypothyroidism and hyperthyroidism. Hyperthyroidism causes diarrhea, which prevents adequate absorption of nutrients from food. Hypothyroidism inhibits adequate secretion of hydrochloric acid (stomach acid) and digestive enzymes. When the hydrochloric acid level in the stomach is low, indigestion and dyspepsia result. Digestive enzymes are needed to break down large food molecules for proper absorption. Brittle nails, lusterless hair, constipation, and similar symptoms can be the result.

With constipation comes an increased likelihood of unwanted microorganisms building up in the colon (which you'll learn more about in Chapter 9). These organisms can create toxins that have local and systemic effects. For example, the intestinal bacteria *Clostridia* converts bile acids to a carcinogenic substance that can lead to colorectal cancer.

Hypothyroidism also results in poor utilization and conversion of essential fatty acids, leading to an overproduction of inflammatory prostaglandins and dry skin. If the gut lining is compromised by micro-inflammation of the colon lining, it causes the absorption of undigested food particles into the bloodstream, which the immune system "attacks" by manufacturing antibodies. This phenomenon is known as leaky gut syndrome. It leads to food allergies and sensitivities and can trigger autoimmune thyroid disturbances and generally has a negative impact on immune function.

KEY INFLUENCES ON THYROID FUNCTION

Research indicates that thyroid problems are on the rise. This may be due to a combination of factors, such as poor nutritional status/intake and increasing levels of environmental toxins. As we have seen, the endocrine glands are in constant communication not only with each other, but also with the nervous and immune systems. In conjunction with the pituitary gland, thyroid hormones influence almost every function in the body, as metabolism establishes the official temperature at which systems operate. Because the thyroid gland's work involves interaction with many body systems, it is particularly sensitive to influences than can disrupt its proper functioning. These are discussed below.

Diet and Thyroid Function

There is a direct relationship between nutrition status and the impact of hormones. The foods we eat and the vitamins, minerals, and nutrients available to the body regulate the synthesis and utilization of thyroid hormones. At the same time, thyroid hormones influence the rate of metabolism of fuel sources from foods: fats, proteins, and carbohydrates. Thyroid hormones increase the rate of energy released from carbohydrates, increase the rate of protein synthesis, and stimulate the breakdown of fats. Low thyroid function slows the metabolism of these foods, leading to depleted energy and a slower metabolic rate that leads to weight gain.

In the presence of too much thyroid hormone, food is turned to energy with high speed and efficiency, increasing the basal metabolic rate and leading to excessive weight loss.

The digestive and endocrine systems are dependent upon each other for the optimal absorption of nutrients from foods and the utilization of nutrients for hormone synthesis. Hypothyroidism results in weight gain, despite a poor appetite, constipation, pernicious anemia, poor utilization of essential fatty acids, and inadequate conversion of beta-carotene to vitamin A. Hypothyroidism is also associated with insufficient production of hydrochloric acid by the parietal cells of the stomach. Hydrochloric acid provides the proper pH environment for the digestion of proteins by the enzyme pepsin. Without hydrochloric acid, the amino acid phenylalanine (from which tyrosine is derived) cannot be obtained from food, and tyrosine is unavailable in adequate amounts for the production of thyroxine.

A cycle of hypothyroidism can be created in this interplay between digestion and thyroid function. Hyperthyroidism can cause diarrhea, weight loss, and deficiencies in fat-soluble vitamins and calcium. Hyperthyroidism can increase metabolic rates by as much as 200 percent, requiring a proportional intake of calories.

Nutrients and Thyroid Function

Several nutrients are critical for the proper functioning of the thyroid gland. In order for the thyroid gland to produce T4, it needs the trace elements iodine, chromium, and selenium, the mineral zinc, and the amino acid tyrosine. Without sufficient supply of these nutrients in the diet, thyroid function is diminished. Several reasons why a person may be lacking these nutrients include dysbiosis (a disruption in the normal balance of microorganisms in the gastrointestinal mucosa), taking oral contraceptives, which deplete many nutrients, especially selenium and zinc, and consuming a diet high in processed foods (chromium, zinc, and selenium are destroyed very easily in food processing). Without selenium and zinc, the enzyme *iodothyronine deiodinase* cannot do its job of converting T4 to T3.

Enzymes and Thyroid Function

Enzymes are cofactors (catalysts) in almost every metabolic pathway in the body. At the cellular level, enzymes bind with other substances (called substrates), triggering changes in the metabolism of the cell. These changes are recognized as the function of the hormone, but would be impossible without enzymes. Enzymes have important functions related to metabolism, including:

- Enzymes are required by the gastrointestinal tract to digest large food molecules so that they can be properly absorbed into the bloodstream.

- Enzymes regulate the steps of cellular respiration: the way energy from food is converted to molecules that can be used by the cells of the body.

- Enzymes are required by target cells to activate metabolic changes, or "messages" delivered by hormones. Enzymes also mediate the conversion of essential fatty acids (EFAs) to prostaglandins.

- Enzymes can be denatured (destroyed or inactivated) by a variety of chemical toxins, known as toxic inhibitors. These include industrial pollutants, heavy metals, pesticides, cigarette smoke, drugs, household chemicals, and endotoxins created by the body. If enzymes are destroyed by exposure to toxic inhibitors, they cannot catalyze the "messages" delivered to the cells by specific hormones. The effect is that while hormone blood levels appear normal, their influence over cells is inefficient.

One enzyme that is particularly vulnerable to inhibition is *adenylate cyclase.* This enzyme activates the molecule cyclic *adenosine monophosphate* (cAMP). Recall from Figure 2.1 on page 23 that cAMP is the "second messenger" of cells, helping to initiate changes in the cells specific to certain hormones. Hormones whose actions depend on the cAMP mechanism include thyroid-stimulating hormone (TSH), follicle-stimulating hormone (FSH), and luteinizing hormone (LH) from the anterior pituitary, antidiuretic hormone (ADH) from the posterior pituitary, parathyroid hormone (PTH) from the parathyroid, and calcitonin from the thyroid. If adenylate cyclase and the cAMP mechanism are disrupted, all the metabolic processes dependent on them, including thyroid activity, are shut down.

The conversion of T4 to the more active T3 is regulated, in part, by the enzyme *iodothyronine deiodinase.* Studies have shown the inhibitory effect of mercury on this enzyme, resulting in a hypothyroid state in spite of normal serum T4. Toxic compounds such as heavy metals may also inhibit thyroid peroxidase, another enzyme essential to thyroid hormone synthesis. Antithyroid peroxidase antibodies have been detected among those with thyroid diseases. It is suspected that these antibodies are derived from an immune reaction to toxins, metals, or other antigenic substances, and subsequently cross-react with endocrine tissue.

The effect of heavy metal exposure on animal fetuses has lead to some startling conclusions about the role that it plays in infertility and birth defects. One study concluded that the changes in enzymatic activities by mercury led to harmful excesses of T3 in the brain of fetal mice, while maternal serum and brain measures remained normal.

Bowel Terrain and Thyroid Function

Intestinal health influences thyroid function in a number of important ways. Leaky gut syndrome can introduce food and bacterial antigens into the circulatory system. The immune system can produce antibodies that "attack" the antigens and mark them for removal from the body. Autoimmune disorders occur when antibodies

Hypothyroidism and Menopause

The body's estrogen levels play a role in thyroid metabolism. High levels of this hormone interfere with thyroid hormones, especially with the utilization of T3. Although estrogen is not discussed in-depth in this book, it does enter into the discussion of metabolism more than once.

It is important to consider the interplay of the thyroid gland during the menopausal years. Keep in mind that some symptoms associated with menopause are also symptoms of hypothyroidism, including depression, irritability, impaired memory or poor concentration, and insomnia. It is possible to alleviate these symptoms by addressing them as a thyroid issue before rushing to take prescription estrogen. Taking prescription estrogen can create elevated estrogen and increased inflammatory cytokine production and, therefore, interfere with thyroid function, leading to a host of other problems.

Hormone replacement therapy (HRT) had become an all-too-common treatment for menopausal symptoms until recent studies began to prove it to be a risky practice. HRT has been shown to increase the risk of uterine, ovarian, and breast cancer, causing many (if not most) women to abandon its use.

If thyroid issues and other factors in metabolism have been addressed as outlined in this book and you are still experiencing menopausal symptoms, natural hormone therapies may be considered. There are some excellent dietary supplements to use in place of conventional HRT for menopausal and postmenopausal symptoms, which you'll learn about in Chapter 6. If you choose to stop pharmaceutical hormonal replacement therapy and go the natural route (and your doctor agrees), do it slowly. Ask your doctor to explain very carefully how to decrease your dosage and begin the natural supplements.

attach to host tissue and initiate destructive pathways. The thyroid gland can be the subject of this misdirected immune response. When this happens, the thyroid either reduces or increases its activity.

Food Sensitivities

There is mounting evidence that hypothyroidism is linked to the digestive system and food intolerances. Many practitioners of both biological and functional medicine have observed the correlation between food intolerances and weight gain. In some individuals, consuming certain foods may trigger an autoimmune response that targets the thyroid gland. Several tests have been developed to detect sensitivities to foods and chemicals, (which we'll discuss in Chapter 9). Avoiding reactive foods and chemicals has a reported 97 percent success rate in weight loss among those who test positive for food sensitivities.

Yeast Toxins

Yeast endotoxins represent another threat to normal thyroid function. Yeast produces highly toxic compounds called endotoxins during the process of reproduction or dying off. These yeast toxins can bind with receptor sites on cells, tricking the cells into believing they have bound with a hormone. The negative feedback mechanism is initiated, which slows the release of the hormone from its originating gland, but no hormone has actually reached the cells. This is known as *hormone masking.* Thyroid hormone receptor sites are vulnerable to masking by yeast toxins. The failure of thyroid hormone to reach its target cells creates a state of hypothyroidism.

Many of the symptoms of yeast toxicity parallel those of hypothyroidism, including weight gain, fatigue, low body temperature, and imbalances of neurotransmitters (including serotonin, epinephrine and norepinephrine, and dopamine), constipation, an inability to concentrate, and dry skin.

Environmental Toxins and Thyroid Function

The thyroid gland is especially vulnerable to three types of toxins: *halogens* (a group of nonmetallic elements), *heavy metals,* and, as mentioned above, *yeast* (fungal) endotoxins.

Halogens like fluorine and chlorine are commonly found in our water supplies. These elements are similar in nature to iodine and can interfere with thyroid hormone formation. Heavy metals such as mercury and lead can interfere with the action of T4 at the cellular level by destroying or binding with enzymes needed to catalyze reactions. Mercury is also known to alter thyroid function first by stimulating the thyroid gland directly, then by decreasing the uptake of iodine, which suppresses the synthesis of thyroid hormone. Mercury toxicity can therefore create both hyperthyroid and hypothyroid conditions.

Heavy metals may contribute to thyroid malignancies and interfere with the uptake of iodine by the thyroid cells. In one study, the thyroid glands of 135 patients and 65 control subjects were evaluated for concentrations of several trace elements. It was found that mercury (along with cobalt, silver, and rubidium) was consistently higher in thyroid glands with cancerous nodules, while iodine concentrations were fifteen times lower. Lack of iodine can result in insufficient T4 production and hypothyroidism.

Many epidemiological studies have explored the relationship between maternal iodine and thyroid hormone levels and the neurological development of the fetus. Maternal iodine deficiency and thyroid dysfunction, especially in the last trimester of pregnancy, is a serious threat to fetal brain development. A pregnant woman exposed to high levels of mercury, therefore, may be placing her unborn child at greater risk for congenital neurological defects. In their book on this topic, *Infertility and Birth Defects: Is Mercury from Silver Dental Fillings an Unsuspected Cause* (Bio-Probe, 1988), researchers Ziff and Ziff conclude: "If we put all the information related to the thyroid together, it appears very plausible to conclude that chronic inhalation of mercury vapor . . . together with mercury and lead dietary intakes, may constitute one of the most serious threats to fetal brain development."

Mercury has been associated with elevated T3 and hyperthyroidism. In another study, direct administration of mercury chloride into the muscles of rabbits caused immediate elevation of T3 and a dramatic drop in T4. The study concluded that measurement of T3 to T4 ratio changes could be considered a reliable marker of heavy metal toxicity.

Center of Science and the Public Interest (CSPI), a nutrition advocacy organization in Washington, D.C., issued a warning that pregnant women should not eat more than two 6-ounce servings of canned tuna per month since tuna contains high levels of mercury. My suggestion is to avoid eating tuna more than once a month—especially fresh tuna steaks—in addition to other fish particularly high in mercury such as pike, swordfish, shark, and walleye.

Stress and Thyroid Function

In the next chapter, we delve into the metabolic effects of stress and alteration in your adrenal function. But for now, you should realize that chronic stress affects the thyroid and endocrine function in a number of ways.

The pituitary gland, the body's "master gland," stimulates and controls the function of the adrenal cortex by secreting adrenocorticotropic hormone (ACTH). If required to maintain a constant level of the major stress hormone cortisol in response to stress, the pituitary gland may overwork. Too much production of ACTH may divert the pituitary from manufacturing other tropic hormones such as TSH, FSH, and LH.

Cortisol production requires tyrosine, the same amino acid needed for the synthesis of thyroxine. Excess cortisol production can deplete tyrosine levels, making it unavailable to the thyroid gland to make thyroid hormones. Stress depletes other important nutrients required for T4 production, namely chromium and zinc. Excessive cortisol production from chronic stress also inhibits the conversion from T4 to T3 and the secretion of TSH. This, in effect, slows metabolism to a screeching halt. Finally, chronic stress and weakened immunity can initiate or aggravate autoimmune disorders such as Hashimoto's thyroiditis.

LAB TESTS FOR THYROID FUNCTION

Although I think that the best test for most people is the Barnes basal temperature test, several laboratory tests are available to help clinicians assess thyroid function. Many of these tests, however, are inherently difficult to interpret and sometimes misleading. Furthermore, the tests themselves are not always accurate. The problem lies in the fact that the exact amount of thyroid hormone entering the cells is impossible to determine with a laboratory test. And there is no exact way to measure what takes place inside the billions of cells, where thyroid hormone controls the rate of metabolism.

The basal metabolic rate (BMR) was long considered the most reliable reference of thyroid hormone activity. The BMR is calculated based on the amount of oxygen utilized by the body at a "resting" state. The difficulty with this test is that it is almost impossible to control all internal (for example, digestive) and external (for example, stress and exercise) influences over basal metabolism. This has led to widespread inaccuracy and false interpretation of test results.

Today, the blood tests discussed below are standard fare for initial screening of thyroid activity.

Classic "Thyroid Panel"

The classic thyroid panel consists of three tests: *Total Serum T4, T3 Uptake,* and *Free Thyroxine Index.* (Remember that T3 is the more metabolically active form of thyroid hormone. T4 is converted to T3 before being taken up by the cells.) The tests in the thyroid panel are taken and interpreted together. Individually, these tests are inconclusive. Collectively, they can provide a primary screening measure of thyroid function.

Total Serum T4 measures the circulating level of T4 bound to its carrier proteins (mostly thyroid binding globulin and albumin). This reflects the amount of T4 secreted by the thyroid and released into circulation. It does not measure the amount of T4 that reaches or enters the target cells.

The value of this test is influenced by the availability of carrier proteins, which is affected by factors such as the use of birth control pills, drugs, pregnancy, and estrogen replacement therapy. This test is more sensitive to hyperthyroidism than to hypothyroidism due to a decreasing sensitivity to T4 at lower values.

T3 Uptake is a tool used to estimate the amount of thyroid binding globulin (TBG) unsaturated by T4. It measures the amount of T3 absorbed by those sites on the TBG that T4 does not occupy. Since TBG has a much higher affinity for T4 than for T3, this is considered a fair estimate of the amount of T4 released from the thyroid relative to the available carrier proteins. If most of the TBG sites are occupied by T4, then less T3 will be absorbed. What T3 remains is "taken up" by a special resin, which is the *uptake value.* Thus, high T3 Uptake would reflect a hyperthyroid state, due to the saturation of TBG by T4. This test has a lesser sensitivity to hypothyroid states.

Free Thyroxine Index is calculated based on the results of Total T4 and T3 Uptake (Total T4 x T3 Uptake = FTI). This test, by correcting for fluctuations in carrier proteins relative to T4 values, reflects the general trend of both T4 and TBG.

There is, however, a wide range of what constitutes "normal" thyroid levels. In many cases, values may be "off the charts" before abnormalities are evident, especially in hypothyroidism.

Other tests that appear to assess thyroid function with more accuracy and correlate more strongly with the clinical signs and symptoms are available. These include tests for *Thyroid Stimulating Hormone, Free T4,* and *basal body temperature* (see the inset "Testing Your Thyroid Function" on page 70). Together, these tests are often sensitive enough to assess thyroid function without the interpretive problems associated with the standard thyroid panel. They are also more sensitive to hypothyroid and subclinical hypothyroid conditions.

Thyroid-Stimulating Hormone Test

Thyroid-stimulating hormone (TSH) measures the activity of the pituitary gland in response to circulating T4. The pituitary releases TSH when T4 is low, stimulating the thyroid gland to produce more. In overt hypothyroidism, for example, TSH values can be double the normal reference range as the pituitary attempts to stimulate the thyroid gland.

This test is a fair measure of early hypothyroidism, where the thyroid may still be producing normal levels of T4, but only with increased stimulation from the pituitary. This will produce an elevated TSH with a thyroid panel that is within normal limits. The drawback to this test is that it does not accurately indicate how much T4 has been converted to T3, which as you now know is the much more active thyroid hormone. There is a wide variety of influences that reduce the ability of T4 to convert to T3, such as deficiencies of zinc and selenium, environmental toxins, stress, and birth control pills and hormone replacement. Any of these factors could skew your blood thyroid test with regard to evaluating your true metabolic rate. Moreover, the American Society of Endocrinology recently released a memorandum stating that normal values ranges for TSH are too wide; therefore, as a result of this test many people whose thyroid was considered normal may now be diagnosed with hypothyroidism if retested.

Free T4 Test

Free T4 measures the metabolically active, unbound T4, which under normal condi-

Testing Your Thyroid Function

The basal body temperature (BBT) is a highly sensitive and accurate measure of low thyroid function, perhaps exceeding the reliability of available blood tests. The late Broda Barnes, M.D., a pioneer in the diagnosis and treatment of thyroid disorders, developed this test and successfully diagnosed and treated many patients based on its results.

The BBT test was developed as a simple measure of detecting hypothyroid conditions. It is based on the observation that hypothyroid patients typically run lower than normal body temperatures. This makes sense, since body temperature (heat output) is a direct measure of the amount of fuel (food and oxygen) being burned by the cells.

In terms of the ultimate objective of measuring thyroid function—that is, determining the ability of thyroxine to enter the cells and influence metabolism—the BBT test is the most logical assessment tool. Unlike the basal metabolic rate (discussed below), this test can be performed at home, which naturally controls for the influence of stress associated with an invasive, in-office procedure. Also, the BBT is taken immediately upon awakening; this is difficult to arrange when taking the basal metabolic test.

To check your basal body temperature, follow these simple steps:

1. Keep a thermometer by your bedside so you can take your temperature before getting out of bed in the morning. (It is important to move as little as possible while taking your temperature.)

2. Shake down the thermometer to read less than 92.0°F.

3. Upon waking in the morning, take your axillary (armpit) temperature for at least ten minutes.

4. Record your temperature.

Repeat these steps for four days. (Menstruating women should record their temperatures on the second, third, fourth, and fifth days of their periods.) Calculate your average temperature for the four days. A normal metabolic rate will produce a waking temperature of between 97.8°F and 98.2°F. Temperatures below 97.8°F may indicate, at the very least, subclinical hypothyroidism. Temperatures higher than 98.6°F may reflect hyperthyroidism.

---

tions is in proportion with bound T4. Under abnormal thyroid conditions, the ratio of bound to unbound T4 is altered. The TSH and Free T4 tests together often provide enough information for an experienced clinician to assess thyroid function.

Reverse T3 Test

Reverse T3 (rT3) is another thyroid hormone that circulates in the blood. Reverse T3's chemical structure differs from normal T3 thyroid hormone. It has no effect on metabolic rate because it is biologically inactive. However, an rT3 assay can be done to shed more light on the status of your thyroid function. In healthy individuals, 40 percent of the T4 will eventually be used for conversion to T3 and 45 percent will go to rT3. In healthy individuals with normal thyroid function, levels of all three hormones tend to change together. However, in metabolic disorders, there will be a decreased conversion of T4 to T3 and increased percentages of T4 to rT3.

An rT3 assay measures the amount of the hormone in the blood and compares it to levels of T4 and T3. This test is usually done to distinguish between hypothyroidism and a condition known as Euthyroid sick syndrome—a change in thyroid function that occurs as a result of an acute illness. In cases of severe physical stress that can occur from an infection or a trauma, the rT3 level will be elevated while T3 will be low. In hypothyroidism, rT3 and T3 will both be low.

When a person experiences prolonged stress, the adrenal glands respond by manufacturing a large amount of the stress hormone cortisol. Cortisol inhibits the conversion of T4 to T3 and favors the conversion of T4 to rT3. If stress is prolonged, a condition called *reverse T3 dominance* (also called Wilson's syndrome) occurs and persists even after the stress passes and cortisol levels fall. Abnormally elevated rT3 levels indicate the presence of this condition. There are other conditions that will cause variations in serum rT3 levels, including caloric deprivation (from fasting or starvation), which results in higher concentrations of rT3, as do other conditions that cause a high fever such as infections. These conditions cause the conversion of T4 to rT3 at the expense of T3 production. Most drugs that affect thyroid function also change rT3 levels.

Hyperthyroidism, illnesses that cause high fever, administration of the intravenous heart drug amiodarone (Cordarone), fasting, and administration of radiographic contrast agents may also increase rT3 values. Hypothyroidism, administration of estrogens or progestogens, and administration of antithyroid drugs are associated with decreased rT3 levels.

TREATING THYROID CONDITIONS

There is some debate over the recommended course of treatment and symptom management for thyroid disorders. There is a discrepancy between what blood levels report in laboratory tests and how the patient feels and presents symptoms. This is another case in which your system can be going down the wrong path of metabolic function; even though you're exhibiting a wide range of low thyroid symptoms, nothing out of the ordinary shows up on your blood tests. If the laboratory tests are not out of the normal ranges, physicians generally don't treat the problem.

Conventional Treatments

The conventional treatment for hypothyroidism is thyroid hormone replacement, in which the patient takes a prescription drug that acts similarly to T4.

The vast majority of doctors prescribe the synthetic drug known as levothyroxine (Synthroid, Levoxyl, Levothroid, Unithroid) for thyroid hormone replacement. Levothyroxine provides a synthetic version of T4. Some people with hypothyroidism find that levothyroxine therapy is sufficient. However, some doctors treat hypothyroidism using liothyronine (Cytomel), a synthetic version of T3, in addition to levothyroxine. Nevertheless, for many people, the symptoms of low thyroid function never fully go away, even if they are on thyroid hormone replacement.

Natural thyroid is *desiccated thyroid,* derived from the gland of pigs. It was the standard thyroid drug until levothyroxine came on the market in the second half of the twentieth century. The most popular brand of this type of thyroid is Armour Desiccated Thyroid Tablets (available by prescription). Modern physicians are using this natural treatment more and more often. The rationale is that the natural thyroid provides the full range of thyroid hormones that are needed to replace deficiency patterns (although critics argue that it is not consistent in dosage amounts).

One of the biggest problems with metabolism probably lies in the conversion of T4 to T3. As mentioned earlier, chronic stress may be one of the biggest influencing factors. During chronic stress, the body's stores of tyrosine and other nutrients are diverted from thyroid hormone production in favor of cortisol production. A high cortisol level prevents the conversion of T4 to T3. Therefore, although some people take prescriptions for T4, their symptoms persist. In this case, some people may get T3 prescribed for them. Other people will opt for using Armour thyroid, which contains both T3 and T4. There are also some people who have taken natural thyroid without good results—most likely because they still are not getting enough T3 and are starting to get way too much T4. So it's important to look at all the factors, including trace minerals, amino acids, and stress that influence thyroid metabolism, and take control of as many aspects as you can.

Hyperthyroid Medications

Antithyroid drugs such as methimazole (Tapazole) and propylthiouracil are used for the treatment of an overactive thyroid (hyperthyroidism). The conventional wisdom is that these drugs should be used only for limited periods, after which, if the hyperthyroidism has not gone into remission, other treatments such as *radioactive iodine* (iodine 131, or I-131) should be pursued. Check with your health practitioner for the precautions to follow when taking radioactive iodine. Some alternative practitioners, however, have maintained patients for years on antithyroid drugs with no adverse effects.

Also, radioactive iodine may be used to "ablate" or destroy the overactive thyroid. This procedure may be necessary in some cases; however, ablation may have long-lasting consequences on the body such as permanent hypothyroidism. If you are experiencing a hyperthyroid state, find a practitioner who will be able to investigate the factors that may be driving your immune system toward an autoimmune situation. Heavy metals, bacterial and yeast toxins, and food intolerance can all be culprits.

Natural Therapies

Although thyroid prescription drugs work in some cases, I often find that they are incomplete in the desired effects. In my experience, the patient will usually achieve only limited weight loss and will still display many of the other symptoms of hypothyroidism, including cold hands and feet, dry skin and hair, and low energy. Of course, if the person's stress levels are not managed, and if he or she has "leaky gut," high insulin resistance, and toxin-binding activity on thyroid receptors, prescription thyroid medication may not be able to do the job.

The use of nutritional and herbal supplements, which support thyroid function naturally, may be the most appropriate therapeutic intervention for subclinical hypothyroidism because it addresses so many of the factors that are the cause of the suboptimal functioning of the thyroid to begin with. By correcting the underlying factors and supporting the thyroid gland with good nutrition, you allow the thyroid

Amy's Story

A few years ago I was experiencing many unusual symptoms, which my medical doctor diagnosed as hypothyroidism. I was always tired even after eight to nine hours of sleep. I had a difficult time getting out of bed in the morning—a crane couldn't have helped! I didn't have the energy to do anything. I didn't have an appetite, so I ate very little. Yet I had gained more than twenty pounds and had gone up three sizes. I had been on the thyroid medication Synthroid for several months, but noticed no difference in my symptoms. In fact, I kept feeling worse. A coworker recommended I go to Dr. LaValle. Because I had seen significant positive changes in my coworker, even though she had seen Dr. LaValle for another type of problem, I decided to try it. Since my first appointment my life has certainly changed for the better. My body responded to the nutritional supplements and modified eating habits. A year and a half later, I feel wonderful. I've even had to buy smaller clothes! Had I not been fortunate enough to find out about "cracking my metabolic code" and how I could support my body with nutrition and supplements, I am not sure in what state my health would be.

Amy is a clear-cut case of low thyroid function brought on by excessive stress and adrenal exhaustion. We began by providing nutritional support for the adrenals, and not long after, the thyroid medication she was taking started working effectively. Amy also needed some coaching on the type of food selections that she was making. Lots of carbohydrates and refined sugars were not helping her metabolism work efficiently. And of course, the cortisol that her adrenals were releasing due to the chronic stress was making her body store fat more efficiently.

gland to rejuvenate and you allow the hormones to be made and properly utilized. In Chapter 6, I'll give you a specific plan of action for treating subclinical hypothyroidism naturally.

THYROID BALANCE IS KEY

As you can see, thyroid function plays a pivotal role in the optimization of your personal metabolic code. The thyroid gland releases hormones that increase the rate at which your cells release energy from carbohydrates, while promoting protein synthesis and the use of fatty acids. Even slight decreases in thyroid hormones, far more common than increases in thyroid hormones, can negatively affect the body. As you have seen, when your thyroid function is out of balance and not functioning up to par, a host of health problems may occur.

In the chapter ahead, we will take an in-depth look at the adrenals and their activities, before putting forth a plan of action through which you can begin to enjoy optimal thyroid activity in balance with the activity of the other endocrine glands.

Now, onward for Key Three . . .

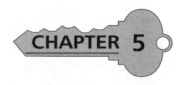

CHAPTER 5

KEY THREE:
Balancing Your Adrenals—
Relieving Symptoms of Chronic
Stress (Cravings, Low Energy,
Memory Loss, and Insomnia)

Are you feeling exhausted, emotionally flat, and just plain burned out? Are you unable to respond to stressful situations without feeling wiped out or emotional? Are you tired of looking at those blue circles under your eyes every time you look in the mirror? Does your energy plummet midday? Are you easily brought to tears? Have you gained weight around the waist since entering your thirties and forties—weight that you cannot seem to lose?

If your metabolism is not what it used to be and you are gaining weight for no apparent reason, if your cholesterol and triglycerides are increasing steadily with age, and if you're craving carbohydrates or sugars uncontrollably—if you're going for that cookie or chips as soon as you enter the door—there may be a fairly simple explanation.

Further, if you seem to always be feeling either irritable or anxious, and your memory is failing, if you are suffering from insomnia—and, by this, I mean that you are waking in the middle of the night worrying about the day's events, there may be just one cause for your multiple woes. Finally, if you seem to be less and less resistant to infection as the years go on, then I wrote this chapter just for you.

What is it that can relate all of these symptoms? It's the functioning of your adrenal glands. Believe it or not, because they are the glands that control our reaction to stress and because they interact with other hormones in the body, the adrenals can affect all these areas. Some other symptoms of adrenal distress are headaches, environmental sensitivities, fatigue, dizziness upon rising, excessive perspiration, salt cravings, and alcohol intolerance. The adrenal glands regulate stress, blood pressure, and blood mineral content through the secretion of various hormones. Along with the thyroid, it could be argued that adrenal function is one of the two *most* important of all the nine keys of your metabolic code (but then all of the keys influence one another).

And yet, adrenal gland function is likely the least understood. In terms of medical understanding and treatment, adrenal dysfunction is probably the least recognized contributor to why people feel fatigued. In fact, typically adrenal stress, depletion, and exhaustion are rarely acknowledged until the function of the glands have become so compromised that it has led to Addison's disease or Cushing's syndrome. Unfortunately, the patient will have, in the meantime, suffered years of distress from poorly functioning adrenal glands. Interestingly, with so many people affected by the many stressors of modern living, I work with adrenal exhaustion, in varying stages, probably more than any other health issue.

The concept of adrenal exhaustion has just started to make its way into the public's eye through the media during the last couple of years. For years, the response to nutritional supplements and lifestyle changes never fails to amaze me. In fact, it can seem downright miraculous. You see, usually, by the time people come into my office, they have been suffering from adrenal exhaustion for years—years with blue rings under their eyes, years of being hypoglycemic, and years of suffering from midday fatigue. They've gone from doctor to doctor, without relief; they may even be told, "You're just getting old." But one look at the blue rings and one glance at their nutritional intake report, and I know that some adrenal nutrient support will perk them right up. It works almost every time. Patients respond so well to adrenal support that their whole outlook changes for the better as their bodies become more and more resilient to stress. They lose weight. Their eyes take on the gleam of health. And, most of all, they get energy back that lasts throughout the day.

You see, adrenal dysfunction is, for the most part, a byproduct of modern living. Adrenal stress is one of the significant problems that often go unnoticed, and it triggers other health troubles—so it is one of the biggest factors leading to that downward spiral toward metabolic syndrome and a host of other illnesses. Modern living subjects us to unprecedented levels and types of stress. At one time, our ability to respond to physical stress *defined* our ability to survive. Today, our ability to cope with the effects of stress *challenges* our health and happiness. The human body's built-in response to stress has not changed. It is the type of stress that has changed. The stress of being chased by a saber-toothed tiger, for example, is altogether different from fourteen-hour workdays, red-eye flights, road rage, and dual-income families, but our bodies react as if it is the same.

Perhaps I can state this better when I say that our bodies are more adept at coping with *danger* than with *pressure*. Danger is resolved quickly, whereas pressure is sustained. The chronicity of pressure—the stress that wears away at our bodies and minds day after day—is what ultimately wears down our metabolism. This is no small thing. It is estimated today that 85 percent of diseases have stress-related factors. In fact, more than three-quarters of visits to a doctor are related to stress and stress-related factors. For this reason, it is essential to understand how the adrenal glands work and what happens to your body under prolonged stress.

HOW THE ADRENAL GLANDS FUNCTION

The adrenals are pyramid-shaped glands that sit on top of each kidney. They are embedded in the same protective layer of fat that surrounds the kidneys. Because of their nearness, the adrenals and kidneys are closely associated physically, although they have different functions.

The adrenal glands contain an inner medulla and an outer cortex, each with its own distinct hormonal influence. The interior or central portions of the adrenal glands house the *adrenal medulla.* The adrenal medulla secretes *epinephrine* (adrenaline) and *norepinephrine* (noradrenaline), two chemicals called *catecholamines* that travel through the sympathetic nervous system, one of two divisions of the autonomic nervous system (the part of nervous system that controls actions of the body that are beyond conscious control like pupil dilation, heartbeat, digestion, and secretions of glands). Impulses transmitted through sympathetic nerve fibers stimulate the brain to release its chemical messengers. These impulses are generated by the hypothalamus in response to stress. The impulses travel through the sympathetic nervous system to the adrenal glands and cause the adrenal cells to release epinephrine and norepinephrine. Because of these hormonal changes, the body is able to respond physiologically to threat. These responses include increased heart rate and force of contraction, dilation of skeletal muscle blood vessels, dilation of airway passages, the conversion of glycogen to glucose by the liver, and increased metabolism.

The exterior or outer portions of the adrenal glands contain the *adrenal cortex.* The cortex secretes more than thirty different steroids and hormones (known as *corticosteroids*). The most important corticosteroids are *cortisol, aldosterone,* and the *adrenal androgens* (sex hormones). Cortisol is the principal hormone secreted in reaction to stress, and it is necessary for many functions in the body.

Aldosterone (termed a *mineralocorticoid*) helps to regulate mineral electrolytes by signaling the conservation of sodium ions and excretion of potassium ions in the urine. In times of dehydration (detected by increasing sodium ion concentration) or falling blood pressure, aldosterone signals the kidneys to reduce urine output and conserve water. This reduces the sodium ion concentration and increases blood volume.

Adrenal Response to Stress

Stress of any kind requires an adaptive response from the body. This response is directed by the nervous system but played out, primarily, by the adrenals. The best known of these adaptive responses is the *fight-or-flight mechanism,* first identified by Walter Canon, M.D., in 1932.

The fight-or-flight mechanism is an autonomic nervous system response that allows for important physiologic adjustments in the face of danger.

The stress response begins in the hypothalamus, where nerve impulses from the central nervous system communicate environmental changes to the brain. The hypothalamus, in turn, sends a message to the anterior pituitary gland to secrete *adreno-*

corticotropic hormone (ACTH). ACTH stimulates the adrenals to release epinephrine, norepinephrine, DHEA (the precursor for the production of both male and female hormones [testosterone and estrogen]), and cortisol.

Cortisol, epinephrine, and norepinephrine released from the adrenal glands provide heightened energy, endurance, and perception needed during the alarm mode. DHEA balances some of the effects of cortisol, the adrenal's principal stress hormone.

Norepinephrine and epinephrine are primarily responsible for the physical changes related to acute stress, which are designed to enhance survival in the face of physical danger. Pupil dilation enhances visual perception. An increased heart rate, as well as an increase in the force of contractions and in breathing, supplies the major organs with blood and oxygen. Blood flow to the brain increases and perception is heightened. Constriction of peripheral blood vessels diverts blood flow from "nonvital" organs, including the stomach and digestive tract. Cortisol increases blood sugar levels by converting noncarbohydrate sources of fuel into glucose.

An increased supply of glucose to the central nervous system enhances brain activity. Cellular metabolism and the production of adenosine triphosphate (ATP) are stepped up, increasing the production of energy in all the cells. So, as you can see, stressful events have quite an impact on your body physically.

Stress can occur at all levels of life. There are nutritional, physical, emotional, mental, psychological, and spiritual stress factors. Even exercise is a type of physical stress. Anxiety, fear, depression, perfectionism, grief, and frustration are stressful. Medical conditions such as infection, chronic illness, or surgery cause tremendous metabolic stress. Change—even seemingly good change like moving into a new home or starting a new job—can be stressful. Environmental and chemical exposure to pesticides, cleaning agents, drugs, and excessive alcohol use can place stress on the body.

Further, the overuse of over-the-counter and prescription stimulants, including the Chinese herb *ma huang* (*Ephedra*) and pseudoephedrine (a chemical used in many diet, sinus, and cold pills) can place stress on adrenal function. For example, thermogenic aids, substances that increase metabolism, containing ma huang have become popular weight-loss tools and are relied on heavily by people for an "energy boost." Unfortunately, without adequate adrenal support, these aids have the opposite effect in the long term. The energy boost they provide today may ultimately exhaust the adrenals, leading to chronic exhaustion years down the road. I have seen this problem caused by the long-term use of stimulants consistently over the last two decades. Other stimulant abuse, such as excessive caffeine intake, can produce similar results.

In 1967, researchers Homes and Rahe were among the first to study the role of stress in health and wellness. You may already have heard of their "Social Readjustment Rating Scale." It identifies major life events and their impact on health status by assigning a point value to recently experienced life events. The totalled points give a score that indicates the relative risk of becoming ill from stress-related causes.

Social Readjustment Rating Scale

LIFE EVENT	POINT VALUE	LIFE EVENT	POINT VALUE
Death of a spouse	100	Change in work responsibilities	29
Divorce	73	Son or daughter leaving home	29
Marital separation	65	Trouble with in-laws	29
Jail term	63	Outstanding personal achievement	28
Death of a close family member	63	Spouse begins or stops work	26
Personal illness or injury	53	Starting or finishing school	26
Marriage	50	Change in living conditions	25
Fired from work	47	Revision of personal habits	24
Marital reconciliation	45	Trouble with boss	23
Retirement	45	Change in work hours or conditions	20
Change in family member's health	44	Change in residence	20
Pregnancy	40	Change in schools	20
Sex difficulties	39	Change in recreational habits	24
Addition to family	39	Change in church activities	18
Business readjustment	39	Mortgage or loan under $10,000	18
Change in financial status	38	Change in sleeping habits	16
Death of a close friend	37	Change in number of family gatherings	15
Change to a different line of work	36	Change in eating habits	15
Change in number of marital arguments	35	Vacation	13
Mortgage or loan over $10,000	31	Christmas season	12
Foreclosure of mortgage or loan	30	Minor violation of the law	11

SCORING

150 or less   =   37 percent chance of becoming ill within two years
151–299   =   50 percent change of becoming ill within two years
300 and more   =   80 percent chance of becoming ill within two years

The Health Effects of Long-Term Stress

Over the last few years several books have been published on the effects of elevated cortisol in your body. From *Fight Fat Over Forty: The Revolutionary Three-Pronged Approach That Will Break Your Stress-Fat Cycle and Make You Healthy, Fit, and Trim for Life* by Pamela Peeke (Penguin, 2001) to *The Cortisol Connection: Why Stress Makes You Fat and Ruins Your Health—and What You Can Do about It* by Shawn Talbott (Hunter House, 2002), these books are popular and for a good reason. People are recognizing the effects of chronic stress on their health and are looking for answers.

Cortisol is released in response to the secretion of ACTH from the pituitary gland. The anterior pituitary is signaled by the release of corticotropin releasing hormone (CRH) from the hypothalamus in response to changing conditions. Conditions of stress, including illness and injury, stimulate the hypothalamus and the eventual release of cortisol. Cortisol production is also controlled by what is known as a negative feedback system, when blood levels become low (due to normal cycling), the hypothalamus is stimulated to release more CRH.

Cortisol (termed a *glucocorticoid*) serves two primary functions: energy production and anti-inflammation. It also causes the constriction of blood vessels. These actions are the means by which they help the body to survive. Cortisol has significant effects on glucose metabolism by influencing fat and protein metabolism. Cortisol increases the blood concentration of amino acids by inhibiting protein synthesis and by stimulating the release of proteins from the muscles if necessary. It also increases the release of fatty acids from adipose tissue for use as a fuel source and stimulates the conversion of noncarbohydrates to glucose. All of these actions serve to regulate the concentration of glucose in the blood to ensure a ready source of fuel for the cells under any type of stress.

Glucocorticoids (95 percent of glucocorticoid production is cortisol) also reduce inflammation and allergic response. For instance, certain cells known as mast cells produce a substance called histamine, a compound in the body that causes an inflammation response. (Any allergy sufferer can tell you about the troublesome effects of histamine.) Cortisol inhibits this production. Other effects of cortisol include decreased permeability of the capillaries and decreased activity of white blood cells. These effects are all life-saving if you are in a traumatic accident or undergoing surgery. However, the continued release of cortisol has some major implications on health.

Although we need cortisol to help the body carry on the function of energy production and to control inflammatory responses, when the hormone is chronically elevated under consistent daily pressures (versus occasional stress or an isolated event), it can cause unwanted effects. One of the functions of cortisol is to help the body produce blood sugar from proteins. This causes an increase in blood sugar levels. If the glucose is not needed for some action such as running or for bodily responses to a trauma, for instance, the excess glucose is then used for *lipogenesis* (fat production). Numerous studies have linked oversecretion of cortisol with obesity and increased storage of abdominal fat.

Yes, it is true that a basic mechanism of weight gain is an imbalance between caloric intake and energy expenditure. But that is not the total story behind why people gain weight and have trouble losing it. Increasing physiologic, biochemical, and genetic evidence suggests that being overweight is a complex disorder of appetite regulation, energy metabolism, and immune-neuroendocrine miscommunication, involving imbalances in the secretion of regulatory hormones, such as in the thyroid, pituitary, and adrenal glands.

Elevated stress hormones contribute to the breakdown of lean muscle tissue, an increase in blood sugar (causing a problem termed "hyperinsulinemia," which can lead to insulin resistance and diabetes) and an increase in the storage of abdominal fat. The breakdown of muscle tissue that can occur from stress hormones is very detrimental because muscle tissue is metabolically much more active than fat, meaning it burns more calories. The more muscle tissue you have, the higher your metabolic rate will be. When muscle tissue is lost, metabolic rate decreases, and it becomes much harder to lose weight or to maintain weight loss.

The increase in cortisol release from the adrenal glands causes food cravings, especially for high-fat, high-sugar, high-carbohydrate foods such as cookies, candy, chips, and ice cream. Even though these foods act as a temporary mood "boost," they in turn feed a vicious cycle, causing additional blood sugar problems, leading to swings in energy and blood sugar, which fuels the stress-cortisol release cycle. Eventually, by stimulating excess insulin release, the body is driven to become more insulin resistant, and with more insulin resistance, more fat is stored than the body needs. Sixty to seventy percent of American adults are overweight or obese, and stress-driven food cravings play an ever-increasing role in this weight gain. Even if sufficient exercise is in place to compensate for the extra calories, or the stress is reduced, you may still find yourself in a vicious cycle.

As if the loss of muscle tissue and food cravings were not enough to deal with, adrenal exhaustion can lead to subclinical or overt hypothyroidism and yet another factor that can lead to a lowered metabolism and weight gain.

Another unwanted side effect of too much cortisol production is that it retards regeneration of connective tissue, resulting in slow wound healing. As you may recall, cortisol causes the blood vessels to constrict. This is a desired effect if there has been blood loss; however, if there has not, the constricted blood vessels can lead to increased blood pressure and increased risk of cardiovascular disease.

So chronic stress can virtually set in motion the chemistry to make you gain weight and continue to pile it on. Over time, in severe cases, you may even begin to have the appearance of a person with Cushing's syndrome, which includes a rounded "moon" face, puffiness, buffalo hump or rounding of the upper back, and obesity.

Cortisol competes with thyroid hormone for the amino acid tyrosine, which is also involved in thyroid hormone formation. Excessive cortisol production therefore limits the amount of thyroid hormone that can be produced. Diminished thyroid hormone decreases energy and increases body fat. At the same time cortisol production rises, more and more of the body's store of DHEA is used up to make more cortisol. As DHEA levels decrease, the effects of the changes in sex hormone levels occur, including reduced libido and increased PMS symptoms. Moreover, cortisol also decreases insulin sensitivity of receptor cells, which decreases the glucose uptake by cells and increases blood sugar. This reduces the energy available to cells, forcing the body to break down muscle tissue for glucose.

Cortisol may also alter immune function. This effect comes from the overall suppression of white blood cell activity, thymus gland dysfunction, and a decrease in natural killer (NK) cell activity in the immune system—hence, reduced immune response. This means that the immune cells responsible for patrolling for foreign agents or cancer cells cannot attack as efficiently. This invites significant risks to your future health. Simultaneously, cortisol will overactivate another part of your immune response, increasing tumor necrosis factor (TNF alpha) and interleukin-6 (IL-6), cytokines that can make the body's defense system become overactive and lead to autoimmune disorders. It is a tedious balance that the immune system relies on, and cortisol wreaks havoc on that balance. Figure 5.1 on page 83 illustrates the route through which this extensive metabolic damage occurs.

The results of chronic stress include exhaustion, lowered thyroid function, cardiovascular stress, alterations in blood sugar, weight gain, muscle breakdown, altered immune function, and more. If you don't think the effects of stress are that big of a deal, just look at the following list to see just some of the effects of increased release of cortisol in your system:

- Decreases insulin sensitivity of receptor cells due to increased TNF alpha, thereby stimulating excess insulin release, and increases blood sugar (leading to insulin resistance, hyperinsulinemia, and even diabetes).

- Increases cravings of high-caloric, high-fat, high-sugar, high-carbohydrate foods—even salty foods.

- Increases weight gain, contributes to the breakdown of lean muscle tissue, and increases the storage of belly fat (via increased insulin resistance and lowered thyroid function).

- Causes decreased production of the thyroid gland, leading to subclinical or overt hypothyroidism and a lowered metabolism, increased weight gain, and decreased fatty acid utilization.

- Increases cholesterol and triglycerides, which, in turn, increases cardiovascular risks.

- Increases blood pressure.

- Causes a loss of sex drive.

- Causes sleep disturbances, marked by an inability to "turn off" the day and wake in the middle of the night typically around 2:00 to 3:00 A.M. because of alterations in blood sugar and decreases in serotonin and melatonin production.

- Contributes to tension, complacency, depression, and irritability (by depleting the "calming" brain chemical serotonin).

- Causes destruction of neurological and brain tissue.

Figure 5.1. Chronic Stress Pathway

ADRENAL

THYROID

- Increase in cortisol uses available tyrosine, making less available for production of thyroid hormone and lowers the conversion of T4 to T3
- Decreases basal metabolic rate
- Cold hands and feet
- Dry skin, nails peel
- Depression
- Fatigue
- Decreases fuel (glucose) burning abilities
- Decreases number of mitochondria in cells
- Slow to start in morning
- Stiffness in morning
- Weight gain
- Decreases ATP production

END RESULTS

- Anxiousness, nervousness
- Cravings for carbohydrates and sugar
- Exercise intolerance
- Fatigue, tired, lowered endurance
- Inflammation chemistry
- Lack of zest, melancholy
- Mid-day crash
- Short-term memory loss
- Sleep problems
- Weight gain, belly fat

FUEL BURNING ALTERED

CORTISOL

ELEVATED CORTISOL:

- Decreases DHEA resulting in:
  — Decreased sex drive
  — Lower metabolism
  — Immune dysfunction

LEADS TO:

- Anxiousness, nervousness
- Increases cravings for carbohydrates and sugar
- Increases cholesterol and triglycerides
- Mid-day fatigue
- Increases Night Eating Syndrome (NES)
- Decreases serotonin
- Short-term memory loss
- Sleep disturbances
- Increases TNF alpha, IL-6, aromatase, and estrogen
- Weight gain

PANCREAS

- Increases cardiovascular disease risk
- Increases insulin resistance
- Increases isoprostanes
- Increases belly fat
- Increases water retention

- Causes loss of memory through shrinkage of the hypothalamus and reduced circulation.

- Depresses the immune system by increasing neuropeptide Y, which tells the body to turn off natural killer (NK) cells of the immune system and causes thymus gland atrophy and an inability to produce mature T killer cells.

- Increases IL-6 and TNF alpha, messengers that cause a systemic inflammatory response and overactivates the immune system. In addition, this leads to increased free-radical damage and causes a destructive force in the arteries.

- Increases bone loss.

- Increases water retention.

- Increases catecholamine (epinephrine) production.

Everyone adapts to stress differently, and the healthier your adrenal function is the better you will respond to stress. Inherently strong adrenal glands can withstand longer periods of stress without adverse effects. Conversely, if the adrenals are weakened, the effects of stress will appear more acutely and more quickly. Once again, the adrenal glands are an endocrine gland that can basically wear out with overuse. This is what can lead to adrenal exhaustion, which can then lead to a different set of symptoms, such as low blood pressure, hypoglycemia, mental lethargy, muscle weakness, and weight loss.

But how, once we've gotten ourselves into the pit of exhaustion known as adrenal "burnout," can we climb back out? How can we set things right? The rest of this chapter examines the factors influencing the health of the adrenals, as well as ways to strengthen your resistance to stress.

KEY INFLUENCES ON ADRENAL FUNCTION

The key factors that most influence the adrenal glands are stress, thyroid function, nutrients, the pancreas, toxicity, and intestinal or bowel terrain. The following section describes the relationship between each of these key factors and the adrenal response to stress.

Diet and Adrenal Function

Nutrition has a profound impact on all operating systems of the body, and the adrenal glands are no exception. We have seen the role of nutrients in thyroid and pancreatic function. Like these, the adrenals are dependent on certain vital nutrients to maintain healthy output of adrenal hormones and adequate response to stress.

One of the most important nutrients for healthy adrenal function is salt (sodium). Sodium is needed to drive the synthesis of adrenal hormones. While it is well known that unrestricted salt in the diet can lead to water retention, the adoption of low-sodium diets by many people to control water-weight gain can disrupt the normal functioning of the adrenals. You should consider using reasonable amounts (light salting) of sea salt to provide a broad range of minerals and support the synthesis of important adrenal hormones. People who are chronically adrenal exhausted will crave salt, sometimes uncontrollably.

Those experiencing unavoidable stress, whether acute or chronic, should pay particular attention to nutrition. Stressful times often result in the increased use of caffeine, nicotine, alcohol, and prescription drugs. All of these substances can further compound adrenal stress and may deplete nutrients. Aggravating lifestyle factors, such as excess caffeine, alcohol, the excessive use of stimulants, and/or tobacco should all be curtailed. (I know that this is sometimes easier said than done. But you have to try to make the first step.)

Nutrients and Adrenal Function

Nutritional deficiencies can lead to physical and emotional stress. Conversely, stress can deplete nutrients. Common nutrients depleted by stress are the antioxidant vitamins C and E, the B vitamins, and the minerals selenium, zinc, magnesium, iron, and sulfur. Carbohydrates, fat, and protein metabolism are all increased during acute stress. And essential fatty acids (EFAs), especially omega-3s, can be depleted through the body's efforts to dampen the inflammation of stress chemistry. Stress activates inflammatory chemistry cascades; omega-3 fatty acids are our natural defense to dampening our inflammatory response.

Vitamin C

Vitamin C, or ascorbic acid, is critical for adrenal function. The adrenal glands have a higher content of vitamin C than any other organ. Vitamin C directly supports the adrenal production of stress hormones. Vitamin C is a potent antioxidant, protecting cells from free-radical damage. (Remember, during times of stress, free-radical damage increases.) Vitamin C also improves resistance to infection by mobilizing white blood cells. It may have a cardioprotective benefit by increasing HDL, or "good," cholesterol and reducing LDL, or "bad," cholesterol, which increases in the presence of cortisol.

B Vitamins

The B vitamins are known as the "antistress" vitamins. Of these, the most important may be vitamin B_5, or pantothenic acid. Vitamin B_5 depletion is associated with stress, nervous irritability, and adrenal exhaustion. Vitamin B_5 is involved in the production of adrenal hormones, and B_5 deficiency causes a progressive decline in the production of adrenal hormones.

Along with folic acid and niacin, vitamin B_5 is necessary for proper adrenal and nervous system function. Niacin can help counteract some of the biochemical effects of stress, including blood sugar fluctuations and digestive irritation. Vitamin B_2 (riboflavin) aids in the production of adrenal hormones. Vitamins B_1 (thiamine), B_6 (pyridoxine), biotin, and B_{12} (cyanocobalamin) support the nervous system and can have a calming effect during stressful times.

Vitamin B_6 is actually a needed cofactor (catalyst) for serotonin metabolism. Inadequate intake of vitamin B_6 can lead to the following:

- Low serotonin levels, which can lead to feelings of anxiousness, carbohydrate cravings, and depression.

- If serotonin levels go low enough, falling asleep is difficult or impossible because serotonin is needed to make melatonin (a hormone needed for sleep that also functions as an antioxidant in the body.)

- Low melatonin interferes with the ability to develop a significant REM (deep) sleep pattern at night, which leads to lighter sleep and to being less rested in the morning, which compounds the impact of stress on the body.

All of the B vitamins are water soluble, which means they cannot be stored by the body. They must be replenished regularly by the diet or by nutritional supplements. Now, don't kid yourself, if your diet is not that great and you are having some of the problems just listed, you may want to consider finding and taking a multiple vitamin that can give you your full spectrum of needed nutrients. (See Table 16.1 on page 407 for the essential requirements of a good multivitamin and mineral formula.) Most multivitamins include a full spectrum of the B vitamins.

Night Eating Syndrome and Stress

Have you ever tried to get to sleep and then, without warning, your stomach tells you it's time to eat? If you have difficulty sleeping at night or awaken often with an intense need to eat, then you may have developed a disorder known as night-eating syndrome (NES). This condition, which is not yet clearly understood, is characterized by a lack of appetite for breakfast, low daytime appetite and calorie consumption, increased appetite in the evening with over 50 percent of calories consumed after 8 P.M., and waking up at least once a night with intense food cravings, usually for high carbohydrate foods. While NES is thought to be uncommon in the general population—estimates are it affects between 1 and 2 percent of adults—some studies report that it may occur in up to approximately one-fourth of obese persons. I find people with this behavior in my practice all the time and believe that it is a much bigger problem than previously recognized.

NES was initially thought to be a sleeping disorder because it is also characterized by insomnia. However, the tendency of the night eating is almost binge-like, which is associated with eating disorders. Though NES was first described in 1955, the true roots of this disorder are just being discovered.

Researchers studied the brain chemical patterns and stress hormone levels in a group of people with NES and compared these to normal control subjects. Scientists found that levels of *melatonin*—the hormone that helps us fall asleep and stay asleep at night—were significantly reduced in NES sufferers. Similarly, *leptin*—the hormone that suppresses appetite—didn't rise to normal levels in night-eaters, suggesting that their hunger pangs may be extreme enough to disturb sleep. Finally, cortisol was ele-

Minerals

Calcium and magnesium are important antistress minerals. Magnesium slows the release of epinephrine and norepinephrine from the adrenal medulla, which makes it a critical mineral for balancing the sympathetic (excitory) nervous system response.

Magnesium helps decrease insulin resistance and stabilizes blood sugar, which is important in counteracting the effects of cortisol. Magnesium increases HDL cholesterol concentration of the blood and balances the cellular absorption of calcium.

Symptoms of magnesium deficiency include anxiety, constipation, fatigue, leg cramps, heart palpitations, insomnia, restlessness, nervousness, and muscle weakness. Severe magnesium loss can result in heart arrhythmias or disruptions in the natural rhythm of the heartbeat.

Because statistics show that 75 percent of Americans are low in magnesium or are getting below the recommended dietary allowances (RDA) for magnesium, I counsel almost all of my patients to start with a magnesium supplement especially

vated at night in the group with NES, further enticing them to wake up and head to the kitchen.

The study findings suggest that NES is a result of a disordered stress response in individuals. Clearly, the physiology of these patients suggests that those who suffer from NES are in a state of adrenal exhaustion.

NES creates a big roadblock for weight management and sustaining your vitality. In general, NES sufferers report feeling miserable due to their lack of sleep and their weight gain due to the out of control night eating. If, upon reading this, it sounds as if you have NES, implementing the nine keys to cracking the metabolic code will help. With the proper plan of action, you can overcome NES and put your metabolism in order.

In order to help patients with NES get some sleep, I most often recommend 100 milligrams (mg) of 5-HTP with 250 mg of Relora®, and 3 mg of melatonin—all taken at bedtime. As my patients begin to sleep better and better, I slowly wean them off the melatonin and the 5-HTP, and depending on their stress levels, the Relora®. The melatonin replenishes what the body is probably not making, while the 5-HTP builds up serotonin levels. The Relora® lowers cortisol levels and reduces the impact of the stressful day. As the levels of serotonin and melatonin begin to rise in my patients (as evidenced by the improved ability to sleep), they can slowly wean themselves off the melatonin and the 5-HTP, and eventually the Relora®, depending on their chronic stress levels.

It is estimated that almost half of all Americans will experience some insomnia this year. One of the greatly overlooked causes of insomnia, in my opinion, is stress.

since the inadequate intakes are happening at the same time that they are having increased needs (under chronic stress).

Zinc, selenium, copper, and manganese are important for the support of enzymes. Zinc alone is involved in hundreds of enzymatic reactions, including those involved in adrenal activity. Zinc is critical for immune function, specifically the production of T cells from the thymus. High levels of cortisol can deplete zinc status. Excess cortisol and ACTH have been linked to thymus atrophy and shrinkage and suppression of T-cell production. Corticosteroid therapy increases the need for zinc supplementation. (This is also true of a host of other nutrients so check Appendix 3 "Prescription and Nonprescription Nutrient Depletions" on page 512 if you have been or are on prednisone or other corticosteroid therapy.)

Iron deficiency is associated with reduction of T and B cells (lymphocytes that stimulate and produce antibodies). Iron absorption can be depleted by insufficient hydrochloric acid in the stomach, a symptom of chronic stress. Iron depletion can be a result of extreme physical stress such as exercise. But you shouldn't take iron unless you have a known iron deficiency or unless you are still menstruating.

Amino Acids

One of the most frequent tests I perform in my office is a simple test called a blood spot amino acid profile. It's usually a surprise to patients when I show them just how low they are in essential amino acids. Amino acids are needed to replenish protein catabolism initiated by chronic cortisol elevations and metabolic challenges. Increasing protein intake during stress is important to maintain adequate amino acid availability. Amino acids are used to synthesize hormones and enzymes crucial for their activities. They are the building blocks of literally all your tissues and the cells needed for metabolic processes.

Tyrosine, an amino acid contained in protein-rich foods, is especially important for endocrine function, and is required for synthesis of epinephrine and norepinephrine, thyroid hormones, and cortisol.

Tryptophan, another amino acid, is needed for the production of serotonin. Eating a high-carbohydrate meal leads to increased tryptophan absorption into the brain where it is made into serotonin. However, as we have mentioned, continually eating too many high-carbohydrate meals can lead to chronically high insulin levels. You can enhance tryptophan absorption by alternating meals that include some complex carbohydrates with high-protein meals. You can also take 5-hydroxytryptophan (5-HTP) to stimulate the production of serotonin. It also is a big help to curb your cravings for carbohydrates and sugar. Often I will recommend 50 mg of 5-HTP in the mid-afternoon and early evening with Relora®. Relora® is a proprietary formula of a patented extract from *Magnolia officinalis* and a patent-pending extract from *Phellodendron amurense,* two plant species that have been used in traditional Chinese medicine (TCM) for over 1,500 years. Both supplements help to reduce excessive stress hormone response and to cut carbohydrate-craving behavior. (See "Supplements and Nutritional Support for the Adrenals" in Chapter 6.)

The craving for carbohydrates feeds into a vicious cycle of insulin resistance, which fuels further cravings. In addition, the craving pattern associated with elevated cortisol levels can also lead to *night eating syndrome* (NES) where people will consume 50 percent or more of their calories in the evening. In this syndrome, people will have a lack of appetite during the day. This is most likely due to the effect of stress hormones. NES is characterized by an increased appetite at night and rising up from sleep to eat. This is in part due to poor glycemic or blood sugar regulation and to elevations in cortisol.

Stress and Adrenal Function

Although the adrenals secrete hormones in response to stress, all the endocrine glands are impaired by stress. And as they are all closely linked in their function, the repercussions of stress impact them all.

The Thyroid

Thyroid and adrenal functions are closely linked. Both endocrine glands are under the control of the hypothalamus and tropic hormones (hormones that control the levels of other hormones), including thyroid-stimulating hormone (TSH), adrenocorticotropic hormone (ACTH), follicle-stimulating hormone (FSH), and luteinizing hormone (LH).

High levels of stress decrease the pituitary secretion of TSH and diminish the production of thyroid hormone. Stress also slows the conversion of thyroid hormone (T4) to its active form (T3). This is an adaptive mechanism designed to conserve fuel during stress by slowing metabolism, but this condition sometimes does not reverse itself when the immediate stress is resolved. It is critical to understand that this is a significant way that stress impairs optimal metabolic function.

If you are under stress, the amino acid tyrosine may help, as tyrosine helps in the production of serotonin. As mentioned earlier, an increase in stress hormones may cause a decrease in serotonin due to decreased tyrosine. When your body's pool of tyrosine is drained to make cortisol under stress, not enough tyrosine remains from which to make thyroid hormones.

Other amino acids play an important role in serotonin production as well. Tryptophan, along with vitamin B$_6$, is needed to make serotonin. 5-HTP is available on the market and is well absorbed across the blood-brain barrier. It easily converts to serotonin.

Since the symptoms of adrenal insufficiency and hypothyroidism (fatigue, poor regulation of body temperature, elevated lipids, depression, constipation, dry skin, sleep disturbances) overlap, they are sometimes confused or dealt with separately. Addressing a low-functioning thyroid without supporting adrenal function may leave you with only half the answer. Worse, it may leave you still feeling fatigued.

The Pancreas

The adrenal glands and the pancreas are both endocrine glands. The pancreas secretes insulin and glucagon from the islets of Langerhans. When blood sugar is high, insulin helps deliver glucose to the cells, driving the content of sugar in the blood down. When blood sugar is low, glucagon is released and stores of glucose (glycogen) are released from the liver. However, the maintenance of blood sugar is not isolated to the pancreas. The adrenals, the pituitary gland, the intestines, and the pancreas work in synchrony to achieve this important balance, supplying the cells with glucose needed for energy, while ensuring enough blood sugar for the brain to function.

The adrenals are called into action when blood sugar levels drop too quickly. The adrenals secrete cortisol and epinephrine, which antagonize the action of insulin and help preserve blood sugar levels. Cortisol also helps to convert glycogen to glucose in the liver. Adrenals that are under the influence of chronic stress cannot respond adequately to drops in blood sugar. For this reason, adrenal insufficiency and exhaustion can produce symptoms of hypoglycemia (low blood sugar, dizziness on standing) and, with time, contribute to the development of diabetes. Hypoglycemia produces irritability, headaches, fatigue, and anxiety, which signal the already-exhausted adrenals to produce more stress hormones.

Conditions of chronic stress and elevated cortisol production have the reverse effect. Because cortisol antagonizes the effect of insulin and helps to release glycogen stores from the liver, chronic stress and the elevation of cortisol produce excess blood sugar, or hyperglycemia. The pancreas responds to elevated blood sugar by producing more insulin, causing hyperinsulinemia and insulin resistance.

There is some evidence that DHEA plays a role in controlling some of the detrimental effects of insulin resistance and hyperinsulinemia—both conditions that cause

Polycystic Ovary Disease

If you are a woman with polycystic ovarian syndrome (PCOS), a hormonal disorder characterized by menstrual regulatory problems, infertility, increased hair growth, and obesity, and you are taking medications to decrease your blood sugar levels, you should evaluate the stress levels in your life using the Social Readjustment Rating Scale on page 79.

If you are experiencing insulin resistance because of chronic stress, you may not be getting the full advantage of the medications that your doctor has prescribed for you. Chronic stress could be negating or hampering the ability of the blood sugar-lowering medications you may be taking. If you suffer from PCOS, I highly recommend using the nutritional recommendations (diet and supplements) and the stress reduction measures given in this book. They may help you control any stress-induced insulin issues and lead to better blood sugar control.

an overproduction of insulin. Just as insulin output by the pancreas appears to increase with age, DHEA production from the adrenal cortex declines with age. One theory is that an increase in insulin causes a decline in DHEA. It is thought that DHEA may have a cardioprotective benefit, shielding the heart from the damaging effects of hyperinsulinemia. Without the protective benefits of DHEA, elevated insulin is even more damaging to the cardiovascular system.

Environmental Toxicity and Adrenal Function

Environmental toxins, particularly mercury and lead, are thought to have a devastating impact on adrenal function. (Mercury and other heavy metal intoxication are discussed in more detail in Chapter 10.) However, it is a little known fact that mercury concentrates in the adrenal cortex causing increased oxidative stress, leading to increased damaging of cellular DNA and mitochondrial DNA. As the mitochondrial DNA are destroyed, the adrenal glands have less energy reserve to generate the new blueprint for healthy cells and do not have the energy reserve to function at full capacity.

It has been demonstrated that mercury vapor accumulates in the adrenal cortex of animals. The adrenal cortex is the site of most of the oxidation of vapor (which comes from environmental contaminants, chemicals on food, and mercury amalgam dental fillings) to the biochemically active ions.

Mercury depletes both vitamin B_5 (pantothenic acid) and vitamin C, weakening the immune response and interfering with the production of adrenal hormones. Large accumulations of mercury have been found in the adrenal medulla (part of the adrenal glands). Mercury also accumulates in the pituitary gland, which directs the activity of the adrenals through the secretion of ACTH.

The production of steroid hormones from the adrenal glands is mediated, in part, by enzymes. Heavy metals are known to interfere with the action of many critical enzymes, including those involved in adrenal steroid production. The enzyme system cytochrome P-450 helps to convert cholesterol into pregnenolone, a hormone used to make cortisol, aldosterone, and DHEA. Research indicates that mercury can impair adrenal function by reducing the concentration of intact cytochrome P-450, as well as another enzyme, 21 alpha-hydroxylase, which adversely affects the function and homeostatic control of the adrenal cortex. A deficiency in 21-alpha-hydroxylase impairs normal cortisol production, which leads to an increase in ACTH. The result is an overproduction of adrenal androgens (male sex hormones).

Another enzyme affected by heavy metals is adenyl cyclase. Adenylate cyclase catalyzes the production of cyclic adenosine monophosphate (cAMP) from ATP. CAMP is a critical cofactor for enzymes in the adrenal cortex, as well as for the production of ACTH in the pituitary. With decreased activity of cAMP, poor output of ACTH and adrenal insufficiency are likely. One study reported that lead, mercury, and cadmium inhibited adenylate cyclase activity in the brain.

Cadmium is a byproduct of zinc refining. It is used in welding and in the production of paints, plastics, fungicides, and fertilizers. Rice and shellfish are sources of dietary cadmium. Smokers acquire cadmium through contaminated tobacco.

In today's world, I think that it is impossible to escape some intoxication from these agents; they have powerful disruptive effects on metabolic function. That is why it is important to take a proactive approach to detoxification.

Bowel Terrain and Adrenal Function

The relationship between the adrenals and the intestine is one of mutual influence. When the human body is in a healthy state, the adrenal glands help regulate blood glucose from food absorbed by the digestive tract. The adrenal hormones help regulate hydrochloric acid secretion and motility of the gastrointestinal tract. Stress and excess cortisol production can result in insufficient hydrochloric acid secretion and poor digestion and gastrointestinal motility. The result may be constipation, heartburn, gas, bloating, and poor digestion of food.

Excess cortisol impairs the function of secretory IgA (an antibody) in the mucosal cells of the intestine, leaving it vulnerable to antigens ("foreign invaders"). This can lead to a chronic heightened immune response, where intestinal microorganisms and even food can trigger allergic or intolerant reactions. Furthermore, cortisol increases blood sugar concentration, which feeds yeast growth and dysbiosis. Cortisol also weakens immune regulation and therefore allows for growth of pathogens, harmful bacteria, and yeast toxins that would normally be held in check. Chronic inflammation and immune response alert the adrenals to produce more stress hormones, ultimately worsening the condition.

As mentioned earlier, stress can lead to decreased production of hydrochloric acid. Hydrochloric acid is one of the factors that controls a naturally occurring organism in the body—*Candida albicans,* a type of yeast. If not controlled, these yeast organisms overgow in the system and can lead to a wide variety of problems (for more information, see Chapter 9). Yeast mycotoxins (harmful byproducts of yeast proliferation) can impair the tissue response to hormones by "masking" the hormone at the receptor cell. Because the hormone is never getting to the intended site, it will appear that the person has the symptoms of impaired adrenal function. Should this occur while a patient is simultaneously under chronic stress, the result is that the patient's system is getting the signals of immune and endocrine disruption from a variety of inputs simultaneously.

LAB TESTS FOR ADRENAL FUNCTION

Besides using the self-test method described above, there is another good method of determining if your adrenals are functioning properly. As we've discussed, when the adrenals are overstressed, cortisol levels are elevated. A salivary cortisol measurement test can be easily performed by your healthcare provider. It is a reliable indicator for elevated cortisol and, therefore, for adrenal function.

Testing Your Adrenal Function

When your adrenal glands are functioning at peak performance, your systolic blood pressure (the top number in the measurement of blood pressure—120/80) is about ten points higher when you are upright than when you are lying prone.

To determine how well your adrenal glands are coping with your lifestyle, you will need to purchase a blood pressure cuff from your local pharmacy. A wrist cuff is easiest to manipulate. The cost of a quality blood pressure cuff is around $30.

Take two blood pressure readings according to the instructions in the kit. Take the first reading while you are lying down and the second immediately upon rising. Rest for five minutes before taking the first reading. Then, take the reading, get up, and quickly take another reading. If you are dizzy when standing up and the second reading produces a lower number, suspect adrenal dysfunction. Then follow the recommendations in Chapter 6 for adrenal support.

MANAGING STRESS

In our world today, stress seems to be compounding like a high-yield bond. I wish I could say that it is easy to manage stress. But it takes a plan of action. And it takes the support of friends, family, and healthcare professionals to do a continual check in and to make sure that you are still working with the plan.

I don't think that it is realistic to tell my patients to simply "avoid stress." After all, how do you do that? Stress is everywhere; it's a part of our daily lives. No, you can't really avoid stress, but you can and should try to establish and maintain your nutritional needs and sharpen your coping strategies.

Determining and then dealing with sources of stress in life is paramount to an adrenal restoration program. The following questionnaire "How Stressed Are You?" is designed to help you determine your general level of stress. (Sources of stress include work performance, physical symptoms, and interpersonal relationships.)

HOW STRESSED ARE YOU?

Indicate how often your feelings agree with the statements below. Scoring for each item is based on the following scale:

1 = Never   2 = Seldom   3 = Sometimes   4 = Frequently   5 = Always

General Feelings
____ I worry a lot.
____ I feel unhappy.

____ All kinds of worrisome thoughts run through my mind.

____ I feel like crying for no reason.

____ I am so irritable: I don't know what is the matter with me.

____ I have lost the ability to sit around and do nothing.

____ I feel like I live in a pressure cooker, always ready to explode.

____ I have been bored with my life, job, friends, and loved ones.

____ I am dissatisfied and I don't know why.

____ I forget things.

_____ TOTAL

Work Performance

____ I have trouble concentrating on my work.

____ I take forever to make decisions.

____ I can't seem to stick to a job.

____ I am restless all day.

____ I overreact to situations.

____ I let minor issues get to me.

____ I procrastinate.

____ I can't seem to get organized.

____ I am unclear about my role.

____ I do a lot of paper shuffling.

_____ TOTAL

Physical Symptoms

____ My heart races or pounds.

____ I have trouble catching my breath.

____ I get diarrhea.

____ I have headaches.

____ I have to urinate frequently.

____ I get dizzy for no apparent reason.

____ I takes me forever to fall asleep at night.

____ I am tired.

____ I have a dry mouth/throat.

____ My stomach is tense.

____ I have no energy.

____ I am chilly.

____ I have pain in my neck/shoulders/eyes/chest/lower back/throat/or hands.

____ I seem to catch every cold or bug that is going around.

____ I run out of energy in the afternoon.

____ My posture is terrible.

____ I crave carbohydrates/sugars and eat them uncontrollably.

_____ **TOTAL**

Interpersonal Relationships

____ I startle easily.

____ I can't speak correctly when around other people.

____ I can't stand to be around a particular person or group.

____ I can't stand to be around other people when they are emotional.

____ I can't tell anyone how I feel.

____ I don't feel anything.

____ I can't laugh at myself.

____ I am not happy with my sex life.

____ I don't trust anybody.

____ I need help (food or drink) to be social.

_____ **TOTAL**

TOTAL SCORE First determine your average score for each section. To do this, add up the items in each section and divide by the number of items for the *section* average score. Second, determine your *overall* average score by adding the totals together from each of the sections and divide by 46. Average scores should be in the 20s or low 30s. Section scores reflect the following:

General Feelings and Work Performance	Physical Symptoms	Interpersonal Relationships
10–20 = Low stress	20–34 = Low stress	10–14 = Low stress
20–30 = Moderate stress	35–49 = Moderate stress	15–30 = Moderate stress
30–40 = High stress	50–64 = High stress	31–40 = High stress
40–50 = Very high stress	65–80 = Very high stress	41–50 = Very high stress

This score, plus your score from the Social Readjustment Rating Scale question-naire, should give you an accurate assessment of the overall stress in your life.

If you scored in the low-stress range, congratulations, you are managing pretty well. You can stay ahead of the game by continuing to practice good nutritional habits and stress-reduction techniques. You may want to take a multivitamin and mineral supplement with a broad spectrum of nutrients just to make sure your intake is adequate to meet all of the body's demands.

If you scored in the moderate-stress range, you should also be very diligent to practice good nutritional habits, including taking a multivitamin and mineral sup-plement, and to incorporate exercise and stress-reduction techniques into your daily routine. However, if you are feeling fairly anxious, you may want to consider adding a stress-reducing supplement, such as Relora®. (See the inset "Relora®: A Special Sup-plement for Adrenal Stress" on page 127.)

If you scored in the high-stress or very high-stress range, you will need to do all of the above, and from my experience, you will need to utilize more nutritional supple-ments to effectively deal with the results of adrenal depletion that occur under stress. More details on nutrition and supplements for stress are outlined in the next chapter. Seeking out the advice of a healthcare practitioner who is experienced in natural med-icine can help you decide which supplements would be most beneficial for you.

In addition, I would highly recommend seeking out professional psychological counseling to help you evaluate whether lifestyle measures will be enough or whether you may need additional support. There is no harm in using medications to help under conditions of severe stress as long as the lifestyle and nutrition issues are also addressed. This will provide immediate help and will address the physiological needs of the body as well, which will help you deal better with the stress. Moreover, it would be a good idea to see your medical doctor to get a full physical evaluation. This will reveal if your stress has gotten to potentially dangerous levels and may help prevent a truly catastrophic result such as heart attack.

Regardless of your score, it is always a good idea to nutritionally support your adrenal glands to either maintain or restore them to optimal function. Restoring weakened, overburdened adrenal glands to their optimal condition requires dietary changes and nutritional support, which we'll address in depth in the next chapter.

LIFESTYLE SUPPORT

In addition to supporting yourself nutritionally, there are many techniques and lifestyle practices that will improve your ability to deal with stress and to prevent and/or improve the physical effects that result from it. Here are several ways to strengthen your resistance to stress.

Stress and Time Management

To put it simply, one of the most stress-inducing factors today is "trying to do too may things with too little time." These days, managing our time is perhaps the hardest part of daily life. As a rule, we expect too much from ourselves in the time that we actually have available on a daily basis. But time management remains a crucial element of stress management. The two most important components of time management are simplifying the demands on our time and organizing the time that we actually have.

As difficult as it may seem, it is essential to allocate our time to things that are rewarding and fruitful in our lives. Simplifying demands means saying *no* to things that are not important, necessary, or fun. Organizing time requires examining the areas of our lives in which time is wasted. This may require a detailed assessment of where your time is spent.

Keep a log of things that cause stress and disorganization in your life for a few days. Doing this won't help you avoid the hustle and bustle of daily life, but you will better understand it and learn from it. Then, you can begin to take the steps needed to get your schedule under control. Just the act of identifying the sticking points in your day and your stress response can allow you to take the first step toward trying to develop a time-management strategy. I admit that this is an area that I still struggle with, but once we all acknowledge the problems we have taking control of our time, it becomes much easier to begin making the changes that will lead to solutions.

Relaxation

Stress often manifests itself as muscle tension and tightness. This is a manifestation of the sympathetic nervous system, which dominates during times of stress. Even if stress is unavoidable, it is possible to reduce the tension built up in your muscles. You can do this by engaging the parasympathetic nervous system, which controls normal body functions such as breathing, heartbeat, blood flow, and proper bowel function.

Relaxation is the opposing force to stress. When you become relaxed, the parasympathetic nervous system, which is designed to also promote repair, maintenance, and restoration, takes charge.

Two modes of relaxation that offer wonderful exercise, as well, are yoga and tai chi. Yoga, a product of ancient India, will improve your breathing, strength, and flexibility. Tai chi, a product of ancient China, will do much the same. For those of you who want even more active exercise, I suggest you explore martial arts.

There are, however, infinite ways to begin to relax; you just have to make the effort. Relaxation exercises, meditation, and massage can also promote the parasympathetic response and assist in relieving the physical signs of stress. Gardening calms people, as does spending time with pets, reading a good book, or watching favorite old movies. Laughter is often an important aspect of relaxation. I find that my patients who create some time each day for relaxation and for things that they enjoy are the patients who regain their health sooner.

If you are experiencing significant muscular aches and pains from stress, seek out a cranial-sacral therapist, who uses a form of therapy that emphasizes improving cranial fluid flow, which promotes muscle relaxation and is effective for a wide range of pain and dysfunction. Or find a massage or physical therapist who specializes in myofascial (massage-oriented) release. Acupuncture, the practice of traditional Chinese medicine using acupuncture needles to free energy blocks in the body, is also effective in relieving muscular aches and pains. All of these techniques are specialized forms of physical medicine.

If stress is getting so bad that you aren't coping well, get yourself into counseling or, at the very least, pick up a self-help book that speaks to your particular situation. Life has its hard times. Work, family crises, and even our own aging process can create stress. But one thing is certain, it is impossible to be relaxed and stressed at the same time. By guiding yourself into a state of relaxation, you are forcing your stress to subside. As a starting point, let me suggest the book *Meditation as Medicine* by Dharma Singh Khalsa, M.D. (Atria Books, 2001). It contains an excellent explanation of the physiologic benefits of stress reduction, as well as a practical, down-to-earth plan of action.

Adequate Sleep

Poor sleep habits add to stress, irritability, depression, and alterations in growth hormone. New evidence actually links sleep deprivation with diabetes, obesity, reduced growth hormone release, increased inflammatory cytokine activity, and other health conditions. Sleep deprivation interferes with productivity, which can further aggravate stress. Inadequate sleep can also interfere with immune function and lead to the physical stress of illness.

The most restful sleep is between roughly 9:00 P.M. and 9:00 A.M. This means that eight hours of sleep (give or take a few hours) between 10:00 P.M. and 6:00 A.M. are more restorative than from 3:00 A.M. to 11:00 A.M. Napping during the day can help make up for sleep deprivation, but it may interfere with falling asleep in the evening. Ultimately, you are cheating yourself if you try to beat the sleep clock. Those who fall prey to deadlines and commitments, slipping into bad sleep habits, inevitably pay the price.

Moderate Exercise

Once again, this book focuses more on the biochemical means to gain control of your metabolism rather than on basic behaviors, such as exercise. Certainly, a discussion of exercise would need to encompass many more chapters than there is room for in this book. Although only a brief discussion of exercise in maintaining health is included here, I cannot emphasize enough the importance of consistent and moderate exercise in helping to regain control of your metabolism.

Deep Breathing: A Quick Fix

The following relaxation technique is simple but it can be used anytime. Find a quiet place to sit. Begin by taking a few deep, slow breaths. Breathe from your abdomen. Next, starting with your hands and arms, tense the muscle to about three-quarters of their maximum tension, then relax; then progress to the shoulders, face, torso, and down through the legs and feet. Inhale and exhale slowly during this exercise.

The exercise can be completed in less than fifteen minutes and the effect is remarkable. You should structure time to complete a relaxation exercise a few times a day if possible. If this does not realistically fit your lifestyle, make sure that you have time to do activities that serve no other purpose than to provide joy and laughter in your life.

Most experts will agree that light to moderate exercise such as walking twenty to thirty minutes, three to four times a week, or gardening and swimming can diminish mental and emotional stress and have a positive impact on your metabolism without heightening risk of injury.

Moderate exercise reduces the effects of stress hormones by providing a physical outlet for stressful feelings. Aerobic exercise stimulates the release of endorphins from the pituitary and hypothalamus. Endorphins are neuropeptides, which bind with opiate receptors in the brain. They function to relieve pain and promote a sense of well-being. There is some evidence that exercise training increases circulating DHEA, even while at rest, which burns off stress hormones and reduces cortisol levels.

Exercise also has a significant impact on blood sugar. By controlling blood sugar more effectively, you are managing a key factor in the development of insulin resistance, diabetes, and obesity. In addition, proper exercise and stretching will keep you limber as you age, build bone density, and just make you feel so much better mentally.

Regular exercise has even been reported to help people who are depressed to overcome their depression. The physiological changes associated with exercise contribute to an overall sense of control, health promotion, and ability to cope with stress. If you have been sedentary for some time, consult with your healthcare practitioner before beginning any new exercise program.

Faith, Spirituality, and Healing

There is a recent renewed interest in the effects of spirituality on health. Faith and religious practices are currently being studied and are being found to play a critical role in people's health and in their relationships. Numerous medical and epidemiological studies support that spiritual or religious life is statistically associated with improvements in cardiovascular disease, hypertension, stroke, colitis, and cancer. Whether that spirituality is expressed through the Christian, Buddhist, Hindu, Muslim, Native American faiths, or of any other faith, spirituality and medicine have long intertwined in health.

The separation between medicine and spirituality that Western medicine created at the brink of the twentieth century was a departure from thousands of years of faith-based healing—healing that took place in most cultures, including our own. While most people will turn to prayer during serious illness or impending death, our healthcare system has tended to downgrade prayer and spirituality as a part of healthcare. Despite recent research that demonstrates a relationship between prayerful practices and health benefits, the reintegration of spirituality into the practice of medicine is just now being examined.

The extent of the healing benefits of spirituality and prayer are a matter of speculation and may differ with the individual. Some researchers attribute the benefits to the release of neurochemicals that protect the heart and immune functions; others point to the placebo effect and the influence of healthier lifestyles associated with religious conviction.

With the resurgence in complementary and alternative medicine in recent years, spirituality and healing have once again become important in the health of our population. Wholistic healing honors the integration and interplay of mind, body, spirit, and emotions. Although stress is a threat to health as we've discussed in this chapter, the implications of stress go well beyond physical well-being. In the words of the noted philosopher Carl Jung, "Every crisis is a spiritual crisis."

Stress that roams uncontrolled chokes the human spirit—the vital force of human energy—which ultimately affects your physical body. Although we can learn and grow from the stressful events in life, the reality remains that most stress is a waste: a waste of time, a waste of energy.

The principles, practices, and ethics of Native American healing have long been regarded as a model for spirituality and healing. Native American healing, spirituality, and culture can be a model for modern healing. Intuition and spiritual awareness are diagnostic tools to native healers. Music, ritual, and ceremony are all part of healing. A community of friends, family, and helpers often participate in the healing intervention. A healthy person has a healthy relationship with his or her community and, ultimately, with all of Nature. The goal of spiritual healing is to find wholeness, balance, harmony, beauty, and meaning, in other words, a truly "wholistic" approach.

I have found in my practice that many older adults, in particular, believe in a higher power, one that supports them constantly, protecting, guiding, teaching, helping, and healing. They believe that prayer can heal both physical and mental illness, if it is "God's will" to do so. In fact, for many of us, having a relationship with God forms the foundation of our total well-being.

The placebo effect—healing based on one's *belief* that a treatment measure will be effective—should not be underestimated. It is thought that the placebo effect carries significant weight in the self-healing process by mobilizing the power of the body to move toward life. Even if the placebo effect is fractional, it highlights the power of the body to repair itself under the right influences. Rather than trying to control the placebo effect of treatment measures, it should be embraced and cultivated as a force of wellness. For this reason, those who have witnessed its phenomenal results encourage prayer and spirituality as important aspects of the healing process.

Perception and Attitude

Stress is a function of perception and attitude as much as circumstance. As difficult as it may be, changing the way a situation is perceived can profoundly influence its effect. Take, for example, a minor car accident. Losing control of a vehicle is one of the most terrifying and stressful experiences in modern life. In most cases, a car accident will elicit a full-blown stress response. The perception of this experience as bad luck, inconvenience, and loss of control will merely exaggerate the stress response. However, seeing it from the perspective of gratitude, feeling fortunate that no one was hurt or killed, and possibly as a learning tool ("I was traveling too fast for these conditions") can ameliorate some of the stressful feelings.

Growth is rarely achieved without struggle. In every challenge, there is opportunity. Managing challenges and crisis effectively requires focusing on what there is to learn and overcome, and the personal growth attached to difficult circumstances. Seeking professional counseling can help manage unresolved issues, fears, or conflicts. Keeping your body metabolically able to cope with stress can help you to cope better, and hopefully reduce the profound impact that stress has on us all.

ADRENAL BALANCE IS KEY

Controlling the stress in your life as it happens is one of the most important measures in optimizing metabolic function. We have all become so accustomed to ongoing stress and the physiological changes that accompany it, that we have failed to recognize its impact on aging and disease processes that are affecting us.

Under conditions of chronic stress, the adrenal glands move through phases of activity, first becoming overactive and over time, exhausted, and devoid of adrenal gland reserve.

Stress can negatively affect metabolism, blood sugar balance, immunity, cardiovascular health, and even memory. Eighty-five percent of diseases are estimated to have stress-related factors. Although stress is a byproduct of living in our modern world, you can and should try to maintain your nutritional needs and sharpen your coping strategies with the suggestions offered in this chapter. Also, if you have environmental stressors in your life (and who doesn't?), you need to detoxify your body as outlined in Chapter 11. In addition, you must take action to balance your hor-

Michael's Story

After a referral by my family physician to Dr. LaValle, my overall health has improved noticeably. Before seeing Dr. LaValle, I had no energy, I was depressed, I had constant lower back pain, and I was twenty-five pounds overweight. Everything was getting worse. After a complete evaluation of my health, Dr. LaValle recommended nutritional supplements and the Healthy Living Guidelines, which were very achievable. I followed his recommendations and was soon back to my old self. I lost the extra pounds and am maintaining the weight loss. Even the pain in my back has diminished to a manageable level. My friends all comment on how great I look. I always tell them of my experience with Dr. LaValle.

Michael is an example of how metabolic dysfunction can lead to chronic pain. When the adrenals become weak, mood lowers, comfort foods are desired, stress taxes the other endocrine glands, and the thyroid begins slowing down. The result is chronic depression, low energy, and low tolerance to pain. Mike exemplifies what can happen when someone decides that he wants to change the path that his health is headed down.

mones, most especially those put forth by your pancreas, your thyroid, and your adrenal glands.

My experience has shown me that sometimes giving the right natural therapeutics to support the effects of stress can go a long way to literally turning your life around. Nutritional supplements, including vitamins and minerals (which were likely depleted by stress in the first place), can be of significant help in managing stress response.

Mild adrenal insufficiency may be corrected within a few months. More severe cases of adrenal exhaustion may take up to several years. In almost twenty years of practice, I can think of only a handful of people who did not benefit significantly from a regimen designed to support the adrenal glands. The majority of patients, however, notice initial improvement in just a few days—sometimes even sooner. Adrenal support often provides the most significant impact on the way a person is feeling. In other words, you really feel the difference.

Restoring weakened, overburdened adrenal glands to their optimal condition requires dietary and lifestyle changes, and adrenal support. Next, let's see if we can formulate a plan by which our adrenals can be balanced in their function so that we can let go of our chronic "fight-or-flight" strategy and learn to relax our way into health.

CHAPTER 6

Key Supplements and Strategies for Balancing Your Metabolism

If after having read about the first three keys, you are finding yourself described within them—that is, you have signs of blood sugar dysregulation, symptoms of adrenal stress, or low thyroid function—you may be coming to understand some of the underlying factors that might be affecting your metabolism. In other words, you are beginning to "crack your metabolic code."

This chapter introduces you to some of the nutraceuticals, vitamins, minerals, and diet and lifestyle changes that will help to support and normalize your endocrine function. Remember, the goal is to get your body chemistry working in harmony. Addressing one area of your endocrine system will help to achieve harmony with the other areas. Balancing adrenal function can greatly improve blood sugar control and can help the thyroid to begin functioning more optimally. Improving blood sugar control and thyroid function can greatly improve weight-loss efforts and make it much easier to maintain your ideal body weight.

Now, let's look at the pivotal dietary supplements and nutritional practices that can help you achieve this harmony of health for the first three keys.

SUPPLEMENT SUPPORT FOR THE ENDOCRINE GLANDS

In my practice, I counsel clients on the use of supplements, as well as on lifestyle and dietary changes, to help them achieve endocrine balance, as well as balance in all their body systems. It is always appropriate to include nutritional and lifestyle changes in any health program. However, it is important to recognize that nutritional approaches and lifestyle changes *alone* aren't always enough to address the health problems at hand.

Let me emphasize this again. Sometimes people wait until their systems are so far out of balance that using nutritional approaches alone not only won't be enough to adequately address their health problems, but also could be dangerous if they don't also seek medical care. In some cases, the addition of drug therapy may be needed to maintain endocrine balance. Many of my clients are already under the care of a medical doctor; therefore, our work on balancing their bodies through supplements and lifestyle *enhances* the medical care they are receiving by improving nutritional status and, therefore, quality of life.

The information on the following supplements is supplied to enhance and support proper medical care—*not* to replace it. If you try some of these supplements, but find that you're not feeling any better, do not put off seeing a healthcare professional. I do not recommend or endorse undertaking any nutritional program as a means of self-treatment for any diagnosed medical condition you may have. If you feel, however, that you may be suffering unnecessarily due to possible nutritional imbalances or lack of attention to nutritional support for your endocrine function, seek the help of a healthcare professional who is experienced in the use of natural medicine. Such a doctor can make sure that any medical conditions you have are being properly addressed, as well as guide you in your nutritional program.

SUPPLEMENTS AND NUTRIENTS FOR SUPPORTING HEALTHY BLOOD SUGAR AND INSULIN LEVELS

The following supplements and key nutrients have known roles in supporting blood sugar balance and regulation in the body. Following this list is an explanation of each supplement or nutrient and how it supports endocrine function, including a suggested dosage range.

The dosages in the bulleted items below are specifically recommended for blood sugar regulation in *insulin-resistant people.* Dosages for those who have *poor blood sugar regulation,* but are not yet insulin-resistant, are addressed in the discussion on each nutrient.

- Alpha lipoic acid: 300–600 milligrams (mg) a day

- Omega-3 EFA (fish oils): 2–6 grams (g) a day

- Omega-6 EFA (primrose or borage oil): 500–1,000 mg a day

The vitamins and minerals listed below can sometimes be found in one multivitamin/mineral supplement. If not, you may need to find a separate single nutrient tablet to get the full amounts recommended.

- B Complex: (See discussion below for specific amounts)

- Chromium: 200–600 micrograms (mcg) a day

- Vanadium: 750 mcg–1.5 mg a day

- Magnesium: 600–1,000 mg a day

- Zinc: 30–50 mg a day

Other nutraceuticals to consider include:

- Relora®: 250 mg, three times a day, if anxiety is a problem (anxiety may aggravate hypoglycemia, and high stress levels may increase carbohydrate and sugar cravings)

- Glucosol: 32–48 mg a day, if you are trying to lose weight

- 5-HTP: 150–300 mg a day helps reduce sugar cravings and is a great combination with Relora® for reducing stress, improving sleep (and therefore insulin regulation), and stopping carbohydrate and sugar cravings

- Cyclo-hispro: 300-mg capsules, three to four times a day, for type 2 diabetics or those with known insulin resistance

- Herbal extracts that help with blood sugar control and to reduce cravings, including:

  Bitter melon: 200 mg, two to three times a day

  Cinnamon extract: 250–500 mg, three times daily

  Gymnema sylvestre: 250–500 mg, three times a day

The following discussions address specifics on some of the key nutrients mentioned above.

Alpha Lipoic Acid

This antioxidant, sometimes called lipoic acid, increases insulin-receptor sensitivity, which means that it can improve the ability of insulin to bind to cells and then carry fuel into the cell to be burned as fuel. This is important for anyone who suspects or knows that he or she is insulin resistant. Alpha lipoic acid also has been reported to improve nerve blood flow, reduce oxidative stress, and improve nerve conduction in diabetic neuropathy. As an added bonus, it helps to reduce the rate of wrinkle formation and helps prevent cataracts.

An important fact about alpha lipoic acid is that it is one of the most powerful antioxidants known. It can neutralize some of the most harmful free radicals known as the *peroxyl* and *peroxynitrite* free radicals. Alpha lipoic acid can get into virtually all body compartments making it a stealth free-radical fighter. Alpha lipoic acid enhances other free-radical fighters in the body, including vitamins C and E, and glutathione.

Recommended dose. Doses of alpha lipoic acid range widely from 50 mg, two times a day for general antioxidant activity, to 300 mg, two times a day for people who are diabetic, insulin resistant, or have metabolic syndrome.

B-Complex Vitamins

All of the B vitamins are water-soluble vitamins that are discussed in detail in Chapter 16. However, they are included here for support of healthy blood sugar and insulin levels because so many of them play a role in proper carbohydrate, fat, and protein metabolism. A B-complex supplement and many multivitamins will typically include all of the B vitamins in the following amounts: B_1 (thiamine, 5 mg), B_2 (riboflavin, 10 mg), B_3 (niacin, 50 mg), B_6 (pyridoxine, 20 mg), B_{12} (cyanocobalamin, 100 mcg), pantothenic acid (15 mg), folic acid (400 mcg), and sometimes other lesser known members of the B vitamins choline (300 mg), inositol (250 mg), biotin (900 mcg), and PABA (12–50 mg). Although some manufacturers include PABA in small amounts, this B vitamin has not been shown to be an essential nutrient in humans.

Chromium

The influence of chromium (also called glucose tolerance factor, or GTF) on blood sugar regulation was first recognized in animal studies in the 1950s. Later, in the 1970s, it was discovered that hospital patients receiving intravenous feedings deficient in chromium had poor insulin regulation and hyperglycemia. Since then there continues to be solid data documenting the success of chromium in maintaining healthy blood sugar levels.

Chromium is believed to facilitate insulin by activating the *protein kinase molecules* on receptor cells, thereby enhancing the uptake of glucose and other nutrients. By aiding insulin in the body, chromium helps to prevent the breakdown of muscle during periods of fasting. Chromium is thought to stimulate fat metabolism and to have a lowering effect on cholesterol and triglyceride levels.

Chromium products, or supplements including chromium in their formulation, are often marketed as weight-loss agents; however, studies have not proven it to contribute to significant weight loss. Nevertheless, if you are low in chromium and crave carbohydrates, you may find that taking chromium will help to improve blood sugar regulation by *down-regulating insulin production*—that is, the insulin that is being produced works more efficiently in the presence of chromium, which spares the pancreas from having to produce as much insulin, and therefore can help some with weight loss. Although some of my patients have lost weight while taking chromium supplements, my experience has shown that the majority of people lose only a few pounds. So, although chromium has an indirect effect on weight loss, marketing it as a weight-loss supplement is somewhat misleading.

As discussed below, several groups of people are at risk for chromium depletion, including those who eat high-carbohydrates, athletes, the elderly, and women with gestational diabetes.

Those with diets high in refined carbohydrates may have up to 300 percent more chromium loss in their urine than those who eat diets that include whole grains. With chromium loss comes the potential for increased insulin resistance. Food processing and cooking destroys the chromium content of food. Since the average American diet is highly refined and processed, most Americans are at risk for a functional chromium deficiency. In fact, one study reported that approximately 90 percent of Americans ingest less than the suggested minimum of 50 mcg of chromium daily. With cardiovascular disease as the number-one killer in our country, it is interesting that cultures with naturally high levels of chromium in the diet have lower rates of cardiovascular disease and diabetes.

At particular risk for chromium deficiency are athletes, who excrete between two and six times the normal amount of chromium in their urine on days of vigorous exercise. This problem is intensified by the pre- and post-exercise consumption of high-carbohydrate foods and beverages that are eaten to improve recovery. The combination of increased metabolic rate, poor diet, and infusion of high carbohydrates makes hypoglycemia a common problem among athletes.

The elderly are also at risk for decreased absorption and intake of adequate chromium. This is particularly significant because of the high incidence of type 2 diabetes among this group. One study involving 47,000 people showed that there was a direct correlation between aging and a reduction in chromium levels.

Women who develop gestational diabetes are often deficient in chromium. This is not surprising, given the rate at which the developing fetus extracts minerals from the mother. In some cases, I have seen gestational diabetes reverse itself with the addition of 200 mcg of chromium added to the mother's daily diet. However, if you are pregnant check with your doctor before adding any supplements to your regimen.

The symptoms of chromium deficiency can include elevated levels of blood sugar, insulin, "bad" cholesterol, and triglycerides, and decreased levels of the high-density lipoproteins, or "good" cholesterol.

Food sources abundant in chromium include beer, brewer's yeast, broccoli, brown rice, cheese, organ meat, oysters, mushrooms, and whole grains.

Recommended dose. The amount of chromium that people need depends primarily on their state of health. The Recommended Daily Allowance (RDA) recommends 50–200 mcg of chromium per day; however, higher amounts may be needed for people with many conditions involving insulin resistance. Supplemental chromium is best taken in the form of *chromium polynicotinate* (200–600 mcg per day).

The picolinate form of chromium, popularized in the media, has been under some scrutiny for its potential carcinogenic properties. In a 1995 study, researchers at Dartmouth College and George Washington Medical discovered that exposing ovarian cells of laboratory animals to certain doses of chromium picolinate resulted in chromosomal damage. However, given the extensive studies documenting the safety and effectiveness of chromium picolinate, this one study is not enough evidence to suggest that it be avoided.

Organically bound *glucose tolerance factor* chromium, or GTF chromium, in a dose of 200–600 mcg daily, is thought to be safe and well tolerated. Diabetics may need higher doses (up to 1,000 mcg daily), but they should be monitored by a healthcare professional for changes in blood sugar levels, which may result in an adjustment of medication.

Magnesium

In my practice, I probably recommend magnesium more than any other supplement. Magnesium is involved in several hundred chemical reactions in the body and is required by every cell. Magnesium status among most Americans is compromised. This mineral has many important functions, including its ability to decrease insulin resistance in diabetics, increase the pancreatic beta cell response in hyperglycemia, and improve the action of insulin.

A study conducted by the Department of Epidemiology at Johns Hopkins University concluded that low serum (blood) magnesium is a strong, independent predictor of type 2 diabetes. Since low dietary intake of magnesium was not a predictor of diabetes, researchers concluded that absorption of magnesium by the kidneys might be one influential factor. Since it is well known that magnesium levels tend to be low among diabetics, and that plasma magnesium levels have an inverse relationship to insulin resistance—that is, as you become more insulin resistant, magnesium levels decrease—magnesium supplementation may play a role in the prevention of type 2 diabetes and its complications. However, while magnesium supplementation has been shown to improve insulin sensitivity among people with type 2 diabetes, there is no associated improvement in glycemic (blood sugar) control. So even though magnesium has shown itself to help insulin function, it has not been proven yet to directly effect blood sugar levels.

Magnesium is also an important therapeutic agent in the treatment of cardiovascular disease. It can reduce platelet aggregation, stabilize abnormal heart rhythms, and raise HDL cholesterol. It is also required for healthy nerve function and bone formation.

Symptoms of low magnesium include anxiety, insomnia, nervousness, leg cramps, and heaviness in the legs, fatigue, palpitations, and arrhythmia (irregular heartbeat). I have recommended magnesium extensively for sleep disturbances, and have had so many patients report much improved sleep just by taking magnesium. And for restless leg syndrome, I find that the use of magnesium reduces the symptoms, over time, *dramatically.*

Magnesium is depleted by excessive intake of phosphorus, calcium, saturated fat, sugar, caffeine, and alcohol. There are several medications such as antibiotics, corticosteroids, and cardiovascular drugs that also deplete magnesium (for more information, see Appendix 3: "Prescription and Nonprescription Nutrient Depletions" on page 512).

Some of the richest sources of magnesium are vegetables and fruits, which coincidentally many Americans avoid eating. Nuts and seeds are also good dietary sources of magnesium. With today's agricultural practices, even if you are eating the recommended five to nine servings of vegetables and fruits a day, variances in food quality could mean that you are not getting enough in your diet.

Recommended dose. The average American diet is deficient in magnesium by at least 70–80 mg. The current RDA for magnesium is 350 mg. As mentioned, however, many experts believe that the RDA is inadequate and recommend therapeutic doses of at least 600 mg daily.

Cyclo-hispro

It has been documented that people with diabetes have impaired intestinal zinc absorption and low plasma zinc levels. Animal and human studies suggest that this nutraceutical positively influences intestinal zinc absorption mechanisms.

Zinc deficiency has been associated with reduced availability of insulin in the pancreas, decreased insulin potency, impaired glucose tolerance (IGT), and increased insulin degradation.

Cyclo-hispro not only contains zinc, but also several cofactors known to stimulate intestinal zinc absorption. It has been proven to reduce blood sugar levels, urinary sugar levels, and hemoglobin A_1C, a marker used for long-term determination of blood sugar levels.

Recommended dose. 200–300 mg (found in a powdered protein extract containing cyclo–hispro), two to four times a day.

Essential Fatty Acids (EFAs)

Essential fatty acids (EFAs) are critical for the proper functioning of cellular membranes, to strengthen immune cells, and to help lubricate joints. Cellular membranes are responsible for maintaining the integrity of the cell, as well as allowing substances to bind with and permeate the cell. Without a healthy cell membrane, insulin binding at receptor cells may be impaired, triggering impaired glucose intolerance (IGT), insulin resistance, and hyperinsulinemia. Therefore, EFAs are among the most important supplements you can take.

The most important fatty acids are omega-3 and omega-6. Omega-3 EFAs, which include eicosapentaenoic acid (EPA) and docosahexaenoic acid (DHA), are found in cold-water fish (salmon, mackerel, tuna, trout, haddock), and other northern marine animals; there are also plant sources of EFAs such as flaxseed oil. Most people do not get the recommended amounts of the EFAs, especially omega-3s. For this reason, and also because it is important to get EFAs in the right ratios (that is, 1:3 ratio of omega-3 to omega-6), taking an EFA supplement is a good way to insure optimal intakes.

Recommended dose. 1–4 fish-oil capsules a day to achieve an intake of about 850–1,600 mg per day. If taking fish oils, check with the manufacturer to ensure that the source fish has been tested for mercury, which is sometimes a problem contaminant in these supplements. Reputable manufacturers often state on their labels whether they distill their oils or not.

For diabetics and people with insulin resistance, borage oil or evening primrose oil (both of which contain omega-6 fatty acids) may be an essential supplement.

Evening primrose oil and borage oil are high in the omega-6 fatty acid gamma-linolenic acid (GLA). In addition to its beneficial effects on insulin, GLA is also needed for cushioning joints and acts as a hormone building block. Consider taking at least one 500-mg capsule daily.

5-HTP

5-hydroxytryptophan (5-HTP) is the immediate precursor of the neurotransmitter serotonin. The body converts that essential amino acid tryptophan to 5-HTP, which is then converted to serotonin.

5-HTP has been reported to enhance serotonin synthesis, aiding the body in sleep, mood disorders, and weight loss. Because it helps to build up serotonin stores, 5-HTP may improve stress, depression, anxiety, sleep disturbances, fibromyalgia, carbohydrate/sweets cravings, or any other condition associated with reduced serotonin levels.

Although conventional literature suggests that 5-HTP should not be taken together with the antidepressants known as SSRIs such as fluoxetine (Prozac) or sertraline (Zoloft), small doses of 5-HTP may actually help the SSRIs work better. This should only be done under a doctor's supervision, however.

Recommended dose. If you are taking antidepressants and choose to supplement with 5-HTP for its beneficial effects on carbohydrate/sugar cravings, make sure that you are being monitored by your healthcare practitioner. Otherwise, a dose of 50–100 mg of 5-HTP, one to three times a day, is the range I recommend. If someone is having trouble sleeping at night and craves carbohydrates during the day, I usually recommend 100 mg of 5-HTP at bedtime, 50–75 mg before lunch (to reduce the midday craving), and 50–75 mg, if needed for late-afternoon snack cravings. A possible side effect of 5-HTP is drowsiness, so use caution when taking it. Therefore, start by taking it at bedtime; then add in daytime dosages as you build up a tolerance.

Glucosol

This formulation contains extracts from queen's crape myrtle tree (*Lagerstroemia speciosa*). Corosolic acid, a constituent found in this plant, has been reported to enhance the utilization of glucose in the body. Research suggests that extracts of *L. speciosa* may be effective in helping the body control plasma glucose levels in those with type 2 diabetes. This extract helps the body to transport glucose into the cells to be burned as fuel. One study showed that people who took 48 mg of Glucosol and exercised, as well as dieted, lost twice the weight compared with people who used exercise and diet alone.

Recommended dose. The suggested dose is 24 mg per day in divided doses. If you are diabetic, it is recommended that blood glucose levels be monitored closely while using Glucosol.

Relora®

This herbal agent is developed by plant-based extraction from the magnolia and phellodendron family. (See the inset "Relora®: A Special Supplement for Adrenal Stress" on page 127.) Relora® has particular efficacy at helping the body reduce feelings of anxiety (and subsequent levels of cortisol), irritability, and nervousness. I have used this agent extensively in my practice, and I find that it also helps with mood (mild depression) and with sleep.

With regard to blood sugar, Relora® is especially helpful if blood sugar instability is being highly influenced by stress, excess cortisol, and carbohydrate/sugar cravings. By influencing cortisol, reducing stress, and helping people get a better night's sleep, there can be some significant benefits on blood sugar. Poor sleep is now associated with reduced growth hormone release, insulin resistance, and increasing inflammatory cytokines in the blood. This adds up to a shift in your chemistry toward metabolic syndrome and away from vital health. So even though Relora® has an indirect effect, my belief is that for many people stress is a significant contributor to disruption in blood sugar cycles and craving behavior. Therefore, Relora® will show itself to be an invaluable supplement in weight loss and blood sugar regulation, and in helping to improve satiety and mood.

Recommended dose. 250 mg of Relora®, two to three times a day. *Caution:* Relora® is not recommended for people under age eighteen. If you are pregnant, nursing, or taking a prescription drug, consult a healthcare practitioner prior to use. Excessive consumption of Relora® may impair ability to drive or operate heavy equipment, and it is not recommended for consumption with alcoholic beverages.

Vanadium

Vanadium is a trace mineral known to be essential in extremely small quantities to plants and animals, yet debate exists over whether it is essential to humans. Research on vanadium, whose biochemical properties are similar to chromium's, indicates that it may produce insulinlike activities in the body, making it of potential value for those with diabetes, insulin resistance, and metabolic syndrome. Oral doses of vanadyl sulfate (the active form of vanadium) were shown to decrease fasting blood glucose levels (glucose levels obtained after no calories are consumed for at least eight hours prior to drawing levels) by 20 percent among people with type 2 diabetes. Vanadium has been reported in some studies to increase insulin sensitivity among patients with type 2 diabetes.

Due to its insulin-enhancing properties, vanadium is also popular among weightlifters and other fitness and bodybuilding enthusiasts. (It is thought that having optimal insulin function will improve muscle building and maintenance.) However, many bodybuilders take vanadium in high dosages, up to 50 mg a day, which is an excessive dose in my opinion. Remember, vanadium is a *trace mineral* not a *macronutrient* (a basic nutrient such as water, carbohydrates, proteins, and fats). Potential for toxicity exists in these doses.

Recommended dose. Dosages range widely from 250 mcg–1 mg, three times a day. I recommend staying with a conservative dosing of vanadyl sulfate since it is meant to be a trace mineral in the body.

Gymnema sylvestre

Gymnema is a vine indigenous to the rain forests of central and southern India. Ayurvedic medical texts dating back 2,000 years document the use of gymnema in the treatment of "sweet urine," or diabetes. Although the exact mechanism is not known, the hypoglycemic or blood sugar-lowering action of the plant may be due to its ability to stimulate the release of insulin stores in the body. Gymnema reportedly increases the activity of enzymes involved in the utilization of glucose by insulin-dependent pathways. Studies with gymnema have suggested that it may also help in weight loss and in suppressing sweets cravings. So, if you are trying to get your carbohydrate-craving and weight-storing chemistry under control, gymnema may be of benefit.

Recommended dose. 250–500 mg of *Gymnema sylvestre,* one to three times a day, standardized to 25 percent gymnemic acids per dosage. Standardized extracts are herbal products guaranteed to contain a specific amount of the herb's primary active ingredients.

Bitter Melon Fruit (Momordica charantia)

Bitter melon fruit has been reported to significantly improve the body's natural ability to regulate glucose in humans and animals. Research indicates that molecules with insulinlike bioactivity may be present in bitter melon seeds. A few studies suggest that the mechanism of bitter melon could be partly attributed to an ability to aid the body in increasing glucose utilization in the liver.

Either way, bitter melon has long been used in South America and the Orient, not only as a food, but also as a medicinal agent used to support the whole system of those with diabetes. Bitter melon helps by improving blood sugar balance and reducing the amount of sugars in the blood. This supplement should find an important role in reducing insulin resistance.

Recommended dose. 200–400 mg, two to three times a day, standardized to 7 percent bitter acids and 0.5 percent charantin. As with any dietary supplement, check with your healthcare practitioner before taking bitter melon fruit. Since taking this supplement may lower your need for medication, this is especially true if you are on antidiabetic prescription drugs.

Cinnamon Extract (Cinnamomum spp.)

Cinnamon is among the world's most frequently consumed spices. Current research suggests that this much-loved spice may have a beneficial impact on our health, as well as on our palates. A compound in cinnamon bark—*methylhydroxy chalcone polymer* (MHCP)—has been shown to increase glucose metabolism (the process in which cells convert glucose to energy) roughly twentyfold in a laboratory test conducted by the U.S. Department of Agriculture (USDA). Researchers tested approximately fifty plant extracts and found that none of them came close to MHCP's level of affecting glucose metabolism. What's more, MHCP prevented the formation of oxygen radicals in a blood platelet test, proving it to be a valuable antioxidant.

Recommended dose. 1–2 teaspoons of cinnamon daily for people with symptoms of insulin resistance. If you are taking antidiabetic prescription drugs, your blood sugar levels should be monitored closely since taking this supplement may lower your need for medication.

Supplement and Nutrient Support for the Thyroid

Several nutrients are critical for the proper functioning of the thyroid gland. In order for the thyroid gland to produce the hormone thyroxine, it needs the trace elements iodine and selenium, and the amino acid tyrosine. Without sufficient supply of these nutrients in the diet, thyroid function is diminished. A typical regimen of dietary supplements I recommend to my patients in support of thyroid function include those discussed below:

Bladderwrack (Fucus vesiculosus)

Bladderwrack, or fucus, consists of the marine plant *Fucus vesiculosus.* Marine algae have been used in Europe and Asia as medicinal agents for thousands of years. Bladderwrack is a rich source of iodine and is traditionally used for weight loss and hypothyroidism. The low incidence of goiter in maritime people has been attributed to the iodine content in bladderwrack, as they use it as a food source. Bladderwrack is thought to stimulate the thyroid gland, thus increasing basal metabolism. Bladderwrack also contains potassium, magnesium, calcium, iron, zinc, and other minerals.

Recommended dose. 300–600 mg, standardized to contain not more than 150 mcg of iodine daily, one to three times a day.

Coleus (Coleus forskohlii)

Coleus has been extensively researched in India over the last twenty years as a medicinal agent useful for thyroid support and for conditions such as high blood pressure, asthma, and weight loss, among others.

Coleus is also thought to activate the enzyme adenylate cyclase. In doing so, it increases the level of cyclic adenosine monophosphate (cAMP) within cells (cAMP, as you may recall, is important in the activation of several biochemical pathways). This catalyst is formed when neurotransmitters bind to the cell membrane and stimulate the formation of adenylate cyclase. Specific hormonal messengers bind to receptor sites to create the release of cAMP. Therefore, while coleus is involved in hormonal regulation, it doesn't increase hormone levels. Instead, it helps improve the efficiency of binding to target receptor sites.

The stimulation of cAMP has an impact on body chemistry in several ways. It stimulates thyroid function, increases insulin secretion, inhibits histamine release (involved in allergic reactions), and increases the burning of fats as fuels. Coleus is claimed to inhibit *platelet activating factor* (PAF)—that is, the formation of blood clots—by possibly directly binding to PAF receptor sites.

Recommended dose. 250 mg of a 1 percent extract of coleus, twice a day. *Caution:* People with ulcers or who are taking blood pressure medications and anticoagulant medications should check with their healthcare professional before taking coleus.

Cordyceps (Cordyceps sinensis)

Cordyceps is a unique black mushroom that extracts nutrients from and grows in the wild only on a caterpillar found in the high altitudes of Tibet and China. Cordyceps is now grown and cultivated under controlled conditions. One of the most valued medicinal agents mentioned in the Chinese *Materia Medica,* cordyceps has been used in traditional Chinese medicine (TCM) for lung and kidney problems, and as a general tonic for promoting longevity, vitality, and endurance. Cordyceps is beneficial in helping people with decreased energy restore their capacity to function at a greater level of activity. It is also important for individuals with improperly functioning thyroid glands because people with low thyroid function have reduced oxygen utilization and increased oxidative stress. Cordyceps acts as an antioxidant, improves oxygen utilization by 9 to 13 percent, improves stamina, and reduces fatigue—all critical issues for people with poor thyroid regulation.

Cordyceps has been used in humans for centuries as a tonic for improving performance and vitality, with the proposed mechanism of action being improved oxygen consumption by the cardiovascular and respiratory systems under stress and decreased energy levels by 9 to 13 percent. Cordyceps also has been reported to alter sex hormone release, controlled by the hypothalamo-pituitary-adrenocortical axis, which is responsible for regulating hormonal balance in the body, and is invaluable for people undergoing chemotherapy.

Recommended dose. 525 mg of cordyceps, standardized to contain .14 to .28 percent adenosine and 5 percent mannitol, two to three times a day.

Essential Fatty Acids (EFAs)

Low thyroid function leads to poor conversion and utilization of essential fatty acids (EFAs). Without *quality* sources of dietary fat, particularly the omega-3 fatty acid alpha-linoleic acid (ALA) and the omega-6 fatty acid gamma-linolenic acid (GLA), the body is unable to regulate hormonal influence over certain cells. EFAs are the building blocks of eicosanoids, a group of "superhormones" that act as hormonal gatekeepers of the cells. EFA deficiency and overproduction of inflammatory prostaglandins (PGE2, thromboxane, and leukotrienes) are associated with a variety of illnesses, including slowed metabolism and increased storage of body fat.

As mentioned on pages 109–110, the best sources of GLA are borage and evening primrose oils. Sources of omega-3 fatty acids are cold-water fish (salmon, mackerel, tuna, trout, haddock), and flaxseeds and flax oil. Although both EFAs are essential to our health, the ratio of omega-3 to omega-6 oils in our diet should be 1:3.

Guggul (Commiphora mukul)

The Hindu medical system of India has used guggul for centuries to treat many illnesses. Guggul has been described in Indian medical literature as an agent for treating obesity and other eating disorders.

These historic uses prompted modern scientists to study guggul. After years of research and scientific studies, guggul was approved for marketing in India in the late 1980s as a lipid-lowering agent. Guggul has been reported in studies to stimulate thyroid function, which may lead to blood lipid lowering and weight loss, as well as improved thyroid function in hypothyroidism.

Recommended dose. 500 mg, three times a day, standardized to contain 5 percent guggulsterones. *Caution:* People taking prescription medications for cardiovascular disease such as calcium channel blockers or beta-blockers, as well as those with hyperthyroidism, should check with their physician before taking guggul.

Iodine

Sources of iodine include sea vegetables (nori, hijiki, wakame, kombu, and kelp), sea salt, and all seafood and saltwater fish. Iodized salt is another source, but it contains significant amounts of aluminum, which is added as an anticaking agent. Iodized *sea salt*, however, supplies iodine without unwanted aluminum.

Recommended dose. 225–1,000 mcg of iodine daily. Typically, I do not recommend supplementing with iodine other than what may be in a multiple vitamin; however, it is always good to try to include good dietary sources.

L-tyrosine

The central nervous system is critically dependent on adequate amino acids to form neurotransmitters, the chemical messengers of the brain. The amino acid tyrosine is a precursor to dopamine, norepinephrine, and epinephrine. These neurotransmitters are produced and stored in the adrenal glands and are released in response to stress signals from the sympathetic nervous system.

Without sufficient available tyrosine, the adrenal glands have a sluggish or inadequate response to stress: heart rate, blood pressure, airway, and metabolism are diminished. And when the tyrosine pool is drained to make stress hormones, there is less available to make adequate levels of thyroid hormones.

Tyrosine is synthesized during the conversion of the amino acid phenylalanine to norepinephrine. It is considered a nonessential amino acid, because it is synthesized in the body and not obtained directly in the diet. The best sources of phenylalanine are soy products, meat, fish, and poultry. Adequate protein in the diet usually provides an adequate supply of phenylalanine, but I do frequently recommend supplements containing tyrosine.

Tyrosine supplements have been used as nutritional or adjunctive support for the treatment of depression, anxiety, sleep disorders, and weight gain, all of which are associated with hypothyroidism.

Recommended dose. 250–750 mg of L-tyrosine daily. You can check the status of your amino acids with testing, but if you're under significant stress, your body temperature is low, and you have other symptoms of low thyroid efficiency, consider taking at least 250 mg a day. *Caution:* Do not take tyrosine if you are currently taking a monoamine oxidase inhibitor (MAOI), a type of antidepressant as dangerously high blood pressure may result.

Thyroid Bovine (Beef) Glandular

Thyroid glandular is a bovine-derived thyroid substance that may boost the human thyroid system when the gland is not functioning optimally. Glandular supplements are carefully processed animal gland tissue; thyroid glandulars contain extremely low levels of thyroid hormone. It is theorized that glandular tissues contain proteins that help the thyroid gland to rebuild itself.

"Glandular therapy" refers to the use of these animal tissues to try to nutritionally support or enhance the function of, or mimic the effect of, the corresponding human tissue. Other glandular tissues that are available are taken from sheep and pig. In my practice, I use bovine thyroid nutritional support regularly, and based on my own observations, I have found it to be very helpful for people with subclinical hypothyroid function.

Recommended dose. 60–400 mg of bovine glandular daily. Use only New Zealand glandular extracts due to superior quality and safety of the raw material. *Caution:* Thyroid glandulars should not be taken in addition to thyroid medication. If you are currently on thyroid medication and would like to try glandular therapy, do not do so without consulting a practitioner experienced in natural therapeutics. Under the supervision of an experienced healthcare professional, it is possible to be weaned off the thyroid medication. This will involve a comprehensive nutritional and natural therapeutics program that addresses the underlying imbalances associated with suboptimal thyroid function.

Trace Minerals

Chromium depletion may influence thyroid function. Chromium is a necessary mineral for the conversion of carbohydrates to energy, and helps maintain a stable blood sugar level. It is also an essential component to enzyme function that supports the conversion of T4 (the less metabolically active form of thyroid hormone) to T3 (the more active thyroid hormone). So chromium can indirectly impact your basal metabolic rate and how you are going to burn fat, use nutrients, and generate energy.

Selenium has also been linked to subclinical hypothyroid symptoms. Selenium is found in selenoproteins, many of which have known roles in the prevention of cellular oxidative damage and thyroid hormone regulation. Selenium is an essential component of the enzyme iodothyronine deiodinase, the enzyme that converts thyroxine (T4) to the active triiodothyronine (T3). It is also found in the enzyme glutathione peroxidase, an important antioxidant. As with zinc, selenium supplementation has been reported to improve thyroid function and regulate symptoms of hypothyroidism. Poor selenium intake is common in the average diet. Low levels of selenium have been linked to an increased risk of cardiovascular disease and cancer.

Other nutrients important for optimum thyroid function include zinc and copper. These trace minerals are also required for the synthesis of iodothyronine deiodinase. Animal and human studies have concluded that zinc supplementation can restore normal thyroid function among patients with low serum zinc, and signs of subclinical hypothyroidism. Zinc is required for the activity of more than 200 different enzymes in the body. It is recognized that zinc deficiencies are common throughout the world, including the United States.

Supplementing with extra zinc requires the addition of copper to maintain healthy zinc to copper ratio. Since the two elements antagonize one another, supplementing with one can lead to a deficiency in the other.

Recommended dose. 200 mcg of chromium daily as part of a multivitamin/mineral supplement; 200 mcg of selenium daily; and 15 parts zinc to 1 part copper, or approximately 20–50 mg of zinc to 2 mg of copper.

A Final Note on Thyroid Function

Many physicians now recognize the problems with thyroid regulation. In fact, the window for acceptable TSH levels has just recently been changed by the American Society of Endocrinologists so that millions more people may get diagnosed with hypothyroidism and get the help they need. Hopefully the use of T3 *and* T4 as drug therapy will become more popular, and in addition, the various influencers of thyroid metabolism such as stress and nutrient abnormalities will begin to become more recognized in the coming decade. Healthy thyroid function is crucial to graceful and vital aging.

So whether you try Armour thyroid, nutritional approaches, get compounded customized thyroid therapy, or use traditional drugs, keep one thing in mind: If there's no relief of low-thyroid symptoms, you are probably still missing a piece of the metabolic puzzle.

Supplements and Nutrients for Regulating Female Hormones

As alluded to in Chapter 4, regulation of the female hormones can play a valuable role in cracking your metabolic code. Oftentimes, secondary sex hormones such as estrogen, progesterone, and testosterone may correct themselves naturally when the nine key components of metabolism are balanced. However, in many instances, additional herbal, nutritional, and hormonal therapy may be necessary to supplement these sex hormones in women (especially menopausal women) and men. Sex hormone deficiencies can decrease thyroid function, increase weight gain, and cause a host of metabolic imbalances. A typical regimen of dietary supplements to support female hormonal regulation includes the supplements discussed below:

Black Cohosh (Actaea racemosa, Cimicifuga racemosa)

This plant has been reported to have phytoestrogenic properties. Phytoestrogens are plant estrogens. Clinical studies have reported positive effects on menopausal, as well as premenopausal and postmenopausal, complaints when subjects used standardized extracts of black cohosh.

Two compounds found in black cohosh may be responsible for its reported uses in relieving menopausal complaints. The isoflavone *formononetin* has been reported to have estrogenic activity in laboratory rats. Formononetin is reported to act as a competitor with estrogen in binding to uterine cells *ex vivo* (a biological process that takes place outside a living cell). The other compound, triterpenoid 27-deoxyactein, has also been reported to produce estrogenlike effects in humans.

In a controlled study, black cohosh tablets, standardized to 1 mg of 27-deoxyactein, were given to 110 female patients in a university gynecological clinic. Patients received two tablets twice daily for two months. Half the patients took the black cohosh tablet and half took a placebo. At the end of the required treatment period, both groups were tested for luteinizing hormone (LH) and follicle-stimulating hormone (FSH) levels. There was no significant effect on the FSH serum concentration in either group. This study reported positive effects of black cohosh on LH suppression in menopausal women, with estrogenlike function.

It should be noted, however, that naturally occurring estrogen in the body also affects the release of FSH through receptor binding. So even though black cohosh has estrogenic properties in the body, it does not have the exact same pharmacology as does naturally occurring estrogen.

Recommended dose. 20–40 mg, two times a day, standardized to contain 1 mg of triterpenes (27-deoxyactein) per dose. *Caution:* Black cohosh should be used with caution in individuals on hormone replacement therapy (HRT) or oral contraceptives. High doses may cause nausea, vomiting, and headache. Many women with a history of breast cancer ask if black cohosh is safe to use. Although it seems that it is safe and may help them to control their hot flashes, there is still conflicting data on this issue. Black cohosh should not be used in pregnancy, due to reported uterine stimulatory activity in human and animal studies.

Diindolylmethane (DIM)

Probably one of the most promising and exciting supplements for estrogen balance is diindolylmethane (DIM). It is the most active cruciferous substance for promoting beneficial estrogen metabolism in women and men. DIM is found in cruciferous vegetables, such as broccoli, cauliflower, cabbage, and Brussels sprouts.

The supplemental use of DIM began with early experiments that demonstrated the prevention of chemically induced cancer in animals that were fed diets with added DIM. Pure DIM was first used in 1987 as a dietary supplement in animals. It was shown to be nontoxic and to prevent breast cancer caused by the carcinogen dimethylbenz(a)anthracene. Similarly, the initiation pathway to chemically induced colon cancer was inhibited with the DIM precursor, I3C. The mechanisms by which DIM prevents cancer in animals has subsequently been shown to involve a reduction in activity of the estrogen receptor system, promotion of beneficial estrogen metabolism, and support for selective *apoptosis,* or "programmed cell death," which removes damaged cells.

In several case-control studies, supplemental use of DIM in humans effectively adjusted the pathways of estrogen metabolism to favor the production of the beneficial estrogens 2-hydroxy estrogen metabolites. These shifts showed an approximate 75 percent increase in the production of 2-hydroxyestrone and a 50 percent decrease in the production of 16-hydroxyestrone. This increased proportion of 2-hydroxy metabolites to 16-hydroxyestrone is correlated with breast cancer protection. Case-control studies have also documented that low levels of 2-hydroxy metabolites are associated with breast cancer in women and men, familial risk of breast cancer, uterine cancer, cervical cancer, and lupus.

Several established risk factors for breast cancer, including obesity and diets high in trans fats and saturated fat, contribute to alterations in estrogen metabolism. Diets deficient in omega-3 fatty acids have also been correlated with low 2-hydroxyestrone production. DIM is unique among all phytonutrients with regard to its ability to favorably modify estrogen metabolism in the direction of greater 2-hydroxy estrogen production.

Recommended dose. 120–360 mg daily. Generally, I start women on 75 mg of DIM, twice a day, unless they have a history of estrogen-dependent health issues such as breast or uterine cancer, fibroid formation, or cyst formation, in which case, I recommend 150 mg, twice a day. It may take several months to notice beneficial results.

Kudzu (Pueraria lobata)

Kudzu is well known in the southeastern United States as a pesky aggressive vine that can cover large areas in a short period. However, in traditional Chinese medicine (TCM), kudzu root is used for its many medicinal and powerful antioxidant qualities. In the Chinese culture, kudzu is also used as a food. Kudzu is rich in isoflavones (phytoestrogens), and is therefore considered similar to soy.

A few studies support kudzu's traditional use as nutritional support for people with alcoholism and addictive behavior. Kudzu also has been shown to promote the

production of the "good" 2-hydroxyestrones in estrogen metabolism. Additionally, it may help in maintaining balance in female hormonal cycles.
Recommended dose. 100–400 mg, two times a day.

Progesterone

The use of progesterone in menopausal women may decrease the risk of uterine and cervical dysplasia (abnormal cell growth considered a precancerous condition) in women taking estrogen replacement therapy. It may also help to prevent osteoporosis by increasing bone density in postmenopausal women. In one study, all of the subjects who used topical progesterone (2 percent cream or 475 mg of progesterone per ounce) reported an increase in bone density. It also helps with the regulation of thyroid hormones. Moreover, it has been reported to benefit women with mild to moderate endometriosis (abnormal growth of cells that form the lining of the uterus).

If you decide to use progesterone cream, it's important to first have your blood levels of progesterone checked. (Once you begin using progesterone cream, saliva tests are not an accurate method for monitoring progesterone levels, but it is a good idea to periodically check your blood levels.)

Transdermal progesterone cream is considered an effective route of administration. An increasing number of physicians are recommending compounded natural hormone replacement therapy, including bio-identical estrogen, progesterone, testosterone, pregnenolone, and DHEA depending upon the needs of the individual. At our clinic, we usually attempt to balance gastrointestinal function (Key Five) and endocrine function before jumping into regulating secondary sex hormones, as this approach can have a positive effect on reestablishing normal hormonal regulation. However, if this is still not enough to balance hormonal function, then individualized natural hormone replacement therapy can be of huge benefit.

In addition to the above supplements for hormonal regulation, I occasionally recommend the following supplements, depending upon an individual's symptoms. Be sure to check with your healthcare practitioner to see which of these supplements might be appropriate for you.

Vitex or Chasteberry *(Vitex agnus-castus)*

The actual activity of the constituents of chasteberry is not yet fully established. Studies have reported it to have a significant effect on the pituitary. Studies also point to a progesteronelike component and effect. Studies report that vitex stimulates luteinizing hormone (LH) and inhibits follicle-stimulating hormone (FSH). Because of this activity, vitex has been recommended for a variety of female complaints, such as PMS, amenorrhea, menopausal symptoms, endometriosis, and hyperprolactinemia (excessive production of prolactin hormone).
Recommended dose. 200–400 mg daily of a standardized extract.

Soy Isoflavones

Isoflavones are phytoestrogens (plant estrogens). These weak estrogens are chemically similar in structure to naturally produced estrogen. Isoflavones are known to provide protection from certain types of cancer and against the formation of plague in the arteries. They enhance bone density and help to alleviate symptoms of menopause. Isoflavones are found in soy foods and are also available in supplement form.

The two primary isoflavones in soybeans are *daidzein* and *genistein* and their respective glucosides, *genistin* and *daidzin,* which have a glucose molecule attached. While some of the benefits of isoflavones are related to their mild estrogen activity, some isoflavones reportedly exhibit effects that are also not related to estrogen activity. In vitro studies have reported that genistein inhibits the growth of a wide range of cancer cells, including those that are not hormone-dependent. It has been hypothesized that genistein's anticancer effect is due to its ability to deactivate the enzymes that control cell growth and regulation.

Raw soybeans contain between 2–4 mg of total isoflavones per gram by dry weight. Due to different processing methods, not all soy foods are reliable sources of isoflavones. Although some research suggests that a single serving of soy foods (such as soymilk or tofu) contains enough isoflavones to exert clinical effect. There is also some controversy about whether soy foods are beneficial or harmful to health. Soy's goitrogen content competes with thyroid hormone. However, studies to date have shown no harm to thyroid function in infants fed soymilk. In my opinion, there is sufficient evidence proving the benefits of soy in the diet, but like anything else, include soy in your diet in moderation. Soy isoflavones are available in supplement form, however, it is preferable to get them from food. Some manufacturers include information on the soy isoflavone content on their labels.

Recommended dose. 60 mg daily.

Supplements and Nutritional Support for the Adrenals

If there is one area that natural therapeutics can play a significant role in prevention, it is in adrenal support. This is not a new concept. In Chinese medicine, adaptogen compounds such as ginseng were highly regarded because of their restorative abilities. By supporting adrenal function, your body becomes more resilient to the physiologic and psychological effects of stress on your chemistry. By reestablishing balance in adrenal function, we can fortify and protect ourselves from our chronic "fight-or-flight" mode of responding to stress, which is disrupting our metabolic patterns.

Substances that increase nonspecific resistance of the body to a wide range of stressors are known as *adaptogens.* Adaptogens modulate, or balance the response induced by stress. Adaptogens have the unique ability to either stimulate or sedate, depending on the needs of the body.

Signs of improvement include the elimination of the need for a midday nap, the end of brutal fatigue, the disappearance of the blue circles under the eyes; less anxiousness, nervousness, and tendency toward depression; and reduced carbohydrate cravings. In addition, I have found that as your stamina and endurance increases, a better outlook toward life and improved resistance to stress begins to settle in.

I recommend a wide variety of nutraceutical and herbal compounds to support adrenal function. However, the following agents are those that I find almost always work. Many times you will see a combination of these compounds in a single formula. Obviously, if you are not feeling the effects of chronic stress, some of these agents may not apply. I typically start off many of my patients with an adrenal extract, rhodiola root (*Rhodiola rosea*), and holy basil (*Ocimum sanctum*), adding other agents to their regimens as needed.

- Adrenal New Zealand glandular: 200–300 mg, two to three times a day, or adrenal cortex New Zealand glandular: 250 mg, two to four times a day.

- Rhodiola root: 50–250 mg, two times a day, standardized to 3 to 5 percent rosavins.

- Holy basil: 400–800 mg, one to two times a day, standardized to 1 percent ursolic acid.

- Relora®: 250 mg, two to three times a day if needed for anxiety or nervousness, chronic stress, or sleep patterns disturbed by stress.

- L-theanine: 50–200 mg, one to three times a day if needed for chronic stress or anxiety.

- Moducare®: Three doses of 20–40 mg, three times a day for the first thirty days between meals; thereafter, one 20–40 mg dose, three times per day if needed to support immunity during stressful times.

- DHEA: An initial dose of 5–50 mg of DHEA daily if needed to help balance adrenal hormone production recommended by a healthcare provider based on lab studies.

- Magnesium: 600–1,000 mg a day if needed to slow the release of stress hormones.

- B vitamins, especially vitamin B_6 or pyridoxal 5 phosphate (an activated form of B_6): (Vitamin B_6 is essential for production of adrenal hormones and energy function. Pyridoxal 5 phosphate an activated form of B_6 used more readily by the body.) If using B_6: 50 mg a day; if using pyridoxal 5 phosphate: 10–15 mg a day.

- Vitamin C: 500–1,000 mg a day for production of adrenal hormones.

Adrenal Glandular

I use adrenal glandular products from New Zealand exclusively in my practice. It works fast. In just a few days or weeks, my patients report feeling like they have more consistent energy without feeling stimulated and that their daily energy swings have leveled off. This especially seems to be the case if the patient is also taking supplements to balance blood sugar.

In many cases, adrenal extracts are combined with other botanical substances to give a broader range of effect. (If you are feeling extremely anxious or have palpitations, I would not recommend an adrenal extract in the initial phase of your rejuvenation program. Instead I would suggest the use of *Cordyceps sinensis,* magnesium citrate or aspartate, and rhodiola root, Relora®, or holy basil.)

Recommended dose. 100–300 mg, two to three times a day, with meals.

Rhodiola Root (Rhodiola rosea)

This herb has been used in Russia for performance enhancement with promising results on improving endurance and stamina. In addition to its effects on athletes, there are several other interesting benefits that are emerging from this herb. Rhodiola seems to have the ability to improve cognition and audio-visual perception in people under stress. A study involving night-shift physicians showed a significant improvement in memory and audio-visual perception and fewer errors. It is well established that chronic stress leads to short-term memory impairment and even shrinkage of the hippocampus area of the brain. Rhodiola also seems to have an impact on immune function in animal models. One of the more devastating effects of chronic stress is that it impairs immune function, leading to the development of cancer and other immune disorders. Supporting immune regulation through adaptogenic compounds can provide lasting health benefits.

Recommended dose. 50–250 mg twice daily, standardized to 3 to 5 percent rosavins.

Holy Basil (Ocimum sanctum)

This herb has emerged from traditional cultures in Thailand, as well as in India. Holy basil has been reported to decrease cortisol production and to help regulate blood sugar. Where I have found holy basil of particular value is in people who have stress-induced hypertension. As cortisol is lowered, the other stress-induced neurotransmitters that place stress on circulation begin to diminish, allowing for a more relaxed circulation.

Helping with blood sugar regulation is a secondary benefit of holy basil. As I discussed in Chapter 3, blood sugar regulation is heavily influenced by chronic stress. Occasionally people report feeling tired after starting on holy basil, but that is typically because they are so used to functioning on a high output of stress hormones. How many times have you heard someone say the phrase, "I thrive on stress"? Yet people who say that are literally playing with "fire," the fire of chronic inflammation, restricted blood flow, increased oxidative stress, memory loss, and insulin resistance.

Recommended dose. 400–800 mg, one to two daily, standardized to 1 percent ursolic acid.

Moducare®

A supplement on the forefront of immune system support, Moducare is a supplement that can provide benefit for protecting the immune system from the effects of chronic stress. The stress can be from physiologic (such as heavy exercise) or psychological causes. Moducare has been reported to increase natural killer cell (NK) activity and improve the activity of T cells.

Moducare is a patented, unique blend of sterols and sterolins derived from plants that involves a specialized process of extraction. Sterols and sterolins occur naturally in fruit, vegetables, seeds, and nuts. After more than two decades of clinical research and double-blind studies, research indicates that it may be effective in supporting HIV patients, benign prostatic hyperplasia (enlargement of the prostate that leads to a pinching off of the urethra), pulmonary tuberculosis, autoimmune disorders such as rheumatoid arthritis, seasonal allergies, and stress-induced immune suppression in marathon runners. The plant sterols and sterolins have been shown to have anti-inflammatory properties by lowering the release of cortisol, interleukin-6 (IL-6), and tumor necrosis factor (TNF alpha). This property found in Moducare may be important in the management of a wide variety of chronic conditions since many disease states are being linked to these inflammatory markers in the blood.

Moducare also has been reported to increase levels of DHEA, fighting the stress-related hormonal issues discussed earlier in the chapter. This is an invaluable naturally extracted agent that not only supports immune function, but also has significant effects on cortisol.

I find Moducare to be a significant agent for maintaining the health of the immune system. It is also great when used to improve recovery time from extensive exercise. Further, it helps with immune function and calms the inflammatory cascade, which is implicated in so many of the conditions discussed in this book.

Watch out for similar products that claim to be 14,000 times more active than Moducare. (Think of that, your immune system would be out of control if that were the case!) This is the brand that is backed by science and is the one that I recommend. **Recommended dose.** The dose is typically three doses of 20–40 mg taken three times a day for the first thirty days between meals; then one 20–40 mg dose three times per day thereafter. As symptoms improve, the need for this supplement may be reduced. *Caution:* If you are diabetic or have an autoimmune disorder, take Moducare under the guidance of your healthcare professional, as it can lower your need for blood sugar-regulating drugs.

DHEA

Adrenal androgens (17-ketosteroids) are sex hormones produced by the cortex. Although they are released as androgens, some are converted to estrogens by the skin, liver, and adipose tissue. The adrenal androgens function to supplement the primary sex hormones of the reproductive glands in males and females.

The most important of these is *DHEA* (dehydroepiandrosterone). DHEA is synthesized by the adrenals and, in small amounts, by the brain and skin. It is a precursor for the production of sex hormones, most notably estrogen and testosterone. For this reason, it is best to get your DHEA levels tested before taking it as a supplement. It can have a powerful effect on your hormones and shift their production and relationships if it is used in excess.

While the primary role of DHEA is to maintain normal sex hormone levels, it is also thought to combat the effects of stress by balancing cortisol and having a protective effect on the immune system. In addition, DHEA increases insulin sensitivity, enhances fat metabolism, increases antioxidant enzyme synthesis in the liver, and protects against free-radical damage.

Recommended dose. 5–50 mg daily. (However, ask your healthcare practitioner what dose is best for you. Use this supplement only under the supervision of a qualified healthcare professional.) DHEA is also sometimes used for people with autoimmune disorders. In such circumstances, the dosage is typically 50–100 mg a day, or as suggested by your healthcare practitioner.

Theanine

L-theanine is a unique amino acid found only in the tea plant, in the mushroom *Xerocomus badius,* and in certain species of the *Camellia* (green tea) plant. It is a relaxant that increases brain alpha waves, producing mental and physical relaxation, and decreasing stress and anxiety, without inducing drowsiness. Studies have shown that women taking L-theanine in doses of 200 mg per day have lower incidence of PMS symptoms, including physical, mental, and social symptoms associated with this condition. Overall, a significant alleviation of PMS symptoms by L-theanine has been observed.

Recommended dose. Based on the results of clinical studies, it has been established that L-theanine is effective in single dosages in the range of 50–200 mg, one to three times a day. It is suggested that individuals with higher levels of anxiety take a dose at the higher end of the effective range (100–200 mg) for best results.

Magnesium and Calcium

Magnesium and calcium are important antistress minerals. Magnesium slows the release of epinephrine and norepinephrine from the adrenal medulla, which makes it a critical mineral for balancing the sympathetic nervous system response. Symptoms of magnesium deficiency include fatigue, anxiety and nervousness, palpitations, restless legs, arrhythmias, and insomnia. Having some of these symptoms can result in your taking several pharmaceutical agents, some of which you could end up dependent upon. Magnesium deficits that go unnoticed often end up steering you toward significant drug therapy. For magnesium supplementation, I recommend magnesium *citrate, aspartate,* or *glycinate* for the best-absorbed forms.

Calcium is important for its role in healthy nerve function, although it has many other important functions, which are discussed throughout this book. In addition, some literature suggests that under conditions of stress, calcium may be lost by being rapidly absorbed into the intestinal tract and quickly excreted in the feces, which makes it even more important to insure that intake is sufficient. The best-absorbed forms of calcium are amino acid chelates, such as calcium citrate, or micro-crystalline hydroxyapatite (MCHC).

Recommended dose. 600–1,000 mg a day of magnesium and 1,000–1,500 mg of calcium.

Relora®

If there is an exciting new agent on the market to combat the chronic effects of stress, it is Relora®. Studies have shown this exciting newcomer to effectively help control mild anxiety and the symptoms associated with anxiety, such as irritability, emotional ups and downs, restlessness, tense muscles, poor sleep, fatigue, and difficulty concentrating. In addition, it has another important benefit: Relora® is non-sedating. Relora® seems not only to treat anxiety effectively, but also to display qualities that enable it to enhance well-being.

Studies indicate that Relora® helps the body normalize cortisol and DHEA levels in stressed individuals, induce relaxation, and act as an aid in controlling weight and stress-related eating or drinking. Most people do not realize that the effects of chronic stress that go unchecked can have a wide-ranging destructive force on their metabolism. Cravings for carbohydrates, night eating syndrome (NES), weight gain, immune disruption, sleep disorders, and depression can all be triggered by chronic stress and anxiety.

In my practice, I have observed that most people feel a significant difference within just two weeks of taking Relora®. This is one of the more promising nutraceuticals to be designed and put on the market over the last decade. As more people become aware of the wide-ranging effects of stress, they will be searching for options such as Relora®.

Recommended dose. 250 mg, two to three times a day. *Caution:* Relora® is not recommended for people under age eighteen. If you are pregnant, nursing, or taking a prescription drug, consult a healthcare practitioner prior to use. Excessive consumption of Relora® may impair ability to drive or operate heavy equipment, and it is not recommended for consumption with alcoholic beverages.

NUTRITIONAL AND LIFESTYLE SUPPORT
OF THE ENDOCRINE GLANDS

I believe that dietary supplements are essential for supporting metabolism and defending against day-to-day environmental stressors. But the true foundations for insulin, thyroid, and adrenal balance, long-term weight control, and reducing the

Relora®: A Special Supplement for Adrenal Stress

Are you frustrated with trying to lose and manage your weight even though you are careful with your diet and you exercise regularly? Are you anxious or nervous and not sleeping well? Do you have night eating syndrome (NES) or just crave carbohydrates and sugar. If you answered "yes" to any of these questions, what you will gain by using this dietary supplement may revolutionize your entire way of thinking about stress, diet, and weight control for the rest of your life.

This supplement, known as Relora®, is the result of an extensive, four-year, worldwide effort by Next Pharmaceuticals, Inc.—a research and development company based in Irvine, California, that specializes in natural ingredients for dietary supplements and functional foods—to find a phytochemical or constituent in plants with anti-anxiety properties but no significant sedative effects.

Because of the in-depth knowledge of phytochemistry, pharmacology, bioavailability, toxicology, and chemistry, scientists at this company have been able to take this vast amount of knowledge and hone in on a manageable number of plants that can be developed into safe and effective natural remedies.

Relora® contains patent-pending ingredients extracted from two plant species that have been used in traditional Chinese medicine (TCM) for more than 1,500 years: *Phellodendron amurense* and *Magnolia officinalis*. Researchers tested and screened more than 100 traditional medicinal ingredients over a four-year period before discovering Relora®. Tests showed that Relora® bound to central nervous system receptor sites associated with anxiety and therefore reduced stress signals in the body.

As you now know, stress is being reported to play a significant role in a wide variety of conditions and disease states. Recent work from the National Institutes of Health (NIH) and other major research centers has demonstrated that stress is a significant contributor to immune dysfunction, Alzheimer's disease, cardiovascular disease, diabetes, age-related disorders, and excess body fat leading to obesity. These conditions are metabolic imbalances that are related to stress-induced hormone imbalances, especially imbalances of the hormones cortisol and DHEA.

The increase in cortisol levels signals the brain that the body is in stress causing food cravings, especially high-fat, high-sugar foods. These foods, in turn, cause additional stress, thereby fueling the stress-cortisol cycle. Eventually, more fat is stored than the body needs unless sufficient exercise is in place to compensate, or the stress is reduced. These hormones not only affect your perception of stress and well-being, but also have a major impact on stress-related eating and drinking and on how the body stores and metabolizes fat.

Relora® works with the body's natural chemistry to normalize levels of cortisol and DHEA, which skyrocket and plunge, respectively, when the body is under chronic stress. By working to reestablish a stable relationship between these hormones, Relora® can play a significant role in the health of anyone faced with chronic stress.

Studies have shown it to be a safe, effective, rapid-acting, non-sedating dietary supplement that helps control occasional mild anxiety.

In phase one of a three-phase trial, fifty subjects were treated with Relora® for two weeks. The dosage was 250 mg of Relora®, three times daily. Based on preclinical studies, Relora® was designed and evaluated against the following concepts; "Relora helps control occasional mild anxiety or mild depression and the associated symptoms: irritability; emotional ups and downs; restlessness; tense muscles; poor sleep; concentration difficulties." Post-trial analysis revealed an excellent agreement (82 percent) with the pretrial concept. Relaxation was reported by 78 percent of the patients. Though the product did not cause significant sedation, 74 percent of the patients had a restful sleep. No significant side effects were reported. When subjects were asked about drowsiness, only 24 percent reported that they were drowsy. Relora® was gentle on the stomach in 94 percent of the subjects, with only mild and transient gastrointestinal problems in the other 6 percent.

A second trial was undertaken at the Living Longer Institute in Cincinnati, Ohio, to measure cortisol and DHEA levels in patients with mild to moderate stress. A two-week regimen of Relora® caused a significant increase (227 percent) in salivary DHEA and a significant decrease (37 percent) in morning salivary cortisol levels. These significant findings support Relora's ability to relieve stress and its potential role in weight control and stress-related eating and drinking behavior.

A third study was completed in late 2002 that evaluated the final formulation of Relora's ability to improve the snacking habits in people who snack on sweets or eat salty snacks when they are under excessive stress. In this study, Relora® cut sweet snacking in the sweet cravers by 75 percent. It cut snacking on salty snacks by 50 percent. Seventy-three percent of all individuals in the study reported feeling less stressed while taking Relora®.

For additional information on Relora® as well as a list of brands available, visit www.Relora.com.

risk of developing chronic conditions, such as diabetes and cardiovascular disease, are sensible food selection, lifestyle and behavioral changes, and regular exercise. Initiating behavioral changes one step at a time leads to overall lifestyle changes that can permanently change your dietary habits. With the right changes, you can improve your own metabolic efficiency.

Nutritional Support

The ideal diet provides adequate protein to maintain anabolic activity (repair and maintenance) without stressing the liver and kidneys or depleting water and minerals. It also contains complex, unrefined carbohydrates, in amounts appropriate for individual level of activity, to maintain a stable blood sugar level without inducing excessive insulin response. And it provides enough quality fat to fuel energy and to supply essential fatty acids vital to the brain, immune system, and cellular membranes.

Not everyone needs the exact same diet. Depending on the need for weight loss or individual comfort, I may recommend a diet that varies between 20 to 40 percent protein, 30 to 50 percent carbohydrates, and 20 to 30 percent fat. Nutrition and diet are discussed in Chapters 12 and 13, but for now, suffice it to say that for day-to day maintenance, I generally recommend that people consume 50 percent of their diet as carbohydrates (of which the majority comes from vegetables), 30 percent as protein, and 20 percent as fat.

In general, it is a good idea to reduce your intake of refined carbohydrates and refined sugar. As a matter of fact, I consider the severe restriction of sugar and other refined sweeteners to be one of the most important dietary changes most people need to make. These foods can exacerbate fluctuations in blood glucose and that means you will stimulate cortisol release and other stress hormones.

You may need to avoid, or at least limit, stimulants such as caffeine. People have different tolerances for caffeine. Some people can do fine with two cups of coffee a day but two cups may make others feel edgy and irritable, and eventually it can even drive the adrenals to the point of exhaustion. Caffeine directly stimulates the central nervous system, which aggravates anxiety and irritability and sleep patterns. It is also aggravating to the adrenals because it elevates blood sugar and cortisol production. Excess caffeine, alcohol, the excessive use of stimulants, and/or tobacco should all be curtailed.

Caffeine sources such as soft drinks, coffee, and even tea can affect sensitive individuals. Many people use caffeine to "pull them" through their day. I do it at times, as well. However, it is important to remember that caffeine taxes adrenal output, and we need to alleviate the stress on the glands, not increase it.

Special Nutritional Considerations for Thyroid Function

In order for the thyroid gland to produce thyroxine, it needs the trace element iodine. Sources of iodine include sea vegetables (nori, hijiki, wakame, kombu, and kelp), sea salt, and all seafood and saltwater fish. Although iodized salt is another source, it is not recommended since it contains significant amounts of aluminum.

Some foods, known as goitrogens, interfere with proper iodine absorption and utilization by combining with iodine and making it unavailable to the thyroid gland. Goitrogens are found among cruciferous vegetables (cabbage, turnips, broccoli, kale, mustard greens, and radishes) and in soybeans, peanuts, pine nuts, and millet. However, it should be fine to eat these foods in moderation.

Despite many of the recently discovered benefits of soy *isoflavones* (a type of plant estrogen), excessive dietary intake of soy products may interfere with healthy thyroid function. Soy-rich diets have been implicated in the development of goiter in several studies, and should be avoided by people with hypothyroidism and hyperthyroidism.

Special Nutritional Considerations for the Adrenals

Attention to good nutrition is especially important during times of stress. Here's why:

- Stress hormones are stimulated by a diet high in carbohydrates and low in protein. An excessive intake of sugar triggers the release of adrenal hormones. Stress increases cellular metabolism, and depletes nutrients more quickly.

- Three to five small meals a day are recommended during periods of stress. This may be better tolerated if you are experiencing a poor appetite or upset stomach. Another reality is that many of us eat on the run—in our cars, on the phone, and at our desks. Try snacks such as a handful of nuts chewed thoroughly and cut vegetables; these are healthy alternatives to fast foods.

- Remember to *chew* your food. Saliva begins the process of digestion so chewing helps to digest your food.

- Protein requirements increase under conditions of ongoing stress, especially physical stress and illness. You may want to consider drinking a protein drink. There are several kinds of protein drinks on the market, but I recommend making your own, simply to suit your personal tastes and because many of these products contain hidden sugars. (See page 332 for recipes.) Look for a protein powder that is composed of whey, egg whites, rice, or even split pea if you are allergic to egg or whey.

- Consume adequate liquids (usually six to eight 8-ounce glasses a day) between meals to help maintain proper digestion and hydration. Try to make pure water your drink of choice whenever possible.

- Avoid overeating as this creates too much demand on the body and digestive tract.

- Detection of food allergies is important for adrenal support. Food allergies elicit an immune response, alter thyroid function, may induce fatigue, and place additional stress on adrenal function.

- The bottom line is that under stress your metabolism will crave more carbohydrates and sugar, store them more efficiently as belly fat, and your metabolism will slow down so you burn your fuel less effectively.

Lifestyle Support

Because proper functioning of the entire endocrine system is dependent on the health of each of its organs, it is not surprising that any lifestyle change that benefits one will benefit the other. In Chapter 13, I present specific details for a lifelong, comprehensive, healthy eating program. A diet that restricts certain foods like refined sugars and emphasizes others like fruits and vegetables will go a long way to restoring metabolic control and therefore overall health. In addition to this eating plan, there are some special lifestyle concerns for the pancreas and blood sugar regulation.

People with poor blood sugar regulation and those who are dieting should pay special attention to what they eat and when. One of the mistakes often made is to eat small, carbohydrate-dense meals early in the day and a high-protein meal in the evening. This schedule is not the most effective way to control insulin or energy.

It is much better to start the day with a high-protein meal, which stabilizes blood sugar through mid-afternoon. For instance, many of you feel that 2:00 P.M. "slump," which can also be traced back to dips in low glucose availability to the cells and poor adrenal performance. With more protein and fewer carbohydrates during the earlier part of the day, the 2:00 P.M. low can be avoided. Around that time, a shift should be made toward increasing the carbohydrate content of meals. A dinner consisting of a modest portion of complex carbohydrates from whole grains (generally wheat free), and generous amounts of vegetables along with a protein source maintains nutrient and fiber needs, stimulates a rise in serotonin production (which helps you to sleep), and promotes healthier digestion. But don't eat a large meal at 9:00 P.M. when you are going to be in bed at 10:00 P.M.

When people try to eat protein at night as their only source of fuel, it can be maddening for them if they are susceptible to night eating syndrome (NES). In this instance, their brains are compelling them to eat more carbohydrates to fuel serotonin and melatonin production. They don't achieve satiety and, many times, end up compelled to eat excessive carbohydrates in the evening. So the potato chip bag "mysteriously disappears." (See the inset "Night Eating Syndrome and Stress" on page 86.) By eating a good mixed meal as described above, chances are your blood sugar will be more stable through the night, as well.

The amount of carbohydrate intake in your diet will vary. Some people may need to restrict carbohydrate foods until their metabolism more or less jump-starts and they begin to lose weight. Others may eat a nearly normal load of carbohydrates, if they are eaten at the correct times and they do not overindulge in refined sugars and grains on a regular basis. My initial suggestion is that you first try using a ratio of 50 percent carbohydrates to 30 percent protein to 20 percent fats and oils— the percents I generally recommend for day-to-day maintenance. However, if you find yourself not breaking your insulin resistance patterns (in other words, losing your belly fat), then you may need to change these percentages to consuming 40 percent of your diet from carbohydrates with the elimination of all grains and 40 percent from protein. Only in rare instances have I resorted to asking people to eat a nearly 0 percent carbohydrate diet. In fact, when I do, it is a four-week diet only.

The most important point to remember is that not all carbohydrates are bad. In fact, carbohydrates serve to fill your glycogen stores for running your chemistry. It is your personal chemistry and health history that will dictate your sensitivity to carbohydrates. In addition to managing your stress and making dietary improvements, one of the best ways to fight insulin resistance is exercise.

Exercise

Only 22 percent of adults in the United States get the recommended regular physical activity (five times a week for at least thirty minutes) of any intensity during leisure time. About 15 percent get the recommended amount of vigorous activity (three times a week for at least twenty minutes). About 25 percent of adults say they do no physical activity at all in their leisure time.

About 25 percent of young people (ages twelve to twenty-one) participate in light to moderate activity such as walking or bicycling nearly every day. About 50 percent of young people regularly engage in vigorous physical activity. Approximately 25 percent report no vigorous physical activity, and 14 percent report no recent vigorous or light to moderate physical activity.

Lack of physical activity contributes to the high prevalence of overweight and obesity in the United States. In addition to helping to burn fat, reduce insulin resistance, and control weight, physical activity improves digestion, increases energy, and reduces stress and anxiety, which are contributing factors to many illnesses and diseases. Exercise has been shown to decrease the risk of dying from coronary cardiovascular disease and of developing diabetes, hypertension, and colon cancer. In addition to these benefits, exercise can relieve depression and improve our sense of well-being.

Incorporating regular exercise into your daily life doesn't have to be drudgery. It is important to select physical activities that you enjoy. If your life is so overcommitted that you can't take an hour a day to exercise, start with fifteen minutes. Just begin to move! Be creative. For example, park further away in parking lots and use stairs instead of escalators or elevators whenever possible. Move that body!

Detoxification: The Keys to Rejuvenating Your Body

CHAPTER 7

The Organs of Detoxification: Why You Need to Cleanse Your Body

Many people think detoxification is something special that you do to your body by taking certain supplements or following a special program. However, detoxification is a process that the body does all the time without your knowing it. While there are measures we can take to aid our bodies in the processes of detoxification, the body has built-in systems designed to remove toxins from the bloodstream and tissues.

Unfortunately, there are many toxins that are stored in fatty tissues for which the body has no removal mechanisms—these are the toxins that many "detoxification programs" are designed to target. In addition, the capacity of the body's detoxification processes is not endless. There may come a time when the immune system just can't handle any more insults and can become completely overwhelmed. At some point, a specific toxin can become the straw that breaks the camel's back. And when the toxic threshold is reached, defenses begin to crumble. The poisons and microbes, with nothing to stop them, start influencing metabolic pathways.

We ingest these toxins, breathe them in, and absorb them through our skin. Their effects on our bodies are no different from that caused by the pollution that destroys lake ecology—killing the fish and negatively influencing the microecology of the water.

Toxins can originate from external sources or internally from inside the body. External toxins include chemical pollutants, heavy metals, electricity, radiation, and infectious agents. Pesticides and additives found in food are external toxins, as are substances in tobacco, drugs, and alcohol. The waste products of bacteria or fungi in the intestinal tract are examples of internally produced toxins. Just as the liver and kidneys have the primary role in detoxifying external toxins, the intestines play a primary role in preventing the production of internal toxins and preventing illnesses from bacterial and other microorganisms.

Some toxins are more damaging than others. For example, trace amounts of mercury (a heavy metal) can cause extensive damage to the central nervous system, whereas a healthy intestinal tract can typically defend the body from numerous bacterial invasions. While it is impossible to abolish all toxins, there are steps you can take to reduce unnecessary exposure and improve the efficiency of your bodies' ability to eliminate them. Knowing where these toxins reside in our environment and their impact on health provides important information to help minimize the health effects of toxic overload.

In this section, we begin an in-depth look at toxins—what they are and how they affect our bodies. We will also learn about how our bodies detoxify themselves and how we can help this process along. The body's ability to deal with the many environmental exposures and its ability to keep a balanced metabolism are intricately linked to the proper and effective functioning of the organs of detoxification and a balanced intestinal tract. While the goal of this section is to help you achieve better health by supporting your organs of detoxification, I hope that it will also inspire you to become more active in helping to clean up our environment.

TOXINS AND DETOXIFICATION

A *toxin* is anything that causes irritation, harm, or destruction in the body. Toxins can come from external and internal sources. *Detoxification* is the process of removing and metabolizing unwanted chemical compounds that can disrupt normal bodily functions. Its goal is to neutralize or eliminate these toxins so that normal function may begin to return to the organs or systems being affected.

Our ability to dismantle and excrete toxins is a critical process, and without it, toxins capable of destroying cells, tissue, and organs would surely overcome us. Understanding how toxins impact our bodies and how we can strengthen our bodies' ability to fight them enables us to strengthen our efforts toward achieving better health, and live longer, better lives as a result.

To understand the process of overcoming the effects of toxins on body chemistry, it helps to look at the body as a terrain—an unproductive garden of sorts that you are trying to restore. Detoxification is like taking soil that has laid barren for years and then working it to produce a healthy harvest. You have to add nutrients, till the soil to aerate it, get healthful microorganisms growing in the soil, and constantly weed out the pests—natural enemies that are always trying to destroy the healthy harvest. It takes a great deal of work to produce a great harvest.

Toxins can alter genetic expression and damage the endocrine (hormonal) system. They can also destroy or disrupt enzymes, negatively alter cellular metabolism and energy production, and/or cause direct neurological damage. Moreover, they can permanently impair the immune system. Lastly, the effects of toxins can accelerate the aging process, causing biological age to exceed chronological age.

Many of the common symptoms listed below can be linked to the environment and the potential for toxic overload:

- Insulin resistance (a prediabetic condition)

- Hypothyroidism (underproduction of thyroid hormone)

- Poor digestion (malabsorption of food and nutrition)

- Fatigue

- Obesity

- Reduced cognitive function (decline in memory and recall)

- Impaired immune function

- Atherosclerosis and cardiovascular disease

- Accelerated aging

- Alzheimer's disease

- Cancer

Exotoxins—The Toxins Outside Us

Toxins that enter the body from without, products of our external environment, are called *exotoxins*. (The prefix *exo-* means "outside.")

You can choose the food you eat, whether or not to exercise, and even how you are going to cope with stress. But the one thing that you are stuck with (for now) is your external environment. There is no getting around it: We live in an increasingly industrialized world, and that world has had significant impact on the environment in which we live, as well as on the environment inside us. We are inextricably bound to the environment! We are constantly exposed to a wide array of compounds, which are then stored in our bodies. And, as you've learned, some of these compounds are quite toxic.

Toxins pervade our environment. We are assaulted daily by radiation from global warming, ozone-layer depletion, and exposure to the sun; by toxic metals such as lead, aluminum, cadmium, and mercury found in pesticides, herbicides, insecticides, fungicides, fumigants, and fertilizers that leak into our soil and food; by thousands of food additives, preservatives, and artificial colorings that pervade the products on grocery store shelves; and even from fresh fruits and vegetables, which are protected by sprays, treated with agents to speed ripening, and then preserved with waxes. Hazardous chemicals and toxic waste contaminate our water and air.

Studies report that our bodies store toxins from a lifetime of accumulated exposures. These studies measure substances—such as those that would be in the body from environmental pollution, pesticides, and preservatives from our foods—in human tissues. Most people would be shocked to know, for instance, that studies conducted by the Environmental Protection Agency (EPA) show that 100 percent of the people studied had fat stores containing chemicals such as styrene from Styrofoam, dioxin from pesticides, and xylene, a solvent. Indoor pollution poses as great a health threat as outdoor pollution levels. Additional studies conducted by the EPA have found that levels of air pollution inside our houses, schools, and offices are typically two to three times greater than levels beyond these walls.

Asbestos, bedding, carbon monoxide, disinfectants, electromagnetic fields, formaldehyde, household cleaners, low-level radiation from computer monitors and television screens, and radon are only a few of the substances to which we are exposed daily. Even house dust may carry dozens of cancer-causing chemicals. And worse, if you work in a corporate environment, complete with wall-to-wall carpeting and floor-to-ceiling windows that do not open, or you live in a new energy-efficient home with modern insulation, you are existing within an environment in which chemicals are out-gassing (emitting) constantly from the carpets, the wall paint, and from cleaning chemicals, into the air you breath. Worse still are molds and fungi such as *Aspergillus* that can infiltrate a house and become trapped within the sealed environment or central air conditioning and central heat. These mold and fungi are known to be a major threat to the human immune system. Chronic or even acute exposure to any of these substances can compromise your health.

Endotoxins—The Toxins Within Us

Internal toxins, called *endotoxins* (*endo-* means "inside" or "within") are poisons that are naturally produced by the body as a result of biochemical processes such as metabolites (metabolic byproducts), hormones, antibodies, or bacterial waste. But, although they are internally produced, they are still toxins and need to be dealt with by the body before they can create havoc.

As you will learn in Chapter 9, one of the principal sources of internal toxins is a poorly functioning digestive system. Toxins are produced in the bowel from several sources. First, they are created by fermentation and the putrefaction of poorly digested foods in the intestinal tract. Second, if the healthy flora that occurs naturally in the digestive system has been disturbed, and unfriendly fungi, parasites, or bacteria have taken hold, the byproducts (excretions) of those parasites' metabolisms can be toxic to the human metabolism.

Many toxins from our external environment become part of our internal environment, as we eat them, drink them, and breathe them in. Thus, our intestines, once organs designed to take nutrients from a natural world, have become organs of self-defense, our bodies' first line of defense, as they attempt to protect us from the poisons that are everywhere in the environment.

A LIFETIME OF TOXIC EXPOSURE

The effects of exposure to toxins vary from individual to individual, based to a certain extent on each person's genetic uniqueness. Some people might be extremely sensitive to internal and environmental toxins and quickly develop chronic symptoms.

Others might be quite hardy either because their bodies' defensive barriers (such as the digestive tract) are strong enough to prevent the absorption of substances from the external environment, or because their organs of detoxification (liver, gastrointestinal tract, and kidneys, lymph, lungs, and skin) have high metabolic reserves and are capable of detoxifying and eliminating those substances.

There is a high cancer rate in Cincinnati, which is where I live. It also has a big industrial basin. I love Cincinnati, and have no intention of leaving, but I also know that I have to work at keeping my body resilient in order to reduce risks to my health posed by the environment. My practice is filled with cancer patients. These cases run the gamut—they are men and women, young people and old, wealthy people and poor, fat and thin. When I meet these patients, many times they tell me the same sad story: "This came out of nowhere. I can't understand how this happened to me." Truly, they do not comprehend what has happened to them. They do not see that their illness is the result of a lifetime of accumulation of metabolic toxicity. They do not understand the price we each pay for living in an industrial world. They do not see its effects on their bodies and their unique chemistry. They do not see that their illness is a result of many factors: the food they ate, the air they breathed, the water they drank, the drugs they took, or the stress they were under. Moreover, they do not understand that the amount of time it took for them to fall into the clutches of their disease depended greatly upon their own unique genetic code, as it was written first by their parents and ancestors and the environment in which they were brought up, and later by the environment in which they surrounded themselves.

The balance between exposure to toxins and the speed with which those toxins are detoxified and eliminated determines one's susceptibility to the metabolic dysfunction that can lead to chronic symptoms of ill health. Wherever you search, whatever you read on the major diseases affecting us, invariably toxic influences—both internal and external—are being linked to the problem. Some reports suggest that 80 percent of all cancer is due to environmental exposure. These studies are being reported in major journals, such as the *New England Journal of Medicine*.

Fortunately, there are laboratory tests we can use to measure the type and extent of the damage the toxins have produced. From that point of discovery, we can work rationally to aid our bodies' detoxification processes and to reclaim our health.

Detoxification is not a one-time event. It is a process that should be part of everyone's lifelong health practices. These practices can be gentle and, in fact, as regular as maintaining the oil levels in your car. You can take time for that, right? Instead of passively waiting for disease to strike, take action now to get healthy and to create an internal and external environment in which you can stay healthy.

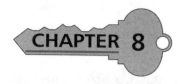

CHAPTER 8

KEY FOUR:
Detoxifying Your Liver—
The Body's Garbage Collector
and Recycler

Although detoxification takes place in a number of body systems, the principal organ of detoxification is the liver. Your life depends on the liver's functions as the primary defense against toxins that enter from the bloodstream. If your liver ceased to function, you would quickly become very ill from the accumulation of toxic substances.

The liver is the body's largest internal organ. An adult liver weighs approximately three pounds. It is located in the upper right quadrant of the abdominal cavity and extends beyond the midline. Anatomically, the liver consists of four lobes: a large right lobe, a smaller left lobe, and two inferior (bottom) lobes. The portal vein supplies the liver with blood from the gastrointestinal tract (including the stomach, and small and large intestines), spleen, and pancreas, while the hepatic artery supplies the liver with blood from the heart. Arteries take blood that has received oxygen to the organs, while veins take the "used" blood back to the lungs to get more oxygen. Together, the portal vein and hepatic artery pump about 1,400 ml (about 1.5 quarts) per minute into the liver. Because blood enters the liver faster than it is removed, the liver is able to store about 300 ml (a little less than one pint) of blood at any given time.

In addition to filtering and detoxifying the blood, the liver contributes to the body's *anabolic* and *catabolic* functions—that is, the reformation or building of new cells, tissues, and organs, and its opposite, the breakdown of cellular structure. The liver also functions as storage for glycogen, a stored form of glucose. The astonishing capacities of the liver make it among the most functionally important organs in the body. It performs hundreds of different functions involving decontamination and recycling substances within the body. These functions include the following:

- Detoxifies chemicals from the environment

- Converts ammonia to urea

- Converts carbohydrates and proteins to fat

- Breaks down proteins

- Eliminates bilirubin (a substance secreted in the bile)

- Filters and detoxifies blood

- Forms ketones (waste products of partially metabolized fat) and phospholipids (fat molecules) from fatty acids

- Forms lipoproteins

- Metabolizes drugs

- Metabolizes hormones

- Produces bile salts

- Produces lymphatic fluid (lymph nourishes and cleanses tissue cells)

- Stores glycogen and converts it to glucose for fuel

- Stores vitamins A, D, B_{12}, and the mineral iron

- Synthesizes cholesterol and enzymes

- Synthesizes blood-clotting factors

- Synthesizes plasma proteins (including globulin needed for antibody formation)

HOW THE LIVER DETOXIFIES

The liver contains cells called "Kupffer cells," which are capable of removing dead cells, bacteria, and foreign substances from the blood. While the Kupffer cells are responsible for filtering about 99 percent of the bacterial and food contaminants from the blood, other important cells in the liver, termed hepatocytes, are active in the detoxification of drugs, heavy metals, chemicals, alcohol, and hormones. These processes of detoxification require two important steps, known as phase one (oxidation-reduction) and phase two (conjugation-elimination).

The liver removes toxic and metabolic waste products from the body by converting them to water-soluble compounds that can be excreted in the urine. Those substances that are not water-soluble are transformed by the liver and excreted in the bile, a substance used for this purpose and for the digestion of fats. The bile is then transported into the intestines where it is eliminated in the feces. Toxins not completely removed by either one of these processes may be eliminated through the skin (fat-soluble compounds are excreted in sweat), or lungs. Toxins that remain in the body accumulate in the adipose (fat) tissue and nerve cells, contributing to a wide range of degenerative conditions.

Phase-one detoxification serves to transform endotoxins (toxins produced within the body) and exotoxins (those taken into the body from the outside) through chemical methods termed *oxidation, reduction,* or *hydrolysis,* by utilizing a complex net-work of detoxification enzymes known as the *cytochrome P-450 enzyme system.* The cytochrome P-450 system is important also because it is where drug interactions take place (whether these be drug/drug, drug/herb, and drug/nutrient interactions).

Phase-one detoxification prepares substances for phase-two detoxification, which further transforms toxic agents so that they can be excreted in the urine and feces. The following is a brief description of this two-step process as depicted in Figure 8.1 below.

Figure 8.1. Pathways of Liver Detoxification

The goal of liver detoxification is to make compounds more water soluble and able to be excreted. This function is very dependent on adequate nutrient status.

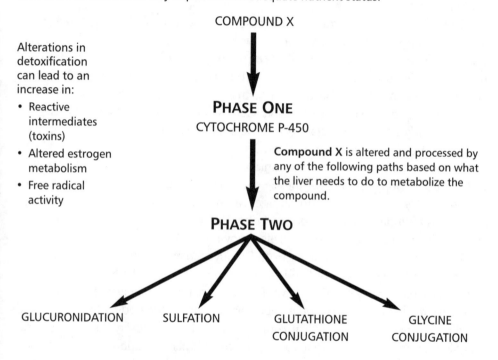

COMPOUND X

Alterations in detoxification can lead to an increase in:

• Reactive intermediates (toxins)

• Altered estrogen metabolism

• Free radical activity

PHASE ONE
CYTOCHROME P-450

Compound **X** is altered and processed by any of the following paths based on what the liver needs to do to metabolize the compound.

PHASE TWO

GLUCURONIDATION   SULFATION   GLUTATHIONE CONJUGATION   GLYCINE CONJUGATION

Phase-One Detoxification

Phase one of the detoxification system is dependent on a group of fifty or so enzymes in the cytochrome P-450 system. Cytochrome P-450 enzymes work primarily by oxi-dizing, or breaking down, toxins that effect our bodies. *Oxidation* is a biochemical reaction that inactivates or destroys chemicals by the transfer of oxygen and loss of electrons. The result is that for every atom destroyed by oxidation a free radical is generated. Management of free-radical damage is a critical concept too in our quest for health, longevity, and prevention of diseases.

Free radicals are a highly reactive species of oxygen and can damage protein, fats, cholesterol (lipids), and nucleic acids (compounds which make up our DNA and RNA—the building blocks or blueprint of who we are).

Free-radical production is normally held in balance by *antioxidants.* Antioxidants that block destructive oxidation reactions include vitamins C and E, carotenoids, and the mineral selenium. Environmental pollution, infections, pesticides, eating the wrong foods, smoking, radiation, and even exposure to sunlight are some of the causes of free-radical formation.

For this reason, the *hepatocyte* cells in the liver require a continuous supply of antioxidant nutrients to neutralize the potentially damaging free radicals. The most important antioxidant required by the liver for detoxification is the chemical *glutathione.* Glutathione is used in both phase one and phase two of the liver's detoxification process.

Glutathione is a short protein chain (called a "tripeptide" containing three amino acids) consisting of L-glutamic acid, L-cysteine, and glycine. Glutathione is an important antioxidant used by every cell in the body. Usually the liver produces glutathione in sufficient quantities to keep "check" on the free radicals produced. But the problems that cause free-radical production, such as pollution, pesticides, smoking, poor food choices, and even disease processes such as diabetes or Parkinson's disease, can cause the body's stores of glutathione to be depleted and not able to keep up with the onslaught of free-radical production.

Important dietary sources of glutathione include fresh fruits and vegetables, fish, and meat. The body can also synthesize glutathione from the amino acids methionine, N-acetylcysteine (NAC), and glycine. Methionine, the primary source for glutathione, is abundant in a well-rounded diet. One excellent supplemental source of methionine is S-adenosylmethionine, also known as SAM-e.

Two other supplements that can significantly increase glutathione levels are milk thistle and alpha lipoic acid. Milk thistle is a preparation from the fruit of milk thistle (*Silybum marianum*). Milk thistle's liver protective action is mainly due to its antioxidant capacity, which helps maintain glutathione levels in the body. Alpha lipoic acid is a glutathione-boosting and antiaging nutrient. Lester Packer, Ph.D., a leading antioxidant scientist, reports that adding alpha lipoic acid to various human and animal tissue cultures resulted in a remarkable 30 percent increase in cellular glutathione levels. Subsequent animal studies also reveal the important role alpha lipoic acid plays in supporting glutathione activity.

Other key nutrients required by the liver for phase-one detoxification include beta-carotene, vitamins C, E, B_3 (niacin), and choline (a form of B vitamin), the minerals copper, magnesium and zinc, and the essential fatty acids omega-3 and omega-6.

Reduction (the opposite of oxidation), *hydrolysis* (breaking a compound into smaller fragments by the addition of water), and *hydration* (the addition of water) are the other processes used in phase-one detoxification. All prepare compounds to be introduced to our bodies and used if needed and/or eliminated.

If the compounds introduced to the liver's phase one metabolism are to be used by the body, they must be converted to active compounds in phase one before moving on to phase-two metabolism. If they are not to be used, they are converted to water-soluble compounds that can be eliminated immediately. This pathway requires a synchronicity between the systems controlling both phase-one and phase-two detoxification. If phase-two metabolism, or processing, cannot meet the output of phase one, then free radicals can accumulate. And, in many cases, these metabolites—compounds created during phase one—are more toxic than the original compound. These compounds are called *reactive intermediates.*

When your liver cannot process these intermediates efficiently, they begin to build up. They are in "limbo," because of the liver's inability to process them. Therefore, an imbalance in the breakdown processes of chemicals in the body can lead to the buildup of reactive intermediate metabolites or chemicals that have not been fully processed. Simply put, the liver does all it can to keep the body healthy, but if overloaded with toxins, it cannot keep up with the challenge, and toxins accumulate in our bodies.

Think of this process as an assembly line—like the one in the *I Love Lucy* episode when Lucy and Ethel go to work in a candy factory. Amusingly, the chocolates kept coming down the conveyer belt, faster and faster. If Lucy and Ethel couldn't keep up with wrapping them, they were going to lose their jobs. That's just like the process of liver detoxification. If the liver can't keep up with processing toxins, pandemonium occurs. In the episode, Lucy began shoving the chocolates in her mouth, in her dress, and in her hat. She simply couldn't keep up with the conveyer belt's speed. That is what your body starts to do with reactive intermediates and toxic compounds when the liver can't process them. To try to keep things normal, these chemicals quickly get stored somewhere in your body, where they begin wreaking havoc on your body chemistry and begin leading you to a continuum of disease and poor health.

Many people have compromised phase-one detoxification systems. They are referred to as *slow detoxifiers.* Liver disease or damage from excessive alcohol, certain drugs, or even birth control pills can interfere with phase-one detoxification. Other factors that may slow phase-one detoxification are fasting, a vegetarian or low-animal protein diet, the intake of partially hydrogenated vegetable oils (semi-solid fats that contain harmful trans-fatty acids), grapefruit (possibly due to a chemical called *naringin*), methyl xanthine from tea, and an overload of iron in the system. Phase one may also be inhibited by a lack of nutrients, vitamins, or minerals. Some inhibitors of phase-one detoxification include:

- Age
- Antidepressants
- Antihistamines
- Grapefruit juice
- H2 blockers
- Hydrogenated fats
- Intestinal imbalances
- Iron overload
- Oral contraceptives

Some substances speed up phase-one detoxification, causing a build up of reactive intermediates if not processed at the same rate by phase two. Some inducers that accelerate phase-one detoxification include:

- Alcohol

- Caffeine

- Cruciferous vegetables (broccoli, cabbage, cauliflower, Brussels sprouts, and others)

- Fumes (from exhaust and paint)

- Some herbal supplements (including St. John's wort, garlic, schisandra berry)

- Some medications (including sulfonamides, steroids, phenobarbital, and other barbiturates)

- Nicotine

- Pesticides

- Protein

Key nutrients required in phase-one detoxification include:

- Beta-carotene
- Choline
- Copper
- Lecithin
- Magnesium
- Glutathione
- Omega-3 and omega-6 fatty acids
- Sulfur
- Vitamins B_3 (niacin), C, and E
- Zinc

Phase-Two Detoxification

Phase-two detoxification relies primarily on a biochemical process known as *conjugation*. Conjugation involves the binding of a toxin with a substance that makes it water-soluble. Once it is water soluble, it can be excreted from the body. There are several different conjugating substances used during this process:

The most important of these substances is the antioxidant glutathione. In the liver, glutathione conjugates by attaching its own sulfur group compounds with toxins, thus creating water-soluble compounds that can be excreted in the urine. In the presence of oxidative substances, glutathione is readily oxidized and is able to protect cellular proteins from free-radical damage.

Other substances used in phase-two detoxification are *glycine, cysteine,* and *glucuronic acid.* The amino acid glycine is important for the conjugation of chemicals like the food additive benzoate. Cysteine is crucial for the process of *sulfation.* In this process, sulfur molecules from cysteine conjugate substances like bacterial toxins from the gut, heavy metals, and hormones. In a similar process, known as *methyla-*

tion, methyl groups conjugate circulating estrogens. Therefore, slow methylation can lead to an increase in estrogen-related disorders such as premenstrual syndrome (PMS), fibrocystic breasts (noncancerous cysts, or lumps, in the breasts), ovarian cysts, and endometriosis (an abnormal growth of cells that form in the lining of the uterus), or may even trigger estrogen-related cancers. The amino acid *methionine* is a major source of methyl groups used for methylation.

Glucuronic acid conjugates drugs such as aspirin and menthol, food additives, and hormones, especially estrogen. An inherited weakness in the glucuronidation process is known as *Gilbert's syndrome.* This condition may be more common than realized. It is characterized by yellowing of the skin, loss of appetite, abdominal pain, weakness, and fatigue, among other symptoms. Studies have demonstrated that prolonged jaundice in newborns is associated with the same genetic mutation, and manifests as Gilbert's syndrome in adulthood. The mutation is found in the genetic code for the *UDP-glucuronyl transferase* enzyme, which catalyzes glucuronidation. For women, this process is especially important, because if glucuronidation is poor, then estrogen is recirculated in the body, and over time, elevations of estrogen in the body can lead to the wide array of problems previously mentioned.

There are several variables that influence glucuronidation. Insufficient levels of beneficial bacteria in the gut, the presence of unfriendly flora in the gut, or a low-fiber diet can all contribute to increasing the enzyme beta-glucuronidase, which cleaves (removes) the glucuronide molecule from its target (estrogen). For example, glucuronide attaches itself to estrogen to be excreted. If it is cleaved off, then the estrogen is free to be reabsorbed into the system. Calcium D-glucarate is a nutraceutical developed that inhibits beta glucuronidase and therefore enhances the binding and elimination of estrogen. I commonly recommend 600–1,000 mg a day of calcium D-glucarate to women who are breast cancer survivors or have estrogen dominant chemistries.

Acetyl coenzyme-A (acetyl-CoA) is a compound that detoxifies substances in a process known as *acetylation,* a chemical process of detoxification. For example, acetyl-CoA conjugates sulfa drugs. An inherited weakness in the ability to acetylate can lead to an intolerance of sulfa drugs. Another cause of sensitivities to sulfur-containing foods (such as sulfites) and drugs is a weakness in the phase two process of sulfation. This detoxification pathway requires the enzyme sulfite oxidase to metabolize sulfur compounds. Sulfites are compounds found naturally in some foods, but added to others like wine, dried fruits, and frozen French fries for preserving the food. Sulfites can be particularly dangerous to those with weak *sulfoxidation,* inducing severe migraine headaches and asthma attacks in sensitive individuals.

Most of the phase-two detoxification pathways are dependent on two groups of substances: amino acids and properly functioning enzymes. Each pathway requires its own unique enzymes. For example, the enzyme required to catalyze the transfer of sulfate groups in sulfation is called *sulfotransferase* (s-transferase). The enzyme needed for methylation is *methyltransferase*. *UDP-glucuronyl transferase* is needed for glucuronidation and *sulfite oxidase* is necessary for sulfoxidation.

If these enzymes are in short supply or are functioning poorly, phase-two detoxification will be inhibited. These enzymes can be thought of as the keys that start the engine to your detoxification processes. Unfortunately, the effects of being exposed to several toxic substances simultaneously are magnified by the damage they inflict on enzymes. Not only do these compounds induce toxic and free-radical damage, but they also linger in the body longer due to slowed phase-two detoxification and can even bind to enzymes to alter their activity.

In my practice, I routinely perform an inexpensive amino acid testing on people by the use of a simple blood sample from a finger stick, and almost always find there are deficiencies. When I feel that people are in need of a very sensitive analysis, such as in cases of cancer or autoimmune disorders, I recommend more thorough amino acid testing. They have developed significant proprietary technologies to peer into your amino acid and peptide imbalances. When a person is low in certain amino acids such as glycine, methionine, or cysteine, the bodies' abilities to perform detoxification processes is compromised. Other amino acid imbalances can influence immune function, metabolism, mood, blood sugar regulation, and neurological function.

Anything that impairs enzymes, or their pathways, in phase-two detoxification results in what is known as *pathological detoxification*. In cases of pathological detoxification, phase two cannot detoxify compounds at the same rate that phase one metabolizes them. As was mentioned earlier, some of the metabolites generated from phase-one detoxification, known as reactive intermediate metabolites, are highly toxic. If not cleared by phase two, these metabolites can accumulate and generate extensive damage. A low-protein diet (which fails to provide adequate amino acids), nutrient deficiencies, and the use of nonsteroidal, anti-inflammatory drugs (NSAIDs), which include ibuprofen (Motrin) indomethacin (Indocin), fenoprofen (Nalfon), sulindac (Clinoril), and many others, can all lead to pathological detoxification.

Some inhibitors of phase-two detoxification include:

- Low-protein diets
- Nonsteroidal anti-inflammatory drugs

Some inducers that enhance phase-two detoxification include:

- Cruciferous vegetables (broccoli, cabbage, cauliflower, Brussels sprouts, and others)
- Eggs
- Fish oils
- Leeks
- Limonene (from lemons)
- Milk thistle seed (*Silybum marianum*)

- Onions
- Raw garlic

Key nutrients required in phase-two detoxification include:
- Alpha lipoic acid
- Folic acid
- Magnesium
- Manganese
- Methionine
- N-acetylcysteine (NAC)
- Selenium
- Taurine
- Vitamins B_2 (riboflavin), B_5 (pantothenic acid), B_{12} (cyanocobalamin), and C
- Zinc

When the liver is operating optimally, phase one and phase two work efficiently at protecting the body against foreign substances. The system breaks down, however, when the rate of exposure to toxins is greater than it can handle. The more toxins that build up in the body, the greater the demand will be on the liver to detoxify them. The more these toxins hang around, the greater the chance to start damaging our cellular structures such as our *mitochondria* (small cellular components known as the powerhouse of the cell responsible for energy production and cellular respiration) and DNA. If the liver doesn't receive the necessary nutrients it needs to detoxify and excrete these substances as nontoxic products, it can become overwhelmed. When it is unable to manage toxins effectively, the liver may release them to other organs and tissues and adversely impair them.

Bile: The Detoxifier of Fat-Soluble Compounds

Bile is a yellow-green fluid consisting of bile salts, cholesterol, water, bilirubin (a waste product that results from the breakdown of old red blood cells), and acidic compounds. Once synthesized by the liver, bile is transported to the gallbladder where it is concentrated and stored. Bile is critical for the proper digestion of fats and the absorption of fat-soluble vitamins. If bile synthesis is compromised, fat-soluble vitamin and essential fatty acid deficiencies can develop. When fats are present in the small intestine, a hormone called *cholecystokinin* (CCK) is released, which triggers the gallbladder to secrete bile and tells your brain that you have eaten enough. Bile and pancreatic enzymes emulsify large fat molecules in the small intestine, forming smaller *chylomicrons.* These smaller particles can then pass through the intestinal mucosa into the lymphatic circulation. (Blood transports water-soluble compounds and lymph carries fat-soluble compounds.)

Bile also plays a significant role in the detoxification process. Bile is a carrier of excess calcium, cholesterol, hormones, dead red blood cells, and toxic substances.

In the lower part of the small intestine, most of the bile salts are reabsorbed and carried back to the liver. The remaining bile is carried to the large intestine where it is bound with fiber and excreted in the feces. A diet lacking in fiber will promote the stagnation and reabsorption of toxic compounds from the bowel. Furthermore, unconjugated bile is irritating to the intestinal mucosa and can contribute to *leaky gut syndrome* (a condition in which minute particles of undigested or partially digested protein pass through the intestinal wall into the bloodstream, which can cause allergic reactions). In some instances, enzymes from bacterial flora can convert bile to carcinogenic compounds. Rice bran, which can be found in various protein drinks and meal replacements, actually binds to toxins and "soaks them up" before they can be absorbed into your system.

LIVER SUPPORT: THE SECONDARY ORGANS OF DETOXIFICATION

Although the liver represents the most critical pathway of detoxification, it could not function optimally without the support of the kidneys, lungs, skin, and lymph system, and the intestines, which are discussed briefly below and more in depth in later chapters. Together, these waste-removing organs have about one-third the detoxification capacity of the liver. They have the important job of metabolizing and excreting toxins that have bypassed the liver.

The Kidneys

The primary function of the kidneys is to filter and excrete metabolic waste from the blood. An extraordinary amount of blood flow passes through the kidneys. At rest, the arteries leading to the kidneys carry from 15 to 30 percent of the total blood volume through the kidneys. Every twenty-four hours, about 180 liters (almost 45 gallons!) circulate through the kidneys. Most of the blood is reabsorbed and goes back to the body for reuse. A fraction of it becomes urine, the primary pathway of elimination. Urine removes water, toxic waste products of metabolism, and inorganic salts from the body.

The kidney consists of an outer cortex and an inner medulla. Each kidney contains about one million *nephrons*—the functional units of the kidney that contain tiny filters that are used in detoxification. Tubes in the nephrons either reabsorb water and salt to go back in the body or send them to be eliminated in the urine.

Our bodies' cellular functions are dependent upon the ability of the kidneys to excrete waste. Without the constant removal of metabolic waste from the cells, waste products accumulate and cells begin to malfunction. When the kidneys fail, our bodies are thrown out of balance and fluids and electrolytes (such as potassium, sodium, and other minerals) are disrupted. Heavy metals are particularly damaging to the kidneys.

The Skin

The skin is the body's largest organ. It consists of the outer *epidermis,* which contains epithelial cells, and the inner *dermis,* which is composed of connective tissue. The dermal layer contains collagen and elastin. These are structural components, which give the skin firmness and elasticity. The dermis also contains sweat glands, hair follicles, and sebaceous glands. Sweat glands help to eliminate water-soluble toxins, while sebaceous glands transport fat-soluble toxins for elimination through the skin.

The skin contains many of the cytochrome P-450 detoxification enzymes. It can metabolize some drugs by converting them to more water-soluble form for easier elimination. That's why certain prescription and over-the-counter products are available as transdermal patches, such as nicotine patches for smoking cessation and progesterone patches for hormone replacement.

If you have chronic skin problems or conditions, such as eczema, psoriasis, or dermatitis, more than likely your detoxification processes are impaired. If the kidneys and liver are not eliminating toxins, the body tries to shove them out through the skin, as was shown in some studies. In one study, people were placed in saunas and their sweat was collected. In evaluating the compounds in the sweat, it was found that a wide variety of toxic chemicals (such as solvents, pesticides, and fertilizers) from the environment were present. In fact, low-temperature infrared saunas are recommended by many environmental health practitioners (experts in food safety and public health) because of their ability to detoxify the skin by gently sweating out the toxins.

The Lungs

The lungs are spongy, triangular organs suspended in the thoracic (chest) cavity. The right lung is larger than the left and contains three lobes. The left lung has two lobes. The lobes are divided into lobules, which are divided by connective tissue. Lobules contain bronchioles, alveoli, blood, and lymphatic vessels. The bronchial tree is the passage through which air is taken in and expired. It begins in the trachea (windpipe), branching further and further until it becomes tiny alveolar ducts within the lobules.

Breathing is the process of moving air from outside the body into the bronchial tree and alveoli (*inspiration*) and out again (*expiration*). The alveolar membranes allow carbon dioxide and other gases to diffuse from the blood into the lungs. These gases are released into the air during exhalation. In this way, the lungs are pathways through which toxic gases are eliminated from the body. The lungs also contain cytochrome P-450 detoxification enzymes, which allows them to convert some drugs to water-soluble compounds that can be excreted in the urine. The antioxidant enzymes superoxide dismutase (SOD) and glutathione peroxidase are important free-radical scavengers that are found in the lungs.

The Lymph

The lymphatic system is an elaborate system of organs (including the spleen, the thymus, the tonsils, and the lymph nodes) composed of lymphatic vessels that run parallel to the veins in the body. The vessels of the lymph system are filled with a fluid called *lymph,* which is collected from the space between the cells. The lymph fluids feed the cells of the body by transporting various nutrients such as salts, minerals, and proteins to every cell of the body. Likewise, lymph fluid carries cell wastes and debris that accumulate from normal cell function away from the cells and turns them over to the blood. The blood shuttles the wastes to the kidneys, lungs, colon, and skin for elimination. The lymph system can be thought of as the cellular toxin disposal system.

Lymph fluid travels to nodes, also called lymph glands, found in various places in the lymph system. There are more than 600 lymph nodes in our bodies, with a particularly large concentration found in the neck, groin, armpits, and abdomen. The immune system's scavenger cells called macrophages *are found in the lymph nodes.* They engulf and destroy many foreign and toxic particles. Lymph nodes also contain *B-lymphocytes,* a group of white blood cells that are manufactured by and matured in the bone marrow, and produce antibodies to protect the body from future viruses, bacteria, yeast, and other organisms.

CONDITIONS OF THE LIVER

There are many health practitioners who believe that most diseases are rooted in a poorly functioning liver. Traditional Chinese medicine (TCM) views the liver as the "General" of all organs, mobilizing the forces of the blood to support the "qi", which is the life force itself. In ancient Greece, many diseases were characterized under the general description of "melancholia," which translated literally means "black bile." Clearly, the ancient Greeks understood the detrimental effects of a stagnant liver.

Liver dysfunction has been linked to diseases not commonly associated with digestion or detoxification. Given its incredible scope of activity in the body, its role in a multitude of disease processes should not be surprising. For example, in a recent study of twenty autistic children, 100 percent were found to have abnormal liver detoxification profiles. Sixteen of the children showed levels of toxic chemicals that exceeded the maximum adult tolerance. This study suggests that autism may be in part rooted in neurological damage caused by an inability of the liver to metabolize toxins and sensitivity of the child to these exposures. There is also a growing correlation being observed between the buildup of certain *neurotoxic* metabolites (substances toxic to the nervous system) such as *arabinose* (a yeast metabolite) and autism.

Another theory suggests that phases one and two of the liver's detoxification process may have a role in the progression of HIV to full-blown AIDS. This theory states that enhancing the liver's ability to clear toxins from the gut should be a part of the therapeutic protocol for those with HIV infection. Also, there is compelling evidence that chronic fatigue syndrome, fibromyalgia, and multiple chemical sensitivity all have associations with compromised detoxification processes in the liver, as well as a poorly functioning gut.

LAB TESTS FOR LIVER DYSFUNCTION

Laboratory analysis of the liver includes liver function tests (LFTs). LFTs are derived from a blood sample. They measure liver enzymes, cholesterol, and bilirubin levels in the serum, and may include prothrombin time (the time it takes for blood to clot), dye clearance, blood ammonia levels, and total plasma proteins.

The clinically normal ranges for these levels are broad. In many cases, illness has established a strong foothold before LFTs show any abnormalities. Some clinicians report that one of the earliest signs of liver or biliary dysfunction is the presence of bilirubin in the first morning urine (bilirubinuria).

Salivary Caffeine Clearance

More subtle alterations in liver function can be detected by the *salivary caffeine clearance test*. This test can be done at home and the results interpreted by a qualified practitioner or laboratory. Caffeine clearance is used to measure the efficiency of several cytochrome P-450 enzymes in phase-one detoxification.

Saliva samples are taken a few hours after drinking a known amount of caffeine. Caffeine is almost exclusively eliminated by phase one cytochrome P-450 enzymes. If the caffeine in saliva remains high after several hours (low clearance), this indicates dysfunctional P-450 enzyme activity. If the caffeine is very low (high clearance), it indicates overactive phase-one detoxification.

Increased phase-one detoxification, not matched by phase two elimination, may lead to a high toxic burden. To measure the four phase two liver detoxification pathways—acetylation, glucuronidation, methylation, and sulfation—a dose of aspirin and acetaminophen is given. Likewise, this can tell whether this portion of detoxification is sluggish.

In addition, it may be useful to compare a ratio of phase one to phase two. Environmental exposure to toxins leads to increased free-radical activity, which in turn depletes antioxidant capacity. This can be linked to disorders such as fibromyalgia, cardiovascular disease, and inflammatory processes that are now being recognized as markers in such conditions as diabetes, autoimmune disorders, and obesity.

Urinary Hippurate

Hippurate is the metabolic byproduct of benzoic acid conjugation. Benzoic acid (benzoate) is a common food additive. Measuring hippurate in the urine is a way to gauge the efficiency of phase two conjugation of benzoic acid. Slow conversion of benzoic acid to hippurate suggests impaired phase-two detoxification. High hippurate in the urine indicates that phase two is functioning strongly.

Comparisons between salivary caffeine clearance and urinary hippurate by a qualified practitioner or laboratory provide information about how the detoxification pathways are functioning relative to one another. Low caffeine clearance relative to hippurate indicates slow detoxification (phase one decreased relative to phase two).

The Power of Detoxification: A Case History

This is a real life story about the biochemical importance of detoxification and how it can impact a person's life—in this case a child's life. A nine-year-old girl was brought to me as a patient a few years ago. She had been battling a condition labeled *idiopathic nephropathy,* a kidney disorder (*idiopathic* meaning of "unknown origin"). She'd had a strep infection several months earlier and had been on multiple rounds of antibiotics. She was spilling significant amounts of proteins and blood into her urine, and was on the border of some serious medical treatments. Unfortunately, the next medical step would be to biopsy her kidney, and, if the results were as anticipated, she would be placed on steroids. In acute situations, steroids have significant benefits. However, chronic use of steroids in a child may present significant risks and side effects.

I initiated some liver support, *probiotics* (supplemental beneficial bacteria) to put healthy flora normally back into the gut, a kidney drainage remedy (a combination herbal or low-dose homeopathic remedy that helps fortify kidney function), some N-acetyl cysteine, and the mushroom *Cordyceps sinensis,* which is known for its kidney-protective properties. The end result? No biopsy, no more blood in the urine, and no more spillage of proteins. The doctors were happy, the child's mother was ecstatic, and the girl was spared some tough treatment.

In this case, metabolic toxins had overrun the young patient's chemistry, most likely caused by the multiple rounds of antibiotics that her body couldn't process. In addition, the antibiotics destroyed the good intestinal bacteria, reducing her ability to detoxify intermediate reactive metabolites. When beneficial flora is diminished, fungi can "take over the neighborhood," producing mycotoxins (metabolic waste) that can damage tissues and increase oxidative stress to cells. In this case, the patient's intestines, liver, and kidneys were playing out this vicious destructive cycle that needed to be broken.

Increased caffeine clearance relative to urinary hippurate indicates pathological detoxification (phase one increased relative to phase two).

A WELL-BALANCED DETOXIFICATION SYSTEM IS KEY

Because the liver is the primary organ in charge of the body's detoxification system, it plays a vital role in helping you to achieve optimal health. It not only collects the toxic garbage from the blood and converts it to nontoxic substances that can be eliminated in urine and feces, but also processes foods from which it recycles important substances for use throughout the body.

When you are in good health, phase one and phase two of liver detoxification are balanced, and the process works efficiently to protect you against harmful toxins to which you are exposed in the environment or from those generated by the body's own biochemical activity.

Liver function is jeopardized, however, when the quantity of toxins within you is greater than it can process. This may be caused by toxic overload, by poor nutrition, and by the absence of nutrients required for the two phases of detoxification, or as a consequence of illness or disease.

Chapter 11 will give you information about how to help your liver function at its best with periodic cleanings and supplement support, and later in Chapter 13, you'll learn how to use diet to support optimal liver function. In the next chapter, let's look at another extremely important part of the detoxification system as well as of the immune system—the intestines.

Now, onward for Key Five . . .

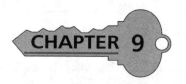

CHAPTER 9

KEY FIVE:
Detoxifying Your Intestines—From Managing Toxins to Improving Immunity

When I first began to study the principles of natural medicine, a consistent theme I encountered was that "illness begins in the gut." I considered this peculiar, since my concept of the intestines was limited to that of a food-processing factory. I had little awareness of the important role the intestines play in immune function. (More than half of our immune system is located in the intestinal tract!) I also knew little about the role the intestines play in any number of chronic diseases. I did not understand that, when the intestinal environment is altered, it can lead to dramatic symptoms (often, seemingly unrelated symptoms)—that eventually can lead to significant health problems.

In most systems of natural or traditional medicine, the health of the gastrointestinal tract (GI) is a central focus. Disturbances in intestinal chemistry can dramatically influence the metabolic code and are a principal cause of why people are spiraling away from health. Staying in tune with your GI tract and being proactive in taking care of it can reduce the chances of future diseases and conditions, and can, at the very least, help you avoid serious discomfort.

If most people were asked how to tell whether their intestines are functioning well, they would be hard pressed to answer. Many people define bowel health by the number of daily bowel movements. Usually once a day is considered adequate, but this is not the only indicator of a healthy bowel. You can have one healthy bowel movement daily, but still have unhealthy intestinal function.

Another problem with assessing whether we are intestinally healthy is the wide range of conditions that are accepted as fairly normal. Many patients experience uncomfortable GI symptoms after eating, and believe these signs are a normal part of their digestive process. They tell me matter-of-factly that after a meal, they get heartburn, feel tired, or need to unbuckle their belts due to bloating. These are the people who often seek out over-the-counter solutions for their discomfort with only modest results.

Finally, many people do know their intestines are out of balance. These are the people who suffer from intestinal disorders, such as irritable bowel syndrome, Crohn's disease, colitis, and diverticulitis. Many times, the intestinal symptoms these folks suffer occur alongside other disorders such as fibromyalgia, mood swings, diabetes, autoimmune disorders, skin disruptions, obesity, and weight gain. These patients have never had it explained to them that their intestinal symptoms could be a central factor in their struggle for health. Or that their intestinal complaints could be directly related to these other conditions, or even to a disease process that is just beginning to unfold.

It is not normal to feel bloated and gassy after meals, to fall asleep after eating, to have difficult bowel movements or chronic constipation. For many people, there is nothing more disruptive than chronic GI distress, but they are not being taught how to balance their intestinal function to alleviate the problems.

A healthy gastrointestinal tract affects all other body systems. The gut and its function are so important in attaining and maintaining health that if it is not healthy, it is not possible for the rest of the body to be healthy. In the case of the gut, *form* (or condition) truly follows *function*. If you had to pick a starting place on your journey toward health, intestinal health is a great place to start. Because of its impact on the rest of the body, most people experience significant benefits very quickly.

This chapter describes the many ways in which the intestines influence overall health and provides you with the tools to assess your own intestinal well-being.

MEET THE INTESTINES

Your gastrointestinal tract is truly amazing. It is a twenty-five to thirty foot hoselike organ that runs from the mouth to the anus, whose function is to acidify, liquefy, neutralize, and homogenize the foods we eat into microscopic particles that the cells can use for energy, maintenance, growth, and repair. This is the function of the intestines with which most people are familiar—the breakdown and processing of foods so that the body can utilize their nutrients.

The vitamins and minerals that the intestines physically and chemically unlock from food virtually run every aspect of body chemistry. These nutrients contribute to detoxification, controlling systemic inflammation, managing levels of homocysteine (an amino acid normally present in the blood), regulating insulin, maturing immune cells, and protecting arteries from becoming clogged with plaque—and that's just for starters. So, by compromising the body's ability to absorb the nutrients it needs, a challenged intestinal tract can have far-reaching, body-wide effects.

The intestines are also involved in the detoxification process. In a healthy digestive tract, there are a variety of *nonpathogenic bacteria* (often called friendly flora or microflora) that, along with the mucosal linings in the intestines, serve as the first line of defense between a fairly dangerous external world and our bodies. A balanced intestinal lining can maintain growth of billions of the friendly bacteria. A variety of potentially disease-causing bacteria (the bad "bugs") can get carried into our bodies on the foods we eat. These friendly bacteria provide a physical barrier to keep these bad bugs and other potentially harmful substances from causing havoc in the body. In addition, the friendly flora aid in the production of some vitamins. They can also change toxic compounds that are formed as a result of digestive processes into benign substances. They also help to keep a common fungi or yeast found in the gut known as *Candida albicans* from overcolonizing.

This leads to another role that the friendly microflora play: protection from *endotoxins* (internally produced toxins). Both yeast and some pathogenic bacteria produce waste products that are toxic to humans. For example, bacteria secrete endotoxins as part of their metabolic processes during their normal life cycle. During the process of reproduction or dying off, some emit highly toxic compounds. These toxins can be absorbed into the bloodstream and carried throughout the body, contributing to a range of both chronic and acute health problems. Also, they can make the intestinal tract permeable or leaky, which allows substances not normally allowed through to enter the bloodstream. In such cases, the immune system may produce an allergic response to an organism or its metabolic byproducts. Additional damage to the intestinal tissues can result from the production of free radicals that occurs when the bacterial balance is lost in the intestines.

The intestines affect hormone metabolism as well. The strong presence of unhealthy bacteria in the gut is but one example of how the intestines can affect this metabolism. The intestines, along with the liver, are the principal areas responsible for estrogen processing and elimination. Unfriendly bacteria may produce an enzyme called *beta glucuronidase.* This enzyme causes estrogen to be released from its estrogen-glucuronide bond, a bond created by the liver in phase-two detoxification. As estrogen is freed up in the intestine and reabsorbed into the body, chronic elevations in this freed estrogen can lead to an increase in estrogen-related disorders such as fibrocystic breast, ovarian cysts, endometriosis, or even to certain cancers such as breast cancer. While this process may not create problems overnight, it has a snowballing effect on body chemistry. The longer it goes on, the greater its influence.

IMMUNITY AND THE INTESTINES

The immune system is a complex system of responses that help to protect the body from toxic metabolites and the daily onslaught of bacterial, viral, and other infectious agents. In fighting off microbes, the immune system must be able to recognize them as invaders and to respond quickly. It does this by developing a "memory" of the invaders so that any future attacks from the same invaders can be responded to even more quickly.

Certain conditions can make for an immune system that begins to mistake harmless substances (such as plant pollens) or even body tissue as invaders, and will attack them as such, creating painful and annoying conditions such as hay fever and sometimes deadly autoimmune diseases. An unhealthy intestinal environment can also cause overstimulation of the immune system.

There are two general categories of immunity: *nonspecific* and *specific*. Nonspecific immunity involves the natural physical and chemical barriers to infection. Some of the barriers are the skin, the small hairs (cilia) inside the nose and lungs, stomach acid, and the mucous membrane linings. The GI tract also contains large amounts of lymph tissue. This, combined with the important role of the microflora, has led many to propose that at least 50 percent of the body's immunity is in the intestines with the remaining 50 percent in the lymph and thymus glands, the blood, and the spleen.

The process of phagocytosis is also part of nonspecific immunity. Phagocytes are cells that engulf and destroy foreign bodies, particularly antibody-antigen complexes, which are explained below. *Macrophages, neutrophils,* and *monocytes* are all phagocytic cells. Monocytes and neutrophils are mobile and are attracted to sites of inflammation. Macrophages are typically stationary and are found in the blood vessels, liver, spleen, lungs, lymph nodes, gut, and kidneys.

Specific immunity is the immune response to specific agents. This type of immunity is acquired by exposure to a substance. Substances that produce specific responses, which are unique to them and are forever imprinted in the "memory" of immune cells, are called *antigens*. Antigens can be bacteria, parasites, yeast, or other microbes, but in an unbalanced gut, antigens can also be organic compounds not usually considered harmful, such as carbohydrates, lipids, and proteins. Thus, if factors are out of balance in the gut and/or if digestion is not complete, not only does our immune system have to deal with excessive bacteria, it may have to deal with our foods.

The cells responsible for neutralizing antigens are *lymphocytes.* Lymphocytes originate in the marrow of long bones throughout the body. As they mature, some remain in the bone marrow and become B cells, while others are transported through the blood and lymphatic fluid to the thymus gland, where they eventually become T cells. T cells regulate cell-mediated immune responses to infection. This means the cell has the ability to attach to the foreign agent and destroy it. The three major types of T cells are *cytotoxic T cells, helper T cells,* and *suppressor T cells.*

Cytotoxic T cells travel throughout the body, attaching themselves to infected and cancerous cells. They secrete *interferons,* which prevent viruses from replicating. Cytotoxic T cells assist macrophages in their ability to engulf and digest infectious agents. Helper T cells help the cytotoxic T cells by secreting a substance called interleukin-2, which assists the helper T cells in directing the cytotoxic T cells. Helper T cells also secrete proteins called *interleukins* (cytokines) that serve as messengers for the cells of the immune system. They are responsible for changes in immune function that result in allergies and inflammatory and autoimmune reactions. Most important, helper T cells stimulate B cells to produce *antibodies.*

Notice the connection between the gut and inflammation: When immune cells are called into action, so are the cytokines, substances that cause inflammation. When the intestinal linings are not intact, too many bacteria can get through to the bloodstream, causing the immune cells to be overactive, and thereby can cause the oversecretion of inflammatory cytokines. This whole system depends on whether a state of equilibrium can be maintained.

Suppressor T cells balance the activities of cytotoxic and helper T cells. They prevent cytotoxic cells from releasing cytokines, and can inhibit the production of antibodies by suppressing the activity of helper T cells. For the suppressor T cells to work effectively in regulating this balance, the ratio of suppressor T cells to helper T cells should be 1:2.

B cells secrete proteins called *antibodies.* This part of the immune system is called humoral immunity. Antibodies bind with antigens, which mark them for destruction by cells so they can be detoxified and eliminated from the body by circulating phagocytes. This marking by antibodies is what identifies the antigen as a foreign substance (bacteria, toxic substance, or viruses) that needs to be removed from the body.

There are five general classifications of antibodies; they are called immunoglobulins and are classified as follows: IgE, IgM, IgA, IgD, and IgG. Each antibody is unique to the antigen for which it is created and, under normal circumstances, reacts only with that antigen. IgG antibodies are the most abundant and are found in blood, lymph, and the intestines. IgA antibodies are also found in gastrointestinal secretions.

The immune system uses these specialized troops and weapons to constantly remove toxins that have gotten past the GI tract and into the bloodstream. Under ideal conditions, natural body functions create low levels of toxic stress that we are designed to handle without difficulty. However, an imbalance in microflora, stress, pollution, increased free-radical activity, and poor nutrition create conditions that are far from ideal. The cumulative effect of internal toxins depletes our capacity for detoxification, putting greater stress on the immune system. In other words, when the immune system is forced to overwork because of an improperly functioning intestinal tract, the body will eventually become hypersensitized and susceptible to allergy, inflammation, and autoimmune disorders.

Any disruption in normal immune function can lead us down the spiral to immune and cellular deregulation causing our metabolism to be disrupted on a cellular level. It is important to take every measure to not overtax the immune system. It can only work so hard for so long. If the immune system is constantly fighting invaders that get through the intestinal tract, it will become overwhelmed and will not be able to adequately fight disease and infections. As seen by the atrophy that occurs with old age, the thymus gland wears out over time. By keeping the immune system from overworking when possible, we can help to preserve our thymus gland, which helps us to maintain a stronger immune system as we enter old age. By maintaining a healthy gut, we support our immune system.

HOW THE DIGESTIVE TRACT FUNCTIONS

The digestive tract consists of the small and large intestines. The intestines are tube-like structures composed of three layers: the intestinal *mucosa, submucosa,* and muscle. The mucosa is where absorption of nutrients takes place. The submucosa contains the larger blood vessels, and the muscle layer is what provides the contractions of the intestine that moves the food around and through the intestinal tract.

In order to understand what can go wrong in the intestine, it is important to understand what the intestine is, how it is laid out, and how it works. Taking the time to read this section will greatly help your understanding of how to keep your intestines healthy.

The Small Intestine

The small intestine is made up of three components: *the duodenum, the jejunum,* and *the ileum.* The functions of the small intestine are to receive secretions from the pancreas and liver, complete the digestion of the food and other substances from the stomach, absorb nutrients, and transport the remainder to the large intestine.

The duodenum is the first and shortest portion of the small intestine, measuring about ten inches long. It is the part of the intestines that receives the contents from your stomach (called *chyme*) after a meal. It is nestled close to the pancreas, and upon receiving chyme, it also receives secretions of digestive enzymes from the pancreas. This is also where bile enters the intestines to aid digestion of fats. The small intestine also secretes digestive enzymes of its own, including *peptidases, sucrase, maltase, lactase,* and *intestinal lipase,* which help to complete digestion of proteins, different types of sugars, and fats.

The midsection of the small intestine is the jejunum. While some digestion of foods start in the mouth and in the stomach, most digestion takes place and is completed in the duodenum and the first part of the jejunum. Absorption of the broken down carbohydrates, fats, and proteins, along with most vitamins and minerals, takes place primarily in the first twenty to forty inches of the jejunum.

The ileum is the last section of the small intestine. It carries what remains of the chyme to the large intestine, and is the part of the intestines that absorbs vitamin B_{12} (cyanocobalamin). The ileum is capable of absorbing other nutrients, but apparently absorption is so efficient in the first few feet that not much is left for the ileum. The ileum is where most of the reabsorption of bile salts takes place, however. The ileum is similar to the jejunum and duodenum in appearance, except that more lymphatic tissue is present. Groups of lymphatic nodules (large enough to be seen with the naked eye) called *Peyer's patches* are present in lining of the ileum. The increased concentration of lymphatic tissue toward the end of the small intestine reflects the fact that the large intestine contains huge numbers of bacteria that must be prevented from entering the bloodstream.

The inner wall of the small intestine contains billions of tiny fingerlike projections called *villi*. It is through these villi that the nutrients must pass before becoming absorbed by the blood or the lymph. The intestinal villi serve to increase the total surface area of the intestines and therefore increase absorptive surface for maximum absorption of nutrients.

The outer layer of each *villus* consists of a single layer of *epithelial cells*. This is where most nutrients actually pass into the blood, through the absorptive cells of the epithelial lining. These cells are continuously shed and replaced by new cells, which migrate from the inner lining. The epithelial lining is renewed approximately every four days. (Interestingly, chemotherapy drugs attack rapidly dividing cells, including the epithelial cells in the gut. This is the reason for the intestinal disturbances that occur during chemotherapy.) The surface of each epithelial cell is covered with *microvilli,* hairlike extensions that serve to further increase the digestive surface area.

Within each villus are blood capillaries, a lymphatic capillary, and nerve fibers. The blood and lymph transport the products of digestion, and the nerve fibers stimulate or inhibit the activity within the villi. The lymph capillary is responsible for the absorption of most fats (medium-chain triglycerides are absorbed in the blood) and all the fat-soluble vitamins. In fact, fat-soluble vitamins won't be absorbed unless they are ingested with some fat.

The Large Intestine

The large intestine is divided into four parts: the *ascending, transverse, descending,* and *sigmoid* colon. While the small intestine is more than twenty feet long, the large intestine is only five feet long. It derives its name from its diameter, which is larger than the small intestine.

The ascending colon begins in the lower right quadrant of the abdomen, where it is connected to the lower portion of the small intestine at the *cecum.* The cecum is a pouch with a valve that opens into the large intestine at one end, and the small intestine at the other. Extending from the left side is a closed tube that points downward. The closed tube is the *appendix,* which contains lymphatic tissue. The appendix does not have any known digestive function, but may have some role in immunity. The ascending colon is positioned vertically and travels up the abdominal cavity until it reaches just below the liver, where it turns left and becomes the transverse colon.

The transverse colon moves across the abdomen, just below the stomach, until it reaches the area of the spleen on the left side. There, it turns downward and becomes the descending colon. At the tip of the descending colon, near the pelvic cavity, the sigmoid colon makes a sharp "s" curve and empties into the rectum. The last one or two inches of the large intestine consists of the anal canal, which houses the anal opening.

The lining of the colon is very similar to that of the small intestine. The walls of the small and large intestine have five layers. The innermost layer of the colon is a mucous membrane (known as the intestinal mucosa) that contains *goblet cells.* The goblet cells form glands that secrete mucous. Mucous protects the inside of the colon, controls the pH (acid/alkaline balance), and consolidates the *chyme* from the small intestine. The mucosal surface of the digestive tract is formed of epithelial cells, which have a rapid rate of turnover. These cells usually die, slough off, and regenerate every four to five days. Epithelial cells are quick to regenerate when injured. However, if the rate of injury or irritation exceeds the rate at which the cells can regenerate, the lining can become inflamed, irritated, or broken down. The middle layers of the intestine house blood vessels and nerves, and circular muscle. The outer layers include a layer of longitudinal muscle and the peritoneal wall.

The large intestine's primary functions are to absorb water and electrolytes (the form in which most minerals circulate in the body), to synthesize certain vitamins such as niacin, vitamins B_1 (thiamine), B_2 (riboflavin), B_6 (pyridoxine), B_{12}, as well as folic acid, biotin, and vitamin K, and to store and eliminate waste. It should be noted here that the friendly bacteria mentioned earlier reside mostly in the large intestines where they not only complete the digestion of any remaining carbohydrates, but also synthesize the vitamins referred to above. (The functions of the friendly flora will be discussed in more detail later.)

The chyme that enters the colon from the small intestine contains mostly water, 90 percent of which is absorbed before elimination. It also contains undigested food, bacteria, bile, electrolytes, dead epithelium, and mucus. The movement of this fecal material through the large intestine is powered by muscular contractions known as peristalsis. The large intestine contracts two or three times per day, moving its contents toward the sigmoid colon. The defecation reflex is stimulated when feces enter the rectum. Feces contain mostly water, along with bile pigments, undigested fiber, fat, protein, mucus, electrolytes, and bacteria. The time it takes food to transit the entire gastrointestinal tract (bowel transit time) is approximately fourteen to twenty-four hours.

CONDITIONS OF THE INTESTINAL TRACT

Digestive illnesses are reaching epidemic proportions in the United States. It is estimated that 62 million Americans, or one-third of adults, suffer from diseases and conditions of the gastrointestinal tract. Diseases of the gastrointestinal tract are among the most debilitating and costly conditions afflicting our society. According to some reports, digestive disorders rank *third* in the total economic burden of disease, placing a significant drain on the workforce, personal expense, and the overall economy. The majority of these health problems are far from minor complaints; they often can result in debilitating and even life-threatening disease.

Like many other chronic diseases, gastrointestinal conditions are triggered as a result of dietary assaults, nutritional deficiencies, and lifestyle factors. Other more insidious culprits such as drug use and exposure to various environmental toxins can also alter mucosal membrane integrity, initiate inflammation, and push the gut into creating a metabolic nightmare for the rest of the body. It's no wonder that the numbers of people with intestinal disorders are skyrocketing when you consider all the underlying factors contributing to it. Add to this the general lack of awareness or even interest as to just how important the gut is to your health, and you have an area of the body that is ripe for disease.

Most people do not realize that there are many ways to improve gut function and eliminate so many of the common GI complaints such as gas, heartburn, constipation, and even irritable bowel symptoms. They do not know they can take charge by evaluating their diet and their environment and by understanding what they are doing to their digestive system. Instead, people only know to keep running for an antacid, an H2 (histamine-receptor) blocker such as cimetidine (Tagamet, Zantac), or for some other "Band-Aid" for their gastrointestinal distress. Commonly used pain medications, such as ibuprofen (Motrin, Advil, and Nuprin) and aspirin (Bayer, Ecotrin, and others) may increase damage to the intestinal lining and cause more inflammation, irritation, and pain, and exacerbate the continuation and severity of the problem.

The following are the most common gastrointestinal disorders. Even if you do not suffer from any particular gastrointestinal complaint, this section still pertains to you. By learning how to recognize these conditions before they occur, you'll be protecting your intestinal health and possibly the health of your whole body.

Inflammatory Bowel Disease

Inflammatory bowel disease (IBD) is an autoimmune (self-attacking) condition that is characterized by inflammation of the intestinal lining, abdominal pains, cramps, and diarrhea, which may be accompanied by fever and rectal bleeding. IBD actually refers to two conditions: Crohn's disease and ulcerative colitis. The single term is used because many of the symptoms of these two conditions are similar. However, as you will learn below, there are differences.

It is estimated that IBD affects approximately 50 million Americans. IBD tends to be more prevalent among people of Jewish descent and in those whose immune systems have become overactive due to some sort of chronic toxic exposure, intestinal infection, or imbalanced intestinal flora. Ultimately, the immune system is unable to regulate the overactivity, and the process of chronic inflammation begins to take its toll on the colon lining. Food allergy, stress, dysbiosis, a high-sugar/low-fiber diet, and infection have been implicated as contributing factors.

Crohn's Disease

Crohn's disease is an inflammatory bowel disorder caused by *granulomatous* lesions

(lesions that have large cells that are chronically inflamed). Approximately 150 out of 100,000 people in the United States are affected by Crohn's disease. These lesions cause inflammation that permeates deep into the intestinal wall, frequently causing intermittent diarrhea, weight loss, crampy abdominal pain, low-grade fever, loss of appetite, and gas. In Crohn's disease, the lesions can penetrate through all layers of the intestinal wall and can occur in the small and large intestine and even in some organs. Malabsorption and nutritional deficiencies are common. Although it appears to have a genetic basis, Crohn's disease does not manifest until triggered by the presence of an offending food or bacteria that causes an abnormal response by the immune system. A diet high in sugar and low in fiber exacerbates the symptoms.

Food allergies or intolerances and leaky gut syndrome may also play a role in the development of Crohn's disease, most likely due to the immune-mediated inflammatory response. The inflammation and irritation in the intestinal epithelial cells can eventually lead to increased sensitivity to foods.

Traditional treatment of Crohn's disease includes the use of corticosteroids to control inflammation, antidiarrheals, and anticholinergic drugs to help suppress cramping. Left untreated, this disease may increase the risk of colon cancer.

Ulcerative Colitis

Affecting as many as 400,000 Americans, ulcerative colitis is a chronic disorder, in which the mucous membranes lining the colon become inflamed and develop ulcers, causing bloody diarrhea, lower abdominal pain, fever, and weight loss, and occasionally hard stools. People who suffer from this condition are at high risk for developing colorectal cancer. In comparison to Crohn's disease, the lesions in this disease affect only the inner lining of the colon, and they occur only in the large intestine.

Traditional treatment for ulcerative colitis may vary according to the severity of the case from the use of nonsteroidal anti-inflammatory (NSAIDs) drugs to surgery for removal of the diseased sections of the intestine.

Colorectal Cancer

Colorectal cancer is a carcinoma of either the colon or rectum, or of both, that occurs due to the formation of cytotoxic factors (that is, anything that is toxic to cells and causes damage to the inner lining and overgrowth of intestinal outer lining). When the intestinal lining is irritated, it sheds and replaces cells more quickly. This process, known as *hyperproliferation,* increases the risk of *neoplasms,* or tumors. This indicates that to reduce the risk of colorectal cancer, it is prudent to prevent anything that causes irritation to the lining of the intestine. Colorectal cancer is the *second* most common cause of death from cancer in the United States. Food allergies, stress, a diet low in fiber and high in animal protein and saturated fat, calcium, and folic acid deficiencies increase the risk for this cancer.

Traditional treatment of colorectal cancer includes surgery, radiation, and chemotherapy, or any combination of the three treatments.

Constipation

Constipation is a symptom rather than a disease. It is one of the most frequently reported medical problems in the United States and is estimated to affect approximately 3 million Americans. This number, however, is most likely lower than it really is. One of the problems with tracking the statistics on constipation is that people aren't really sure what it is. I have many patients report to me that they are not constipated, then I find out they are only having a bowel movement every two or three days, one of the indicators of constipation.

Constipation is characterized by hardened stools, difficulty completing a bowel movement, or a decrease in normal frequency of bowel movements. While it's easy to think that constipation is not a serious problem, chronic constipation can have serious health effects. Fecal matter that moves too slowly through the colon can increase the fermentation of foods, feeding undesired bacteria in the gut. These bacteria emit metabolic waste products, which can be absorbed into the bloodstream. Slow transit time can give rise to many different conditions, including allergies, depression, diverticulitis, dysbiosis, fatigue, gallstones, gas, headaches, hemorrhoids, indigestion, obesity, and varicose veins. It may even be involved in serious diseases such as cancers of the colon and breast.

In many cases, constipation is caused by insufficient fiber and water intake. Most doctors first recommend increasing fiber, water intake, and exercise to treat constipation. If these measures are ineffective, laxatives and/or stool softeners may be given. However, they are not a good permanent solution because people can become dependent upon them to have a bowel movement.

Diarrhea

Diarrhea is characterized by frequent and loose, watery stools that may be accompanied by abdominal pain, cramping, vomiting, and, in cases of chronic diarrhea, fever and/or mucus or blood in the stool. This condition affects some 99 million Americans at any given time.

Like constipation, diarrhea is a symptom rather than a disease. It may be an isolated incident or may result as a symptom of many possible factors, including dumping syndrome (the rapid emptying of stomach contents, usually right after a meal); excess alcohol consumption; food allergies; lactase insufficiency (an inability to digest milk proteins); infections; use of laxatives such as magnesium salts, senna, or cascara; undigested carbohydrates in the bowel; and emotional stress. Antibiotics, chronic aspirin or nonsteroidal anti-inflammatories (NSAIDs) use, chemotherapy, radiation, Crohn's disease, food poisoning, and ulcerative colitis, also cause chronic diarrhea.

Diarrhea is treated by removal of the offending food or substance, by replacement of electrolytes and fluids, and by use of anti-diarrheal medications.

Diverticular Disease

Diverticular disease includes *diverticulosis* and *diverticulitis.* Diverticulosis is a condition in which pouchlike formations, called *diverticula,* occur in the colon. These are actually areas where the muscle layer of the colon wall has become weak. Diverticulosis occurs in 10 percent of people over the age of forty and in 50 percent of people over the age of sixty. People with diverticulosis disease often don't know they have the condition. Its symptoms—constipation, intermittent diarrhea, and flatulence—are often dismissed or overlooked. It is associated with a low-fiber diet and is not generally found in less developed countries where refined foods are not eaten. When the intestinal contractions are taking place with hardened stools, they are much harder to move. This apparently creates such pressure that the colon wall bulges into the abdominal cavity, and fecal matter becomes trapped within the folds of the diverticula. Sometimes, the diverticula become inflamed and infected; this is diverticulitis.

If diverticulitis develops, complications can be serious. *Fistulas,* openings between two segments of the intestinal wall may develop. If the diverticula burst, penetrating the wall, the result can be a potentially fatal inflammation of the abdominal cavity wall known as peritonitis. Anything that contributes to a hardened stool, like a low-fiber diet and not staying well hydrated, contributes to development of these conditions.

Typically, diverticulitis is treated with NSAIDs, antibiotics, and a low-fiber diet until inflammation subsides. Afterwards, the fiber content of the diet is increased incrementally until well tolerated.

Irritable Bowel Syndrome

Irritable bowel syndrome (IBS) is the most common digestive disorder treated by physicians. It is estimated that 20 percent of the population suffers from symptoms of IBS, which is also known as spastic colon, spastic bowel, mucous colitis, colitis, and functional bowel disease. In IBS, the normal rhythmic contractions of the digestive tract become uncoordinated, causing irregular peristaltic contractions, which can result in erratic and uncomfortable movements. This disrupts the normal processing of food and waste material, which can accumulate in the intestines, causing obstructions, and accumulation of toxins. Signs of IBS are alternating constipation and diarrhea, including symptoms such as abdominal pain, gas, bloating, and cramping. Nutritional deficiencies are common among IBS sufferers, as the irritable bowel does not optimally absorb nutrients from food.

The cause of this disorder may have a genetic component, but is largely not known. Food allergy or sensitivity, digestive enzyme deficiencies, lactose intolerance, medications such as NSAIDs and aspirin, dysbiosis, bacterial overgrowth, parasites, a low-fiber diet, and stress are all possible contributing factors. In some cases, people may require food allergy testing or a comprehensive digestive stool analysis to further understand other factors that may be contributing to their IBS.

Traditionally, prescription medications are used to control the symptoms of IBS. These include antidiarrheals, antispasmodics, antidepressants, and fiber products depending on the symptoms.

WHERE THE REAL TROUBLE OFTEN BEGINS

Quite often, treatments for problems of the gastrointestinal tract do not address the underlying conditions that cause these ailments. Long before these conditions surface, slight insults to the intestinal lining or small shifts in the numbers of micro-flora are occurring, and immune function is weakening. Gradually, over time, an unhealthy gut becomes an entry point for the slow leaching of toxins.

Dysbiosis, leaky gut syndrome, and food allergies are conditions that, while not often clinically diagnosed, are proving to be underlying, or at least major contributing factors, in many of the common digestive disorders discussed above, as well as a wide variety of complex systemic disorders. Dysbiosis, leaky gut syndrome, food allergies, and a weakened immune system are all interwoven in a labyrinth of intestinal dysfunction and related systemic disorders. Parasites, not often thought about in our culture, are also sometimes an underlying cause of intestinal disturbance.

Let's now look at how these insidious and indirect processes of bowel dysfunction can have devastating effects on total body metabolism and chemistry.

Parasitic Infections

Though not nearly as common in the United States as other parts of the world, parasites can be an underlying cause for digestive disruption and other health problems. Parasitic infections are on the rise in the United States due in part to the increase of foods imported from other countries. One of the problems that we face today in America is that only 1 to 2 percent of the foods that are imported are actually inspected. Sanitation practices vary from country to country. In fact, the Food and Drug Administration (FDA) has just recently changed inspection procedures in order to address this problem because of the drastic rise in parasitic infections in this country.

The symptoms from parasitic infections vary from indigestion, gas, and bloating to headaches, fatigue, and joint pain. Many also cause diarrhea, and if untreated, they can lead to severe damage of the intestinal mucosa, increased permeability of the gut, and subsequent absorption of bacterial toxins, yeast, and undigested food molecules. Typically, the person is either someone who occasionally or regularly eats raw seafood such as sushi or raw oysters, or it is someone who has traveled to another country. Parasites can be transmitted through the fecal-oral route, commonly by contact with unsanitary food and water. This is a polite way of saying that bacteria-laden stool from one person finds its way onto a food and into the mouth of another, which ends up causing an infection.

Intestinal parasitic organisms can be classified as one of three types: protozoa such as *Giardia* (single-celled organisms that constitute the majority of parasitic infections), *Platyhelminthes* such as flukes or tapeworms (flatworms), and *Aschelminthes* also known as nematodes (roundworms). More than one-third of the global population is infected with parasitic worms.

Conventional treatment begins with correctly identifying the intestinal parasite, which is not easily done. Some parasites can be detected by salivary or intestinal IgA antibody testing. Stool cultures for *Giardia* antigens and abnormal bacteria are highly sensitive.

Parasitic infections can remain dormant for months after initial infection. Symptoms can recur after treatment, sometimes differing from the first outbreak. Drug resistance and incomplete treatment are common causes of recurrence. Within a month after treatment, stool cultures should be repeated. Immunologic testing should be done again after three months.

The conventional treatments for parasites tend to disrupt the normal intestinal flora and lead to dysbiosis, discussed below. So, typically in a nutritional approach, therapy focuses on reestablishing a healthy gut lining. This information is not meant to make you paranoid, but to help you realize that parasitic infections are probably a much larger issue in this country than most of us think. In many cultures, the periodic use of herbs to rid the body of parasites is common. Even in our own cultural history, an extract of black walnut (*Juglans nigra,* a vermifuge or parasite-killing substance) was made in the fall and used by people in rural communities.

There are numerous nutraceutical agents that are very effective in and have a long history of use for intestinal parasites. These are discussed in depth in Chapter 11.

Dysbiosis

Dysbiosis is one of the most common underlying issues leading to health problems. Almost every person who walks into my office has some form of dysbiosis. In my estimation, dysbiosis is one of the most important problems that people must deal with to get their metabolism back on track. Also, I believe that it is truly one of the key factors contributing to GI problems; autoimmune disturbances; allergies and asthma; cognitive, neurologic, and behavioral problems; diabetes; cardiovascular disease; and cancer. As mentioned in the beginning of this chapter, disease really can begin in the gut! I always work on this aspect of a person's chemistry as a top priority. The results that people feel are, at times, nothing short of spectacular.

The concept of dysbiosis is not hard to understand. There is an enormous ecosystem of microorganisms in the gut. Simply put, dysbiosis is the disharmony caused when the balance of this ecosystem in the intestine is disrupted, causing an alteration in the number and type of organisms that inhabit it. This differs from a normal state of *symbiosis,* in which both the host and microbes benefit from their relationship. Simple enough, right? Health equals balance when it comes to intestinal flora, and imbalance equals disease.

The number of these microorganisms is staggering. For every gram of feces, there may be as many as a hundred billion microbial cells. The most abundant microflora in the colon are *anaerobic* bacteria (meaning they live without oxygen), followed by *aerobic* bacteria (meaning they live only in the presence of oxygen), yeast, and protozoa. These bacteria live on the mucosal surface of the small intestine and colon and in the lumen (the inside of the colon) in either symbiotic or antagonistic relationships, where they feed off fermented carbohydrates from fiber and simple sugars.

Intestinal bacteria are of three basic types. Most bacteria in the digestive tract are probiotic, meaning they are the "good" or "friendly" types of bacteria. Examples of probiotic bacteria are *Bifidobacteria spp., Lactobacillus spp. (L. acidophilus, L. rhamnosus, L. bifidus, L. casei and L. plantarum*). Probiotic bacteria live in harmony with the intestinal tract by helping in the breakdown and absorption of nutrients, making vitamins the body can use and by detoxifying substances in the gut. We allow them to inhabit us because they provide nutritional and digestive benefits. They also manufacture antibiotics, such as acidophilin, which are effective against many types of bacteria, including *Streptococcus* and *Staphylococcus.* Friendly flora play an important role in our ability to fight infections, providing a front line in our immune defense.

The second type of bacteria that reside in the gastrointestinal tract are the "commensals." They are considered neutral bacteria; they neither help nor harm the body. The third type of bacteria is "unfriendly," or harmful bacteria that can cause illness. Examples of pathogenic bacteria are *Clostridium, Salmonella, Staphylococcus, Proteus, Campylobacter,* and *Listeria.* Bacteria that cause chronic illness are generally weak organisms. They are often found in small quantities in all of us and are harmless in small numbers. Yet, when these organisms are given the opportunity to thrive, they can and do cause illness.

The ecosystem within the intestine is dynamic. It changes constantly in response to variables in the environment, within the host, and among the presence of other microbes. There are a variety of influences that can affect the intestinal microflora. The most common causes of dysbiosis include:

- altered gastrointestinal pH (acid-alkaline balance)
- antibiotic overuse
- birth control pills
- chemicals (pesticides, herbicides, preservatives, solvents)
- chemotherapy and radiation exposure
- chronic stress

- diets high in refined sugars and grains

- excess alcohol consumption (especially, beer, wine, fermented liquors)

- food additives

- *H. pylori* infection (an ulcer-causing bacteria)

- heavy metal exposure (lead, cadmium, and especially mercury)

- pain reliever use (especially NSAIDS, antacids, and corticosteroids)

Dysbiosis most often involves the overcolonization of intestinal flora that can be harmful to the body. Dysbiosis of the small intestine results in *fermentation* (faulty digestion of carbohydrates that results in gases, sugars, and alcohol) whereas the condition in the large intestine is described as *putrefactive* faulty digestion of fats and animal protein that results in gases, sugars, and alcohol. Both forms of dysbiosis can result in problems of metabolic toxicity.

Bacterial and yeast overgrowth in the upper GI tract interferes with carbohydrate digestion, in part by the destruction of pancreatic and intestinal enzymes by proteases. Partially undigested carbohydrates enter the large intestine, where bacteria and yeast feed on them and produce gases. This fermentation results in abdominal distention, bloating, and gas. Some of the metabolic byproducts of carbohydrate metabolism, including ethanol and D-lactic acid, are absorbed systemically. Ethanol causes mental cloudiness and fatigue, like a metabolic intoxication. D-lactic acid can decrease the local pH in cells, leading to disruptions in cellular metabolism and elevations of blood lactate levels. An increase in lactic acid in the cells means less energy produced. Elevated lactate levels are now being linked with severe candida imbalances, anxiety disorders, and fibromyalgia. Damage to the intestinal mucosa, increased intestinal permeability, and malabsorption are other complications associated with fermentation.

Typically, dysbiosis will result in a deficiency of beneficial intestinal flora, which is a problem for several reasons. First, as we've alluded to, in the absence of probiotics, unwanted microbes are able to grow unchecked. Second, an imbalance of intestinal flora can lead to the depletion of essential nutrients. A healthy intestinal ecology has important functions of its own, without which the body cannot operate efficiently. Bacteria synthesize vitamin K, estrogen, and some B vitamins, and help form the short-chain fatty acids butyrate and acetic acid. Butyrate helps to maintain the intestinal lining, and along with acetic acid, may help lower serum cholesterol. Some bacteria improve lactose digestion, and help process environmental and metabolic toxins. Lastly, these probiotic flora help to keep the metabolism of hormones, such as estrogen, on track. Also, they help to guide the genetic expression of the cells of the intestine, making a significant impact on the blueprint for future cells that will line the intestine.

The lining of the gastrointestinal tract is a natural protective barrier against infection. When the lining of the gastrointestinal tract is damaged or irritated, its protective function is impaired. When microorganisms, such as dysbiotic bacteria, yeast, or parasites, contact the damaged mucosa, they can penetrate the barrier and even enter the bloodstream where they do not belong.

Candidiasis

The most common and most insidious form of dysbiosis is *candidiasis,* which is an overgrowth of the yeast *Candida albicans.* (Hereafter, the terms "yeast" and "candida" are used interchangeably.)

Candida is yeast that normally inhabits the mucous membranes of the body, including the gastrointestinal lining, the urinary tract, sinus cavity, and the vagina. *Candida* is harmless when present in small quantities. But, sometimes, conditions arise that permit the yeast to flourish and reproduce beyond what is normally tolerable to the host. Larger numbers of *Candida* produce larger numbers of toxins, which further irritate and break down the intestinal lining, creating toxic conditions in the body that can lead to symptoms in virtually every body system. (See Table 9.1 on page 174.) This effect has been termed *Candida-related complex* (CRC). And once CRC has been established, simply destroying the yeast usually does not alleviate the symptoms.

Considerable attention has been given to CRC because of its growing prevalence, debilitating symptoms, and connection to a multitude of other diseases. Unfortunately, until recently, candidiasis was rarely recognized in standard medical practice. Until now, only two yeast-related conditions have commonly been diagnosed and treated by most clinicians: vaginal yeast infections and the life-threatening infection of the blood, *candidemia.* Candidiasis, as a low-grade systemic imbalance, has usually been overlooked.

Causes of Yeast Overgrowth. The conditions that encourage yeast overgrowth are similar for those that create dysbiosis. The most important variable in *Candida* overgrowth is the immune status of the host. A weak immune system allows unwanted microorganisms, including candida, to overcome the healthy bacteria that would flourish in a normal environment.

Yeast, as an opportunistic organism, is common throughout nature. Whenever a species is weakened or compromised, fungus looms in the shadows awaiting the chance to grow and feed off decaying matter. To understand how debilitating fungus can be, consider, for example, seeing a huge tree that has a very small ring of fungus around its trunk. The forester would tell you that the tree's immune system is compromised and that the tree will be fallen in the next five years. You look at the tree and think, "That little line of fungus will down that big tree? No way." Sure enough, five years later, the tree is fallen and fungus is growing all over it, and a few years from that, it is broken back down in to the earth.

Table 9.1. Major Symptoms Associated with Chronic Candidiasis

EFFECTS ON THE BODY CAUSED BY YEAST TOXINS	PRIMARY SYMPTOMS ASSOCIATED WITH CRC
Cardiovascular	Potential for increased plaque formation, an increase in C-reactive protein and homocysteine
Endocrine	Disturbances in blood glucose, subclinical hypothyroidism (decreased metabolism), hypoadrenal function, PMS, endometriosis, infertility, dysmenorrhea, decreased sex drive
Gastrointestinal	Gas, bloating, constipation, diarrhea, intolerance or reactivity to food, irritable bowel syndrome (IBS)
Immune	Food sensitivities, allergies, intolerance to fumes, odors, chemicals, autoimmune diseases, decreased resistance to infection, decreased immune regulation abilities
Neurological	Difficulty concentrating, short-term memory deficit, chronic fatigue, mental fogginess, neurasthenia
Nutritional	Essential fatty acid, vitamin, protein, mineral deficiencies; intense cravings for carbohydrates and sugar
Other	Impaired oxygen transport by red blood cells, imbalance of proinflammatory prostaglandins leading to joint inflammation, symptoms of fibromyalgia, skin problems (acne, eczema, psoriasis, rosacea), post-nasal drip, sinusitis, asthma, chest congestion, tightness, shortness of breath
Psychological	Depression, anxiety, insomnia, mood swings, reduced attention span, hyperactivity, autism
Urogenital	Chronic vaginal yeast infections, urinary tract infections, cystitis, prostate disorders

You can think of our relationship to fungus in a similar way. Cancer patients, weakened by disease and by multiple rounds of chemotherapy, commonly develop severe opportunistic yeast infections, as do patients with HIV (human immunodeficiency virus). In essence, the weaker your natural defenses are, the more susceptible you become for yeast, as well as any bacteria or fungus, to proliferate in your body and rob you of your vitality. This process can be occurring for a long time in your body, disrupting your immune response and many other aspects of your metabolism. The rising use of antifungal medications in our population and the growing body of research linking yeast to a wide array of symptoms is evidence that this problem is becoming more prevalent.

Candida overgrowth is typically triggered by overuse of antibiotics and other commonly used medications. These drugs disrupt the balance of the intestinal tract, kill the bacteria that keep *Candida* in check, and the yeast infection quickly takes hold. Once considered "magic bullets" with unlimited potential, antibiotics may have, to a certain extent, proven to be the Trojan horse of modern medicine. Certainly, antibiotics have saved millions of lives. However, their overuse has resulted in microbial evolution and a frightening increase in the development of resistant species. In addition, the overuse of antibiotics can lead to a weakened host defense.

Much of the increase in bacterial resistance has been caused by the use of antibiotics for viral infections (for example, bronchitis, colds, or purulent nasal discharge), which usually don't respond to antibiotics unless a bacterial infection is also present, as well as for throat infections, which are not "strep" in nature. Most viral infections are self-limiting. In other words, the treatment should be to wait and to simply let the infection "run its course," while supporting the patient's system with nutritional supplements in order to achieve a positive result. In addition to the misuse of antibiotics, pressure from patients for physicians to prescribe antibiotics has contributed to the rise in antibiotic resistance.

When the problem of resistance to antibiotics first became apparent, the "solution" was to create a new generation of antibiotics with a broader range of antibacterial force. Broad-spectrum antibiotics, by nature, destroy a variety of microorganisms, including beneficial flora. Not everyone who takes these antibiotics will develop candidiasis, but with chronic use, the seed is planted for yeast imbalances. It is the child or person who has been on three, four, and more rounds a year that has the increased risk of disrupting their intestinal health. I have patients who have been on antibiotics continuously for three or more years at a time. Sometimes this is necessary, and if so, steps should be taken to counterbalance the effects of the antibiotic on probiotic flora.

Repeated rounds of antibiotic therapy without replacement of beneficial flora will almost always lead to immune dysfunction. Studies have shown the overuse of antibiotics to be a driving force in the increasing rates not only of fungal infections, but also of allergic asthma, allergies, eczema, attention deficit disorder (ADD), attention deficit hyperactivity disorder (ADHD), and autism.

Other types of medications that encourage the proliferation of *Candida* include corticosteroids, NSAIDs, chemotherapy, and some antacids. Corticosteroids are commonly used to treat inflammation, allergies, and autoimmune diseases such as rheumatoid arthritis, Crohn's disease, and asthma. Synthetic corticosteroids such as prednisone and cortisone mimic the corticosteroids produced by the adrenal glands. Although they can be extremely beneficial, long-term use of corticosteroids suppresses the immune system, making conditions favorable for *Candida* growth, and induces bone loss, diabetes, and muscle wasting.

NSAIDs are a class of pain relievers that include aspirin, ibuprofen, naproxen (Naprosyn), and the newer generation of NSAIDS including rofecoxib (Vioxx) and celecoxib (Celebrex). These medications are frequently prescribed for the control of pain and inflammation associated with rheumatoid arthritis, osteoarthritis, and other chronic inflammatory conditions. Their principal mechanism of action is the inhibition of the enzyme cyclooxygenase, which is necessary for the formation of prostaglandins (hormonelike substances). Prostaglandin E2 (PGE2) is present in large amounts in the synovial fluid of those with rheumatoid arthritis, and is responsible for the swelling, vasodilation, and bone destruction that accompanies this disorder.

PGE2 is also the primary mediator of pain and fever. The therapeutic effect of NSAIDs stems from the nonselective inhibition of PGE2.

Antacids, specifically H2 blockers such as cimetidine, famotidine (Pepcid), and omeprazole (Prilosec) are associated with an increase in fungal overgrowth. H2-blockers increase the pH (acid-alkaline balance) of the stomach by blocking the production of gastric acid. Stomach acid normally plays an important role in destroying unwanted microorganisms before they can enter the intestine. An elevated pH promotes yeast growth in the intestinal tract and contributes to candidiasis in susceptible individuals.

Chronic use of NSAIDs is reported to be damaging to the intestinal lining, leading to inflammation and increased permeability. Not only does chronic use of these drugs weaken the immune system and increase the risk for gastrointestinal bleeding, but it also provides a foothold for opportunistic pathogens like *Candida.*

Chemotherapy also triggers rapid development in yeast symptoms. In fact, it is my belief that most people who are developing cancer already are experiencing a fungal overgrowth. Some of the more common side effects of chemotherapy include oral mucositis or inflammation of the mucosal membrane in the mouth, thrush (*Candida* in the mouth), and constipation and diarrhea, which result from the decline of the beneficial flora. People who are undergoing chemotherapy, at the very least, should be made aware of problems that can occur from the killing off of the friendly flora during chemotherapy, because maintaining nutritional status in cancer patients is already a challenge. A big mistake that cancer patients make, usually because they just don't know better, is that they don't work at balancing their bodies' chemistry after the chemotherapy and radiation is finished.

Diet is another important factor in yeast overgrowth. Yeast thrives on sugar, and any diet that is high in refined sugar and carbohydrates promotes yeast proliferation. Refined sugar, of which Americans eat approximately 150 pounds a year, as well as other refined sweeteners such as corn syrup, has been shown to increase the ability of yeast to adhere to mucous membranes.

Refined carbohydrates are readily converted to glucose and transported in the blood to cells. Yeast cells in the gastrointestinal tract rapidly proliferate in the presence of sugar. Sugar is delivered to all the cells of the body through the circulation, feeding pathogenic yeast along the way. It also alters the pH of the mucous membranes, enhancing the environment for yeast. Also, sugar decreases the ability of white blood cells to fight infection.

If you could look at sugar in your intestine, you would see that it undergoes changes just like hops and grapes do when beer or wine is made. Sugar catalyzes fermentation, which, in your body, means bloating, gas, and abdominal discomfort. Any condition that increases blood sugar, including diabetes, insulin resistance, and stress, decreases the resistance to fungal overgrowth.

Heavy metal exposure, especially chronic mercury toxicity, has a potent influence on yeast proliferation. Yeast growth actually accelerates to trap the mercury within its cell walls. It is trying to help save the organism (you) from a noxious insult. So, if you are struggling to get your chronic *Candida* under control, and you haven't succeeded, you need to look deeper into what is keeping your chemistry out of balance.

Remember, yeast is part of your natural chemistry. When it gets out of control, it can be for any combination of reasons that end up weakening your host defense to the point that a fungal terrain (chemistry) begins to dominate your metabolism. At such a point, major disruptions in your metabolism begin to occur. I believe that, at the very least, a significant portion of our population has minor imbalances in yeast production. Over the last twenty years of my practice, it has been a central component of helping people to reclaim their metabolic code.

It is not simply the yeast that is the problem; it is the metabolic byproducts of yeast metabolism that destroy body chemistry. (See the inset "A Toxic Mix: The Effects of Fungal and Yeast Toxins" on page 179 for more information.)

Nutrient deficiencies, including selenium, zinc, iron, B_{12}, and folic acid are linked to candidiasis, due to the effect of diet on the immune and detoxification systems. Without adequate nutrients, the body cannot make the immune cells needed to keep the balance in the intestines between pathogenic bacteria and yeast. Once an overgrowth of yeast begins to take hold, this gets to be a catch-22, because dysbiosis reduces the ability of the intestines to absorb nutrients.

During pregnancy, *when progesterone* levels are high, many women experience the onset of chronic vaginal yeast infections. Pregnancy can also increase blood sugar, which encourages yeast growth. And many pregnant women suffer from a chronic yeast disturbance. Oral contraceptives can also stimulate yeast disturbances, as does the elevation in progesterone during the premenstrual period (five to fourteen days prior to menstruation). Many women who suffer from PMS have concurrent yeast disturbances. There also appears to be a strong relationship between yeast overgrowth, endometriosis (an abnormal growth of cells that form in the lining of the uterus), and infertility.

Stress is another underlying contributing factor in yeast overgrowth. There are, no doubt, countless mechanisms involved in stress-related *Candida* disturbances. Most notably, chronic stress elevates cortisol release from the adrenal glands with two significant results: altered immune function and alterations in blood sugar control. Cortisol is a natural immunosuppressive agent. It causes the release of *neuropeptide y,* which then sends a message to your natural killer cells to basically turn off. Pharmaceutical derivatives of corticosteroids (those naturally produced by the adrenal glands) are often administered to intentionally suppress the immune system as therapy for autoimmune conditions. In addition to suppressing immune function, cortisol decreases insulin sensitivity by receptor cells (insulin resistance) and, therefore, decreases glucose uptake from the blood. The elevation in blood sugar is intended to provide quick energy to fuel the "stress response." But with a chronic elevation of cortisol, it also stimulates yeast growth, adherence, and virulence.

While the toxic effects of some environmental compounds are becoming well known, their specific effect on *Candida* overgrowth is at best poorly studied. Yeast toxicity and chemical toxicity are sometimes difficult to distinguish from one another and, many times, will affect someone simultaneously. Multiple chemical sensitivity syndrome (MCS) can create a symptom profile that closely resembles candida-related complex (CRC). Patients complain of intolerance to odors, fumes, foods, and mold. Chronic fatigue, depression, gastrointestinal symptoms, and anxiety may also be present. In my practice, improving the ecology of the gut has had dramatic effects on my patients with MCS.

Remember, the more toxic your body becomes, the more compromised your immune system becomes and the more prone you are to grow unfriendly "bugs." By weakening the immune system, toxic exposure increases the susceptibility to *Candida* disturbances. Since they are not conditions that require public reporting, the prevalence of *Candida*-related infections and yeast overgrowth in nonhospitalized people is difficult to estimate. However, some idea can be ascertained from the sales of prescription antifungal preparations. In the first quarter of 2000, reported revenues from the sale of the popular antifungal drug fluconazole (Diflucan), for example, were nearly $250 million worldwide!

Lab Tests for Dysbiosis and Yeast Imbalances

Until a few years ago, it was difficult to identify a patient with a yeast problem. After all, most of the symptoms associated with candidiasis can be linked to other diseases. In the past, the only way to identify a person with candidiasis was with a subjective questionnaire. I still use questionnaires because symptoms alone can sometimes very accurately indicate the presence of dysbiosis. Repeat completions of the questionnaire allow for tracking an individual's success. These days, however, lab tests can help to identify this all too common problem. The following lab tests, when used in conjunction with the symptom profile and clinical picture, can be used to identify yeast-related disturbances.

Candida Antibody Test. This test measures for the presence of antibodies (IgM, IgA, and IgG) to *Candida.* The premise of the test is that if *Candida* is present in the circulation, the immune system will detect it as foreign and form antibodies to attack the yeast. This test is sometimes inaccurate because *Candida* patients have weakened immune function, and therefore do not produce the antibodies. Even among patients with pervasive, chronic Candidiasis, as many as 25 percent lack measurable antibodies in the blood.

CandiSphere Enzyme Immuno Assay Test (CEIA). This is the second most frequently

A Toxic Mix: The Effects of Fungal and Yeast Toxins

There are a number of different types of toxins that are produced by both fungi and yeast in our bodies. These mycotoxins are secreted by yeast and fungus cells in order to destroy competing microorganisms and to secure the invaders a foothold in the host environment.

Mycotoxins are substances produced by the fungal cells as they mature from the bud to mycelial states. *Mycelia* are threadlike filaments that penetrate the surface of the mucosa, enabling the yeast to attach to their hosts and obtain food. Mycotoxins are also generated when yeast cells are destroyed, and their contents spill into the extracellular space.

Well-researched yeast mycotoxins include *ethanol, alloxan, arabinose, acetaldehyde,* and the enzymes *phospholipase* and *proteinase*. Ethanol is the major ingredient in alcoholic beverages. Acetaldehyde is a metabolic product of ethanol. Acetaldehyde is highly irritating to the mucous membranes and has damaging effects on the liver. It is not unheard of for people with candidiasis to experience a "drunken" state after eating large amounts of carbohydrates, which feed the yeast and promote fermentation and ethanol production. It is kind of like having your own "brewery" in your body.

Acetaldehyde interferes with immune function by inhibiting suppressor T-cell function. Consequently, B cells are allowed to overproduce antibodies, even to substances that are harmless. This explains the hypersensitivity to chemicals, fumes, and odors that afflict those who suffer from CRC. It also contributes to food reactions and allergies. In the absence of suppressor T cells, B cells may also produce *autoantibodies* (antibodies that react with an antigen that is a normal component of the body), contributing to autoimmune disorders such as rheumatoid arthritis, systemic lupus erythematosus, myasthenia gravis (disorder in which eye muscles weaken), multiple sclerosis, and scleroderma (an autoimmune skin disorder).

Acetaldehyde readily binds with the amine groups (the nitrogen-containing part) of proteins, interfering with the synthesis and function of neurotransmitters in the brain. Neurotransmitters are chemicals that allow nerve impulses to be delivered smoothly from neurons in the brain. Many people with CRC report mental disturbances including poor concentration, depression, mood swings, short-term memory deficit, and insomnia. Many of these symptoms can be linked to deficiencies of the amino acids required for the synthesis of neurotransmitters. Also, yeast inhibits the action of the enzyme acetaldehyde dehydrogenase so the break down of acetaldehyde in the brain is reduced. Acetaldehyde alters brain chemistry and has a direct toxicity to neurologic tissue.

Two toxic enzymes produced by yeast cells are *phospholipase* and *proteinase*. Phospholipase is an enzyme that initiates the hydrolysis (breakdown) of phospholipids. Proteinase deaminates (removes the amine group) structural proteins and in that way degrades pancreatic and intestinal enzymes (all enzymes are made from proteins). Together, they are responsible for splitting fatty acids in the intestine, creating excess free radicals, and damaging the intestinal mucosa. Without proper fatty acid synthesis, symptoms such as dry skin, fatigue, rashes, and neurological disturbances appear. Serious symptoms of impaired fatty acid metabolism can occur if these enzymes are left unchecked.

Alloxan is a mycotoxin that has a particular affinity for destroying the beta cells in the pancreas over time and contributing to poor blood sugar regulation by causing insulin imbalances. Alloxan is actually used in laboratory animals to kill the beta cells in order to induce experimental diabetes so that the animals can be used to study therapies for this disease. So chronic, low-grade alloxan production in the body could lead to insulin resistance and diabetes by slowly destroying the beta cells. Interestingly, fungal growth on the nails, hands, and skin is common in diabetic individuals.

Other toxins include *glycoprotein* toxins and *polysaccharide protein complexes* such as *arabinose, tyramine, canditoxin,* and *mannan.* These toxins interfere with cellular functions all over the body. They especially have neurotoxic effects that could influence mood, cognitive function, and even cause seizures. These are symptoms commonly seen in children with autism and ADHD, who are known to have elevated arabinose levels as well as other yeast mycotoxins.

Metabolic waste products from yeast organisms and other pathogenic bacteria in the gut are known to be markedly elevated in people with a number of conditions, including autism, seizures, chronic fatigue, migraine, colitis, lupus, depression, fibromyalgia, obsessive compulsive disorder, and inflammatory bowel disease. This indicates that dysbiosis may be an underlying factor in many of these conditions. The damaging effects of yeast toxins are truly the hidden culprits responsible for many of the widespread symptoms associated with candidiasis.

used test. CEIA measures metabolic enzymes from the cytoplasm of *Candida* cells. These molecules are normally found only inside the *Candida* cell. If they are present in measurable form (normal range is 70–100) outside the cells, it is indicative of systemic candidiasis.

This test is more accurate than the Candida antibody test because it does not produce "false negative" results.

Quantitative Candida Stool Culture. This test measures the amount of yeast present in the stool. The yeast appearing in the culture are both live and dead organisms. This limits the accuracy of the test because dead yeast does not grow in a culture medium. For this reason, stool cultures sometimes give false-negative results. Negative stool cultures often appear among patients with the most severe symptomatic candidiasis, while asymptomatic patients sometimes have positive cultures. Stool samples from patients with suspected candidiasis, however, may provide other valuable diagnostic information.

Organic Acid Urine Test. Organic acid urine testing can yield information on the status of many metabolic pathways and allow us to identify problems associated with metabolism. Organic acids are key metabolites of many pathways of metabolism. A number of organic acids are normally excreted in the urine, depending on diet, medication taken, health status, and age. When they are under- or overproduced, it shows alterations in normal metabolism. When candida organisms (yeasts) are present in the body, certain compounds, known as metabolites, formed by the yeast will be present in the urine. A high level of these metabolites indicates yeast overgrowth.

Restoring Bacterial Balance

One of the big mistakes people make is that they try to make *Candida* and CRC the bad "guy" and don't look any deeper into the possible disruption of the immune system that is allowing the yeast to grow. If your immune system is functioning well, yeast will not overmultiply and cause systemic damage. There are many therapeutic programs that people may use to rid themselves of yeast overgrowth. I've found that the one detailed below works best.

1. Starve and eliminate. The most important and effective way to destroy *Candida* is to take away their food. Sugar and refined carbohydrates must be eliminated from the diet. Alcohol consumption should be eliminated or at least decreased. If an alcoholic drink is desired occasionally, vodka is the best choice. Wines, beers, and scotch are fermented. All fermented products are to be avoided. Of all liquors, vodka has the least reactive components and is thought to be the best metabolized of alcohols. In general, have no more than one to two drinks two times a week.

In the most severe situations, antifungal medications may be necessary to destroy yeast, but the results may only be temporary if measures are not taken to restrict future overgrowth. Drug therapy is commonly used for oral *Candida* infections (thrush), such as mycostatin (Nystatin) and Diflucan. Clotrimazole, miconazole, terconazole, and fluconazole (Gyne Lotrimin, Lotrimin, Mycelex, Monistat, and others) are commonly used for vaginal infections. Ketoconazole (Nizoral) is for fungal infections of the skin. (If you resort to taking prescription antifungals, take 300 milligrams [mg] of alpha lipoic acid per day and 300 mg milk thistle daily to protect the liver on days that you take the medication.)

Natural products can be effective in decreasing *Candida* or yeast overgrowths and have less risk for side effects. Some natural antifungal/antibacterial products that are commonly used and found in various combinations include aged garlic (*Allium sativum*); cat's claw root or bark (*Uncaria tomentosa*); grapefruit seed extract (from

Boost and Balance Your Immune Defense

A weak immune system provides the underlying opportunity for yeast overgrowth. Following the general guidelines below will help to strengthen your immune response.

- Learn to manage or reduce stress as much as possible.

- Exercise regularly by finding an activity you enjoy.

- Improve food selection habits (see Chapters 13 and 14 for guidelines).

- Drink plenty of quality water.

- Severely reduce or eliminate refined sugars and carbohydrate intake.

- Take antibiotics only when absolutely needed. Should you need to take antibiotics, be sure to ingest probiotics twice daily while taking the prescription and for two weeks following a course of any antibiotic medication. (*Note:* Take the probiotic two hours apart from the antibiotic).

- Use immune-supporting nutritional supplements, including vitamins C and E, the B-complex vitamins, natural mixed carotenoids, selenium, zinc, Moducare®, and other herbal and nutraceutical agents.

- Assess the toxin levels in your body (this may take the help of an experienced healthcare professional), and take steps to detoxify and rejuvenate.

- Get adequate sleep (six to nine hours are required by most healthy adults).

- Limit your exposure to chemicals as much as possible (use natural alternatives!).

- Have fun and enjoy life!

Citrus paradisi); oregano leaf extract (*Oreganum vulgare*); olive leaf extract (*Olea europaea*); caprylic acid (from the coconut); supplemental colostrum (the pre-milk liquid produced from the mammary glands during the twenty-four to forty-eight hours after giving birth); and plant tannins found in many herbs (the product Tanalbit works well).

2. Control Dietary Sources of Yeast. Those with candidiasis often report intolerance to fermented foods and those containing mold and yeast. These foods feed the yeast already present and introduce new yeast buds into the body. Although dietary yeast is not the same species as *Candida albicans,* there are common features between the two. Increased antibody titers to common baker's yeast have been found among patients with Crohn's disease, suggesting that the immune system reacts to common yeast as a food antigen. In laboratory studies, human cells exposed to baker's yeast show similar immune-reactive sensitivity. Fermented and yeast-containing foods are eliminated as part of the yeast control protocol.

Yeast is found in all manufactured citric acid products; in most fruits; in vinegar, which is made of fermented wines; and in ciders from such fruits as grapes, pears, apples, and some herbs. Vinegar is used as a preservative for mustard, catsup, olives, mayonnaise, many dressings, pickles, horseradish, spices, soy sauce, Worcestershire sauce, and dried fruits. Canned or frozen fruit juices contain yeast, only hand-squeezed and fresh juices are yeast-free. Fruit and fruit products that are canned commercially have higher yeast content than those that are canned at home. The outer skins of melons (especially cantaloupes), grapes, and oranges are loaded with mold and yeast. Fruit should be peeled when possible.

Mushrooms and cheeses of all kinds contain or actually *are* specific types of molds or yeasts. Milk products such as buttermilk, sour cream, cream cheese, ricotta cheese, ice creams, powdered milks, and milk itself contain lactose, which is thought to feed yeast organisms.

Tea, coffee and coffee-substitutes, pepper, and many spices and tobacco can acquire molds or yeast in their drying processes. Though I do not typically require that people eliminate all coffee, tea, or pepper from their diets, some people benefit considerably from reducing their intakes, especially of coffee.

Leftovers from a previous meal should be frozen for future use or be eaten within forty-eight hours, as they can frequently begin to grow mold within twenty-four hours. Foods containing brown spots should be avoided because there is a high probability that the spots are yeasts and molds that have begun their job of breaking down that food's nutrients for their own growth and survival.

Vitamins, such as the B-complex thiamine, niacin, and riboflavin, are usually yeast-grown, although it is possible to obtain them from a brown rice, yeast-free base.

Antibiotics such as penicillin, mycins, tetracyclines, lincomycin, and chloromycetin are drugs that are derived from mold cultures. Malt is used as a flavoring and coloring agent. It is the major ingredient of beer, ale, and malt liquors, as well as some nonalcoholic products. Malt is a sprouted grain that is easily fermented and produces the enzyme diastase, which is important in the development of grain liquors. Most dry cereals contain malt or malt extract. Other foods that encourage fungal growth are baked goods, breads, biscuits and pancake mixes, soda crackers, and any other foods requiring the use of baker's yeast. Ice cream, candy, malted milk drinks, and soft drinks contain sugar, which promotes yeast growth. Restriction of carbohydrates is essential to the success of any program to eliminate *Candida*. Severe restriction of most forms of sugar, including almost all fruit juices, is necessary. Following the phase-one guidelines in Chapter 13 for at least three months will help to starve the yeast and help you to regain control of many of your metabolic processes.

3. Replenish the normal intestinal flora. Supplementation with probiotics, butyric acid, and fructooligosaccharides (FOS) are important measures toward reestablishing healthy intestinal flora. An adequate amount of healthy bowel flora prevents yeast from gaining access to nourishment. Without food, they cannot thrive. Probiotics have other health-promoting functions, including the synthesis of certain B vitamins (biotin, pyridoxine, folic acid, and niacin) and the promotion of healthy bowel function. Probiotic supplements should include *Lactobacillus acidophilus, Bifidobacterium bifidum,* and *Lactobacillus bulgaricus.* Dairy and milk-free products are available for those with allergies.

FOS are carbohydrates that can be utilized by colonic probiotic bacteria, but not yeast. Thus, taking FOS promotes the growth and proliferation of beneficial bacteria, which inhibits yeast. FOS can be taken up to twice a day. I recommend using 500 mg per day for three months, in conjunction with probiotics.

Butyric acid helps several strains of friendly bacteria, including *Lactobacillus acidophilus, L. plantarium, L. Rhamnosus, Bifidobacterium infantis, B. bifidum, B. longum,* adhere to intestinal lining and helps increase the natural healing mechanism of the gut tissue after antifungal treatment for *Candida* overgrowth. Other agents to include such as L-glutamine, SeaCure, ginger, and turmeric help to rebuild gut integrity and reduce inflammation. These agents will be discussed later.

Anticipate Yeast Die-Off

Yeast "die-off" phenomenon is the temporary worsening of yeast-related symptoms during initial phases of treatment. It is caused when the yeast cells rupture and spill their toxins into the surrounding tissue. The die-off reaction can occur one to two days after treatment begins and can last for several days. Die-off symptoms may include headache, body aches, skin rash, and general flulike discomfort. Some patients interpret the symptoms as a negative reaction to the program that they initiated.

If you're undertaking a program for *Candida* on your own, follow phase one of the Healthy Living Guidelines in Chapter 13 for a week or two before beginning a supplement regimen for yeast reduction to minimize the die-off effect. Vitamin C in the form of mixed mineral ascorbates, Alka-Seltzer Gold, and activated charcoal are known to buffer the symptoms of the die-off reaction. If you're working with a healthcare practitioner, he or she should be able to help you control the die-off effect in most cases.

Adequate rest, reduced stress, and proper nutrition are essential to reestablishing normal flora for the gut and to restore healthy immune function.

Leaky Gut Syndrome

A healthy intestinal lining allows only properly digested food particles to pass through so they can be absorbed and distributed. At the same time, it serves as a barrier to keep out bacteria, foreign substances, and large undigested molecules. Leaky gut syndrome describes a condition that results in an alteration in the way nutrients and chemicals are absorbed into the bloodstream.

The syndrome occurs because there has been a change in permeability (filtering ability) of the gastrointestinal lining (barrier). The intestinal mucosa (lining) is a semi-permeable membrane that allows for the selective absorption of hydrogen ions, bicarbonate, and nutrients, including vitamins and minerals, and for the rejection of toxins that can damage the body. It is covered by a lipid layer that prevents the absorption of water-soluble molecules. If the permeability of the mucosa is altered and hydrogen ions are allowed into the tissue, its protective function is disrupted. Think of it as a dam with small cracks in it. At first little, if any, water will seep through, but over time, the integrity of the dam is compromised. As hydrogen ions build up in the tissue, enzymes are destroyed and the tissue begins to break down. Water-soluble molecules are moved more freely and are able to penetrate the intestinal mucosa.

When the intestinal barrier is penetrated, the immune system first reacts by mobilizing nonspecific, local inflammation pathways. The immune system then releases chemicals that create inflammation in the intestinal mucosa, which, in turn, creates space (cracks in the dam) between the normally compacted goblet cells (mucous-secreting cell). These cracks allow larger particles, including phenolic compounds from food, yeast, other endotoxins, bacterial proteins, and other potential allergens to leach into circulation.

Once these substances pass through the intestinal walls into the bloodstream, they become antigens, and the immune system is activated. IgA, IgG, and IgM antibodies (immune compounds) are formed specific to these molecules. The antibodies attach themselves to the circulating antigens marking them for removal (phagocytosis) by monocytes and neutrophils. If these complexes are not eliminated from circulation, they continue to be treated as invaders each time they are encountered. With repeated assaults, the body may begin to react more fiercely, not only generating allergic reactions and triggering inflammation locally, but also triggering responses beyond the digestive system.

The more "leaky" the gut becomes, the more difficult it becomes for the intestinal tract to discriminate between beneficial and harmful substances. This inflammatory response then further worsens gut permeability, contributing to a vicious cycle. Mounting evidence supports that this type of gut dysfunction can lead to a constellation of symptoms and contributes to a wide variety of complex disorders. These conditions include inflammatory bowel diseases, inflammatory joint conditions, inflammatory skin conditions, autoimmune disorders, chronic fatigue, Epstein-Barr virus, fibromyalgia, herpes, multiple sclerosis (a progressive, degenerative disease of the central nervous system), weight gain, neurologic symptoms, cognitive symptoms, and food intolerance.

All of the conditions listed below have inflammatory components that contribute to the metabolic problems of diabetes, weight gain, thyroid conditions, cardiovascular disease, and problems with immunity usually associated with metabolic syndrome. The variety of clinical disorders associated with leaky gut arises from the complex interactions between the gut and the immune system:

- Acne
- Alcoholism
- Celiac disease
- Chronic fatigue syndrome
- Crohn's disease
- Cystic fibrosis
- Dermatitis herpetiformis
- Eczema
- Food allergies

- Hyperactivity
- Irritable bowel syndrome
- Liver dysfunction
- Multiple chemical sensitivities
- Pancreatic insufficiency
- Psoriasis
- Rheumatoid arthritis
- Systemic lupus erythematosus
- Weight gain

Often in my practice, I encounter people who have several diseases and conditions simultaneously and also suffer from a host of other seemingly unrelated symptoms. When one takes a closer look at the common threads of inflammation, flora disturbances, and endocrine weakness, the patterns become very clear. After years of clinical experience, I began to see these patterns over and over, and finally, research is beginning to verify the connections. For instance, certain skin conditions are also associated with gut inflammation. IgA-immune complexes, originating from the gastrointestinal tract, have been found in the circulation of those suffering from *dermatitis herpetiformis,* a chronic and relapsing condition that primarily affects the skin.

Some evidence points to the fact that intestinal microflora play a role in the pathology of the generalized autoimmune condition, systemic lupus erythematosus (SLE). The gut bacteria may have some role in the formation of anti-DNA antibodies, biochemical markers found in individuals with autoimmune diseases.

In exploring this relationship, one study measured the prevalence of antibodies to gut bacteria in subjects with active and inactive forms of SLE. Among those with active SLE, total plasma IgG antibodies were doubled compared with inactive SLE and healthy controls. Antibacterial IgG antibodies were lower among those with active SLE than in subjects with inactive SLE, suggesting that the antibodies may be utilized to form immune complexes that trigger acute episodes of SLE.

Some inflammatory joint conditions can originate from immune-mediated reactions to microorganisms that penetrate the intestinal mucosa. The bacteria *Proteus mirabilis* is thought to have an important role in the pathology of rheumatoid arthritis. In a survey of eighty-nine patients with rheumatoid arthritis, 63 percent of the women and 50 percent of the men had *P. mirabilis* in their urine. Antibodies specific to *P. mirabilis* were higher in rheumatoid arthritis patients than in the healthy control group. IgG antibodies against the bacteria *Klebsiellia pneumoniae* have been found among patients with ankylosing spondylitis (an arthritis of the spine), many of whom also have inflammatory bowel disease. Other microbial infections, such as mycoplasma, may coexist in rheumatoid arthritis and other autoimmune situations.

Mycoplasma, a fungal microorganism once thought to be benign that has become particularly prevalent, has the capacity to invade cells, tissues, and blood, producing systemic infections in numerous organ systems. Because it has the ability to damage the immune system by invading the natural killer cells (NK cells), it weakens them, reduces their numbers, and renders them susceptible to viral infections.

The relationship between leaky gut syndrome and systemic inflammatory disorders and autoimmune conditions is complex. Normally, the immune system has an inherent tolerance to substances produced by the body. Autoimmune reactions occur when the immune system loses its tolerance for "self" and autoantibodies are produced. Most of these are IgG antibodies. Suppressor T cells are inhibited in autoimmune diseases. This means that your body has too many T-helper cells functioning and not a balance of T-suppressor cells present to keep the T-helper cell activity in check.

In many diseases associated with leaky gut syndrome, there is no clearly defined point at which intestinal permeability ends and the inflammatory and autoimmune disorders begin. Leaky gut appears to have both a role in and results from inflammatory disorders and autoimmune disorders.

Crohn's disease, for example, which causes inflammatory lesions in the intestine, increases permeability of the gut and contributes to leaky gut syndrome. Conversely, Crohn's disease is considered an autoimmune disorder that may have its origins in IgG-mediated reactions to food, bacteria, fungus, or parasites. One study demonstrated the presence of IgG antibodies to yeast in 63 percent of patients with Crohn's disease, compared with only 8 percent of the healthy control group. Seventy-five percent of the Crohn's disease patients had detectable IgG antibodies against *E. coli* (bacteria found in the gut) and 42 percent had IgA antibodies specific to yeast. Once the inflammatory cascade is initiated, increased levels of the messengers of inflammation—interleukin-6, C-reactive protein, 5-lipoxygenase, TNF alpha, and arachidonic acid—run rampant through the body accelerating the oxidative stress on cellular health. These inflammatory markers are common in cardiovascular disease, diabetes, and obesity, among many other disease states linked with metabolic syndrome.

Leaky gut syndrome may not necessarily manifest itself in these conditions. It displays a wide variety of not-so-obvious symptoms, including abdominal discomfort or pain, dyspepsia, asthma, bloating, confusion, diarrhea, gas, joint and muscle pain, malaise, mood swings, nervousness, skin rashes, and more. Some of these reactions may occur one to two days after eating an offending food. So you really don't get a feeling for what it is that is causing you to feel the way you do. Other foods and substances can create immediate reactions.

Leaky gut syndrome puts an extra burden on the liver. When large molecules in the gut penetrate the inflamed mucosa, they are transported to the liver for detoxification. The liver passes them through its detoxification process, oxidizing and conjugating toxins, working overtime, before they are excreted in the bile or urine. Oxidation generates free radicals, and conjugation uses up valuable antioxidants such as glutathione. Furthermore, chronic toxin-laden bile can damage and irritate the pancreatic ducts. Increased permeability of the gut is also associated with secondary liver and pancreatic dysfunction.

When inflammatory irritants continuously bombard the liver, the liver becomes less effective at neutralizing harmful chemical substances. The substances that it cannot properly process get stored somewhere in the body. These toxins then become a triggering source of inflammation and dangerous free-radical reactions.

Causes of Leaky Gut Syndrome

There is no single cause of leaky gut syndrome, but the following are some of the most common causes. All can lead to damage and subsequent erosion of the mucosal barrier of the gut. They tend not only to decrease the integrity of the intestinal lining, but they also help in disturbing the delicate balance of the gastrointestinal flora.

- Food allergies and intolerances
- Drugs, including NSAIDs, aspirin, chemotherapy, and H2 blockers (be sure to take glutamine and probiotics if on these medications)
- Excessive alcohol consumption
- Chemical toxicity
- Chronic stress
- Dysbiosis
- Infections
- Injury
- Inadequate digestive enzymes
- Nutritional deficiencies

Lab Tests for Leaky Gut

There is a test to find out just how "leaky" your gut is. This test, which is called the lactulose-mannitol challenge test, directly measures the permeability of the gut. Five grams each of the sugars lactulose and mannitol are taken orally.

Normally, the gut is less than 1 percent permeable to lactulose, while about 14 percent of mannitol, which is a smaller molecule, is transported across the intestinal wall. Once absorbed into circulation, both sugars are fully excreted in the urine within six hours.

The test measures urinary excretion of both sugars, then compares the ratio of lactulose to mannitol excretion. A normal gut will reflect less than a 0.03 ratio of lactulose to mannitol (very low presence of lactulose). A leaky gut will register a higher ratio of lactulose to mannitol, indicating the diffusion of lactulose across the intestinal barrier. Essentially, the gut lets the lactulose through the cracks of the dam.

Decreased mannitol excretion indicates the possibility of malabsorption. This test is performed after fasting and again after ingestion of "challenge foods." Several studies have indicated that this is a reliable and accurate measure of intestinal permeability. Its non-invasive nature makes it a valuable evaluation tool.

Variations of the test include substituting rhamnose (a sugarlike substance) for mannitol, and measuring serum samples instead of urine. Other measures of intestinal permeability include IgG antibody titers, specific to food antigens and bacteria.

Food Allergy and Intolerance

Food allergies or intolerances affect a great deal more Americans than was recognized even as few as ten years ago. One of the reasons is that, as with candidiasis and leaky gut syndrome, the symptoms of this type of allergic reaction can be quite diverse. Food allergy, in the classic sense, is characterized by an immediate and severe reaction by the immune system to an ingested food or substance that is not normally harmful. Food allergies trigger IgE-mediated antibodies that surround the offending substance (antigen). The IgE reaction causes the release of cytokines and histamines that results in rashes, respiratory distress, fainting, or anaphylactic shock. True food allergies are relatively rare. It is estimated that only 1 to 5 percent of the population suffers from these reactions. Foods known to induce severe reactions include tree nuts such as almonds, Brazil nuts, cashews, filberts, pecans, walnuts, shellfish, and strawberries. It is now being discovered that more and more people are gluten- and gliaden-sensitive, which could be leading to life-threatening reactions in some individuals. Gluten is a protein found in many grains, including wheat, rye, barley, and oats. Gliaden, also a protein, makes up gluten along with glutenin and water.

Food intolerances, on the other hand, are delayed hypersensitivity reactions mediated by sensitized T cells of the immune system in response to foreign foods, chemicals, or bacterial toxins. IgG antibodies are cell mediated, rather than immune mediated like IgE antibodies, which means they can induce symptoms in numerous tissues throughout the body. Symptoms of food intolerance are more subtle, insidious, and difficult to identify. They may appear within an hour of ingesting a particular food, or up to several days later. One study determined that close to 60 percent of those with food intolerance had delayed reactions. People may suffer for years from a chronic condition associated with food sensitivity and not be aware of the offending agent(s).

Food intolerances are much more common than true food allergies, affecting as many as 30 percent of the population. Yet they often go unrecognized by health-care professionals for a number of reasons. For one, traditional allergists, until recently, did not acknowledge the association between food sensitivities and chronic diseases.

Although the word "allergy" simply means, "altered reaction," sometime during the early part of the twentieth century, allergists narrowed the definition to include only those reactions that were immediate. Consequently, the delayed reactions that characterize food intolerances are generally not recognized as strict allergies even though an overactive reaction from the immune system does occur.

A second reason food intolerances are often unrecognized is that standard tests for food allergies consist of measuring serum IgE antibodies for common food allergens. Food intolerances that involve cell-mediated inflammatory reactions do not show up in standard antibody titers. It is estimated that 80 percent of food reactions are mediated by IgG antibodies.

A third reason food intolerances are frequently missed is that testing is typically limited to only the most commonly reactive foods. Unfortunately, allergies can involve a multitude of foods and substances such as additives, herbs, and spices. Furthermore, the symptoms associated with food intolerances are extremely varied. No two people with food intolerances have exactly the same clinical profile.

For our purposes, the terms "food allergy" and "food intolerance/sensitivity" will be used interchangeably. In both cases, the immune system is involved in a hypersensitivity reaction to commonly harmless substances, and each term falls well within the context of "altered reactions."

Symptoms of Food Allergy

The symptoms associated with food allergies can be difficult to identify because they are often delayed. Symptoms of food allergies can be different from person to person, at different stages of life, and can manifest in virtually any system of the body, further complicating their identification, as Table 9.2 on page 191 illustrates.

The most common complaints expressed by those with food intolerances are gastrointestinal upset (diarrhea, gas, constipation, irritable bowel syndrome), neurological disturbances (inability to concentrate, hyperactivity), aggravation of autoimmune disorders, joint pain, migraine headaches, weight gain, obesity, and skin eruptions (eczema, acne, urticaria).

Typical signs of food sensitivities, particularly in children, are runny nose; redness of the nose, cheeks, ears or eyes; eczema; wrinkles and dark circles under the eyes; patchy tongue; excessive perspiration; thirst; cold hands and feet; hyperactivity; chronic ear infections; and restless or aching legs. Young children and infants may experience sleep disturbances, colic, and chronic diaper rash. Allergic children often cling and whine excessively.

Table 9.2. Symptoms and Conditions Associated with Food Allergies and Intolerances

AGE GROUP	SYMPTOMS	CONDITIONS
Infants	Spitting up/vomiting	Eczema
	Restlessness/sleeplessness	Chronic ear infections
	Excessive drooling	Chronic upper respiratory infections
	Chronic diaper rash	Esophageal reflux, colic
Children	Hyperactivity, aggression	ADHD
	Red ears, nose, eyes, cheeks	Asthma
	Dark under eye circles, bags	Recurrent infections (allergies)
	Restless legs	Gastrointestinal complaints
	Bed wetting	Hives, dry skin
	Hypersensitivity to medication	Autism
	Weight gain	Obesity, insulin resistance
Adolescents	Failure in school, inability to concentrate	Depression, suicidal thoughts or behavior
	Hypersensitivity to light, sound, touch	Acne
	Inappropriate behavior	Menstrual abnormalities
	Weight gain	Obesity, insulin resistance
Adults	Diarrhea, constipation, gas	Peptic and duodenal ulcers
	Bladder problems	Chronic infections
	Wheezing	Depression, insomnia
	Red, itchy skin, rashes	Dermatitis, eczema, seborrhea
	Irregular heart rate	Asthma
	Edema	Acne, eczema, hives
	Fatigue	Arthritis
	Joint tenderness	Autoimmune disorders
	Headaches	Menstrual abnormalities, food allergies
	Weight gain	Autoimmune disorders, Alzheimer's disease, cancer, cardiovascular disease, insulin resistance/diabetes, obesity

Almost any food or substance can cause a reaction, but the following are the most common food allergens:

- Chocolate
- Citrus fruits
- Coffee
- Corn
- Dairy products, including milk and cheese
- Peanuts and tree nuts
- Pesticide residues on foods
- Refined sugars
- Soy
- Tomatoes

- Eggs
- Food additives

- Wheat
- Yeast

Some of the most significant and devastating effects of food intolerance are neurological. The relationship between brain chemistry and eating patterns has been well established. Researchers have found that some foods, for example, can trigger neurotransmitter loss, like serotonin (a neurotransmitter found primarily in the brain that is considered essential for relaxation, sleep, and concentration), which affect appetite and food cravings. When these foods are eaten, they increase satiety and reduce cravings. People with food allergies often develop addictions to the foods to which they most allergic. (An addictive substance can be any food, chemical, or drug to which a person develops a sensitivity reaction upon exposure, followed by withdrawal symptoms, which can be suppressed by repeated exposure to the substance.)

In the book *Brain Allergies: The Psychonutrient Connection* (Keats Publishing, 1980), William Philpott, M.D., and Dwight Kalita, Ph.D., reveal that in one survey, 92 percent of the patients diagnosed as schizophrenics demonstrated strong maladaptive reactions to foods and chemicals. Of these patients, 64 percent manifested symptoms when exposed to wheat, 51 percent upon exposure to corn, and 51 percent when exposed to cow's milk. Seventy-five percent of the patients reacted to tobacco, 10 percent of which manifested in psychotic symptoms. Some reactions precipitated suicidal or delusional thoughts.

Dr. Philpott has explored the complex neurological reactions to foods and chemicals by conducting controlled dietary experiments. In one such study, patients underwent a strict four-day fast. After this period, foods were reintroduced one at a time and clinical signs and symptoms were observed. These studies led researchers to conclude that any food or chemical is capable of producing strong reactions in susceptible individuals; chronic symptoms are improved after a four to seven-day avoidance of incriminating foods and chemicals; and many chronic physical and mental illnesses are rooted in "addictive reactions to foods and chemicals."

While some foods can produce dramatic neurological symptoms like schizophrenia or suicidal tendencies, manifestations that are more common include depression, hyperactivity, poor attention span, and an inability to concentrate. One of the mechanisms used to explain these changes in mental status is hypoglycemia.

Drs. Philpott and Kalita observed that the blood sugar changes dramatically upon exposure to allergenic substances. It is suggested that the ability of the pancreas to secrete insulin, and therefore to regulate blood sugar, is altered by immunologic pathways. Hypoglycemia is the first stage of becoming insulin resistant, and as you have already read, any health problem that is left unaddressed will only accelerate a person further in the downward spiral toward metabolic syndrome and a host of other problems. The brain and central nervous system, which require a steady supply of glucose in the blood, are particularly sensitive to fluctuations in insulin.

Causes of Food Allergy

The exact origin of allergic reactions is unclear. Some allergies have a genetic component. Children whose parents both have allergies are twice as likely to develop allergies themselves. Such children inherit the tendency toward allergies, but not to one specific form. (It could be hay fever, asthma, eczema, and others.) Also, the propensity to manufacture IgE antibodies (antibodies formed as part of an allergic reaction to a food substance) has been found to be inherited as well.

Another genetic-based theory, proposed by Peter J. D'Adamo, N.D., author of *Eat Right for Your Type* (Putnam Publishing Group, 1996) is that blood type determines both the ability to digest and the specific immune response to certain dietary proteins called *lectins*. According to D'Adamo, some blood types react to certain lectins in the gut by creating nonspecific inflammatory responses (the release of histamines, activation of complementary and secretory IgA). For example, gluten, the lectin in wheat, binds to the intestinal mucosa and induces inflammation most often among those with type O blood. If one's blood type induces such a reaction in the gut, the leaky gut allows lectins to enter the circulation and deposit in tissues. Once in the circulation, IgG antibodies are formed specific to the proteins. In the tissues, lectins cause cells to agglutinate (clump together), which damages the tissues and targets them for destruction by the immune system. Depending on the type of lectin, any number of tissues can be affected. This theory while plausible is unproven so far.

Although heredity plays an important role in the development of allergies, no single system in the body operates in a vacuum. In almost every case, pathology in the body can be traced to a series of breakdowns among systems. Your allergic threshold begins at birth. Before you were born, you inhabited a sterile environment in your mother's womb. You were first exposed to beneficial bacteria as you traveled down your mother's vaginal canal during a normal birthing delivery. These bacteria got into your mouth and traveled into your gut where they proliferated and began forming a healthy bowel microflora.

Babies born by cesarean delivery miss this important initial exposure to beneficial bacteria. Studies report that infants from a vaginal delivery have a much higher fecal microflora than infants who are delivered by cesarean section. Studies also report that infants who are breast-fed have a much greater percentage of beneficial bacteria compared to infants who are bottle fed with infant formulas. Secretory IgA passed from mothers to infants in breast milk prevents allergens from penetrating the infant's gastrointestinal lining. Intestinal microorganisms may help regulate inflammation by enhancing the ability of IgA to distinguish between antigens, and by improving the control of the secretion of type 2 T-helper cells.

These early experiences can set the stage for a healthy immune system and a well-functioning digestive system or for a greater risk of digestive problems, food allergies, and immune system disorders later on. A recent Swedish study evaluated the intestinal microflora of children with low and high prevalence of allergies. Allergic children were found to have less lactobacilli and higher counts of aerobic bacteria, particularly *Staphylococcus aureus,* than nonallergic children. Among allergic children, the proportions of coliforms were higher, and bacteroides lower than in nonallergic children. The study suggests that the administration of probiotic bacteria in infancy may be a primary preventive measure against the development of allergies later in life. (The repeated use of antibiotics by young children will most likely disrupt normal flora.)

Another study demonstrated that lactobacilli supplementation decreased mucosal inflammation and atopic eczema among infants with cow's milk allergy. The study revealed that lactobacilli helps prevent defects in intestinal permeability, promotes antigen specificity, and helps control antigen absorption.

Also, the environment in which a child develops will greatly affect the chances of allergies developing. Repeated exposure to allergens may stimulate the production of IgE antibodies, as may environmental pollutants. For instance, the prevalence of atopic allergies, such as asthma and eczema, has risen steadily since the 1960s. While no single culprit can be held responsible for this increase, it does correlate with increasing levels of pollutants. Another factor to consider is the chronic use of antibiotics, including those used in humans for the treatment of diseases and those contained in our food chain from use in animals.

Repetitive antibiotic use leads to dysbiosis, which disrupts the immune dysfunction and contributes to a leaky gut. As you have learned, food allergies or intolerances can easily result from leaky gut syndrome. Undigested food particles that cross through damaged lining of the intestines into the bloodstream are mistaken for foreign invaders by the immune system, which releases antibodies to fight them.

Most likely, there is no single cause of food allergy or delayed sensitivity. Illness has a domino effect. In the case of allergies, the relationship between toxicity and immune dysfunction is the most critical. Doris Rapp, M.D., author of the best-selling book on childhood and adult allergies *Is This Your Child?* (William Morrow, 1991) describes the relationship between the two in terms of the barrel effect.

The barrel effect proposes that each person has an allergic threshold: a barrel that, when filled, creates an allergic response. The barrel may be filled by any number of insults on the detoxification systems in the body: the liver, gut, lungs, and kidneys. For example, a high pollen count can aggravate one detoxification system (the lungs), while medications or exposure to chemical pollutants can tax another (the liver or kidneys). Pesticides and poor nutrition add to the toxic overload by assaulting the gut. Once the barrel is full, allergic reactions become evident. The only forms of relief are to either decrease the toxic load or increase the size of the barrel. Increasing the barrel size requires strengthening the detoxification systems.

The following conditions are examples of how seemingly unrelated health problems have strong associations with food allergies and a leaky gut. Addressing the underlying imbalance of intestinal flora and gut integrity will go a long way in resolving the symptoms of these conditions.

Food Allergies, Asthma, and Eczema

Atopic dermatitis (eczema) and asthma are hypersensitivity reactions with remarkably similar mechanisms of inflammation, yet different manifestations of disease. Many healthcare professionals have established the correlation between infant eczema and childhood asthma. Eczema is a chronic skin condition, characterized by dry, red, flaky patches of skin. Eczema appears most commonly on the face, neck, elbows, wrists, knees, behind the ears, and the scalp. During acute episodes, the patches become oozing, inflamed, and itchy.

There are currently two recognized classifications of eczema: *atopic* and *contact*. Contact dermatitis is typically aggravated by direct skin contact with an allergen, such as chemicals, wool, lanolin, soap, and cosmetics. Atopic eczema is usually triggered by inhaled or ingested allergens, such as certain foods, pollen, dust, or animal dander.

How are allergies and eczema related? Allergic reactions to certain foods are thought to stimulate T-cell migration to the skin, triggering eczema and other inflammatory skin reactions. Some literature suggests the discussion of a third classification: "dysregulatory microbial eczemas." This category refers to eczema caused by the introduction of microflora into the horny layer of the skin, and subsequent inflammation, caused by a breakdown in the epidermis.

Asthma is a respiratory condition characterized by difficulty breathing. Asthma results from inflammation and constriction of the airway passages. Increased mucous secretion further inhibits the movement of air into the lungs. Like eczema, asthma is a chronic condition that can be triggered by a number of things, including allergens, stress, extreme temperature change, and pollution.

Eczema and asthma are caused by several immune mechanisms. The itching of eczema and the bronchospasms associated with asthma are a result of allergens interacting with IgG on the surface of mast cells and macrophages. Another mechanism is the flooding of histamines—prostaglandins, and other inflammatory components, along with T lymphocytes (type 2 T-helper cells) and macrophages—to the skin (eczema) or bronchioles (asthma).

Food Allergies and Chronic Ear Infections (Otitis Media)

Middle ear infections (otitis media) are responsible for an estimated 40 percent of annual visits to the pediatrician (in children ages two to four). Last year, more than 2 million permanent tubes for ear drainage were inserted at a cost of approximately $2 billion. Antibiotics are prescribed more frequently for ear infections than any other illness. Food allergy (especially dairy) and sugar consumption are the leading culprits that contribute to recurrent otitis media.

Eighty percent of food allergies are delayed IgG-mediated reactions. Antigen-antibody complexes in the circulation eventually deposit in tissue, where they initiate nonspecific, cell-mediated inflammation. These immune complexes commonly deposit in the mucosa of the inner ear, resulting in inflammation, damage to the mucosa, and mucous secretion. As fluid builds up, conditions are favorable for bacterial growth, increasing the possibility of these complexes' being deposited in the inner ear. Antibiotics, rather than helping the underlying problem, often do more to upset overall healthy immune function. Eighty-eight percent of ear infections resolve without antibiotics. Antibiotics complicate the underlying problems associated with otitis media due to their tendency to lead to dysbiosis. Antibiotics disrupt the intestinal flora, increasing the antibody-antigen load in the circulation, and cause the bacteria to eventually become resistant to treatment, adding to the negative effects of the invader.

If you have a child who suffers from middle ear infections, it is extremely important to his or her future health to try to break the reliance on antibiotics. I have used immune-enhancing supplements in my practice for years with great success. Recently, a study conducted at the New York Eye and Ear Infirmary showed similar results. They found that children given a daily dose of cod liver oil (a good source of omega-3 fatty acids, which have anti-inflammatory effects, and of vitamin A, which is needed for immunity) and a chewable multivitamin that contained the trace mineral selenium (an immune-enhancing trace mineral) led to significantly fewer infections and fewer antibiotics were needed. Studies like this are music to my ears—not only do they confirm what I have been seeing "anecdotally" for years, but also they confirm for parents that there are viable nutritional alternatives to antibiotics.

Food Allergies and ADHD

Attention deficit hyperactivity disorder (ADHD) is the most frequently diagnosed childhood psychiatric condition. An estimated 6 to 9 percent of school age children and 2 percent of all adults are affected by this disorder. It is highly unlikely that ADHD results from a single metabolic dysfunction. A genetic predisposition may be "awakened" by a host of nutritional and environmental influences. Many cases of ADHD have been successfully treated by controlling dietary, nutritional, and environmental influences.

A great deal of attention has been given to the consumption of salicylate-based additives, sugar, and allergenic foods as possible triggers of ADHD. During the 1960s, Benjamin Feingold, M.D., a California pediatrician, initiated using a low-salicylate diet for the treatment of ADHD after observing an exacerbation of symptoms among hyperactive children when they ate salicylate-containing foods.

Feingold's observations led to a controlled clinical trial, led by pediatric neurologist Dr. Joseph Edgar, which demonstrated that in addition to artificial colors and preservatives (which contain high amounts of salicylates), 90 percent of the ADHD children in the study had additional food intolerances. Dr. Edgar concluded from this study that the Feingold diet could not successfully treat ADHD if food intolerances were not addressed simultaneously.

The most common allergenic foods among children have been identified as cow's milk, corn, wheat, soy, peanuts, and eggs. An experimental diet among pre-school boys with sleep problems and hyperactive behavior demonstrated that after removal of artificial flavors and colors, dairy products, caffeine, MSG, and chocolate, more than 50 percent of the children improved. One study compared the treatment success of dietary restriction with methylphenidate (Ritalin) and found that while 44 percent responded to the drug treatment, 24 percent had equal success with dietary modifications alone.

Treating food allergies among those affected with ADHD is just the beginning. Assessment of heavy metal toxicity, dysbiosis (look at the history of antibiotic use), and essential fatty acid and mineral deficiencies is critical in the treatment protocol. Supplementing with probiotics and replacing deficient nutrients must be incorporated into the plan of care. (For specific recommendations, see Appendix 4: "Supplement Protocols for Other Common Conditions," page 518.)

All of these conditions are good demonstrations of a "barrel effect" of health. There are many factors that are contributing to what becomes ultimately expressed in certain symptoms. Addressing the underlying causes will strengthen immune response and alleviate symptoms.

Tests for Food Allergies

There are several tests for diagnosing food allergies: skin tests, blood tests, food elimination/challenge, rotation diet, and pulse testing. Both blood and skin tests require the supervision of a healthcare practitioner, while food elimination tests, rotation diets, and pulse testing can be done at home. Although home tests can be very revealing and highly accurate, they are not recommended for children. Some children may have severe and life-threatening reactions to certain foods. Therefore, tests for food allergies in children should be done in a controlled environment under the supervision of a healthcare professional.

Undiagnosed food intolerances are a major source of physical, emotional, and behavioral problems. However, many illnesses are rooted in other physiological disorders. If your symptom profile matches those listed in Table 9.2 on page 191, then proceeding with supervised testing or any of the at-home tests is recommended. If it does not, examining other sections of this book and completing the system discovery assessment questionnaire in Chapter 17 may reveal underlying sources of illness. Food allergies are often found in conjunction with other imbalances in the body.

Skin Tests. Skin tests are frequently used to test allergic reactions to environmental allergens. Scratch tests are done by first making a slight indentation in the skin and then superficially breaking the surface of the skin with a rough instrument. Once the scratch has been made, an extract of the allergen is placed on the broken skin and observed. If redness or swelling erupts within twenty minutes, the test is considered positive. As many as forty different allergens may be tested at one time. The greatest disadvantage is that scratch tests are unreliable for testing food allergens. This type of test measures IgE reactions to allergens, but does not measure the IgG-mediated delayed reactions typical of food intolerances.

Intradermal testing involves injecting diluted solutions of allergens into the outer layers of the skin and observing for reactions similar to those elicited by scratch tests. The advantage of this test is that progressively stronger dilutions can be injected to determine less severe reactions. The disadvantages are the same for scratch tests.

Blood Tests. Blood tests have a high degree of accuracy for detecting delayed IgG-mediated food reactions. Several types of blood tests are available. The most popular is the radioallergosorbent test (RAST). The RAST test measures the presence and amount of IgG and IgE antibodies specific to certain foods. Food allergies are diagnosed based on the detection of high levels of antibodies. Standard RAST tests only measure IgE antibodies, unless otherwise specified. Details about the test should be requested from the laboratory. One advantage of the RAST test is that several foods can be detected at one time. However, the RAST test is expensive, and it can fail to detect some food allergies because the test is standardized to include only the most frequently reactive foods. Entire food categories can be overlooked in the diagnosis.

The enzyme-linked immunoserological assay activated cell test (ELISA-ACT) measures serum antibodies using different detection techniques than the RAST. It measures immediate (IgE-mediated) and delayed (IgG-mediated) antibodies and cell-mediated responses to a wide variety of reactants, including food additives, heavy metals, chemicals, and environmental pollutants. It is considered a sensitive and comprehensive method of analyzing food and chemical sensitivities.

The antigen-leukocyte cellular antibody test (ALCAT), developed in 1983, uses a specially designed hematology analyzer to interpret the changes in white blood cells in response to antigen loading. The test is capable of determining a comprehensive list of reactive foods, as well as those foods considered safe.

Food-Provocation Challenge. The classic self-test for food allergies is the elimination-provocation challenge. The test involves eliminating all potentially reactive foods from the diet, then reintroducing them while noting any reactions. (See the inset "The Do-It-Yourself Allergy Test" on page 199.) Another method for determining (and managing) food allergies is the *Diversified Rotation Diet.*

Rotation Diet. This diet addresses the fact that the typical American diet is fundamentally a monotonous rotation of the same few foods: beef, pork, poultry, eggs,

Do-It-Yourself Food Allergy Test

Self-testing for food allergies has some obvious advantages. Since it is self-directed and takes place at home, it is a cost-effective method for determining food sensitivities. If done correctly, it can be a highly accurate method of testing for a broad range of foods and additives. The major disadvantages are that the methods are time-consuming and require substantial discipline. Since eliminating allergenic foods from the diet involves breaking food addictions, the test can be very difficult. Any variation of the tests or "cheating" can render the results inaccurate.

The classic self-test for food allergies is the elimination-provocation challenge. The test involves eliminating all potentially reactive foods from the diet, then reintroducing them while noting any reactions.

1. Elimination

Eliminate suspected foods for seven to fourteen days. Suspected foods are foods eaten repeatedly, foods that are craved, and foods that produce any unusual changes in the body (good or bad). Eat only foods that you are unlikely to be sensitive to. Typically foods allowed during an elimination diet include non-citrus, fresh fruits; all vegetables (except corn and tomatoes); rice; turkey; white fish (halibut, sole, swordfish); almonds, walnuts, and sunflower seeds. If many foods are suspected, there are many books available that provide guidelines for successfully eliminating these foods.

2. Provocation

Reintroduce suspicious foods one food at a time in small amounts, such as one-quarter to one-half cup, with no more than one suspicious food a day. The less potentially allergenic foods should be introduced first. If there is a reaction to a food, eliminate it from the diet for three to six weeks before retesting. Some reactions to foods are fixed, causing consistent reactions. If you experience the same reaction the next time you reintroduce the food, then you've found the suspect. Carefully note your reactions to other foods in the same food family; it is common to be sensitive to more than one food or food family. These foods should be eliminated permanently.

Take heart, most foods can be tolerated if rotated in the diet and eaten infrequently. This is, somewhat obviously, called the "rotation diet" (see page 198 for details).

Note: Severe reactions to foods can be neutralized by taking about 2,000 mg of vitamin C mixed ascorbate powder every fifteen to thirty minutes until a loose stool occurs, or the symptoms subside. Vitamin C helps to stabilize the immune system and control the release of various immune chemicals that cause inflammation and allergies.

Children can have severe and life-threatening reactions to some foods. It is safer to test these foods in a controlled environment under the supervision of a health-care professional. If possible, consider testing offending foods by one of the blood tests described under "Tests for Food Allergies."

wheat, potatoes, tomatoes, sugar, soy, and corn, as well as a stunning repertoire of food additives. This overeating of the same few foods can contribute to food allergies. Interestingly, most of these foods can be found on the list of common food allergens. Whether these foods are inherently addictive because of their allergenic potential or induce reactions due to their frequent use is a question to ponder.

Rotation diets are still heavily relied upon to identify suspected problematic foods. These diets are typically divided into two phases: the *refractory* phase and the *diversification* phase. During the refractory phase, foods that cause a reaction, or are suspect, are eliminated from the diet for six weeks; the diversification phase involves reincorporating the food into the diet, eating it only once every four days, and observing whether there is any adverse reaction.

Rotation diets require a great deal of discipline and organization to be done correctly. Many good books are available that provide details about how to correctly follow a rotation diet.

Pulse Testing. Another method for identifying food sensitivities at home is *pulse testing.* This method requires establishing a baseline resting pulse rate, as well as accuracy in taking the pulse. If an increase in pulse is detected, a one-hour interval should pass before testing another food. This test is not completely accurate, as some allergic reactions will not always result in an increased heart rate. However, it may serve as a good starting point for choosing foods to eliminate on the elimination-provocation challenge.

Treating Food Allergies

Unlike the standard treatment for environmental allergies (allergy shots), there are no widely administered pharmaceutical treatment measures for food allergies. (Epinephrine injections are available in case of severe anaphylactic reactions to foods.) Antihistamines and immunosuppressive drugs reduce some symptoms, but do not address the underlying causes of allergies.

Cromolyn sodium (Intal) is often used to prevent allergic reactions to environmental and food allergens. Inhaled, it can be effective at reducing the symptoms of asthma. If taken orally, it can block minor reactions to food. Cromolyn sodium inhibits mast cell degranulation and the subsequent release of inflammatory mediators. By this mechanism, it has indirect anti-inflammatory properties. Because it is rapidly excreted, it is virtually nontoxic and can be used by children. Several studies have reported success in using cromolyn sodium for the prevention and symptom management of food reactions.

There is evidence that alkaline preparations like sodium bicarbonate (baking soda), potassium bicarbonate, and over-the-counter combinations like Alka-Seltzer Gold (which is available both with and without an antihistamine) relieve some food allergy symptoms. These preparations, taken immediately after symptoms develop, at times have demonstrated some dramatic results. They should not be taken regularly, only for situations in which symptoms are intolerable or for occasions when avoiding problematic foods will be difficult. (To use sodium or potassium bicarbonate, mix one to two teaspoonfuls in water; for Alka-Seltzer Gold follow directions on package.)

Once you have identified and avoided an allergenic food, you can usually reintroduce it without any adverse reactions, as long as you maintain a rotation diet (see page 198 for details). Rotation diets give a method for working the food back into your diet as you become less sensitive.

The Vicious Cycle of Allergy-Addiction

One aspect of food allergies that makes this condition extremely challenging to treat is the phenomenon of addiction. An addictive substance can be any food, chemical, or drug to which a person develops a sensitivity reaction upon exposure, followed by withdrawal symptoms, which can be suppressed by repeated exposure to the substance.

Those with food allergies often experience intense cravings for the foods to which they are most allergic. Allergic addiction follows predictable reactions in the sensitive person, beginning with the initial sensitivity response. First contact with an allergen produces a typical allergic reaction: the symptoms may vary according to the individual. Once the reaction subsides, withdrawal symptoms begin, marked by an intense craving for the allergenic substance. This is known as the "withdrawal-phase" or "maladaptive reaction." These symptoms can be alleviated by contact with the allergen, and prolonged relief can be obtained by repeated contact. This is the "stimulatory period" or "adaptive" addiction.

In the adaptive phase, it appears that exposure to the allergen is either harmless or even enhances well-being. Allergy symptoms are generally absent during this phase, and there may be a "high" associated with exposure. Narcoticlike substances are released from the brain upon exposure to some allergens, including endorphins and opiate alkaloids.

With repeated exposure, more of the allergen is needed to maintain the adaptive state. Ultimately, the load on the body becomes too great and illness develops. This state of exhaustion, or "chronic maladaption," is the final phase of allergic addiction.

The vicious cycle of allergy-addiction can take place over a lifetime. Masked allergies will slowly erode the health of cells, tissues, and organs until eventually unexplained chronic illness sets in. Examining the foods that produce the most intense cravings, followed by a feeling of well-being after consumption, is a good place to begin identifying possible adaptive addictions.

The treatment of food allergies cannot be addressed without considering the integrity of the gut. I have rarely seen a situation of food intolerance that did not involve dysbiosis, candida-related complex (CRC), and/or leaky gut. Following the supplement guidelines for restoring gut health addressed in Chapter 11 and phase one of the Healthy Living Guidelines in Chapter 13 has often proven adequate for addressing food allergies in my patients. The initial phase of the eating plan in this book addresses the most common food allergies by temporarily eliminating wheat and dairy products. By adding in the supplements for restoring gut integrity, many times the allergic tendency of the gut subsides. (If more specific protocol is

Marriann's Story

I am a twenty-eight-year-old professional woman. For as long as I can remember, I have suffered from irritable bowel syndrome (IBS). As a child, no one had a name for my symptoms, but I had frequent and severe painful constipation. Most of the time the pain was so severe I would just lay in a fetal position until I became so sick I would vomit. I went to a gastroenterologist who recommended Metamucil, but it didn't help. I also had a colonoscopy, but it showed nothing. So I just had to live with the constant pain. Eventually, I noticed if I ate greasy food, it would make me go to the bathroom. I knew this wasn't a healthy solution, but no one else had any solutions. I overheard a coworker recommend Dr. LaValle to other people in our office for other problems. As I listened, I thought he might be able to help me. So I set up an appointment.

That was over a year ago. Since I began taking the supplements that Dr. LaValle recommended and following his Healthy Living Guidelines, I have not had an attack and I've been able to eat foods that formerly had bothered me. I was even able to avoid constipation when I was pregnant, which surprised me. I feel so much healthier. Dr. LaValle's recommendations improved not only the IBS, but also my overall health, enabling me to have a very healthy pregnancy and baby girl. I would recommend Dr. LaValle's teachings for cracking the metabolic code to anyone. You will feel great and your overall health will be vastly improved.

Marriann is a good example of what happens when the intestinal tract develops dysbiosis. She virtually suffered with chronic pain for years, and for her, the solution was fairly simple. She followed the eating plan in the Healthy Living Guidelines, and when she began to reintroduce common allergy-producing foods, she found out that she did not tolerate dairy products. She simply stopped eating dairy products. In addition, she took the supplements needed to balance her intestinal chemistry. The combination of a healthier but individualized diet and supplements gave Marriann back her life.

needed, see Appendix 4: "Supplement Protocols for Other Common Conditions," on page 518.)

INTESTINAL HEALTH IS KEY

A healthy digestive system is fundamental for a healthy body. Somehow, we tend to think of the intestines as bulletproof and self-contained, when in essence, the importance of a healthy gut may well be the most important aspect of health. If your digestive system and intestines are not functioning properly—whether it is due to yeast overgrowth and its many causes, leaky gut syndrome, food allergies, or other intestinal disturbances—a host of problems will arise.

For millions of us, the accumulated challenge on our digestive systems has become greater than our guts can adapt and respond to. Again, let's think of the body as a car. To run, a car requires fuel on a daily basis. If low-quality fuel is used, the car's engine, pipes, valves, and other systems would deteriorate and become clogged and cause the car to breakdown or run poorly.

The body's fuel is quality food. This fuel is effectively broken down and absorbed by the body. If the digestive system and intestines are clogged, slowed, and/or not functioning "up to par," the nutrients and fuels needed to run the body as a well-tuned machine will not be digested and absorbed. This affects every organ in the body—from the lungs, heart, and eyes to the small vessels that carry the necessary oxygen and nutrients to every living cell.

Virtually all of the energy you need to function is obtained from one source—the food you eat. Good nutrition is key to a healthy digestive system. A diet high in fibrous foods, especially fresh fruits and vegetables, is of utmost importance. Not only are these foods chockfull of vitamins, minerals, and invaluable phytonutrients, but they also help to keep the intestines clean and functioning properly. The detox program and gastrointestinal support I use with my patients is presented as a plan of action in Chapter 11. Also, you'll learn more about an optimal diet for supporting intestinal health in Chapter 13. The next chapter focuses on the external toxins in our environment and on the impact those toxins have when they enter our bodies.

Now, onward for Key Six . . .

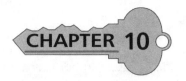

CHAPTER 10

KEY SIX:
Detoxifying Your Environment—
The Effects of Environmental
Toxins on Your Health

According to the Environmental Protection Agency (EPA), approximately 87,000 chemicals are in use today. More than 15,000 of these chemicals are produced in amounts exceeding 10,000 pounds per year. Sixty-two thousand chemicals contain molecules that are able to cross cell membranes and potentially disrupt the cellular function of living organisms. And only a fraction of these substances are screened and tested by the EPA.

Chemicals are found in cleaning agents, fuel, cosmetics, building materials, toys, packaging, and so on. Almost every commercial product in use today contains some form of chemical. Nearly every chemically laden product in use today was developed after the 1960s.

Ours is a generation of consumers exposed to industrial living almost constantly. It is a choice we make, but now it's clear that safer options must be developed to drive our economy without destroying our health. In all honesty, we have no idea what the cumulative effects are when all of these chemicals meet at the cellular crossroads of our mitochondria (our cells' powerhouses) and DNA.

Knowing where these toxins reside in our environment and their impact on health, however, can provide important information to help you minimize the health effects of toxic overload.

PESTICIDES

Pesticides are chemicals used to control pests, including weeds, insects, and rodents. Insecticides, fumigants, fungicides, rodenticides, and herbicides are the most commonly used pesticides. Alarmingly, 90 percent of the pesticides in use today are used in the production of food. However, pesticides are also found in a surprising variety of products, including shampoos, disposable diapers, carpets, paint, mattresses, contact lenses, and so on.

Pesticides are highly toxic in large doses, and there is much concern about the health effects of chronic (long-term) low levels of exposure on humans. Most pesticides work by destroying the central nervous system of insects and rodents. The long-term effects of pesticide exposure in humans are not known and are poorly studied. Moreover, it is unknown what multiple chemicals acting together are doing to our body chemistry. Some researchers, however, have made it clear that there is a need to study the effects of chemical combinations.

Pesticides enter the human body in a number of ways. When pesticides are sprayed on crops, residue remains on the food. In addition to direct consumption from residue on foods, pesticides enter the food chain from the soil and water. Once in the soil, pesticides enter the groundwater and streams from precipitation, erosion, and runoff. Pesticides pollute our drinking water and the water used to grow crops. Groundwater contamination is very difficult to reverse because of the slow rate of flow. Streams and rivers are vulnerable to rapid and widespread contamination from pesticides due to their higher rates of flow. Fish become contaminated from existing in polluted rivers and seas. Predatory animals eat contaminated fish, and humans eat fish and predatory animals, thus pesticides permeate the human food chain.

Consider this seemingly benign manner in which toxins can invade your system. Think of any avid golfer happily playing through on the pristine turf at any country club. Now think about how that turf is kept so very beautiful; it is treated rather heavily with a variety of chemicals for insect and weed control. Now consider that golfer's exposure to chemicals as he plays, breathing in residues, and picking up balls covered with chemical residues.

If you look at breast cancer rates on the women's golf tour it might give you pause for concern. In two years, four players were diagnosed with breast cancer, and 618 golf-course superintendents have contracted various forms of cancer between 1970 and 1992. Interestingly, the Ladies Professional Golf Association (LPGA) has offered mammograms to players since 1991. Women are particularly susceptible to the toxins, many of which act as *xenoestrogens*—chemical toxins that act like estrogen and disrupt hormonal activity in the body.

The suspected role of xenoestrogens as endocrine (hormone) disrupters is, in fact, one of my most serious concerns about the use of pesticides. The EPA estimates that there are 60 million pounds of endocrine disruptors released into the environment each year. The endocrine system regulates hormone synthesis, release, and activity throughout the body. Hormones control metabolism and reproductive function. The thyroid gland, the pancreas, the ovaries, the testes, the pituitary gland, and the adrenal glands are all endocrine glands. The endocrine system is one of two major control systems in the body, the other being the nervous system. And the endocrine, nervous, and immune systems are closely interrelated. In contrast to natural hormones, which are effective at extremely low concentrations, hormone disrupters are found in relatively high concentrations in the body.

Endocrine disrupters can interfere with hormones in three ways: The first is through hormone *mimicry,* in which the chemical mimics the hormone by binding with receptors and stimulating cellular activity. This mimicry tricks the body into thinking it has sufficient levels of certain hormones, which signals the hypothalamus to stop its hormone production. The second is hormone *masking,* in which the chemicals bind with receptor sites and blocks the hormone's activity at the cellular level. In this case, the hypothalamus is stimulated to produce more and more of its hormone. The third way endocrine disrupters alter hormone balance is by *binding* with the hormone itself, thereby rendering it unable to carry out its hormonal message. Through mimicry, masking, and binding, endocrine disrupters can halt or stimulate hormone production, increase or decrease activity at the cellular level, disrupt metabolism, and interfere with immune function. Because of their influence over reproductive hormones, these agents can also alter reproduction and development.

A number of chemicals are known to disrupt the endocrine systems of animals. When these chemicals accumulate in natural ecosystems, reproductive and developmental abnormalities appear among fish and wildlife. Reproductive and developmental defects have been observed in birds, most notably the bald eagle, resulting in lowered reproduction and population decline. Laboratory studies have shown that exposure of animals to hormonally active agents can lead to structural and functional abnormalities of the reproductive systems.

Empirical evidence suggests that *organochlorine* pesticides, known to cause endocrine disruption in birds, fish, and mammals, also interfere with hormone regulation in humans. Women with breast cancer tend to have higher levels of DDE (a metabolite of DDT) residue in their breast tissue. Higher tissue levels of DDE are also associated with diminished milk production during breastfeeding, suggesting that pesticides may interfere with lactation.

In Iowa, elevated levels of the *triazine* herbicides (*atrazine, metolchlor,* and *cyanzinc*) in municipal water were associated with increased rates of low birth weight, prematurity, and intrauterine growth retardation between 1984 and 1990. Further, cases of lupus, which seems to have a strong estrogen component, have risen fourteen-fold in women over the last fifty years, which could be linked to the increased solvent and xenoestrogen exposure.

There is some speculation that endocrine-disrupting chemicals are responsible for some hormone-specific birth trends. For example, during the period of 1970 to 1990, the number of male births declined by 2.2 per 1,000 live births in Canada and 1 per 1,000 in the United States. While these numbers are statistically significant, there is no scientific explanation. The *Journal of the American Medical Association* (JAMA) reported in 1998 that the ratio of male births declined significantly, while the number of male reproductive tract defects are on the rise. According to the Centers for Disease Control and Prevention (CDC), the incidence of *hypospadias* (a congenital defect of the urinary tract) in the United States doubled between 1968 and 1993. The rate of severe cases increased, while the ratio of mild to severe cases decreased.

The 1996 Food Quality Protection Act specifically mandated the EPA to develop an endocrine-disrupter screening program. Recommendations for a screening program were finalized in August 1998 by the Endocrine Disrupter Screening and Testing Advisory Committee (EDSTAC). The Endocrine Disrupter Screening Program is supposed to develop methods and procedures to detect and characterize endocrine activity of pesticides, chemicals, and environmental contaminants. However, the methodology of the screening program appears limited. The initial screening model—the Quantitative Structure Activity Relationship (QSAR)—is only designed to predict a chemical's affinity for estrogen and androgen (male hormone) receptors. The QSAR relies on a computer to compare the structure of a chemical with the structure of the receptors to determine whether there is enough similarity to warrant concern about endocrine disruption. This discounts the myriad of ways that chemicals can influence the endocrine system, including disruption of hormones in the circulation and affinity for other types of receptors (thyroid, insulin, cortisol, and others).

The EPA completed its initial QSAR analysis in January 2000. The foods it listed as most contaminated by pesticides were:

- Apples
- Apricots
- Bell peppers
- Cantaloupe (from Mexico)
- Celery
- Cherries (from the United States)

- Cucumbers
- Grapes (from Chile)
- Green beans
- Peaches
- Spinach
- Strawberries

Pesticides are some of the most difficult toxins to eliminate from the body. They are particularly dangerous because they tend to be lipophilic or lipid (fat) loving. That means they can penetrate body cells and damage nuclear and mitochondrial DNA. This increases the genetic damage and can increase the risk of developing cancers.

Organochlorine Pesticides

Organochlorine pesticides are fat-soluble compounds that are well absorbed orally and topically. Fat-soluble substances mix easily with other fat-soluble substances. In humans, the fat-soluble-containing tissues such as nerve tissues including the brain, cell membranes, and the fat cells themselves are the tissues most likely to be affected by fat-soluble compounds. This also means that they enter the systems of humans and animals easily, but they are difficult to excrete. In the fatty tissue, organochlorines accumulate to unsafe levels potentially causing neurotoxicity (toxic to the nervous system) and cancer.

In addition to human health concerns, organochlorines have documented effects on the health of wildlife. Scientists have known since the 1970s that organochlorines cause eggshell thinning in the bald eagle; and produce hormone and reproductive disturbances in aquatic reptiles, birds, fish, and mammals.

In the 1970s, some organochlorine pesticides (for example, DDT) were banned because of their cumulative impact on the environment. Developed in 1939, DDT was first used during World War II to clear the South Pacific islands of malaria-causing insects for U.S. troops. In Europe, it was used to kill lice. DDT was the most powerful pesticide the world had ever known. Unlike most pesticides, whose effectiveness is limited to destroying one or two types of insects, DDT was capable of killing hundreds of different kinds at once.

At the time DDT was considered revolutionary. Its inventor, the noted Swiss scientist Paul Muller, Ph.D., was awarded the Nobel Prize for its discovery. However, caution was not employed in the use of DDT, and it was a poster child for what can go wrong when a pesticide is used without proper testing and is used indiscriminately. When DDT became available for civilian use in 1945, only a few people expressed concerns about its use. In fact, public safety commercials were made that showed children at lunch tables being sprayed with DDT while they were eating to demonstrate its safety.

One of those who expressed concern about DDT early on was nature writer Edwin Way Teale. He warned, "A spray as indiscriminate as DDT can upset the economy of nature as much as a revolution upsets social economy. Ninety percent of all insects are good, and if they are killed, things go out of kilter right away." Another was Rachel Carson, who wrote the book *Silent Spring* in 1962. This landmark environmental book changed the way Americans viewed the impact of technology on the environment. Rachel Carson is credited with starting the environmental movement.

Despite the warnings of those concerned, DDT was used heavily and extensively for years. As early as the late 1940s, it was discovered that DDT was highly toxic to fish, and many insects were becoming resistant to it. DDT is stored in fat-soluble substances and has a fairly long half-life of eight years, which means that it will take eight years for the body to rid itself of half of the DDT ingested. Many of the effects of DDT weren't seen until years later. However, despite some of the early problems, DDT was not banned in the United States until 1973.

In some cases, the environmental damage caused by pesticide use takes many years to resolve. DDT and DDE have been detected in riverbed sediment and freshwater fish decades after its use was banned. Highlights from a 1996 U.S. Geological Service survey concluded that organochlorine pesticides that have not been used for twenty years could still be found in aquatic ecosystems. The most frequently detected compound is the breakdown product of DDT (known as DDE). A recent survey of the U.S. food supply found detectable residue of DDT in 16 percent of the samples.

Among the alarming facts related to food inspection is that the United States has a great deal of its foods imported from other countries, but only 2 percent of these foods are inspected as they enter the United States. Other countries regularly still use

DDT and other outlawed chemicals. In fact, some of the chemicals are actually made in the United States, shipped abroad, and then reenter our food supply via foreign growers even though it is outlawed here because of safety concerns. It seems as if the problem we shipped overseas has returned to our shores. Think of our children who, by weight, are being overwhelmed with these chemicals. It is no wonder that cancer is the third leading cause of death of children.

All this because American business found it more profitable to sell these chemicals to third-world countries when they were outlawed here, instead of just destroying what they knew to be poisons. And so, pesticides have become a global issue. They

Pesticides and Children

In 1989, the National Resource Defense Council (NRDC) studied eight widely used chemicals and their impact on children's health. The study reported that children on average receive up to four times more exposure to carcinogenic pesticides in food than adults. Children are more exposed to contaminants in food and water because in relation to body weight, they eat and drink more than adults. They are also more physiologically vulnerable to contamination and injury due to their immature systems and developing organs.

There are approximately ninety suspected carcinogenic pesticides in use today. Children are the most vulnerable to these chemicals because of the rapid proliferation of their cells. Several epidemiological studies have examined the relationship between childhood cancers and exposure to pesticides. The Children's Cancer Study Group conducted a case-controlled study of occupational exposure of parents whose children had developed leukemia. The most consistent finding among the 204 cases was an association between prolonged pesticide exposure by the parents and acute nonlymphoblastic leukemia in the children. The risk was significantly increased if the child had direct exposure to pesticides in the home, or if the mother was exposed to household pesticides during pregnancy.

The incidence of all types of childhood cancer increased 10.5 percent between 1973 and 1994, and the incidence of central nervous system and brain cancer increased 35.1 percent. Other childhood conditions, including asthma, are also on the rise. Some research suggests that pesticide exposure may disrupt the autonomic nervous system (the part of the nervous system that governs involuntary actions), leading to respiratory disease in children.

In 1993, the National Academy of Sciences (NAS) report "Pesticides in the Diets of Infants and Children" stated that, despite the fact that children are more vulnerable to effects of pesticides in food, the government does not sufficiently protect them from exposure. The report led to the 1996 Food Quality Protection Act. The act required that the EPA establish the maximum allowable pesticide content in food based on the

are everywhere. Although the highest concentrations of these pesticides are found in the areas of use, low levels have been detected in the remotest parts of the globe.

Organophosphate Pesticides

Organophosphate pesticides (OPs) have mostly replaced organochlorines in U.S. food production. Organophosphates account for approximately half of all the insecticide use in the United States.

Each year, about 60 million pounds of OP are used to treat 60 million acres of agricultural crops. Another 17 million pounds are used for nonagricultural purposes,

sensitivity of children and infants and "a reasonable certainty that no harm will result from aggregate exposure to a pesticide." All new and previously used pesticides must now meet the "10x Safety Factor," in which the EPA retains an additional tenfold margin of safety for any pesticide not specifically shown to be safe for children.

In 1997, the EPA identified the pesticides thought to pose the greatest health risk to both adults and children, including nerve poisons, carcinogens, and endocrine disrupters. The EPA named organophosphates (OPs) and carbamate, another major pesticide, as the insecticides most threatening to public health. Some animal studies indicate that exposure to OPs during the prenatal period and early infancy may result in permanent loss of brain function. No studies have confirmed the safety of neurotoxic pesticides on the developing brains of human children. Levels determined "safe" for adult consumption, therefore, should not be assumed safe for children. Keep in mind that all the other influences can also be working against the child at the same time: nutrient and food quality, stress, prescription drug use (which today is significant in children), and genetic and toxicological load from the mother amongst other factors.

A 1999 risk analysis conducted by the Environmental Working Group (EWG), a nonprofit environmental research group, found that children are even more exposed to dangerous levels of pesticides than recognized in previous data. The EWGs findings report that, "Over 250,000 children aged one through five years consume a combination of twenty different pesticides each day; over 1 million consume at least fifteen pesticides daily; and 20 million ingest an average of eight pesticides daily."

Every day, 610,000 children aged one through five consume amounts of organophosphates pesticides that the EPA considers unsafe. Half of this exposure comes from the OP methyl parathion. Children aged one through five drink thirty times more apple juice, twenty-one times more grape juice, and seven times more orange juice than the average adult. More than one-half of the children who consume unsafe doses of OP pesticides are exposed from apples and apple products. Some apples can deliver unsafe doses of OP pesticides to children younger than five years old in one bite.

including the treatment of livestock, pets, stored foods, and for residential and commercial insect control.

Like some organochlorine pesticides, OPs are broad-spectrum pesticides capable of destroying a multitude of species. This makes OP more convenient and less expensive than using several pesticides. Organophosphate pesticides destroy insects by interfering with *cholinesterase,* an enzyme needed for the proper functioning of the neurotransmitter *acetylcholine.* Acetylcholine regulates nerve impulse transmission between nerve cells and between nerve and muscle cells. Without cholinesterase, muscle weakness or paralysis can result. Acute OP toxicity in humans has the same effect as in insects. The chronic effects of human exposure to organophosphate pesticides are not known, although some research has indicated that chronic exposure can lead to neurological, immune, and endocrine damage.

Two organophosphate pesticides in use today, chlorpyrifos and methyl parathion, are especially problematic. *Chlorpyrifos* (Dursban) is the most widely used insecticide in the United States. It has been registered for use since 1965. There are approximately 822 products containing *chlorpyrifos* on the U.S. market. It is used in residential and commercial applications, including schools, daycare centers, hotels, restaurants, hospitals, and food-manufacturing facilities. Epidemiological data shows that 82 percent of adults and 92 percent of children have measurable concentrations of the primary metabolite of Dursban (3,5,6-TCP) in their urine.

A recent EPA review found that chlorpyrifos poses excessive safety hazards to those who treat their homes and gardens with the product. According to the EPA's review, nearly all of the common home applications of Dursban result in exposure levels that exceed safety levels. For example, hand spreading the granules exposes an individual to 10,000 percent of the safe dose. Application with a hand sprayer indoors exposes one to 811 percent of the maximum safety margin, and use of a hand sprayer outdoors is 435 percent of the maximum safe dose. The review also found unsafe concentrations of chlorpyrifos in groundwater and drinking water.

In addition, researchers at Rutgers University have shown that home flea treatments (aerosol/foggers), another common use of chlorpyrifos, elevate air pesticide levels in excess of legal limits for more than twenty-four hours after application. Levels just above the floor ("the infant breathing zone") were ten times above the legal limit seven hours after application and three times the legal limit after twenty-four hours. The researchers oppose manufacturers' instructions that state that it is safe to return home after several hours following application.

Human studies have revealed that humans may be more sensitive to the toxic effects of chlorpyrifos than animals, rendering animal safety tests insufficient for determining the safety thresholds for humans. Newborns and young children may be especially sensitive to the cholinesterase inhibiting effects of chlorpyrifos. In a Duke University study, newborn rats given the equivalent of 5 milligrams (mg) per kilogram (kg) of body weight of chlorpyrifos for the first four days exhibited severe brain stem cell loss and significantly increased mortality. When chlorpyrifos was administered on days eleven to fourteen, cell loss occurred in the forebrain.

A similar study noted that newborn rats given 2 mg/kg of chlorpyrifos showed significant inhibition of DNA synthesis in all regions of the brain. In both studies, brain changes were detectable at doses that were not considered toxic. One author of the study concludes, "The lower threshold for these cellular effects compared to that for systemic toxicity indicates that the developing brain is a selective target for chlorpyrifos: effects that should be considered in assessing safety thresholds."

Chlorpyrifos has also been associated with immunologic abnormalities. In a California State University study, twelve subjects exposed to chlorpyrifos were found to have a high rate of atopic allergic reactions, antibiotic sensitivity, and autoimmune disorders compared with two control groups. The immunologic changes occurred one to four and a half years after exposure. Autoantibodies were found for smooth muscle, parietal (stomach) cells, brush border (intestinal) cells, thyroid tissue, and myelin (nerve cells).

The Environmental Working Group (EWG) has issued a Dursban advisory to consumers, recommending that any unopened products containing chlorpyrifos be returned to the place of purchase, and opened products be taken to hazardous waste disposal sites. The group states that Dursban home and garden or lawn use is unsafe for children. The EWG has called on the EPA to immediately ban the sale and use of Dursban in the United States.

Another OP product generating considerable concern is *methyl parathion.* Methyl parathion is considered toxic to children in small amounts and is pervasive in the foods commonly eaten by children. Any detectable residue on foods delivers an unsafe dose to children. The EPA has established that the maximum daily exposure should not exceed 0.000026 mg per kilogram of body weight. It is estimated that a substantial number of American children could exceed the safe dose of methyl parathion by 100-fold each day. The foods that put children at the highest risk of exposure are peaches and grapes. Grapes appear to be especially contaminated. According to an EWG analysis, 92 percent of the most exposed children obtained methyl parathion from grapes.

Methyl parathion is considered a Category 1 Acute Toxin (the most dangerous). At acute doses, it is a known neurotoxic agent. Chronic exposure is associated with retinal and sciatic nerve degeneration in animals. The EWG has called on the EPA to impose an emergency ban on methyl parathion. Methyl parathion is currently illegal (or has never been registered) in twenty-seven other countries. Among these countries is Denmark, home of the largest methyl parathion supplier to the United States.

Government Tests for Determining Pesticide Levels

The EPA approves the use of pesticides and established *tolerances.* Tolerances are the maximum amount of residue allowed to remain on or in a food that has been treated with a pesticide. The EPA establishes tolerances based on the toxicity of the pesticide, how much and how often it is used, and how much residue typically remains on the food.

With so many chemicals in use today, the regulation of pesticide safety by the EPA is marginally adequate. In the 1980s, a National Academy of Science (NAS) study found that 78 percent of the most widely used commercial chemicals had not undergone "minimal toxicity testing." The EPA has confessed its own limitations.

According to a former EPA Pesticide office director Daniel Barolo, in the *Newsday* article "EPA Offers Thin Shield of Safety," it is logistically impossible for the EPA to test every chemical in an independent laboratory under strict scientific methodology. Instead, it relies on studies conducted by laboratories hired by chemical manufacturers. This creates a serious conflict of interest and dramatically skews test results.

Between 1989 and 1995, the results of forty-three, industry-funded studies were published in scientific journals. The studies evaluated the safety of several potentially hazardous chemicals (the herbicides atrazine and alachlor, the preservative formaldehyde, and the dry-cleaning agent perchloroethylene). Only six of the forty-three studies negatively assessed the safety of these chemicals. In contrast, during the same period, 118 independent studies (sponsored by nonprofit organizations) were published concerning the safety of these chemicals. Seventy-one studies reported hazards associated with the use of the chemicals.

The current standards for protecting humans and wildlife established by the EPA are based on *maximum acceptable concentrations* of pesticides. There is considerable evidence that these standards fail to protect us from the hazards of pesticide pollution. Maximum acceptable concentrations have not been established for many of the pesticides in use today. Furthermore, most toxicity experiments are conducted on single compounds within a limited range of concentrations. Values do not include the cumulative effect of the pesticide metabolites or the impact of contaminated ecosystems. Nor do they focus on how compounds interact when they are mixed. Chemicals are rarely isolated in the soil, air, or water. For example, pesticides commonly mix with fertilizers in the ground and water.

Under the 1996 Food Quality Protection Act, the EPA is required to review all existing tolerances for pesticides. There are currently 469 pesticides with active or high hazard ingredients, and 9,700 tolerances in effect for chemicals used in the production of food. The law requires the EPA to reassess the safety of these tolerances by August 2006. According to the EPA, "organophosphate pesticides, carbamates, probable carcinogens, reference dose exceeders, and high-hazard inerts" will be the first reviewed.

HEAVY METALS

Heavy metals are particularly dangerous to the body. They can destroy cell membranes, increase cellular free-radical activity, and deplete the body of sulfur-containing enzymes. Heavy metals also directly attack organs, such as the kidneys, which further hinders the ability to excrete toxins. Heavy metals have known neurotoxic, endocrine-disrupting, and *immunotoxic* (toxic to the immune system) effects. Heavy metals also displace enzymes dependent upon zinc as a cofactor (zinc is needed for many biochemical reactions).

Approximately eighty minerals found in nature are classified as metals. They are divided into categories based on physical characteristics and biological activity. Metals are *cations,* meaning that (in water) they give up one electron to form a positive charge. Because they are positively charged, they are highly reactive in the body, and perform several important functions. For example, potassium and sodium serve as conductors of electrical charges, regulating cellular exchanges and controlling nerve impulses. Magnesium and calcium maintain the *concentration gradient* inside cells. (The concentration gradient prevents movement of ions back and forth across the cell membrane.) The metals zinc, iron, copper, and cobalt serve as catalysts of enzymatic reactions.

Most enzymes in the body require metal ions to either activate or stabilize them. These metals are known as *oligo* elements, or trace minerals. For example, iron (a stabilizing ion) is a structural and functional component of the cytochrome P-450 enzyme system. Zinc (an activating ion) forms a temporary bond with alkaline phosphatase (an enzyme needed for bone formation). Once the reaction takes place, zinc is unbound from the enzyme.

Heavy metals are those metals with a high atomic weight and a specific gravity greater than 4.0. While almost any metal can be toxic at high doses, heavy metals are toxic at much smaller doses (some heavy metals are toxic at any dose). The basis of heavy metal poisoning is the destruction of enzymes, which are proteins that make many of the biochemical reactions in the body. Enzymes very often require vitamins and cofactors to be activated. Heavy metals denature (destroy) proteins. They also bind with vitamins and trace minerals, displacing enzymatic cofactors. Enzymes with temporary bonds (such as those bound to zinc) are the most vulnerable to displacement, because these bonds are loose and fragile. A substance that is capable of displacing a metal bond is known as a *chelating agent.*

Heavy metals also inactivate enzymes by oxidation. In this reaction, the heavy metal cation "steals" an electron from the enzyme to stabilize its charge. Enzymes that contain sulfur amino acids, including methionine, glutathione, and cysteine, are most vulnerable to heavy metal oxidation. Destruction of sulfur-containing antioxidant enzymes cripples the detoxification pathways of the liver, leading to toxin overload and widespread free-radical damage.

Heavy metals are known to cause damage to cells by interfering with the fluidity of cell membranes. The fluidity of a cell membrane allows it to be selectively permeable, allowing the entry of only those substances that it needs to thrive. If it loses this capability, it can become damaged or destroyed.

Heavy metals enter the body through contaminated food and water, and by inhalation of fumes or dust particles. Heavy metals can be absorbed from the lungs or digestive tract into the bloodstream. While most heavy metals are excreted through the kidneys, some are eliminated through the gastrointestinal tract.

Heavy metal toxicity can be acute or chronic. Acute poisoning is associated with high levels of exposure over a short period and can be easier to recognize. Chronic toxicity, from low levels of exposure over time, produces vague and widespread symptoms that may be difficult to distinguish.

Once thought of as quackery, laboratory analysis now has validated low-level exposures in people who are facing significant health challenges. And a litany of primary research is being published linking heavy metals to a wide variety of disease states.

The heavy metals of most concern to human health are mercury, cadmium, lead, aluminum, and arsenic.

Mercury

Mercury, also known as quicksilver, is named for the Roman messenger of the Gods. It occurs naturally in three forms: *elemental* (metallic), *inorganic,* and *organic,* as discussed below.

According to one FDA toxicologist, 2,700 to 6,000 tons of mercury is released into the atmosphere annually from degassing of the earth's crusts and oceans. Conservative estimates are that human activities and industry contribute an additional 2,000 to 3,000 tons of mercury to the environment every year. Some experts argue that the number is much higher.

Mercury is found in pesticides and fungicides, is added to cosmetics, and is a component in silver dental fillings (amalgams). Industrial pollutants, particularly the burning of fossil fuels, are a major source of mercury exposure. But what is considered the most influential exposure actually comes from our diet. Common sources of mercury exposure are:

- Amalgam fillings
- Broken thermometers
- Contaminated fish
- Diet
- Fabric softeners
- Film
- Floor waxes and polishes
- Fungicide-treated grains
- Fungicides for lawns and shrubs

- House paint (latex paint)
- Industrial waste
- Latex- and solvent-thinned paints
- Leather tanning products
- Medicines (vaccines, certain injections, and eye preparations)
- Some air-conditioning filters
- Some cosmetics
- Tattoos

Elemental (Metallic) Mercury

Elemental mercury is silver-white and liquid at room temperature. It quickly vaporizes when exposed to air and is readily oxidized to its ionic form. It is insoluble in water, but can be dissolved in organic solvents.

Inhalation of mercury vapors is toxic to the lungs, causing inflammation of the alveoli, bronchi, and bronchioles. Acute (or immediate) toxicity from inhaled vapors results in fever, chills, shortness of breath, and a metallic taste and burning sensation in the mouth. Symptoms can progress to severe cramping pain, vomiting, and excessive salivation. Once inhaled, elemental mercury can cross the blood-brain barrier and accumulate in the brain tissue. Elemental mercury is toxic to the cells of the brain and nervous system.

Chronic inhalation of mercury vapors can lead to insomnia, emotional instability, nervousness, poor appetite, and dementia. Nineteenth-century hatters used mercury nitrate to stiffen hat-making materials, and many suffered from mercury-induced neurological symptoms. The term "mad as a hatter" was derived from their fate.

Inorganic Mercury

One of the most controversial subjects in the dental profession is centered on the use of amalgam fillings. Amalgams are the "silver" fillings used to restore teeth with dental caries, or cavities. Amalgam refers to the alloy of mercury with several other metals. An amalgam typically contains about 50 percent mercury with the remainder consisting of copper, zinc, and tin. Mercury is in a liquid state before the amalgam is sealed, then hardens after placement on the tooth. A bill is now in Congress to phase out all amalgam use by 2006.

Dentists have used amalgams for more than 150 years. It is estimated that at least 40 percent of Americans (about 100 million people) have at least one amalgam filling, and many have multiple fillings. The dental industry in the United States handles approximately 100 tons of mercury each year. Scientific literature shows that there is considerable cause for concern regarding the safety of mercury in amalgam fillings. Several European countries have taken specific action toward banning the use of amalgams. Both the U.S. EPA and the World Health Organization (WHO) have been unable to identify any "harmless" level of exposure to mercury. Yet the American Dental Association (ADA) has not yet developed a policy for dentists that recommends removal of amalgams for health reasons. It is unclear why the ADA continues to support the use of mercury-based amalgams, since there are equally effective and relatively inexpensive methods of tooth restoration.

While the ADA denies that the mercury in amalgams poses a health threat, many dentists and researchers contend that the use of mercury in any amount is toxic. A series of studies conducted by Lorscheider and Vimy from 1985 to 1995 found that mercury from amalgams is continuously released from the mouth as vapor, inhaled, absorbed into body tissue, oxidized to ionic mercury, and then bound to cell proteins. They also discovered that intra-oral (air) mercury of patients with amalgams was nine times that of people without. Chewing increased this level by a factor of six, resulting in a fifty-four-fold increase over control subjects. It was found that mercury exposure from amalgams was as high as 29 micrograms (mcg) per day, exceeding the maximum allowable daily limits established by some countries by as much as eighteen-fold. The limits established by the EPA for a 154-pound person are 30 mcg per day. These and other studies have provided reasonable evidence that mercury-based amalgam fillings substantially increase exposure to mercury vapors.

Research has demonstrated that bacteria in the mouth can corrode amalgams, leading to the conversion of inorganic elemental mercury to vapor. Once in the vapor form, it is inhaled by the lungs and transported across the alveolar membranes to the bloodstream. In the blood, mercury attaches to proteins and lipoproteins. This allows it entry into almost any cell of the body, but appears to accumulate mostly in the central nervous system, gastrointestinal tract, and the kidneys.

Mercury vapor easily crosses the blood-brain barrier (series of semi-permeable partitions monitoring and separating the body and its supply of substances and nutrients from the brain) leading to central nervous system disturbances like tremors, irritability, and depression. In the brain, elemental mercury vapors are oxidized to ionic mercury. Ionic mercury, which is not fat-soluble, accumulates in the central nervous system because it cannot cross back over the blood-brain barrier.

In 1994, researchers Siblerud and Kienholz hypothesized that mercury from amalgams may be related to multiple sclerosis (MS). They found that MS patients with amalgams had higher levels of mercury in their hair; lower red blood cells, hemoglobin, and hematocrit counts; lower thyroxine (hormone produced by the thyroid gland) levels; fewer T lymphocytes; and more exacerbations of symptoms. This in no way implies that all MS is due to mercury toxicity. But it is most likely another neurological irritant that switches on the autoimmune response leading to the downward spiral toward MS.

Bacteria in the gut can also oxidize mercury vapors, forming mercury ions. The ionization of mercury vapors is one step in the biochemical conversion of elemental to organic mercury. Ionic mercury is highly volatile, meaning it is strongly attracted to organic compounds, particularly sulfhydryl protein molecules (molecules with sulfur and hydrogen groups). When this happens, ionic mercury becomes an organic mercury compound. Organic mercury compounds are highly toxic in any form. Interestingly, amalgam fillings are considered safe, yet if mercury had to pass current safety standards for a filling material for the teeth, it would fail. In addition, if an amalgam filling is removed, once out of the mouth it is considered biohazardous material as soon as it exits the mouth. Common sense simply tells us that amalgam fillings are not the best option for teeth restoration.

Organic Mercury

The mercury poisoning of more than 800 people in Minamata, Japan, from the 1950s to the 1970s is a well-known example of the devastating effects of mercury contamination. During that period, a local factory had dumped an estimated 100 tons of mercury waste into Minamata Bay. Unfortunately, the mercury did not simply settle to the bottom of the bay and remain covered in sand, as was originally predicted. Instead, bacteria in the bay transformed the inorganic mercury to methyl (organic) mercury. The algae took up the freshly converted organic mercury, which was consumed by the fish. People who ate the contaminated fish became sick, and many died from subsequent complications. The neurological complications that persist among people of the region today are known as Minamata disease. Between 1952 and 1976, there were more than 100 deaths associated with Minamata mercury poisoning and more than 800 cases of severe brain damage. By 1982, there were approximately 1,700 reported cases of Minamata disease and more than 450 deaths attributed to its complications.

Mercury vapors are also released into the air from power plants and other industries that burn coal, such as metal refineries. Organic mercury compounds have been widely used as fungicides, particularly to increase the storage life of seed grain. In Iraq in 1972, seeds treated with alkyl mercury, intended for planting only, were accidentally ground into flour and made into bread. Consumption of the mercury-treated seed grain was responsible for more than 500 deaths and more than 6,500 hospitalizations. It was the worst case of mercury poisoning recorded in history.

Organic mercury compounds are fat-soluble and can easily cross cell membranes, the placenta, and the blood-brain barrier. Most nonexposed individuals have a blood content of about 8 ppb (parts per billion). Organic mercury is toxic to the brain and nervous system at blood levels of approximately 200 ppb. About 10 percent of the total body content of organic mercury passes into breast milk. Developing fetuses and young infants are highly vulnerable to the toxic effects of organic mercury compounds because of their developing nervous system. Laboratory studies have demonstrated that mercury has a special affinity for fetal neurons and astrocytes (star-shaped cells), as well as fetal hemoglobin. Mercury concentrations in fetal red blood cells can exceed those of the mother by as much as 30 percent

Infants of mothers exposed to mercury during the Japanese and Iraqi incidents have provided some data about the prenatal effects of mercury exposure. In both instances, it was shown that prenatal exposure was more damaging than exposure after birth. Studies following the infants of Minamata Bay mothers have associated methyl mercury poisoning with cerebral palsy, cleft palate, microcephaly, and kidney disease. Twenty-five children born to women poisoned from Minamata Bay had severe mental retardation.

After the Iraqi epidemic, thirty-two infants exposed to methyl mercury *in utero* were followed for a five-year period. Of the thirty-two, fourteen displayed early signs of mercury toxicity. Most of the fourteen children had severely delayed language skills, ten had cerebral palsy (six of those were blind), and four had abnormally small head circumference (microcephaly). Of the remaining eighteen children, half of them developed neurological symptoms after the age of two, although none were debilitating. Nine of the thirty-two children died within three years, a mortality rate of 28 percent compared with 6 percent among the children viewed as controls.

Many experts question the safety of even very low mercury exposure among pregnant women. Most Minamata Bay mothers whose infants displayed signs of congenital mercury toxicity had no outward signs of mercury poisoning. Since safety thresholds have not been established for fetuses, the FDA recommends that pregnant women and women of childbearing age limit their consumption of fish with higher concentrations (> 1 ppm) of mercury to no more than once a month. The National Research Council (NRC) estimates that potentially 60,000 newborns a year in the United States are at risk for neurologic damage due to mercury toxicity just from dietary sources!

Table 10.1 below shows mercury's detrimental effects throughout the entire body in all its forms.

Table 10.1. Symptoms of Chronic Mercury Exposure on Body Systems

Cardiovascular	Blood pressure changes, hypoxia, irregular heartbeat, irregular pulse
Central Nervous	Depression, dizziness, hallucinations, headaches, insomnia, irritability, memory impairment, multiple sclerosis, nervousness, ringing in ears, shyness, tremors
Endocrine	Cool skin, low body temperature, miscarriage, perspiration
Gastrointestinal	Cramps, diarrhea
General	Anemia, anorexia, fatigue, stuttering, muscle weakness, weight loss, weight gain, urological problems
Immune	Allergies, asthma, autoimmune disorders, cancer
Oral	Bleeding gums, halitosis, metallic taste, increased salivation, ulcers
Respiratory	Cough, emphysema

Mercury in the Diet

Most organic mercury exposure comes from the diet, and the most significant source of organic mercury in the food chain is found in fish. When we consume fish, as much as 90 percent of organic mercury is absorbed by the gastrointestinal tract. Nearly all fish contain traces of mercury, and some are more contaminated than others. Mercury content in fish is measured the same way it is in humans, in parts per million (ppm). The FDA has established a limit for human consumption at 1.0 ppm. Typically, mercury in fish ranges from 0.01 to 0.88 ppm. However, some large predator fish like tuna, swordfish, and shark can exceed 3.0 ppm. (Canned tuna comes from the smaller albacore and skipjack tunas, which have mercury concentrations of about 0.17 ppm.) Freshwater predators like walleye and pike have high mercury content, especially if caught near areas of high mercury pollution, such as coal mining, coal-burning power plants, gold mining, construction work, and battery and thermometer manufacturers. Mercury accumulates in fish by binding to the protein and muscle tissue. Mercury cannot be "cooked out."

The FDA advises that pregnant women and women of childbearing age limit their consumption of shark and swordfish to less than once a month. For others in the population, the FDA recommends that fish with mercury levels exceeding 1.0 ppm should not be consumed more than once a week. One serving is approximately 7 ounces. It should be noted that there is considerable difference in the fish advisories from state to state, depending on the various departments of health in the areas. You can contact your department of health to obtain advisories on the safety of fish in rivers, lakes, and streams in your area. States that share bodies of water have been known to provide conflicting information based on different criteria and risk approaches. Some states have advised to avoid certain fish species altogether.

From 1992 to 1994, the FDA conducted a sampling of at least five fish from each species, caught from a variety of waters. Table 10.2 below indicates the results of the survey. Note that the results are *average* values. Some of the larger fish exceeded the 1.0-ppm limit by a wide margin. For example, the range of values for shark was 0.30 to 3.52 ppm.

Table 10.2. Average Mercury Content in Fish

DOMESTIC FISH	CONTENT (PPM)	IMPORTED FISH	CONTENT (PPM)
Catfish	<.10	Pollock	0.16
Cod	0.13	Shark	0.36
Crab	0.13	Tuna (canned)	0.14
Flounder	<.10	Tuna (fresh)	0.27
Hake	<.10		
Halibut	0.24		
Pollock	<.10		
Salmon (canned)	<.10		
Salmon (fresh)	<.10		
Shark	0.84		
Swordfish	0.88		
Tuna (canned)	0.20		
Tuna (fresh)	0.38		

Inorganic mercury is the product of elemental mercury combined with inorganic substances. The result is a mercuric salt. Mercuric salts are highly corrosive and extremely irritating to the mucous membranes of the gastrointestinal tract. Inorganic mercury is a constituent of batteries and can be used in explosive devices. The most well-known inorganic mercury compound is *mercurous chloride* (calomel), a cathartic once used widely in general medicine but is not in use anymore.

Symptoms of acute poisoning from inorganic mercury include severe gastroenteritis, with bloody diarrhea, vomiting, and abdominal pain. Later symptoms may include neurological damage and kidney failure.

Mercury in the Body

Several biochemical pathways are altered in the presence of mercury. In order to comprehend the scope of influence mercury has on health, it is important to review its effect on biological function. In terms of understanding how mercury influences the chemistry of the body, the most important characteristic is the attraction between mercury and sulfur. This means that, all things being equal, mercury will bind most readily with any molecule that contains sulfur (including sulfur and hydrogen complexes known as sulfhydryl groups). The result is known as a chelated metal.

Chelation is one way the body rids itself of heavy metals. It can also deprive the body of critical sulfur-containing compounds. One of the most abundant sulfur-containing substances in the body is the enzyme *glutathione.* Glutathione functions as a potent detoxifier, protecting cells from free-radical damage. One of its critical roles is the removal of heavy metals. By attaching its sulfur molecule to mercury, glutathione chelates mercury and dumps it in the bile for excretion. In this way, mercury (and other heavy metals) depletes the body of glutathione. Paradoxically, as mercury in the body and the demand for glutathione increase, the supply is diminished. The trace mineral selenium is also a significant protector from mercury toxicity; one reason is it is a component of glutathione.

A 1993 study highlights the important protective benefits of glutathione. In the experiment, mice were supplemented with N-acetylcysteine (NAC), a precursor to glutathione, after acute exposure to methyl mercury. A single dose of NAC ameliorated the lethal effects of mercury on the mice embryos, and subsequent doses significantly reduced the incidence of low birth weight and cleft palate.

As previously discussed, glutathione is probably the most important antioxidant in the body. It is also very important for immune system function. When glutathione stores are depleted, the activation of lymphocytes is reduced. Preliminary data suggests that mercury and nickel from amalgams can directly affect the production of T lymphocytes. Animal research indicates that mercury causes atrophy of the thymus gland, thereby reducing T-cell production and the ability of the body to fight infections.

Glutathione is abundant in red blood cells. There is evidence that mercury interferes with the permeability of cell membranes by inactivating cellular enzymes. In the case of red blood cells, inhibition of glutathione and the enzyme glucose-6-dehydrogenase by mercury has been shown to induce alterations in the activity of the cells and changes in red blood cell counts.

The sulfur-containing amino acids are cysteine, methionine, and taurine. Since amino acids are the building blocks of proteins, virtually every protein contains sulfur. Other sulfur-containing complexes in the body include the hormones insulin, prolactin, growth hormone, and vasopressin. When mercury binds with these molecules, it reduces their ability to carry out their normal metabolic functions.

In addition to its attraction to sulfur, mercury has a tendency to bind with certain nutrients. Among these are selenium, zinc, calcium, magnesium, vitamins C and E, and the B vitamins. By binding and interfering with these nutrients, mercury toxicity mimics the symptoms associated with nutrient deficiencies. For example, anemia, a symptom of mercury toxicity, is also a symptom of folic acid and vitamin B_{12} deficiencies.

Mercury toxicity can interfere with biological function on many levels. Unfortunately, this obscures a direct association between mercury and certain clinical observations, making a diagnosis of chronic mercury toxicity difficult. From PMS, infertility, and birth defects to cancer and multiple sclerosis, more studies are needed to explore the insidious ways that mercury influences illness and disease.

Thimerosal, a commonly used preservative in vaccines and contact lens solutions, is a water-soluble, cream-colored crystalline powder. It is 49.6 percent mercury by weight and adds formaldehyde to top it off. In the human body, thimerosal is metabolized to *ethylmercury* and *thiosalicylate.* There is a potential for the amount of mercury in vaccines to be toxic to children, especially of the vaccination age, and hair analysis of children has revealed low levels of mercury exposure after vaccination.

Given that exposure to low levels of mercury during critical stages of development has been associated with neurological disorders in children, including attention deficit disorder (ADD) and autism, learning difficulties, and speech delays, the predicted hair Hg concentration resulting from childhood immunizations is cause for concern. Based on these findings and the impact that vaccinal mercury has had on the health of American children, preservative-free vaccines are now on the market and preservative-based vaccines are being banned. The preservative-free vaccination may also cause immune-inflammatory response in the glial cells in the brain leading to inflammation and neurologic damage. But at least *monovalent* (single dose) vaccinations with no preservatives are a giant step in the interest of public health.

Lead

Lead is the most common toxic heavy metal. Although it is not as toxic as mercury, it is more pervasive in the environment and therefore the risk of contamination is greater. Lead originates in the earth's crust, and, once removed, it cannot be returned to its source. Extracted lead therefore accumulates in the air, soil, and water over time. Lead is the principal element in commonly occurring compounds such as lead acetate, lead arsenate, lead chromate, lead nitrate, and lead oxide.

Lead exposure was first documented about 5,000 years ago. Because of its low melting point, it was used extensively for silver smelting. The ancient Romans used leaded water pipes, and some historians have theorized that lead poisoning contributed to the demise of that civilization. Today, some amount of lead can be detected in all humans. Lead exposure has increased 500 to 1,000-fold since the industrial revolution. North America has the highest lead exposure in the world. The United States uses 1.3 million tons of lead a year, and pumps 400,000 to 600,000 tons of that into the environment. The Agency for Toxic Substances and Disease Registry (ATSDR) and the EPA have ranked lead as the number-one priority hazardous substance found at sites on the EPA's National Priorities List.

The most common sources of lead exposure include:

- Batteries
- Bone meal (unless from New Zealand)
- Car batteries
- Cigarette ash and tobacco
- Contaminated food and water supplies
- Exhaust fumes
- Imported dietary supplements (mainly from China)
- Improperly glazed pottery
- Lead shot from firing ranges
- Lead-based paints
- Organ meats
- Painted glassware
- Pesticide additives (lead arsenate)
- Plumbing (soldered pipes)
- Putty
- Rain, water, and snow
- Soldering (electrical)
- Tin cans (prior to the banning of lead use in)

The majority of daily lead exposure comes from contaminated food and exhaust fumes. Lead is also found in stationary sources (for example, mines and smelter sites), soil, dust, and water. Prior to the 1970s, tetraethyl lead, a combination of lead and petroleum distillates, was added to gasoline to increase its octane level and improve the performance of cars. Although unleaded gasoline is now used in most cars, some older vehicles still require the lead additive. Tetraethyl lead contaminates the surrounding air, soil, and vegetation. Food grown near heavily traveled roads is more contaminated with lead.

Food is also contaminated by the use of lead arsenate. This compound, which contains lead and arsenic, serves as a ripening agent when applied to crops. An estimated 30 percent of grapefruit crops in Florida are treated with lead arsenate to extend their growing season by a few months. The EPA is in the process of conducting a "special review" of the use of lead arsenate, and is awaiting study results.

Food processing and storage in tin cans with lead solder was once a source of contamination, although in 1979, the U.S. government banned the use of lead in food storage cans. Water stored or transported in lead soldered pipes can increase lead intake. Some glazes make pottery unsafe for the storage of food and water.

Even exercising caution when selecting a mineral supplement is advised. Some mineral supplements, particularly calcium and magnesium supplements from bone meal or dolomite, can contain significant amounts of lead. As much as 25 percent of the supplements in one study were found to contain levels of lead that would be considered unsafe for children under six years old.

Also of concern is lead content in herbal supplements, particularly those manufactured in China. Over the past few years, some herbal supplements purchased from China have been reported to contain high levels of lead. However, if you are purchasing an herbal supplement manufactured in the United States, you need not worry, as reputable companies test for heavy metals.

Nutritional factors can influence the degree of lead toxicity. Deficiencies of protein, calcium, phosphorus, vitamin E, iron, selenium, and zinc can increase the absorption of lead.

One of the most abundant sources of lead is paint. Lead paint can be found in approximately 64 million homes, or about 75 percent of those built before 1978. In 1978, Congress passed the Lead Paint Act, which banned the use of lead-based paint in homes. Unfortunately, many homes still have lead paint either exposed or hidden underneath newer paint. This is especially a problem in public housing, which tends to be older and less frequently maintained.

Sadly, the number of children poisoned by lead paint is inversely related to their economic status. Young children, attracted to the sweet taste of lead paint chips, frequently ingest them. Teething children can be exposed to lead by mouthing and chewing objects painted with lead-based paint. The absorption rate of lead in children is higher than that of adults.

In 1992, Congress passed the Residential Lead-Based Paint Hazard Reduction Act (also known as Title X). The law was designed to help inform potential renters and buyers by requiring disclosures of *known* information on the use of lead-based paint. The enforcement of such a law is somewhat ludicrous, however, given the difficulty of *proving* prior knowledge of the paint history. The law does not require any testing or removal of lead-based paint by sellers or landlords. Nor does it cover housing built after 1977, lofts, efficiencies, dormitories, or housing for the elderly or handicapped.

Lead in the Body

Lead is toxic to the brain and nervous system. Chronic exposure can lead to fatigue, anemia, insomnia, depression, high blood pressure, headaches, and cognitive impairment. Acute exposure can result in kidney failure, gastrointestinal distress, and impaired brain function.

Lead exposure among women has been associated with infertility, miscarriage, and higher infant mortality. Decreased sperm quality and loss of sex drive are attrib-

Lead and Children

Exposure to lead poses a "serious public health problem," especially for children. The number of children annually exposed to lead-based paint at potentially toxic levels is estimated to be about 12 million. Another 5.6 million are exposed to lead from gasoline, while an additional 5.9 to 11.7 million children may be exposed to lead-contaminated dust and soil. Contaminated drinking water reaches an estimated 3.8 million children.

Preschool-aged children and developing fetuses are the populations most at risk for the damaging effects of lead exposure. This is due to a number of factors: 1) The developing brains and nervous systems of fetuses and small children are highly susceptible to the neurotoxic effects of lead; 2) Children and infants are much more likely than adults to put things in their mouths, which increases the risk of ingestion of contaminated soil and paint; 3) Lead is absorbed through the intestinal tract of children more readily than adults; and 4) Nutritional deficiencies (calcium and iron, for example) are more common among children and increase the absorption of lead.

In 1990, the EPA estimated that approximately 3 million children had blood lead levels greater than 10 μg/dL (micrograms per deciliter). Blood levels around 10 μg/dL have been linked to decreased intelligence, impaired school performance, and behavioral abnormalities in children.

Although elevated blood lead levels do not always correspond with diagnosed attention deficit hyperactivity disorder (ADHD), Tuthill reported in 1996 that hair lead levels strongly correlated with physician-diagnosed ADD and negative teacher ratings among 277 first graders. Experimental animals exposed to lead exhibit behaviors described as "inability to inhibit inappropriate responses," characterized by impulsive behavior and diminished ability to wait for rewards. Some researchers propose that an inability to manage postponed reinforcement, also known as reward deficiency syndrome, is linked to attention deficits and addictive behavior.

According to a 1999 study conducted by the CDC, lead exposure can affect the physical growth of children. An analysis of data from more than 4,000 children aged one to seven years old showed that for every 10 μg/dL of blood lead; there was a predicted 1.57 cm reduction in stature and 0.52 cm reduction in head circumference.

Most children are exposed to lead in their homes. The remnants of lead-based paint, lead dust, and contaminated dirt are the major sources of their exposure. The environmental damage from lead paint was not eradicated by the 1978 ban. When homes or buildings with lead paint are torn down or burned, lead contaminates the surrounding soil.

In 1991, the CDC revised its policy statement on lead exposure in children, lowering the safety threshold from 25 μg/dL to 10 μg/dL, a level associated with health risks, and recommended the universal screening of all children for elevated blood levels.

uted to even moderate exposure to lead in males. There is also compelling evidence that lead can contribute to certain birth defects.

The EPA classifies lead as a Group B_2 substance, or "probable human" carcinogen. While human studies are inconclusive, animal trials indicate an association between oral lead exposure and kidney cancer. The animal tumors induced by lead are similar to those that occur spontaneously in man.

Until the 1970s, blood lead levels of 80 µg/dL (micrograms per deciliter) were considered acceptable. Although the EPA has yet to establish a reference dose for lead, today, blood levels greater than 10 µg/dL in children and 25 µg/dL in adults are considered dangerous. Blood lead levels as low as 10 µg/dL have been associated with impaired intelligence and behavioral complications in children, pre-term birth, and low birth weight. The CDC reported in 1994 that the overall mean blood levels for the U.S. population was 2.8 µg/dL, with consistently higher levels among young children, central city residents, low-income families, and minorities.

Some of the health effects associated with elevated blood lead are listed in Table 10.3. below

Table 10.3. Health Effects Associated with Elevated Lead Levels

EFFECTS OF LEAD	BLOOD LEVELS
Brain and kidney damage (adults)	100 µg/dL
Brain and kidney damage (children)	80 µg/dL
Death (children)	125 µg/dL
Decreased IQ and growth in young children	20 µg/dL
Increased blood pressure	40 µg/dL
Pre-term birth, low birth weight	10–15 µg/dL
Slowed nerve conduction velocity	30 µg/dL

Lead is stored in the bones and teeth, with smaller amounts in the liver and kidneys. It also crosses the placenta and into breast milk. Modern levels of lead in the body typically range from 125–200 mg. Daily exposure of up to 2 mg is considered within "acceptable" limits, although even very low levels of chronic exposure are associated with health problems, particularly hypertension, poor hemoglobin (oxygen-carrying component of red blood cells) production, and anemia.

The following conditions are those most commonly associated with long-term exposure to lead.

Hypertension. Research shows that the odds of developing hypertension are heightened with increased bone lead levels, suggesting that long-term lead accumulation is an independent risk factor for developing the disease. In recent years, researchers have found that, among adolescents with normal blood lead levels, those who had elevated bone lead as preschoolers had a higher prevalence of hypertension in young adulthood.

The damage caused by lead appears to be directed at the kidneys, which are partially responsible for regulating blood pressure. The kidneys help regulate blood pressure by secreting the enzyme *renin*. Renin calls on plasma proteins to release a substance called *angiotensin*. Angiotensin causes the blood vessels to constrict, which increases blood pressure. A 1999 Italian study on rats confirmed that chronic exposure to lead dramatically increased plasma angiotensin and, subsequently, systolic and diastolic blood pressure.

In humans, chronic occupational exposure to lead has been linked to a high incidence of kidney dysfunction, characterized by renal failure, hypertension, and gout. Chronic low-level environmental exposure impairs the ability of the kidneys to remove creatinine from the blood. Measurement of creatinine in the urine (the creatinine clearance test) is a benchmark of kidney function. In a 1996 Harvard study, a tenfold increase in blood lead level predicted an increase in serum creatinine that was comparable to the increase predicted by twenty years of aging.

Anemia. Lead poisoning has long been associated with reduced hemoglobin formation and anemia. Common symptoms of anemia are fatigue, pallor, difficulty breathing, heart palpitations, and dizziness. Anemia is characterized by poor oxygen-carrying capacity of red blood cells (RBCs). The oxygen-carrying components of red blood cells are hemoglobin. There are about 200 hemoglobin molecules in each red blood cell. The hemoglobin molecule consists of *heme,* an iron portion, and *globin,* a protein. Iron, a heavy metal, is crucial for the formation of hemoglobin. Some research has found a strong association between iron deficiency and lead poisoning in children. Anything that interferes with hemoglobin synthesis can result in anemia.

Oxygen deficiency stimulates the kidneys to release a hormone called *erythropoietin*. Erythropoietin increases the production of red blood cells in an attempt to increase the oxygen-carrying capacity of the blood. Elevated serum erythropoietin, reduced hemoglobin, decreased red blood cells, and reduced hematocrit (the percentage of red blood cells in plasma) are potential markers of anemia. If the kidneys have been damaged by lead, erythropoietin synthesis may be inhibited. Reduced erythropoietin production can be a primary cause of anemia.

Chronic lead exposure, reflected in bone lead levels, is also associated with reduced hemoglobin levels, even in the absence of elevated blood levels. Although the mechanism is not entirely understood, research has shown that lead inhibits the synthesis of hemoglobin. An early study on experimental animals found that hemoglobin concentration dropped as much as 70 percent in the presence of blood lead.

Children exposed to lead appear to be able to correct for reduced hemoglobin formation by increasing erythropoietin and RBC synthesis. With advancing age, this compensatory mechanism gradually fails.

Oxidative Damage. Lead is a significant environmental source of free-radical dam-age. Oxidative stress, or free-radical damage, has become a familiar term in recent years. Oxidative stress is thought to be a basic underlying mechanism in a wide vari-ety of pathological conditions, including cardiovascular disease, cancer, autoimmune diseases, diabetes, premature aging, and neurologic degeneration.

A free radical is a molecule that has a free or unpaired electron. The missing elec-tron creates a positive charge, which makes the molecule highly reactive. A free rad-ical will react with just about any molecule. The reaction, known as oxidation, removes electrons from a "donor" molecule in order to stabilize the free radical. The oxidation of the donor molecule transforms it into a free radical in search of an elec-tron, thus establishing a chain reaction.

William Pryor, Ph.D., a leading expert of free radicals and author of *Free Radicals in Biology* (Academic Press, 1984), likens the free radical to a lone bachelor in a room full of dancing couples. Once the bachelor cuts in and obtains a dancing partner, another lone dancer is created. However, it is not a simple one-to-one relationship. One free radical can initiate a chain reaction, which results in the production of hun-dreds of thousands of additional destructive free radicals.

Lead appears to exercise its damaging properties on two levels: first, by displac-ing antioxidant minerals and interfering with antioxidant enzymes, and second, by oxidizing cell membranes, protein enzymes, DNA, and RNA. For example, lead dis-places zinc in the brain, leading to neurotoxic effects and interferes with zinc-dependent enzymes throughout the body. It is also thought that lead destroys cell membranes directly through oxidation, generating widespread free-radical tissue damage. Researchers have found that lead-exposed rats showed signs of oxidative stress to red blood cells as evidenced by *lipid peroxidation* (damaging oxidation by free radicals on fatty substances in the body) and reduced glutathione. Other studies show an increase in oxidative stress in the brains of lead-intoxicated rats.

The belief that oxidative stress is a major mechanism of lead toxicity indicates that antioxidants may have a promising role in treatment. Study findings demon-strated that treatment with an antioxidant (N-acetylcysteine) and a chelating agent reversed the effects of oxidative stress on red blood cells. Later research indicated that alpha lipoic acid increased cellular glutathione in lead-treated rats. In another study, pretreatment with the pineal hormone melatonin protected rats against lipid peroxidation and the depletion of antioxidants.

Testing for Lead in the Body

Conclusions made about the health effects of lead are frequently based on blood analysis, which are measured in µg/dL. However, blood measurements reflect only recent exposure. After about twelve hours, most lead is excreted in the urine or trans-ported to the bones and tissue. Within twenty-four hours after exposure, blood lev-els decline while bone and hair levels begin to rise. Acute exposure to lead can also be assessed by measuring erythrocyte protoporphyrin (EP), a component of red blood cells that increases with blood lead concentration.

Some experts consider hair analysis a more accurate and reliable method of determining body lead burden. Hair analysis can determine the lead deposition in soft tissue, as well as the ability of the body to excrete heavy metals. The reference range for hair lead is 0–30 ppm for adults and 0–10 ppm for children (see page 235 for more details). Another method for assessment of lead is to measure the amount of lead excreted by the kidneys through the urine, after a single injection or an oral dose of a substance (EDTA, DMSA, or DMPS), which pulls heavy metals from the body.

Measurements of bone lead using x-ray fluorescence have become a new standard for measuring toxicity. A 1994 Harvard study, published in the *Journal of the American Medical Association* (JAMA) reported "the first epidemiological evidence that bone lead may be an important biological marker of ongoing chronic (lead) toxicity." Since lead accumulates in the bones, they are an accurate gage of chronic exposure and retained body burden. Bone lead measurements have become a useful tool for studying the long-term health effects of lead accumulation.

Cadmium

Pure cadmium is a soft, silver-white metal. In nature, cadmium is usually combined with other elements to form compounds like cadmium sulfate or cadmium oxide. Cadmium is extracted from the earth during the production of other metals such as zinc, lead, and copper. Like lead, cadmium was virtually nonexistent in the environment until the early 1900s. Between 1900 and 1975, the use of cadmium has increased to an estimated 15,000 tons per year. Environmental contamination first came from zinc mining. Later, cadmium appeared in tobacco, coffee, and refined grains, as these plants readily absorb cadmium from the soil.

Food and cigarette smoke are the largest sources of cadmium exposure to the general public. The average person consumes 30 mcg daily in food. Shellfish and foods grown in water, like rice, absorb cadmium from the water. Some other sources of cadmium include fertilizer and plastics. Cadmium is found in nickel-cadmium batteries and is used to rustproof tools. Some water pipes contain cadmium, as it is used to inhibit corrosion of other metals. Soft, acidic water tends to break down the metals in water pipes, allowing cadmium to leach into drinking water. Tire erosion and coal combustion contribute to environmental cadmium. Each year approximately 90,000 people are exposed to cadmium in the workplace. Welders, construction workers, electricians, miners, workers in the paint and battery industries, and wrecking/demolition crews are among those who are exposed to cadmium in their jobs.

Cadmium is poorly absorbed from the gastrointestinal tract and lungs. An estimated 2 percent from the intestinal tract and 10 to 50 percent from the lungs make it to the general circulation. However, the elimination of cadmium is very slow. The half-life of cadmium averages approximately sixteen years, which means that after sixteen years, half of the body burden will remain. Smokers have four to five times more cadmium in their blood than nonsmokers and twice the kidney cortex concentration.

The EPA reference dose (RfD—or the maximum dose that would not likely result in significant health effects) for cadmium is 0.0005 mg/kg daily from food and 0.001 mg/kg daily from water. For an average 175-pound man, this equates to approximately 40 mcg from food and 80 mcg from water daily. A daily intake of 40 to 50 mcg is considered acceptable by more conservative standards. Some experts recommend maintaining blood levels below 0.15 ppm or hair levels less than 2 ppm.

In the early 1990s, a cross-sectional study of residents in Belgium was conducted to investigate the health effects of cadmium in the environment. Belgium is the largest European producer of cadmium, and parts of the country have been polluted by industrial emissions. A total number of 2,327 subjects from areas of different environmental pollution were randomly sampled. It was estimated that the cadmium body burden of those subjects from polluted areas was 50 to 85 percent higher. The results of the study demonstrated that cadmium exposure increased the risk of kidney dysfunction and impaired calcium homeostasis.

Cadmium in the Body

Once cadmium is absorbed from the gastrointestinal tract or lungs, it is bound to a protein called *metallothionein* and carried in the blood to the liver and kidneys. Once in the kidneys, protein-bound cadmium is absorbed by the renal tubules. There, a series of catabolic and anabolic reactions prevent the excretion of cadmium. Cadmium is toxic to the kidneys, specifically to the renal tubules (the portion of the kidneys that form, collect, and transport urine).

Chronic inhalation and ingestion of cadmium reduces proper kidney filtration and function, increases the frequency of kidney stones, and increases the amount of protein in the urine. The EPA reports that 200 mcg of cadmium per gram of wet weight is the toxic threshold of cadmium for the kidneys. The RfD for cadmium is based on this threshold, although some studies have demonstrated a lower range of toxicity.

In addition to kidney damage, symptoms of acute exposure to cadmium can result in anemia, brittle bones, low back pain, restricted spinal movement, and shrinking of the testes. Symptoms of acute cadmium toxicity may include abdominal pain, cramping, diarrhea, lung irritation, and nausea. The following conditions are those that are most commonly associated with chronic exposure to cadmium.

Hypertension. Although human evidence is inconclusive, hypertension has been linked to cadmium exposure in animal studies. Several mechanisms have been proposed. Kidney toxicity is the most compelling explanation for a hypertensive response to cadmium. The kidneys regulate blood pressure by controlling the fluid volume of blood. Cadmium has been shown to interfere with sodium excretion in the urine, increasing blood volume and blood pressure. A little known fact is that up to 40 percent of hypertension begins in the kidneys. It makes sense then that cadmium is implicated in hypertension since it affects the kidneys. Moreover, smoking is not only one of the risk factors for developing hypertension, but also is a primary source of cadmium exposure.

Cancer. There is substantial evidence that cadmium causes cancer in humans. The EPA considers cadmium a Group B1 substance, or "probable human carcinogen." One study followed 602 cadmium smelter workers in a longitudinal study and found that the risk of lung cancer increased twofold for those exposed six months or longer. Urine cadmium levels among the workers reflected a high level of exposure.

Several studies support that cadmium exposure induces prostate cancer in animals, but human data is limited. The interaction between cadmium and zinc is a possible explanation for injury to the prostate and other tissue.

The relationship between zinc and cadmium is an important factor in cadmium toxicity. Structurally, they share many qualities. In the body, cadmium can displace zinc, interfering with a multitude of important zinc-dependent processes. For example, zinc is abundant in normal prostate tissue, but there is evidence that it decreases with prostatic carcinoma. Cadmium concentration appears higher in prostate cancer and *prostatitis* (inflammation of the prostate) than in normal tissue. Depletion of zinc has been used as a model to explain increased susceptibility to cadmium-induced free-radical damage in the testes. Many enzymes require zinc as a catalyst or as part of their structure. Zinc controls cadmium absorption; therefore, a zinc deficiency can increase cadmium levels. Likewise, supplementing with zinc has been shown to reduce cadmium accumulation in tissue.

Iron also influences absorption of cadmium. A 1994 Swedish study found that reduced iron stores were strongly associated with elevated blood cadmium levels. Dietary fiber also reduced the gastrointestinal absorption of cadmium. Another interesting relationship is that of cadmium and calcium. Some research indicates that low calcium intake increases the absorption and accumulation of cadmium. Cadmium may also interfere with the important functions of calcium throughout the body. Both human and animal studies indicate that osteoporosis may be a critical effect of cadmium exposure.

Oxidative Damage. Like lead, cadmium has been shown to induce free-radical damage in experimental animals, as marked by lipid peroxidation and depletion of glutathione. In one study, oxidative damage to kidney and liver tissue was controlled when the rats were given antioxidants (either NAC or vitamin E). In another study, cadmium administration increased lipid peroxidation by more than 200 percent in treated mice. Lipid peroxidation, but not glutathione depletion, was prevented by coadministration with alpha lipoic acid. (The Japanese drug Neo-Minophagen C, which contains glycine, glycyrrhizin, and cysteine, is reported to protect against cadmium-induced oxidative stress.)

Another study reported that rats exposed to toxic levels of cadmium exhibited exaggerated anxiety and startle responses. In addition to increasing stress and anxiety, cadmium also reduces resistance to infection. This may be associated with increased cortisol production by the adrenal glands in response to stress.

Aluminum

Aluminum like all heavy metals comes from the earth's crust. It has many uses in industry, but has no known biological function. Workers can be exposed to aluminum during production or processing of this metal and its alloys. Workplace exposures have well-known health risks and workplaces must follow strict guidelines to prevent their workers from being exposed. In addition to workplace exposure, people can come into contact with aluminum in many other ways. Aluminum is found in food, drinking water, and in some over-the-counter and prescription drugs. Aluminum is used to conduct heat in cookware, to inhibit sweat in deodorants and antiperspirants, and as a food additive to keep powders from clumping.

Aluminum has been a known toxin to the nervous system for many years. The first laboratory animal study linking aluminum to brain damage was published in 1937. One of the ways some of the side effects of aluminum became known was through dialysis patients who developed side effects such as *encephalopathy* (also referred to as dialysis dementia), bone disease, and anemia. Furthermore, aluminum in infant formulas and in solutions for home parenteral (intravenous) nutrition was associated with neurological damage and metabolic bone disease.

Most recently, aluminum along with mercury has been implicated in Alzheimer's disease, a type of senile dementia. Senile dementia is a progressive brain disease; symptoms include short-term memory loss, slowness in thought, confusion, disorientation, difficulty in communicating thoughts, as well as slowness in movement and other loss of physical function. Aluminum is found in the lesions of the brain tissue of Alzheimer's patients. Although researchers have yet to conclude that aluminum causes Alzheimer's disease (initially they felt that the accumulation of aluminum in the brain may be a result from the disease), studies continue to emerge showing an association between aluminum and Alzheimer's. Aluminum exacerbates oxidation and inflammation, which may be the link between aluminum and the tissue damage that occurs in nerve tissue.

Because research is still implicating aluminum in Alzheimer's disease, it is recommended that you limit your intake of aluminum as much as possible. Experts seem to believe that even though we can increase aluminum intake by cooking in pots and pans made from it, the body does not absorb this form of aluminum readily. Apparently, aluminum enters the body most readily in drinking water and through the skin. While there has been considerable debate about the contribution

Minimizing Your Exposure to Aluminum

It may be a while before all the factors between aluminum and Alzheimer's disease are known. In the meantime, it is wise to limit your aluminum intake. The following information includes recommendations from the First International Conference on Metals and the Brain (Italy, September 2000).

1. Monitor aluminum in drinking water. Aluminum in drinking water should be less than 50 mg/L. Some bottled-water companies provide an analysis of the aluminum content of their water. You should also be able to obtain this information from your public water company. Aluminum is not present in distilled water or in water filtered by reverse osmosis.

2. Consumers should monitor aluminum contents of foods and any over-the-counter or prescription drugs. The aluminum content should be declared in all food preparations and pharmacological products. Aluminum is contained in many antacids. Aluminum is also a common ingredient in baking powder and flour, so many baked goods could potentially contain aluminum. Aluminum-free baking powders are available at natural food stores. Consult with your pharmacist for the aluminum content of over-the-counter or prescription drugs.

3. Do not take aluminum-containing drugs, such as antacids, with citric acid. Citrate-containing compounds (commonly found in medicines and some supplements such as calcium citrate) appear to increase the absorption of ingested aluminum.

4. Acidic foods, for example, acid cabbage (sauerkraut), tomatoes, and others, should not be cooked or stored in aluminum ware. Researchers have found aluminum content up to 20 mg/L in sauerkraut that was cooked in aluminum. Be sure to cook acidic foods in nonaluminum cookware. Pickles and cheese, which contain aluminum, should not be eaten in excessive amounts.

5. Infants, the elderly, and those with renal failure are more susceptible to aluminum toxicity and should pay special attention to aluminum intake.

6. Make sure to get adequate magnesium and iron intake. Aluminum may be more easily absorbed in the presence of magnesium and iron deficiencies. Getting at least the RDA for these minerals, as well as for calcium and zinc, should help protect you against aluminum accumulation.

of drinking water containing aluminum to Alzheimer's disease, eighteen studies on drinking water have linked aluminum levels to elevated risks of this disease and elderly cognitive impairment. (For supplemental protocol for improving cognitive disorders, see Appendix 4: "Supplement Protocols for Other Common Conditions," page 518.)

Arsenic

Arsenic is a naturally occurring element that is used industrially to mine iron ore, to preserve wood, and as an agent in some pesticides. Arsenic is also found in fossil fuels. In addition to industrial emissions, the greatest threat to health is from arsenic in drinking water. The EPA has recently lowered the acceptable levels of arsenic in drinking water from 50 ppb to 10 ppb.

Some people in the United States have recently become aware of arsenic toxicity due to the recent change in preservatives used for outdoor woods. People were becoming sick using arsenic-treated wood for building decks and play sets.

While breathing or ingesting high levels of arsenic can lead to death, lower levels of arsenic can cause nausea and vomiting, abnormal heart rhythm, a numbing sensation in the hands and feet, darkening of the skin, and small corns or warts on the palms of the hands, soles of the feet, or on the torso. Also, long-term ingestion of arsenic is associated with an increased risk of lung and bladder cancer. In addition, the American Heart Association (AMA) has reported that arsenic exposure is a risk factor for the development of atherosclerosis.

Because of the many health risks of arsenic, it is extremely important to reduce one's exposure. Reverse osmosis water filtration systems remove arsenic, as well as other heavy metals like aluminum, from drinking water. You can also avoid contact with arsenic by using arsenic-free woods for home-building projects.

Testing for Heavy Metal in Your Body

As a whole, heavy metals present many problems for human health, yet so many people are not aware of them. Not only are they associated with many chronic diseases, including cardiovascular disease and cancer, but some are also known endocrine disrupters. Naturopathic healers have acknowledged the role of heavy metals as an underlying cause of disease for years, and recently more medical doctors are becoming aware of the health effects of heavy metals. Heavy metals can and do cause health problems; therefore, it is good to be aware of the testing available to determine heavy metal toxicity and ways to support the detoxification of them from your body.

A heavy metal test with urine and/or hair analysis can determine how extensive heavy metal toxicity is and whether EDTA or another chelating agent is needed and if so, how much. Although some practitioners use hair analysis, I have found that heavy metals may not show up in hair until some thing has been done to push them out of fat cells. A urine heavy metal test, also known as a provocative urine test, will show them right away.

Hair analysis. Hair is formed in the dermal layer of the skin, within the hair follicle. During its growth, the hair is exposed to a variety of metabolic substances, including extracellular fluids, blood, and lymph. As it reaches the surface of the skin, the hair shaft hardens and seals in whatever metabolic products it was in contact with during growth. The first one to one and one-half inches of new hair growth is considered a reliable record of metabolic activity, nutrient status, and heavy metal exposure that has occurred over the previous six to eight weeks.

The process involves removal of a small amount of hair near the nape of the neck. The hair sample is then sent to a laboratory where it is chemically washed, stripped of all substances found on it, and dissolved in acid. Using a method of chemical analysis called *atomic absorption photospectrometry,* each metal is isolated and measured on a ppm scale. Hair analysis is simple, noninvasive, and relatively inexpensive, but it may not show stored levels of heavy metals.

Your healthcare professional should be able to help you obtain an analysis from a reputable laboratory. I use Great Smokies Diagnostic Laboratories for this test, but there are other qualified labs. Great Smokies Diagnostic Laboratories is located at 63 Zillicoa Street, Asheville, NC 28801. The laboratory can be reached at (800) 522–4762, or visit their website at www.greatsmokies-lab.com.

Provocative heavy metal urine test. In this test, an agent (usually DMSA, dimercapto-succinic acid, or DMPS, dimercaptopropane sulfonate) that removes heavy metals from the body tissues is given. If metals are present they will be excreted in the urine. The amount of each metal is measured and correlated to the severity of the problem. Your healthcare practitioner can then recommend an appropriate treatment for detoxification of the metals.

Detoxifying Heavy Metals

Chelation therapy is the intravenous infusion of a proteinlike agent that binds with metals in the body, making them soluble in blood. The metals are then excreted in the urine. The most common chelating agent is *ethylenediaminetetraacetic acid* (EDTA). EDTA is an effective chelator of most heavy metals, including lead and cadmium. EDTA helps to reduce the free-radical activity of these heavy metals in the body. Also, EDTA binds with calcium, reducing plaque formation and atherosclerosis. Other agents like DMPS or DMSA are also used because they bind to mercury much more effectively. These agents can be used orally as well with good clinical results. If you decide to use oral DMSA or EDTA, do so under the guidance of a healthcare professional who is familiar with their use.

According to Leon Chaitow, D.O., N.D., EDTA can decrease free-radical production as much as a million-fold and increase the efficiency of mitochondrial energy production. Free radicals diminish cellular energy production by interfering with the 500 or so oxidative enzymes required by the mitochondria. Oxidative enzymes help convert inorganic adenosine diphosphate (ADP), sugar, and glucose into adenosine triphosphate (ATP), the universal energy molecule used by the body. Calcium also inhibits enzyme activity and decreases cellular energy production. When cells are depleted of energy, they become increasingly acidic, drawing in more calcium ions. Increased calcium in the cells, free-radical activity, and reduced cellular energy are consistent with the clinical profile of cardiovascular disease.

By binding with calcium, reducing plaque, removing free radicals, and improving oxygen content in the cells, chelation therapy can improve many conditions associated with poor blood flow and reduced oxygen. These conditions include cardiovascular disease, diabetes, emphysema, macular degeneration, varicose veins, gallstones, cataracts, arthritis, Parkinson's disease, psoriasis, and kidney disease.

Oral chelating agents consist of nutritional supplements and certain foods that have mild chelating properties, which we'll discuss in Chapter 11.

HOUSEHOLD POLLUTANTS

Pollution is a problem of growing concern for many of us, and justifiably so. Pollution is the most significant source of chemical exposures inside our homes. In fact, the same pollutants restricted by environmental laws are typically found at much higher levels *inside* average American residences than are found outside. This is of major concern, because chemical residue from volatile organic compounds (VOCs) are linked to 3,000 cases of cancer every year. Household products such as deodorizers, dry-cleaned clothing, particleboard, and carpets, as well as fumes from gas burners, are responsible for the growing problem of indoor air pollution. Factors that influence the effects of indoor pollution include ventilation, time spent indoors, and degree of exposure. Currently, manufacturers of household products are not required to identify hazardous chemicals on labels.

Most people are unaware of the risks associated with household pollutants. Education and risk management are essential for control of this problem. (See the inset "Additional Indoor Air Polluters.")

Carbon Monoxide

Of all sources of indoor pollution, carbon monoxide poses probably the greatest threat. Any amount is harmful, and it can build to fatal levels if it goes undetected. Carbon monoxide is a colorless, odorless gas that is a byproduct of fuel combustion. Oxygen and fuel generate energy (in the form of heat) and carbon monoxide. When fuel (wood, gas, and others) is burned inside a home that is tightly sealed, oxygen inside the home is used faster than it is replaced by outdoor air. This creates a negative pressure inside the home, known as a back draft. The back draft draws the carbon monoxide and exhaust fumes back into the home. Carbon monoxide is taken up by the lungs and transported throughout the body in place of oxygen. Carbon monoxide can also enter a home from an improperly burning gas furnace, gas leaks, gas fireplaces and stoves, dryers, and from kerosene heaters.

Carbon monoxide poisoning causes headaches, shortness of breath, and fatigue

Additional Indoor Air Polluters

Here are just a few other substances that cause indoor air pollution. Outgassing from plastics, mold, and chemicals used in cosmetic and personal-care products are also a concern. With more and more research emerging on the effects of these chemicals, it makes sense to educate yourself and to take every measure possible to reduce your risk.

Cigarette smoke: Cigarette smoke contains many toxic chemicals, including acetaldehyde, formaldehyde, benzene, cadmium, lead, and toluene (some of which are discussed below). These chemicals greatly increase your risk of cancer; they also aggravate allergies, asthmas, and upper respiratory infections. To reduce risks, don't smoke indoors, or smoke only near an exhaust fan. Room-air filtering devices remove some of the particles from smoke, but not the gases.

Home chemicals: Cleaning solutions, lawn-care products, and use of pesticides can release toxic chemicals into and around the home. Pesticide use in the home is unmistakably correlated with increased cancer risk in children. Many home-cleaning products contain chemicals such as naptha, benzene, petroleum distillates, butoxyethanol, and propylene glycol, which are known or suspected carcinogens, neurotoxins, and/or immune system depressors. To reduce risks from home pesticides, never spray or apply pesticides when children are present. Find natural alternatives such as using cedar chips instead of mothballs. There are many non-chemically based cleaners available now in stores. If using chemical-based cleaners, always ventilate the area by opening windows and running exhaust fans.

Home decorating: Most items used to finish and decorate a home emit harmful gasses; the release of chemicals from home decorating items like carpet, paints, or paneling is known as *outgassing*. One such chemical is formaldehyde, which is found in plywood and any pressed wood product such as furniture, glues and adhesives, permanent press textiles, and unvented gas stoves or kerosene heaters. Formaldehyde can be irritating to the eyes and throat, but more important, it is carcinogenic. To reduce risks, use low outgassing building materials, carpeting, paints, and furniture products. If you have recently built a home with conventional materials or installed new carpeting, open windows and run exhaust fans to reduce your exposure to the chemicals.

Radon: Radon is a gas that occurs naturally as a result of the breakdown of uranium that is found in rocks and soil. Radon seeps into homes through cracks in foundation walls, sewer openings, or joints between walls and floors of buildings. Prolonged exposure to radon is associated with an increased risk of lung cancer. In fact, radon is thought to be the second leading cause of lung cancer. Radon is undetectable, however, there are home-testing kits available at most hardware and building supply stores. If your home is found to have a radon problem, call the EPA radon hotline at (800) 767–7236 for guidance on how to keep radon out of your home.

(all symptoms of oxygen deprivation), and if prolonged, death. Make sure that all gas appliances are in good working condition and install carbon monoxide detectors.

Solvents

A solvent is a substance that is capable of dissolving another substance (called a *solute*). A solute dissolved in a solvent forms a solution. Organic solvents (carbon-containing) are usually highly toxic and flammable. Many household products contain organic solvents. Cleaners and degreasers typically contain petroleum distillate or *trichloroethylene*. Improper use and disposal of these chemicals can result in widespread environmental damage. For example, one cup of trichloroethylene can contaminate approximately 3 million gallons of water. They can cause fires, poison children and animals, damage the skin, injure eyes, and contribute to allergies. Long-term exposure can damage the lungs, kidneys, liver, and nervous system.

To identify solvent-containing products, look for label warnings that include "flammable," "combustible," "harmful if swallowed," or "use only in well ventilated areas." Products that typically contain 99 percent or more organic solvents include furniture stripper, nail-polish remover, lighter fluid, dry-cleaning agents, paint thinner, degreasers, fuel (kerosene, gasoline), lubricating agents, and turpentine. Other products that contain organic solvents include furniture polish, shoe polish, spot removers, glue, wood cleaner, paint, and wood stains.

Benzene

Benzene is a highly toxic organic solvent used in household cleaning products, paint thinner, some art supplies, and adhesives. It is also found in gasoline and tobacco smoke. Benzene is produced naturally by active volcanoes and as a product of forest fires. For industrial purposes, it is extracted from coal and oil. Oil refineries, chemical plants, gasoline storage, shipping and retail stations, shoe manufacturing, and the rubber industry contribute to the environmental contamination of benzene. The most common exposure to benzene is inhalation of polluted air.

Acute exposure to benzene can result in drowsiness, headaches, dizziness, and death. Chronic exposure may interfere with normal blood production, resulting in anemia and bleeding disorders. There is overwhelming human and animal evidence that benzene is carcinogenic. Leukemia has occurred in workers exposed to benzene for fewer than five years.

Benzene also appears to affect the immune system, reducing resistance to infection and disease. In addition, genetic changes have been associated with benzene exposure. Reproductive abnormalities in animals indicate that benzene may lead to low birth weight, delayed bone formation, and bone marrow damage. Human reproductive studies are limited.

Benzene is ranked fifth on the EPA's list of its Top Twenty Hazardous Substances (1999). The list, which is revised periodically, is available online through the

CDC home page www.cdc.gov or directly at www.atsdr.cdc.gov/cxcx3.html. The latter includes links to "ToxFAQ Sheets" and "Public Health Statements" for each substance.

Conditions Commonly Associated with Chronic Exposure to Household Toxins

Having considered some of the leading specific toxins that are found in the average American household, let's consider the ailments that chronic exposure to those toxins can cause. The ailments listed here are only a few of the many conditions that have been found to be caused by long-term exposure to common household toxins.

Chronic Fatigue Syndrome (CFS)

Chronic fatigue syndrome (CFS) is a condition characterized by overwhelming exhaustion, fatigue, muscle and joint tenderness, depressed immune function, and mental disturbances. It is estimated that 500,000 people in the United States suffer from CFS. Although the CDC recognizes CFS, and more physicians are increasingly recognizing CFS, not long ago relatively few physicians acknowledged or treated the condition because it was considered to be a psychosomatic illness.

The CDC has established strict criteria that must be met before a diagnosis of CFS can be made. This includes at least six months of severe chronic fatigue in the absence of any other known medical condition. In addition, at least four of the following symptoms must be present: short-term memory impairment; sore throat; tender lymph nodes; muscle pain; multi-joint pain; headaches; nonrestorative sleep; or increased fatigue after exercise, which lasts more than twenty-four hours.

In my opinion, CFS represents a disruption of metabolism involving adrenal exhaustion, low thyroid output (clinical or subclinical hypothyroidism), intestinal disturbances, environmental toxicity, exposure to viral or microbe load, chronic stress, and nutrient deficiencies. Combined, they create a net effect of metabolic cellular failure to generate energy. Evaluating levels of heavy metal and toxin exposure, and improving liver, intestinal, and hormonal health with support from the following nutrients will help to alleviate symptoms of CFS. These agents consist of cordyceps (*Cordyceps sinensis*), N-acetylcysteine (NAC), coenzyme Q_{10}, glandular extracts (adrenal, thyroid, and thymus), NADH (nicotinamide adenine dinucleotide), magnesium malate, a quality, high-potency multivitamin and mineral supplement, and DHEA (when indicated by lab values), and homeopathic nosodes (if viral or microbe load is detected). (For specific dosage recommendations, see Appendix 4: "Supplement Protocols for Other Common Conditions," page 518.)

Fibromyalgia

There appears to be a significant overlap between the symptoms of CFS and fibromyalgia, leading some experts to believe they are the same clinical syndrome.

Fibromyalgia is chronic muscle and joint pain that cannot be traced to any physiological condition. A recent study found that 58 percent of female and 80 percent of male patients with fibromyalgia met the full CDC criteria for CFS. Common underlying problems that exist in both conditions are impaired liver detoxification and altered gut permeability as mentioned.

Characteristics important to fibromyalgia include the presence of elevated lactic acid levels. People with elevated cellular lactic acid levels often feel as if they have exercised vigorously. This is most likely due to the uncoupling of energy production in the cells. When the cells don't burn their fuel completely, lactic acid builds up.

Low serotonin levels are also strongly associated with fibromyalgia, which suggests that chronic stress could be another factor in the gradual disturbances in serotonin levels. When serotonin is low, craving for carbohydrates increases, insulin resistance increases, tyrosine levels decrease, and less thyroid hormone is available.

Researchers have evaluated the effects of liver detoxification and gastrointestinal healing on chronic fatigue, fibromyalgia, and irritable bowel syndrome (IBS). In one study, eighty-four patients were given a food supplement designed to support liver detoxification and gut function. Twenty-two patients served as the control group. Both groups received an allergy-free, calorie-controlled diet. The treatment group experienced a 52 percent reduction in symptoms over a ten-week period, compared with a 22 percent reduction in the control group. The treatment group also demonstrated a normalization in phase-one cytochrome P-450 in relation to phase-two glycine conjugation, improved nutrient absorption, and increased glutathione reserves.

As with CFS, symptoms of fibromyalgia can often be successfully treated by restoring balance to the liver, intestines, and hormones. This can often be accomplished with the bowel terrain program and the following supplements: coenzyme Q_{10}, SAM-e, alpha lipoic acid, magnesium malate, rhodiola, Relora®, 5-HTP, NAC, cordyceps, L(+) lacticum acidum (a homeopathic remedy), a quality, high-potency multiple vitamin and mineral supplement, and thyroid/adrenal glandular support. Screening for heavy metals and microbes, and for women, an evaluation of their hormone levels, is also recommended. (For specific dosage recommendations, see Appendix 4: "Supplement Protocols for Other Common Conditions," page 518.)

Multiple Chemical Sensitivity (MCS)

Many people with CFS and fibromyalgia also have multiple chemical sensitivities. MCS is a chronic disorder characterized by hypersensitivity to environmental pollutants and chemicals that are generally tolerated by the healthy population. Because of the pervasive use of chemicals and widespread pollution, people with MCS are sick most of the time.

Symptoms of MCS include headache (migraine), depression, neurological symptoms (ADHD and hyperactivity), chronic fatigue, chronic respiratory inflammation (rhinitis, asthma, and sinusitis), skin rashes, sore throats, and muscle or joint pain. MCS is associated with a number of conditions, including hypothyroidism, autoimmune thyroiditis (allergy to thyroid hormone), impaired metabolism of essential fatty acids and amino acids, and deficiencies of magnesium and vitamin B_6 (pyridoxine). The etiology of MCS remains unclear. Although some theories propose organic causes of MCS, there is no consensus in the scientific literature. The most likely cause appears to be toxin overload, which activates inflammatory mediators that rev up or create an overactive immune system, which in turn creates immune reactions to irritants; these factors may also be accompanied by neuroendocrine abnormalities.

Direct stimulation of olfactory nerves is another hypothesis behind the dysfunction associated with MCS. Several studies have recognized the link between olfactory stimulation and changes within the central nervous system. MCS individuals are predisposed to exaggerated immune responses upon exposure to various irritants. The immune system triggers neuroendocrine reactions, altering metabolic pathways. When this occurs, the liver must meet the increased metabolic and detoxification demands. Over time, the detoxification pathways of the liver are depleted of vital enzymes and antioxidants. Eventually, the toxic load overcomes the defense systems, leading to exhaustion and illness. One study found that treatment with antioxidants improved symptoms in 43 percent of the MCS patients.

Supporting detoxification of the liver and initiating a bowel terrain program for candida will often alleviate symptoms of MCS. This, along with the following supplements, support the problem areas associated with MCS: Fish oils, methylsulfonylmethane (MSM), ascorbate C, and homeopathic isodes specific for environmental toxins. In addition, adrenal and thyroid function can be supported if needed, in addition to the use of Moducare (a plant sterol and sterolin complex) to modulate the hyperimmune response.

POLLUTANTS IN WATER

All water contains some impurities. As water flows in streams, sits in lakes, and filters through layers of soil and rock in the ground, it dissolves or absorbs the substances that it touches. Some of these substances are harmless, but some are not. Pesticides, heavy metals, and other environmental pollutants can and have contaminated our water supply. You will learn all about the importance of water and the contaminants in it later in Chapter 14.

MINIMIZING EXPOSURE TO ENVIRONMENTAL TOXINS IS KEY

In addition to my work in clinical practice, I do a lot of writing and public speaking on natural medicine. One of the reasons I really enjoy public speaking is the feedback I get from people on all sorts of various topics. Of all the subjects I speak on, the subject of environmental toxins and their effects on our health seems to be met with the most skepticism. This is very perplexing. One has only to do a quick perusal of the

Ryan's Story

In November 2000, our eleven-year-old son Ryan was diagnosed with osteosarcoma, a type of bone cancer. During the next twelve months, Ryan received eighteen chemotherapy treatments and a femur resection along with several other surgeries and numerous tests. The hard work Ryan had done mentally and the tremendous physical abuse he endured during this time seemed to have paid off when he was pronounced cancer-free after the treatments.

Then, in March 2002, scans revealed the cancer had returned with a large area below the previous spot and some unknown spots in his lungs. Ryan's oncologist, who is a terrific man and outstanding doctor, informed us there weren't many options. After much discussion, we decided on one traditional chemotherapy drug and a new experimental drug, along with an alternative drug we had been researching. The new chemotherapy was taking a hard toll on Ryan physically. Little did we know, life was about to change for the better.

We learned about Dr. LaValle and called his office immediately. I have to admit I was somewhat skeptical. My wife, who is what I call "a vitamin pusher," was very excited. I was open minded, but wanted to look and listen. I always studied Ryan's chemotherapy medicines, methods of delivery, and side effects and knew the risks and potential ratios for each drug. The information I was hearing from Dr. LaValle was all new to me. After spending time with Dr. LaValle, I was convinced enough to begin his recommendations along with the other treatments we had already begun.

During the weeks to follow, I was amazed. Ryan was a different boy; he looked and felt much better. He even regained some of his appetite. Dr. LaValle followed Ryan closely during his next five months of chemotherapy and his leg amputation. In October, Ryan had his scans again and I'm happy to report he is cancer-free once again. For anyone battling osteosarcoma, which is recurrent in such a short period, you know what the odds are. Ryan's victory to date is tremendous. To tell you for a fact that I know which one of the many things we did cured him, I can't. But, as a parent, I can tell you what I saw and experienced. Two to three weeks after seeing Dr. LaValle, Ryan felt and looked better than he had in the previous year. Ryan continues his tremendous physical recovery with the help and support of Dr. LaValle. I would like to take this opportunity to thank Dr. Jim for his work and the huge role he played in returning our son to good health.

Even when someone is facing a significant challenge like cancer, I believe that the Healthy Living Guidelines and nutrient support for various systems of the body can play a valuable and supportive role. Our patients who are going through chemotherapy seem to do very well when compared with those who do not incorporate nutritional support into their treatment. Ryan is an inspiration to us all.

EPA website to obtain verification of the health risks posed to humans and to wildlife by chemicals, heavy metals, and other pollutants. Yet some people choose to remain ignorant.

Still, other groups are all too aware. Recently, I was in a meeting with a group of oncologists (cancer specialists) and, to my surprise, they all agreed that cancer is greatly influenced by toxins in the environment and their impact on the body. Statistics, once scant, now back this up. Cancer is the third leading cause of death in children according to the CDC. However, little is being done to clean up our air, our water, and our environment. Indeed, if anything, our government seems to be getting more lenient with what few laws exist to keep our environment clean.

If we are to survive, both as a population and as individuals, it is essential that we understand our survival is in our own hands. We must take charge of our environment—both internal and external—today.

If you read in the newspapers about the environmental challenges facing us and yet you don't think that it is affecting you or your family, ponder these questions: Do you have mercury fillings? Do you have a job that exposes you to various chemicals such as petroleum products and paints? Do you make pottery? Do you live in a very polluted city? Do you drink unfiltered water? Have you just had new carpets laid down in your house? Do you love eating those great-tasting unwashed grapes from the grocery store that unfortunately have pesticide residues on their skin? Do you enjoy eating fish? If you answered yes to any of these questions, then your environment is affecting you and your family.

There are a host of toxins that can be potentially damaging to our bodies. Many are generated from our external environment, and some from inside our own bodies as we learned in the last chapter. We have also learned about the liver and the other organs important for detoxification. A weakness in any one will shift the burden of detoxification to the others, creating stress and imbalance throughout the body. And, as we already know, such an imbalance increases your chances for developing many health problems that could be prevented by appropriate detoxification.

By keeping the organs of detoxification "in tune," and in good working order, we can rid our bodies of the external and internal toxins that can accumulate over time and compromise health. Whether the source of toxins originates outside ourselves or within us, detoxification is important and imperative for "cracking the metabolic code." Ridding these toxins from your body will help you reinvigorate and maintain a balanced metabolism, and lead to the good health that you deserve.

Now we need to take what we have learned and put it into action. In the next chapter, I present the ways in which you can use your second set of keys to lay the foundation for your future state of optimal health.

CHAPTER 11

Key Supplements and Strategies for Detoxification and Rejuvenation

No other generation before ours has been exposed to as many man-made chemicals and toxic substances as we are today. There is now a significant amount of research and published study findings confirming the effects of the environment on our chemistry. Many of our most dreaded diseases such as cancer, Parkinson's disease, Alzheimer's disease, chronic fatigue syndrome, diabetes, cardiovascular disease, and autoimmune disorders to name but a few are being associated with our exposure to toxic compounds.

The air we breathe is polluted. The water we drink is unclean. The food we eat is processed. Unfortunately, avoiding exposure is impossible. Our lifestyles are sedentary in respect to exercise, yet too fast-paced. Our body cells are not receiving the adequate oxygen, vitamins, minerals, and enzymes needed to drive our metabolism. Our organs of detoxification and excretion are overwhelmed. Our bodies are overloaded with waste products and toxins, which render us vulnerable to all sorts of bacteria, viruses, intestinal infections, pollutants, chemical sensitivities, and allergies, all of which can create havoc with our metabolisms and produce chronic inflammation in our bodies. How are we to survive?

Fortunately, the human body possesses regulatory mechanisms that are self-healing. A healthy body is capable of eliminating the toxic substances generated by its normal functioning and some substances imposed upon it from the environment. But, if the production of toxic metabolites and the ingestion of toxic substances overwhelm the organs of detoxification and excretion, the body begins to store these substances in organs, as well as in adipose (fat) and connective tissues, which then begin to change the regulation of the important tasks that runs our metabolism. As these chemicals exert both a direct toxic effect on cells and also alter enzyme function, the metabolic pathways of the body become affected, shifting away from proper function and self-regulation.

The body has many ways of showing the buildup of toxins. Some of the more common complaints include fatigue, digestive distress, mental fogginess, allergic tendencies, chronic inflammation, and most important, weight gain, and metabolic shutdown. We know that an impairment of the basic regulatory processes can lead to a "regulatory freeze," a state that is typical for those experiencing some form of cancer. In the case of "regulatory freeze," the body does not properly react to health challenges. Yet the person is seemingly healthy. Cancer patients have mostly shown no sign of illness for years before their tumors manifest.

All of us, whether or not we suffer from cancer, a chronic degenerative disease, or symptoms of metabolic syndrome should make every effort to improve the function of our liver, gut, kidneys, lung, and skin and lymph system. We can do this by periodic and routine detoxification of our bodies. Detoxification is a decisive step toward restoration of the body's regulatory mechanisms. Most detoxification starts with the liver. When the liver is working efficiently and effectively, the skin, lungs, intestines, lymph, and kidneys usually follow suit. They eliminate toxins processed by the liver. With detoxification, digestion, immune, brain, and endocrine function—all other body systems—tend to work better.

APPROACHES TO DETOXIFICATION

Detoxification comes in many forms. The term is used to refer to many different programs that aid the body's removal of toxins and that help reduce the intake of toxic substances. Fasting, modified fasting, colonic irrigation (a type of cleansing enema to rid the colon of excessive waste), diet, herbal aids, saunas, and others all have therapeutic value. Some detoxification programs work only with the intestines; others may be targeted to cleanse the liver, kidneys, lymph, neuroendocrine tissues, or the skin.

While much can be done to support the body's natural detoxification process,

Why Detoxify?

To understand the importance of detoxification, consider the following research findings:

- Microorganisms found to be contributory factors in chronic degenerative diseases and cancer thrive in a toxic bodily environment.

- Chemical compounds and heavy metals ubiquitous in our food, air, and water are now found in every person. The bioaccumulation of these compounds in some individuals can lead to a variety of metabolic and systemic dysfunctions, and in many people, trigger outright disease states.

- As metabolism starts to enter a downward spiral, it produces greater amounts of toxins that inhibit immune functions and damage tissues (for example, inflammatory markers increase as does free-radical production). These increase the load of toxins, which diminishes the body's ability to control the progression of the disease.

rigorous cleansing programs and rapid detoxification methods should be avoided unless absolutely necessary. Over twenty years in clinical practice, I have heard all sorts of stories about what people did or didn't eat or drink while attempting a detoxification program. I have never been a strong supporter of "heroic" purges. In my opinion, some of these programs (especially those using herbal laxatives) can be dangerous, and others simply painful, expensive, and ineffective.

Some healthcare professionals are advocates of fasting. Fasting can be an effective way to periodically detoxify. But it can be difficult. Moreover, it can initiate an overwhelming release of toxic materials into the system, which, if greater than the body's elimination capabilities, can create a significant challenge to body chemistry. I do not often recommend fasting unless it is a one-day juice fast each week for several consecutive weeks. In which case, various vegetable juices are used in place of solid food to decrease digestive stress load. This type of fast is easy to do and generally causes little discomfort.

Fasts are not appropriate for everyone. Diabetics, pregnant or nursing women, and those with cardiovascular disease, for example, should not fast. Those with chronic illnesses, such as cancer and AIDS, should fast only under strict medical supervision.

The best measures for decreasing the toxic burden are moderate detoxification programs that include the following:

- Learning the source of your toxic exposure

- Avoiding or limiting your exposure to these toxins

- Maintaining adequate nutrition

- Undertaking a proactive nutritional support program for the organs of detoxification, as well as for capturing and eliminating unwanted solvents, metals, and chemicals

Many different approaches to detoxification and wellness work, even though they attack the problem at different levels. Any program that augments detoxification can improve health. You'll find entire books written on the topic of detoxification. In this chapter, I outline the detoxification program that I use every day in my practice. It is simple, gentle acting, yet effective, and you can perform the basics without medical supervision as long as you are not under the care of a physician for a current medical problem. You'll learn how to improve the detoxification abilities of the liver and rejuvenate intestinal function, so that they no longer contribute to your toxin load.

There are also many nutraceuticals you can use to support the body during the detoxification processes. Including vitamins, minerals, herbs, and phytochemicals in your detox program will enhance well-being, improve mental processes, and increase physical stamina. Making time for exercise and a massage or a sauna are some other important and enjoyable ways that we'll discuss for having fun and feeling great while reducing your toxin load.

THREE STEPS TO DETOXIFICATION

For many people, the word "detox" brings up images of heroic and uncomfortable processes. But, for the most part, if it is well planned, it should be a gentle ongoing and gradual process that is a part of your daily life.

The detoxification process is typically broken into three stages: the *elimination*, the *intensive*, and the *reintroduction stages*. The duration of each stage varies with the individual. The detoxification diet presented here is very similar to the diet presented in my Healthy Living Guidelines, except that it eliminates grains at first and limits protein to mostly beans, fish, and poultry. The intensive and reintroduction stages represent the key concepts of phase one and two of the Healthy Living Guidelines. We'll introduce the concepts here and go into details later in Chapter 13.

The most basic step to detoxification usually begins with the foods you eat. My detoxification diet, and most other detox programs, is based on a diet high in fruits and vegetables. Fruits and vegetables not only contain fiber for stimulating good bowel elimination, but also contain vitamins and minerals that feed and nourish the intestines and the liver, as well as other eliminative organs. Also, they include a valuable source of enzymes. Proper food selection helps the body eliminate toxins in many ways.

Step One: The Elimination Stage

Elimination is the first step in the detoxification process. This stage rids the diet of common allergy-provoking foods known to cause many problems with digestion and elimination. These foods include:

- Gluten-containing grains such as wheat, rye, oats, barley and rye (gluten-rich grains), soy, dairy (cow's milk and milk products, and cheese), and citrus fruits.

- Sugar and artificially sweetened foods are eliminated because of their tendency to produce hypoglycemia. Sugar also depresses the immune system and causes the depletion of several minerals.

- Red meats are limited to once a week because they may contain hormones and antibiotics, and require many enzymes for digestion.

- Caffeine and alcohol are removed from the diet, as are refined, processed, high-fat and junk foods due to their many ill effects in digestion.

These substances are omitted in order to provide the best possible support for the liver and gastrointestinal tract as their function improves. During the elimination stage, center your diet on the following basic foods and eating practices. Select organically grown produce whenever possible to avoid adding insult to injury.

- **Fresh Vegetables.** Eat five to seven servings of veggies a day. Artichokes, asparagus, beets, daikon, garlic, onions, radishes, and vegetables of the cruciferous family such as broccoli, cabbage, cauliflower, collards, and kale are especially good for the liver. Beets are also known to cleanse the liver. These vegetables can be eaten cooked or raw. It is not necessary to eat all foods raw (uncooked) as some detox diets emphasize. Attempting to eat only raw vegetables is not only a very difficult adjustment for most people, but also many times their digestive capacity just isn't good enough to take on such a significant change. If you are more adventurous, you can include seaweed and green foods (microalgae) such as chlorella and spirulina, which help with the detoxification of heavy metals. In Chapter 13, Table 13.1 "Vegetables Grouped by Carbohydrate Content" on page 320 lists the most desirable to the least desirable vegetables based on glycemic index. During the elimination stage, limit your intake of the high-glycemic vegetables in groups 4 and 5.

- **Fresh Fruits.** Consume two to three servings a day of fruits such as blueberries, cherries, and peaches. These fruits are rich in vitamins, fiber, and water, and are easy to digest. Avoid fruits that are high in carbohydrates such as bananas, prunes, and figs. In Chapter 13, Table 13.3 "Fruits Grouped by Carbohydrate Content" on page 326 lists the most desirable to the least desirable fruits based on glycemic index.

- **Fats.** Keep harmful saturated-fat intake low. Most saturated fats are of animal origin, although a few, such as coconut oil and palm oil, come from plants. Consume more of the good fats such as fish oils, olive oil, and other sources of omega-3 fats. These fats are crucial for balancing prostaglandin production and for forming healthy brain cells and cell membranes; they are found in cold-water fish such as anchovies, halibut, mackerel, salmon, sardines, and sea bass; in canola, pumpkin, and flaxseed oils; in raw nuts such as walnuts, almonds, and filberts; in seeds such as pumpkin and sesame; and in legumes such as adzuki, pinto, and garbanzo beans.

- **Fiber.** Eat plenty of fiber, including fresh fruits and vegetables. These foods help the body eliminate toxins through the intestines. Try to include two tablespoonfuls of flaxseed meal (ground flax seed) daily. Most of my patients find that blending the meal with a whey- or egg white-, yellow pea- or rice-protein powder drink in the morning is satisfying for hours and helps improve bowel regularity (for recipe, see page 332). In addition, the lignans in flaxseeds have many health benefits.

- **Quality Protein.** Use rice and whey protein powders, high-quality proteins that are free of fat and lactose, or milk sugar. These foods bind to intestinal toxins and help transport them from the body. Other sources of high-quality protein that can be eaten include beans and legumes, fish, chicken, and turkey. I recommend that most people limit their intake of animal protein to one-half gram per pound of body weight in the first phase of the program. People who exercise vigorously or lift weights can increase their protein intake a little beyond this to accommodate the increased muscle maintenance and building.

- **Water.** Try to drink at least eight 8-ounce glasses of water a day. Water is essential during detoxification: It cleanses the internal organs, helps eliminate toxins from the bloodstream, and lubricates and flushes wastes and toxins from all cells. Make sure to use a quality source of water, preferably reverse osmosis (filtration method that forces pressurized water through a contamination-rejecting membrane) or otherwise purified water. Diluted juices are acceptable, but drink no more than two to three 8-ounce glasses per day. Juices should be diluted with one part juice to three parts water. Herbal teas are acceptable as well. If you have had a high caffeine intake, either from coffee or soda, you may need to slowly decrease your intake over a period of a week to limit the withdrawal symptoms. It is common to experience headaches when withdrawing from caffeine.

Weaning yourself off common allergy-provoking foods may seem challenging at first. Making changes to your diet and lifestyle is easier said than done for some people. Many people want to be healthy and will go to any length to improve their health, including dietary changes. Others may need to ease into the process. So, if you have to, go slowly and be gentle with yourself. All I know is the better food selections you make, the better your chemistry will respond. I simply encourage people to keep trying. The old adage "Rome wasn't built in a day" applies here. Changing dietary habits is difficult, but if you stick with it, you will find yourself feeling better and the motivation to stick with it will come.

During the first several days of the elimination stage, you may feel light-headed or mentally foggy, develop a rash, have head or joint aches, or even experience loose stools or constipation. These symptoms generally pass within a few days and are simply an indication that toxins are being flushed out of the body or that the body is going through withdrawal from caffeine, sugar, alcohol, or other substances. But, even in these cases, I have found that after this brief period of discomfort, the person begins to feel better and stronger than they have felt in years. This first phase of detoxification can be done for a period of one to three weeks.

Step Two: The Intensive Stage

In step two, all hypersensitizing substances—wheat, dairy, and yeast, as well as some of the common allergy-producing foods—are still eliminated from the diet; however, now your choice of foods widens. Although some practitioners will screen for a food allergen before reintroducing any food, I have found that most people will begin to better tolerate more foods once they have been on supplements to restore intestinal health, their toxin load is reduced, and their immune system and inflammatory response is reduced. In other words, the sensitivity to foods usually will begin to lessen as the gut begins to heal.

In this stage, you are asked to follow the eating guidelines outlined in phase one of the Healthy Living Guidelines beginning on page 318. This phase involves learning how to eat from each of the five food groups and to integrate wholesome alkaline foods into your diet. The goal is to eat a more alkalinizing diet that has less immune-reactivity potential.

This stage may need to be followed for several months depending on your health situation. Someone who has a significantly compromised digestive system, chronic *Candida* overgrowth, dysbiosis, or immune challenges may need to adhere to this stage of treatment for six months. Whereas an individual who may simply be feeling the pressures of stress and have a few pounds to lose could get by with four to eight weeks. Most people quickly begin to identify the foods that make them feel poorly and to self-regulate how often they can eat these foods.

If you are hungry during this stage of treatment, nuts and seeds such as almonds, sunflower, or pumpkin seeds, which are alkalizing and usually nonallergenic, effectively satisfy hunger.

Step Three: The Reintroduction Stage

The *reintroduction* stage slowly reintroduces foods back into the diet to determine whether they can now be tolerated. In this stage, you are asked to follow the eating guidelines recommended in phase two of the Healthy Living Guidelines beginning on page 333.

You should add only one new food at a time back into the diet to see how your body responds, so, for instance, if you reintroduce dairy, do it alone. Some people will never be able to tolerate dairy foods made from cow's milk again and yet others can consume a moderate dairy intake without a problem. Some practitioners feel that cow's milk in any form should never be eaten by anyone. I have found that once steps are taken to correct intestinal imbalances most people better tolerate moderate intake of dairy products, especially cultured dairy products like yogurt. Common signs of intolerance are constipation, bloating, runny nose, and sinusitis.

If a reintroduced food triggers a reaction, it is once again eliminated from the diet, only to be added one or two weeks later to verify a food sensitivity or allergy. It is helpful to keep a daily log of everything you eat and of your symptoms. Observe your body carefully. Pay attention to how good you feel, and be careful not to overdo it. Keep in mind that food sensitivities often result in delayed reactions, so it may take up to forty-eight hours to feel the effect of a newly introduced food.

At the very beginning of a detoxification program, people appear to become more sensitive to food allergens. This is because the offending food has been eliminated, and the body has been freed from its effect. When reintroduced, the reaction appears more severe.

Often individuals are more aware of their food and behavior addictions during this period. This is the longest phase and often requires reinforcement and ongoing education. Yet it can also be the most rewarding. Many of my patients have gotten rid of their chronic sinusitis and joint pain, have lost weight, and have rid themselves of a host of other symptoms during the detoxification process.

Over years of clinical practice, I have found that this moderate approach to detoxification is the best way to get the maximum benefits with minimum discomfort. In this form of detox, a person's individual needs set the agenda. The unique state of each patient will determine how strict or lax he or she will be in implementing the guidelines. But, in all cases, the goal stays the same: To learn how to eat to be healthy, to learn when to be strict, and also to learn when it is appropriate to give yourself a treat.

The old adage "eat to live, don't live to eat" definitely applies here.

NUTRACEUTICALS AND HERBAL SUPPLEMENTS FOR DETOXIFICATION

Proper supplementation is essential for successful detoxification of the liver, intestines, and other organs of detoxification. The correct supplements can help reduce withdrawal symptoms from caffeine and sugar, maintain energy levels, and stimulate the elimination of collective toxicity. Dietary changes alone will not usually be sufficient to heal the gut and eliminate heavy metals from the body.

The following sections discuss the most influential nutrients in a detoxification program and a recommended dosage range for each.

ANTIOXIDANTS

At the outset of a detoxification program, I put my patients on antioxidants. Sufficient amounts of antioxidants are a necessary part of any ongoing detoxification efforts by your body. The antioxidants such as selenium and vitamin C are essential components to many of the body's biological detoxification processes. If not eliminated, toxins induce excessive free-radical damage, which leads to disease or at the very least accelerated aging. Antioxidants are needed to neutralize free radicals and prevent their damaging effects. The essential antioxidants to include in your program are vitamin C, natural mixed tocopherol (vitamin E), selenium, mixed carotenoids, alpha lipoic acid, and coenzyme Q_{10}. You will learn a great deal more about antioxidants and free radicals and their effects on metabolism in Chapter 15.

All of the following nutrients work together as a team of antioxidants or to support production of antioxidants that the body makes to protect and strengthen the body during a liver detoxification program.

Glutathione

High concentrations of glutathione exist in liver cells. Glutathione attaches to toxic compounds in the liver during the conjugation process and neutralizes them, enabling them to be excreted. Glutathione is too large a molecule to effectively pass through the intestine into cells, so supplementing with glutathione itself is not helpful.

There is a type of glutathione that is "reduced" that some healthcare practitioners feel does get absorbed. Studies to date have been unable to verify this. If you choose to supplement with glutathione, then use "reduced glutathione."

Recommended dose. 250–500 mg daily. 500 mg of vitamin C a day has been found to raise glutathione levels by 50 percent in the blood. Other nutraceuticals and herbals discussed below can improve the production of glutathione as well. Some doctors are resorting to administering intravenous (IV) glutathione to patients with neurologic syndromes such as Parkinson's disease and are getting some promising results in relieving symptoms; while effective, IV glutathione is very expensive and may be financially too costly for many people.

Vitamin C

Vitamin C is a water-soluble antioxidant that aids the detoxification process in several ways. It helps to limit damage to the body from free radicals and recycles other antioxidants such as glutathione and vitamin E. High intakes of vitamin C help detoxify the body, rebalance intestinal flora, and strengthen the immune system. It is especially effective in helping the body rid itself of heavy metal toxins like mercury, lead, cadmium, and nickel. (Some physicians use a 25–50 gram IV drip of vitamin C for support of heavy metal detoxification.)

Recommended oral dose. 1,000–2,000 mg of vitamin C daily.

Vitamin E

Vitamin E is the most important fat-soluble antioxidant in the body. Vitamin E and water-soluble vitamin C recycle one another in the fight against free radicals. Vitamin E insures the stability and integrity of cellular tissues and membranes throughout the body by preventing free-radical damage. Natural vitamin E has a substantially greater ability to be absorbed into the body than synthetic vitamin E.

Recommended dose. At least 400 IU and up to 800 IU (international units) of natural (d-alpha tocopherol or a mixed tocopherol) vitamin E a day. Oral doses of vitamin E up to 3,200 IU a day have shown no evidence of toxicity.

Zinc

Zinc is a mineral that works to protect tissues with the sulfur component of the antioxidant enzyme superoxide dismutase (SOD). It does this by converting damaging superoxide free radicals into hydrogen peroxide, which is further catabolized into water and oxygen. Zinc also works as a cofactor for alcohol dehydrogenase, the

Performing a Vitamin C Flush

If someone has an allergic reaction or has multiple chemical sensitivities, I suggest a "vitamin C flush." When vitamin C has saturated your mast cells, you won't release histamine, and that means you won't trigger an allergic response. A vitamin C flush can also be used to help determine your daily dose of vitamin C.

To do a vitamin C flush, mix one-half teaspoon of a pH-balanced, mixed-mineral vitamin C ascorbate powder in 4–6 ounces of water and drink. Do this every hour until your stools become loose. When you reach this saturation point, count the number of doses it took to produce the loosened stools, and cut back to 70 percent of the final amount given. For example, if it took three and one-half teaspoons of vitamin C powder to cause mild diarrhea, then calculate three and one-half times 70 percent, which equals two and one-half teaspoons (3.5 x 70 percent = 2.5). This amount becomes your new dose for the following day. Continue the next day using the same method until tissue saturation has occurred. It might not take the full 70 percent to reach tissue saturation. Whatever the amount is that produces loose stools, this is the amount to cut back to 70 percent of.

Note: Perform a vitamin C flush only during waking hours. If you feel uncomfortable or too full, you might want to reduce the amount of water that you dissolve the vitamin C in. Also, it is best to drink room temperature water. Adding 10–15 grams of MSM to the vitamin C flush per day will help to neutralize the allergic response. Occasionally, this may upset the stomach; if so, discontinue its use.

---

enzyme that works in the liver to detoxify ethanol, methanol, and other alcohols. Zinc is important for the production of proteins making it very important for the immune system and wound healing. It is also needed for insulin activity.

Recommended dose. 15–30 mg of zinc per day. Take no more than 50–100 mg of zinc each day if using long-term. Large doses of zinc can interfere with copper absorption, although taking copper along with zinc will prevent this.

Selenium

Selenium is a trace mineral with important roles in detoxification. It is a cofactor for the production of glutathione peroxidase, a form of glutathione that enhances the antioxidant protection against lipid peroxidation. Supplementing with 0.03 mg of selenium per kg of body weight was found in studies to significantly stimulate glutathione peroxidase. Selenium also makes zinc more effective and works closely with vitamin E. Selenium is known for its role in preventing cancer, especially skin cancer and stomach cancer. It is also known for its cardioprotective effects. It assists in the detoxification of heavy metals by enhancing the activity of lymphocytes and macrophages.

Recommended dose. 200 micrograms (mcg) daily in selenomethionine form.

High-Potency Multivitamin and Mineral Supplement

When we consider the extra stresses on the body from environmental pollutants, it is difficult to obtain the nutrients that we need for all the extra demands from food alone. I recommend a high-potency multivitamin and mineral supplement to all my patients. When choosing a general nutritional supplement, try to come as close as you can to matching the nutrients levels recommended in Chapter 16, in Table 16.1: "Suggested Optimal Daily Allowances of Important Nutrients in a Multivitamin and Mineral Formula for Healthy Individuals" on page 407. The antioxidants in the dosages described above can often be obtained in a high-potency multivitamin and mineral complex.

Supplements to Support Liver Detoxification

The following is my basic protocol of dietary supplements to support the body during detoxification.

Milk Thistle *(Silybum marianum)*

Milk thistle is an essential detoxifying agent that supports liver function and acts as an antioxidant. Add this herb to your antioxidant program before the intensive phase is undertaken. Milk thistle is beneficial to the liver because silymarin, the active component of the herb, inhibits liver damage and stimulates the growth of new liver cells to replace damaged cells. It protects liver cells from damage due to environmental exposure, as well as from drug use. In addition, it has been shown that milk thistle may inhibit the inflammatory response, thereby dampening the effect of leukotrienes, 5-lipoxygenase, and NF kappa B (a substance that regulates genes in the inflammatory pathways), which play a significant role in acute and chronic inflammatory diseases such as atherosclerosis and autoimmune disease.

If you are a chronic user of prescription or over-the-counter medications, take at least one milk thistle capsule daily. People with hepatitis, alcoholic and nonalcoholic liver disorders, or elevated enzymes should also consider taking 600 mg of milk thistle every day. In general, I recommend all my patients take milk thistle for prevention. I consider it an essential defense against modern industrial living, especially if you live in a city where there is a lot of industry or a known pollutant problem or if you work in an environment that has an added risk of environmental intoxication. Milk thistle can be taken every day, but for general prevention, consider cycling it: five days on, two days off. If you have an active disease process such as hepatitis C or elevated liver enzymes, or are taking it to reduce insulin resistance, take milk thistle daily.

Recommended dose. 300 mg of standardized extract, one to two times a day.

S-adenosylmethionine (SAM-e)

SAM-e is a metabolite of the amino acid methionine. Methionine regulates methylation, a chemical process in which methyl groups conjugate, or bind with, circulating estrogens. It is an excellent antioxidant and promotes glutathione production in the liver, thereby improving phase-two detoxification processes in the liver.

SAM-e also has many other significant effects on the body. It improves cellular membrane function, protects neuronal tissues, supports the remyelization of nerves, as well as enhances levels of the neurotransmitters dopamine and serotonin. Clinical trials have demonstrated its value in the treatment of fibromyalgia, depression, and arthritis. For depression and fibromyalgia, doses should start at 1,600 mg per day. Over a period of a month, reduce the dose gradually until maximum benefits can be maintained with 400 mg. SAM-e's one drawback is its high cost. For this reason, I don't usually include it in my basic list of recommendations during detoxification or prevention. However, if cost is not an issue, this product is very effective. If you take SAM-e, make sure that you are also taking vitamin B_{12}, folic acid, and vitamin B_6 to reduce the chance of forming homocysteine in your body. A high-potency daily multivitamin and mineral supplement easily provides sufficient amounts of these vitamins.

Recommended dose. 200–1,600 mg a day.

Alpha Lipoic Acid

Alpha lipoic acid (ALA) is a vitaminlike sulfur-containing compound that can be synthesized naturally in the body. It is often referred to as the "universal" antioxidant since it is both fat-soluble and water-soluble, which enables it to provide antioxidant protection in virtually every part of your body. ALA is the superstar of antioxidants because it helps to generate the activity of other antioxidants in the body including vitamin E, glutathione, and CoQ_{10}. Once in the body, ALA is converted to dihydrolipoic acid (DHLA), which is efficient at neutralizing two of the nastiest free radicals: singlet oxygen and peroxynitrite. ALA also helps to detoxify and chelate mercury, lead, and cadmium. It has gained popularity for its "anti-aging" effects both internally and for the skin.

In addition, ALA has been shown to help with insulin resistance and blood sugar management. ALA is critical in glycolysis (the conversion of glucose to lactic acid) and the Krebs cycle (the breakdown of carbohydrates into energy), two energy-producing processes that the liver depends on to meet its energy needs. Though ALA can be synthesized in the body, the supply often cannot keep up with the demands placed on the body in today's world. I recommend at least 300 mg of ALA a day as a part of a maintenance plan against modern industrial living.

Recommended dose. 100–300 mg, two times a day.

Phyllanthus *(Phyllanthus niruri, amarus, urinaria)*

Phyllanthus (*Phyllanthus niruri, amarus, urinaria*) is an herb that was first used in ayurvedic and traditional Chinese medicine, and is now becoming popular for liver support. It appears to reduce viral replication and may have particular value in people with hepatitis. I use this herb in cases where a little extra protection for the liver is needed. It is not a first choice unless it is in a combination product that contains milk thistle.

Recommended dose. 200 mg, two to three times a day of a standardized extract.

Picrorhiza *(Picrorhiza kurroa)*

Picrorhiza (*Picrorhiza kurroa*) is also an emerging herbal compound that has promising activity for support of liver function. Like milk thistle, it has antioxidant activity that is similar to superoxide dismutase and is shown to help restore glutathione levels. It appears to have an ability to regenerate liver cells and may be a promising agent for treating hepatitis.

Recommended dose. 400 mg, one to three times a day of a standardized 4 to 10 percent kutkin extract.

Schisandra *(Schisandra chinensis)*

Schisandra (*Schisandra chinensis*) is another herb with liver protective abilities that was first used in traditional Chinese medicine. It is used as an agent for kidney support and as an adaptogen. Typically, I recommend schisandra in combination with other liver or adaptogen compounds. As an added benefit, it improves some people's energy levels.

Recommended dose. 100–200 mg, two times a day.

Artichoke Extract *(Cynara scolymus)*

Artichoke extract (*Cynara scolymus*) can be considered a primary liver detoxification support remedy, but is also beneficial as part of a prevention strategy. It helps to restore the liver, protect against volatile chemicals, and improve the liver's antioxidant capacity. Artichoke extract has the added benefit of improving heartburn and helping with irritable bowel syndrome by breaking down fats and improving bile production. This herbal extract has also proven useful to support cholesterol metabolism. If you have a tendency to belch and take antacids frequently, consider incorporating artichoke extract into your daily maintenance program. Many combination products contain artichoke extract. Make sure the artichoke extract included is standardized to 2 to 5 percent cynarin.

Recommended dose. 250 mg, three times a day.

INTESTINAL SUPPORT (BOWEL TERRAIN PROTOCOL)

The following supplements support the body's natural detoxification processes by working to restore digestive function. I commonly refer to this list as my "bowel terrain protocol." Together, this team of supplements supports gastrointestinal integrity and health, thereby increasing the gut's detoxifying ability. When gut integrity is restored, the overall toxic burden on the body is reduced. And because the gut is no longer leaky, it no longer allows substances into the bloodstream that shouldn't be there.

It is difficult to advise you on how long to stay on these remedies. It really depends on the extent of your dysbiosis. Some people need ongoing nutritional support for their gut as maintenance; others are fine after adhering to the program for just sixty to ninety days. How well you adhere to the Healthy Living Guidelines in Chapter 13 will play a role in the ability of your gut to heal as well. As you see resolution of any constipation, diarrhea, cramping, gas, or any other problems you may have, you can begin to taper off of the supplements. If symptoms begin to return, you know you may need to keep taking the supplements.

Cat's Claw *(Uncaria tomentosa)*

Cat's claw works as an antifungal, anti-inflammatory, antibacterial, and immune-modulating substance. Its antifungal properties are particularly beneficial in helping to overcome overgrowth of *Candida albicans.* It is gentle acting and extremely effective in helping with chronic gut symptoms. There are several different types of cat's claw; one is standardized to *total alkaloids;* the other is more specialized and has a lower level of *tetracyclic oxindole alkaloids* (TOA). There is value to both extracts.

Recommended dose. 500 mg of cat's claw daily standardized to 3 percent total alkaloids, three times a day. For TOA cat's claw containing >1.3 percent pentacyclic oxindole alkaloids and <0.06 percent tetracyclic oxindole alkaloids, use 20 mg, three times a day, for three weeks, then decrease the dose to 20 mg one time a day.

Olive Leaf *(Olea europaea)*

Olive leaf has antifungal, antiparasitic, antiviral, and antibacterial properties, as well as anti-inflammatory and blood pressure regulating activity. If you have hypertension, consult your physician before using olive leaf. Olive leaf can be alternated with cat's claw in six-week intervals for reducing unfriendly flora in the intestine.

Recommended dose. 250–500 mg of olive leaf, one to three times a day, standardized to contain 15 to 23 percent oleuropein per dosage.

Grapefruit Seed Extract

Grapefruit seed extract is an antifungal, antibacterial, antiparasitic substance, which has proven to be especially effective at inhibiting the growth of *H. pylori,* the organism known to cause many ulcers. Grapefruit seed extract is available in capsule or liquid form.

Recommended dose. 100–200 mg of grapefruit seed extract, three times a day with meals, or five to ten drops diluted in a beverage or water, three times a day with meals.

Many times combinations of the intestinal remedies discussed above are contained in one product. Some people have good results with these combination products. However, because each of these agents has certain strengths at which they are most effective, it is best to rotate their use. Other popular antifungal agents include the product Tanalbit, oregano extract (*Origanum vulgare*), and caprylic acid. Other antiparasitic agents include goldenseal (*Hydrastis canadensis*) and other berberine-containing herbals such as wormwood (*Artemisia absinthium*) and cloves (*Syzygium aromaticum*).

Digestive Enzymes

By aiding in proper digestion, enzymes help replenish nutrients needed by the body. Only use enzymes if you are having difficulty digesting your food. Signs and symptoms of poor digestion include belching, bloating, abdominal discomfort, constipation, and even heartburn. First try a product that includes a full-range of digestive enzymes and contains pepsin, papain, and betaine. Once the gut's flora balance is restored and you begin to eat healthfully, many times you do not need to continue with an enzyme supplement. However, when needed, digestive enzymes are very effective. Many people are amazed that their gas and bloating go away in as little as one dose.

Recommended dose. One to three tablets with meals, three times a day.

L-Glutamine

L-glutamine is an amino acid that supports the health of the lining of the gastrointestinal tract. With leaky gut syndrome, the colon lining becomes deficient in L-glutamine. For example, when undergoing chemotherapy, oral mucositis or gastrointestinal problems often result. Taking L-glutamine in water, then swishing and swallowing, can prevent these problems. Why? Because it prevents glutamine deficiency, and the lining of the mucosa doesn't become inflamed and ulcerated. L-glutamine also acts to improve protein anabolism, thereby preventing the breakdown of lean muscle. It helps to facilitate growth hormone release as well.

Recommended dose. When starting a detoxification program, begin with a minimum of 500 mg of L-glutamine, three times a day, and build up to 1,000–4,000 mg, three times a day. Although this supplement is very safe, people undergoing chemotherapy should consult with their medical doctor to determine the best dosage for them, and because it is an amino acid, people with liver failure should not take it.

Seacure

This predigested fish protein has proven helpful for improving gut integrity and for reducing inflammation in the lining of the colon. It was developed to feed malnourished children in third-world countries who could not absorb intact or whole proteins from foods. Studies have found SeaCure also helps accelerate wound healing. It is considered a very high-quality protein supplement that provides the requisite amino acids for tissue repair.

Recommend dose. Two to three 500-mg capsules, three times a day before meals.

Butyrate

Butyrate is an amino acid that supports a healthy intestinal environment, which probiotics can thrive in. It serves as a source of energy or fuel for colonocytes (a type of cell that lines the intestines) and helps the liver to detoxify fat-soluble compounds. Use butyrate periodically throughout your bowel terrain program. Four weeks on and four off, unless you feel significantly improved when adding in the butyrate, in which case, remain on it for several months.

Recommended dose. 250–500 mg, two times a day.

Probiotics

Lactobacillus acidophilus and *Bifidobacterium bifidus* and multiple-culture probiotics support the rebuilding of healthy bowel flora. They are key players in maintaining gastrointestinal function and its interplay with the immune system. When the intestinal flora becomes imbalanced, immune dysregulation and inflammation usually follow. I recommend a steady supply of probiotics as part of maintaining your health. Probiotics help with constipation, diarrhea, and mucus in the stools, and are invaluable if you are going through chemotherapy or radiation. The many different roles of probiotics in health, such as the prevention of infection from different pathogenic bacteria, to detoxification of compounds in the gut, to the synthesis of many vitamins are well documented. Maintaining the gut's flora is an essential component to maintaining health and metabolism.

Recommended dose. 5–10 billion CFU of a dairy-free probiotic, two to three times a day in capsule or powdered form. After six months reduce to once a day. (Refrigerate probiotics after opening to maintain potency.)

Fructooligosaccharides (FOS)

Fructooligosaccharides (FOS) provides food for beneficial flora in the intestines, thereby helping to maintain healthy gut flora. FOS is sometimes used as a sweetener in foods and provides dietary fiber. FOS tends to produce significant gas production when first started, which detracts from its use. FOS is often incorporated into a probiotic formula. If you take FOS singly, use as recommended.

Recommended dose. 500 mg, one to two times a day.

Fiber

Dietary fiber has a number of health-promoting activities. Fiber holds water and provides bulk to stools, which speeds up transit time of food and helps prevent constipation and hemorrhoids. Fiber binds to glucose, which means that it slows absorption of glucose into the bloodstream, helping to improve glycemic index of foods, and is actually thought to lower calorie absorption from foods. Fiber binds to bile acids, helping to lower cholesterol levels. Fiber also binds to toxins, thereby lowering colon cancer risk and helping with general detoxification processes.

Flaxseeds are a great source of fiber, lignans, and essential fatty acids. Lignans are substances that are high in antioxidants and phytochemicals. The lignans in flaxseed are known to bind to estrogen-receptor sites in the body. This renders xenoestrogen substances that enter the body from the environment or circulating hormones in the body less free to act at receptor sites, which reduces the risk of hormonally related cancers such as breast cancer. For all these reasons, it is wise to make sure you eat at least 2 tablespoons of ground flax meal daily. The meal can be added to a protein drink or to any fruit or vegetable juice. Rice protein and bran are other valuable fibers. Rice protein powders are excellent for binding to toxins in the colon and helping to excrete them.

NATURAL REMEDIES FOR INTESTINAL CONDITIONS

The following remedies can be used to treat some of conditions briefly alluded to in Chapter 9. These alternatives may help you avoid turning to antibiotics and other prescription medications for relief, and thereby preserve intestinal integrity. In addition, there are measures to take that can help support and heal the walls of the intestines, especially if you suffer from irritable bowel problems. (Dosage recommendations are provided in Appendix 1: "Nutrient Reference Guide" on page 481 and Appendix 2: "Herbal Reference Guide" on page 498.)

Colds and Flu

The following agents should be ready resources in every medicine cabinet in the event you feel a cold or flu coming on. They are very effective in lessening symptoms or shortening the duration of symptoms, and may help you avoid the need to take antibiotics.

Simple remedies for the common cold include elderberry extract, echinacea, vitamin C, colostrum, and AHCC mushroom extracts (for example, Immpower). In addition, zinc lozenges have been proven effective to lessen severity and shorten the duration of colds.

To ease flu symptoms, try Oscillococcinum (*Anas barbariae*), a homeopathic treatment that has been proven successful for more than sixty years. Oscillococcinum works well if taken at the first signs of the flu; the sooner you start, the better your results will be.

Crohn's Disease

First, remove offending foods from the diet. Many people afflicted with Crohn's disease have been able to identify and eliminate foods that aggravate their symptoms.

Chocolate, cereal grains (especially gluten-containing grains), dairy products, yeast, fats, and artificial sweeteners are common offenders. In one multicenter trial, people with Crohn's disease who ate a diet that eliminated only those foods that precipitated their symptoms remained in remission almost twice as long as those receiving corticosteroid treatments.

Eat a diet high in protein and fiber. Protein provides amino acids needed for healing.

While low-fiber, low-residue diets consisting of foods that are easily digestible and pass easily through the intestinal tract have traditionally been recommended, there is evidence that diets high in refined carbohydrates increase the incidence and severity of acute episodes. Therapeutic regimens that include increased fiber and decreased refined carbohydrates have shown a positive influence. In one study, sixteen of twenty subjects on a sugar-free, fiber-rich diet remained in remission for an average of nineteen months after discontinuing drug therapy. Interestingly, diets high in sugar and fast food correlate with an increased risk of Crohn's disease, whereas diets high in fiber and low in sugar are associated with a reduced risk. Saturated fat and cholesterol have also been identified as dietary risk factors.

Eat the right kind of fats. Saturated fatty acids found primarily in animal products should be minimized, as they can aggravate diarrhea and promote inflammatory pathways in the intestine. However, unsaturated omega-3 fatty acids can reduce and/or reverse the inflammatory response. Supplementation with fish oil, which is high in omega-3 fatty acids, is recommended.

Colorectal Cancer

Eat a nutrient-rich diet. Nutrients such as calcium, omega-3 fats, fiber, and folate (folic acid) may provide protection against some dietary risk factors for colorectal cancer. The Danish Cancer Society recently conducted an epidemiological study on the Faroe Islands where the incidence of colorectal cancer is among the lowest in Northwest Europe and North America. Despite a diet high in fat and low in vegetable intake, there is a large consumption of fish, calcium, and vitamin D. Fish are rich in omega-3 fatty acids, which are thought to suppress the growth of some cancers. Calcium may exert a protective benefit by drawing out fatty acids and bile salts, which are thought to be toxic to the epithelial cells that line the colon wall. A recent study in France also supported the intake of dietary fiber as being protective against cancer.

Folic acid (folate) depletion is the number one nutrient deficiency associated with colorectal cancer. To address this nationwide deficiency, the United States began fortifying foods such as cereals and breads with folate. Although these efforts have been successful, some groups remain at risk for folate deficiencies, including pregnant women, and individuals with excessive alcohol intakes and on certain folate-depleting medications. (For specific medications, see Appendix 3: "Prescription and Nonprescription Nutrient Depletions" on page 512.)

If you are diagnosed with colon cancer, the following nutraceuticals will help support your body at different phases of treatment.

- **Phase one.** Natural cancer-fighting medicines, including the following: AHCC mushroom extracts, which helps to activate T-killer cells and NK cells, and protect against leukopenia (a condition in which the white blood cells in the blood are lower than normal); Moducare, which helps with immune system modulation, NK cell activation, and stress, so there isn't a negative impact on the immune system; lycopene, a carotenoid, which helps to prevent DNA mutations and protects cells from oxidative stress; the herbs green tea, graviola, and N-Tense (combination from rainforest herbs); and maitake, shiitake, and *Coriolis versicolor* mushrooms.

- **Phase two.** Nutraceuticals to reduce the side effects of the chemotherapy, including probiotics, which reduce diarrhea and inflammation of the colon lining; cat's claw, which decreases chances of developing secondary fungal infection; and milk thistle, which supports liver detoxification.

- **Phase three.** Nutraceuticals to improve effectiveness of the chemotherapy, including *Cordyceps sinensis,* which helps to oxygenate cells and prevent fatigue, and improves protection of both white and red blood cells; and L-glutamine (swish with and swallow one teaspoon dissolved in water), which prevents oral mucositis.

Diarrhea

Making sure the digestion of foods is complete often helps in the treatment of diarrhea. Supplementing with a full range of digestive enzymes can assist in complete digestion. Other recommendations vary depending on the type of diarrhea.

For *osmotic diarrhea,* which is watery diarrhea usually associated with sugar and/or lactose intolerance, take either the fruit or leaf of bilberry. Restrict your intake of simple carbohydrates and sip rice water (water that is drained off boiled rice) to help replace fluids, form stools, and to provide B vitamins. The commonly used over-the counter medication polycarbophil (Mitrolan) acts as a fluid absorbent. To prevent dehydration, remember to drink plenty of liquids and replace the body's electrolytes (minerals such as sodium and potassium that are often lost in diarrhea) by sipping vegetable soups or using an electrolyte-replacement formula such as Pedialyte.

Secretory diarrhea is diarrhea that is caused by acute secretions of the mucosal cells. Mucosal secretions are generally a response to bacterial, viral, or parasitic infections, excess bile salts, or fatty acids present in the colon. Treatment consists of treating any underlying infection with cat's claw, olive leaf, or grapefruit seed extract, and balancing the normal intestinal flora with probiotics.

Exudative diarrhea is associated with inflammation of the intestinal lining such as may occur with Crohn's disease, ulcerative colitis, chemotherapy, or food allergies. Diarrhea associated with food allergies is intermittent and often alternates with constipation. Treatment is aimed at restoring fluids and electrolytes and correcting the underlying problem, except in diarrhea induced by chemotherapy.

If you experience chronic or painful diarrhea or loose stools, and/or have alternating constipation, check with your doctor. If a diagnosis cannot be found, begin a detoxification program, follow the Healthy Living Guidelines diet in Chapter 13. And try these three intestinal supplements: probiotics, cat's claw, and butyric acid.

Irritable Bowel Syndrome (IBS)

Overcoming IBS is possible, but it involves lifestyle adjustments such as learning to manage stress more effectively, assessing food habits, and identifying and eliminating irritating foods.

Dairy products and wheat (gluten) are often the offending culprits. IBS sufferers should first try eliminating these foods. Refined sugar and carbohydrates have also been found to aggravate the condition because of the increased fermentation processes that occur when eating these types of foods. Low-fiber diets have been considered a strong contributing factor in IBS. A high-fiber diet is essential to regulate transit time and prevent constipation. Increase your intake of high-fiber foods but do so gradually. Vegetables and salads are often much better tolerated once the intestinal tract has healed.

Fat may also be problematic for IBS sufferers, especially saturated and hydrogenated fats; these foods seem to stimulate peristalsis in IBS sufferers. Fried foods like French fries and fried chicken bites tend to be the worst, and most patients have already learned they can't eat them.

Follow the Healthy Living Guidelines outlined in Chapter 13. Supplementing with probiotics such as *Lactobacillus acidophilus* and *Bifidobacterium bifidum* will decrease the inflammatory response in the mucosal lining and has shown great improvement in symptoms. Also consider including adrenal support supplements to manage stress and to build up the body's serotonin levels. The discovery of serotonin receptors in the gut has lead experts to believe that imbalances in neurotransmitters could be playing a crucial role in IBS. This makes sense since many times IBS is triggered by stressful events.

SUPPLEMENTS THAT SUPPORT ELIMINATION OF ENVIRONMENTAL POLLUTANTS AND HEAVY METALS

While people may think they are immune from the effects of heavy metals and other exposures, it is nearly impossible not to have some level of heavy metal exposure today. Heavy metals wreak havoc on many aspects of our metabolic code. In particular, they are highly neurotoxic.

To evaluate your exposure, you can have a hair analysis done, and then repeat this test after being on the program for three months. A hair analysis will show only the last six weeks of metabolic activity in your body. If you see an initial drop in heavy metal concentrations, take another test twelve weeks later. If your levels rise again, repeat the test every three months until the results show the body is clear of harmful levels of toxic metals. You can also use a provocative urine test to look for heavy metals, but this must be done under the guidance of a healthcare professional. You can help the body eliminate these toxins gently with many of the nutrients listed below. Or, if you need rapid removal because of serious health problems that already exist, then consider IV chelation therapy.

Evidence is mounting that suggests that most cognitive disorders, including autism and attention deficit disorder (ADD), Alzheimer's disease and dementia, neurological conditions, cardiovascular disease, autoimmune disorders, endocrine disruptions, chronic infections, and cancer have heavy metal toxicity as one of the major root causes. In general, I find this to be true; however, bear in mind that heavy metals accumulate over time and may or may not affect a person's health based on their specific chemistry and lifestyle factors. Everyone does not have the same ability to excrete these exposures, so there are variations in the outcome of these chronic exposures.

If you specifically want to rid your body of heavy metals, I suggest using the following supplements in combination with the liver detoxification diet program. Keep in mind that using nutraceuticals to eliminate heavy metals from the body is considered a gentle approach. It does not work overnight, nor did you become toxic overnight, so don't expect to rid your body of these heavy metals overnight. A variety of products on the market contain a combination of several of these nutrients. Check the product's label to ensure it includes amounts close to the dosages recommended below, which are necessary in order to have a beneficial effect in the body.

N-acetylcysteine (NAC)

NAC is a sulfur-containing amino acid that stimulates the production of glutathione, the chief detoxifying molecule in the body. NAC is used to help fight viruses and catalyze detoxification of environmental pollutants, including heavy metals, pesticides, tobacco smoke, and exhaust emissions, by improving phase-two detoxification mechanisms in the liver. NAC also exerts a protective action on kidney tissue, which is prone to heavy-metal damage. I regularly use NAC as part of both the liver and heavy metal detoxification programs. Typically, I begin with a dose of 600 mg, two times a day, and combine it with chlorella or garlic.

Recommended dose. 600 mg of NAC, one to three times a day.

Cilantro Seed *(Coriandrum sativum)*

Few studies have been performed on cilantro seed, known also as coriander, as a heavy metal chelating (binding) agent, but it is a favorite of many healthcare professionals and is gaining the science needed to support its use in the detoxification specifically of mercury, lead, and cadmium. Cilantro is also reported to aid in fat metabolism, thereby helping maintain blood cholesterol levels. Current heavy metal detoxification formulas for such toxins as mercury may contain cilantro.

Recommended dose. One to two 400 mg tablets or capsules of cilantro seed, two to three times a day.

Garlic and Aged Garlic *(Allium sativum)*

In addition to the wide array of garlic's benefits, including its ability to improve blood

Lowering Cholesterol While Detoxifiying

Heavy metal toxicity is known to contribute to risk of cardiovascular disease. Any agent that works to detoxify heavy metals will have a tendency to also lower cholesterol since the presence of heavy metals are known to create inflammation in the linings of the arteries that can lead to the formation of plaque and atherosclerosis. For this reason, aged garlic and artichoke can be effective in lowering cholesterol. Detoxification protocols alone will often begin the process of lowering cholesterol, but the following nutritional supplements, though they do not work as heavy metal chelators, are known to lower cholesterol and improve lipid profiles.

Policosanol

Policosanol is an extract from sugar cane or beeswax. It has been extensively studied and is well known for its cholesterol-lowering properties. Policosanol improves overall lipid profile by decreasing LDL ("harmful" cholesterol) and triglycerides, increasing HDL ("beneficial" cholesterol), and decreasing platelet aggregation. It has no adverse side effects and no toxicity. So if your cholesterol levels are mild to moderately high, consider first trying 15 mg of Policosanol twice a day before moving to more potent "statin" drugs.

Sterols and Sterolins

Sterols and sterolins are substances that are present in all plants, including fruits and vegetables. Also known as phytosterols, sterol and sterolins are actually fats that have chemical structures similar to cholesterol. Phytosterols have anti-inflammatory, anticancer, and immune-enhancing properties. In addition, studies with animals and humans have shown that beta-sitosterol (BSS), one of the primary sterols, can lower cholesterol levels and can be used clinically to lower elevated cholesterol levels. BSS is thought to interfere with cholesterol absorption and to help the liver to more efficiently trap and remove circulating cholesterol. Two capsules containing 20 mg of beta-sitosterol and 200 mcg of beta-sitosterolin may be taken three times daily between meals. Phytosterols are nontoxic and have a high margin of safety. Side effects are rare, although caution should be used in patients with multiple sclerosis.

sugar regulation, lower cholesterol, and exert anticarcinogenic activity, garlic helps protect the liver and is an excellent detoxifier of heavy metals. The sulfur-based compounds in aged-garlic extracts in particular are exceptional at stimulating detoxification processes in the body. Garlic has a direct binding, or chelating, effect on heavy metals. The garlic actually binds to the heavy metal and carries it out of the body. Garlic is highly recommended for treating heavy metal toxicity; in fact, some experts believe that garlic may be the most effective agent for drawing heavy metals such as mercury out of brain tissue.

Recommended dose. 300–1,200 mg of garlic or aged garlic a day.

Chlorella *(Chlorella pyrenoidosa)*

Chlorella is a freshwater species of green algae that has come to be the standard in heavy metal detoxification. Not only does this algae help to detoxify heavy metals, but also it is beneficial for removal of chemical compounds and insecticides. Chlorella contains a wide range of vitamins and minerals in addition to glutathione. It is an important part of heavy metal and toxin elimination programs and is routinely used by healthcare professionals in conjunction with DMSA, EDTA, or D-penacillamine for heavy metal elimination.

Recommended dose. 3–5 grams of chlorella a day, or up to fifteen pills a day. (They are very small tablets, so don't let this scare you out of trying chlorella.) For best results, take chlorella one-half hour before meals. You may experience some bloating or loose stools when first beginning chlorella; however, these side effects should subside within one week.

NUTRACEUTICALS FOR USE UNDER PROFESSIONAL SUPERVISION

There are several potent agents that can be used for the removal of heavy metals. These substances can be taken either orally or by IV if administered by a physician. The physical side effects of oral detoxification can be challenging; these include foggy-headedness, loose stools, and even some body aches. Therefore, it is important that you request to be detoxified in a "mild or conservative" fashion. Be sure to include alpha lipoic acid, chlorella, or cilantro seed in your treatment, in combination with drainage remedies to support the organs of detoxification, principally the liver, lymph, and especially the kidneys. (For more details about drainage remedies, see page 269).

Dimercaptosuccinic Acid (DMSA)

DMSA is a water-soluble amino acid that removes heavy metals such as lead, arsenic, mercury, and cadmium from the body. DMSA is a safe and convenient metal chelator that can be taken orally. When detoxifying with DMSA, some people experience an increase in urination (in fact, it is very important to drink extra water when taking DMSA); it may also loosen stools and increase bowel movements temporarily. DMSA can chelate other needed minerals such as copper and manganese, so it is important to take a high-potency multivitamin and mineral formula to replace these nutrients at the end of the dosing period. Some experts believe that DMSA stresses the kidneys; therefore, on those days when you are using DMSA, take 300 mg of alpha lipoic acid, three times a day.

Recommended dose. 10 mg of DMSA per kilogram of body weight. Use for three days, then stop for eleven days; and repeat. Do not take any minerals or multivitamins containing minerals on days when using DMSA, since most of the minerals will be removed and you will not get the maximum benefit from it. During the eleven DMSA-free days, take fifteen tablets of chlorella and one capsule of aged garlic, twice a day. Also consider using a kidney drainage formula. Many are on the market, but one of the best is the herb goldenrod (*Solidago*), which comes from the goldenrod plant. It is often sold in liquid form. Dilute twenty drops in water, three times a day. Repeat this three-days-on/eleven-days-off schedule for three to six months. After six months, retest yourself for heavy metals. Use DMSA three times a year for one-month periods as a maintenance agent.

Another option is to take one 100-mg capsule of DMSA at night for ninety days, then every third month, take one capsule at bedtime for thirty days. Combine DMSA with other important detoxification agents such as milk thistle, NAC, chlorella, cilantro seed, and aged garlic as a regular part of your health-maintenance regimen.

Ethylenediaminetetraacetic Acid (EDTA)

EDTA is a food preservative that is especially effective at chelating lead from the body. It helps to dissolve calcium-rich plaque in the arteries and to remove lead from tissues. It can be taken orally or administered by IV therapy.

Recommended dose. Generally one-half to one teaspoon (2.5–5 grams) of EDTA is administered one or two times a day in water or juice. Continue taking EDTA until you test clear of lead, at which point it can then be used once or twice a year for one month for maintenance. Some practitioners keep people on a maintenance dose year-round, but I prefer to use a combination of chlorella, alpha lipoic acid, and cilantro seed for maintenance. Like DMSA, EDTA can remove minerals the body needs; therefore, take a high-potency multimineral supplement at least two hours after EDTA. EDTA is commonly taken in the morning, and the multimineral then taken at night. If the minerals are not being replaced adequately, you may begin to notice signs of mineral loss such as muscle cramping.

D-penacillamine

The prescription drug D-penacillamine is an efficient detoxifier of mercury from the body. The typical dose is 7.5 mg of D-penacillamine per kilogram of body weight, four times a day, twice a week, for thirty to sixty days. Antioxidants are usually given simultaneously to help counteract the free-radical damage that heavy metals cause.

Retesting should occur after the first treatment period to determine whether all the mercury is removed.

ADDITIONAL REMEDIES FOR SUPPORT DURING DETOXIFICATION

Detoxification programs should also include the following therapies, which help the body to detoxify and excrete toxins more rapidly.

Drainage Remedies for Liver, Lymph, and Kidneys

Drainage remedies are specialized formulas that are usually herbal or low-dose homeopathic medicines that have been designed to support or facilitate elimination of toxins from the body. Many natural food stores or healthcare professionals who specialize in natural therapeutics will have these types of compounds available.

Treating yourself to a therapeutic massage as often as possible from a therapist who specializes in lymphatic drainage massage will help the body's elimination of waste products from the lymph. This is particularly beneficial if you suffer from lymph edema due to an accumulation of lymphatic fluid.

Unlike the circulatory system, the lymphatic system does not have a pump. Therefore, by taking steps to aid lymphatic drainage, you are helping the immune system, which, especially during times of detoxification, is overloaded with substances to be eliminated.

Jumping on a rebounder (a mini-trampoline), two to three minutes, one to two times daily, contracts the muscles and keeps the lymph fluids flowing as well.

Another way to support lymph drainage is to stimulate the skin and the key lymphatic areas under your arms and down the inside of your thighs with a loofah sponge during your shower or bath. Rubbing outward from the center of these areas will improve drainage of the lymph in these areas.

Low-Temperature or Infrared Sauna

A low-temperature or infrared sauna is lower in temperature than a regular hot-rock heated sauna. This type of sauna uses infrared rays, which causes the body to sweat at lower temperatures and penetrates warmth to mobilize toxins in fat cells so they can be excreted through the skin.

Slow, steady, sweat encourages the release of fat-soluble toxins through the skin from their storage sites in our tissues. Be sure the saunas temperature is set between 110°F and 114°F. Attempt to spend twenty to forty minutes in a sauna, three to five times a week. Releasing toxins cannot be produced using higher heat or shorter amounts of time. An added benefit of low-temperature saunas is that they improve metabolism and basal metabolic rate, so they can actually help you lose weight. Many health clubs now have saunas, or you can seek out a health spa or consider purchasing an inexpensive home unit.

Exercise

Exercise is an essential component of a detoxification program. Regular activity of at least thirty to forty-five minutes, four times a week, helps the body to detoxify and excrete toxins more rapidly. Asking you to devote this amount of time to exercise may seem unrealistic, especially if you are also trying to incorporate therapeutic massage, a sauna, and loofah skin buffing into your detoxification program. Strive to do whatever amount of exercise you can.

By becoming aware of the health problems that can result from environmental and internal toxins and relieving the body from the burden of waste and toxic substances, you will be taking key steps necessary for stopping the downward spiral toward metabolic chaos and encouraging the body's own regulatory self-healing mechanisms to function fully again.

Nutrition: The Keys to Maintaining Peak Metabolism and Optimal Health

CHAPTER 12

Nutrition Basics: Why You Need to Nourish Yourself

In your lifetime, you will consume approximately 70,000 meals and from that food you will eliminate about fifty tons of waste products. The foods you choose to eat in those meals can either build up your health or tear it down. The food choices you make, whether they are good or bad, accumulate over time. The saying "You are what you eat" is absolutely true. The choices you make affect how you feel, what diseases you may or may not get, and consequently even your health-care costs.

When people find out that I am a practitioner of integrative medicine, who uses diet and lifestyle approaches to restore the body to health, I get a variety of responses. The remarks that amuse me most are the ones about eating "rabbit food," meaning vegetables, or "dying young but happy." People tend to think that eating anything they want will kill them, but at least they'll enjoy it while eating it. If I'm around folks who make such comments for any length of time, they'll eventually tell me all about their many health complaints, such as heartburn or arthritis; they don't realize that these conditions are affected by their food choices. When people tell me they don't care if they die young as long as they die happy, I respond by telling them that I just want to feel better while I'm here. That's my primary goal for eating the way I do and for taking the supplements I take: to feel great and have lots of energy.

Keep this in mind, because it can be a source of motivation for improving your nutritional intake. True, nutrition impacts what diseases you may or may not get, but let's forget about that momentarily. How do you feel right now? If you're like most Americans, my guess is you're not feeling that great. Most people are stressed out and exhausted. On top of that they get frequent headaches, have annoying allergies and fungal toenails; they get frequent colds and/or flu, have decreased sexual desires; they're depressed, they have carpal tunnel syndrome, and they can't get a good night's rest.

I see people every day who are suffering needlessly from inadequate nutrition or poor food choices. And most don't realize that by improving their diets they could improve how they feel. Here are a just a few examples:

- If you have nagging skin problems, chronic colds, or seasonal allergies, you may not have an adequate intake of vitamin A and zinc.

- If you have bleeding gums, you may be low in vitamin C.

- If you are nervous or irritable, or if you have tight, tense muscles, you may be deficient in magnesium.

- If you have blood sugar problems, your intake of minerals may be insufficient.

- If you are constipated, you are probably not getting adequate water and fiber intake.

- If you are just plain tired, poor nutrition may be part of your answer.

- And finally, if you are overweight or if you feel you have lost control of your metabolism, your dietary choices and nutritional intake play a primary role.

While all nine keys to optimal health discussed in this book work in synchrony to influence metabolism, if your nutrition is poor and nutritional deficiencies are present, reclaiming your metabolism is not likely. Proper nutrition starts with the building blocks of foods: the macro- and micronutrients. Paying attention to *macronutrition*—the intake of carbohydrates, protein, and fat—is an essential component of getting yourself on the road to optimal health. *Micronutrition*—the intake of vitamins and minerals—is also important, as these nutrients work as cofactors to keep your metabolism running smoothly, making sure that the processing of macronutrients occurs both efficiently and effectively.

In 400 B.C., Hippocrates, the father of medicine, said, "Let food be your medicine, and your medicine be food." Twenty-five hundred years later, we have lost all understanding of this wisdom. Instead, our "medicines" are refined foods and pharmaceutical drugs. The impact of this shift is evident in the diseases and mortality associated with poor diet and nutritional deficiencies. Back in 1988, the U.S. Surgeon General stated, "Approximately two-thirds of all deaths are associated with imbalances in diet and nutrition." More recently, current U.S. Surgeon General, David Satcher, M.D., Ph.D., issued a call to action against epidemic obesity rates in the United States, warning that the health consequences from this one condition alone may overwhelm the healthcare system. How is it that we're unable to control our lifestyles for our own good health?

Until the twentieth century, humans existed almost 100 percent on food from plants and animals. Today, it is estimated that two-thirds of the caloric intake of most Americans comes from processed grains, sugar, fat and oil, and alcohol. The shift from the healthier nutrition intakes of our ancestors to what has become known as the standard American diet (SAD) took place gradually as America transitioned from a society based on agriculture to one based on industry. Today, we are generations removed from the concepts of a truly healthy diet. Yes, it's true that we have longer life expectancies, but does this mean we are actually *healthier* or just that we are living longer with our chronic diseases?

Americans need a wake up call. What is the best way to keep our immune systems strong, to fight chronic disease, and feel healthy and energetic? Good nutrition and exercise. Why do we keep fighting it? Have we become a little lazy and our taste buds spoiled by an unlimited supply of high-fat, high-sugar, flavor-enhanced foods? Hopefully, this chapter and the next will not only help you wake up, but will also give you some practical suggestions and tools for making better nutrition choices on your road to better health.

FACTORS THAT LEAD TO POOR NUTRITIONAL STATUS

If we take a moment to review the diets of our ancestors, we will see how our food supply has been adulterated at the expense of our nutritional status. We don't need to travel very far back in time to find the moment when the human diet began to change from natural to processed. We need only to travel back to the industrial revolution.

Before the industrial revolution, the human diet was still largely plant based. It consisted of foods that could be *hunted* (rabbit, fish, bird, buffalo, deer, and wild game), *gathered* (nuts, seeds, greens, and berries and other fruits), and *grown* (corn, wheat, oats, vegetables, and farm animals for meat, milk, and eggs). Foods were unprocessed and were eaten while very fresh. This was a diet that could support very robust health.

The changes that began to take place with the industrial revolution in the late nineteenth century led to a population shift from farms to factory as more and more people found that they had to leave the land for the city in order to earn a living. They began to rely more on buying food than providing their own.

Population growth and the further industrialization of the twentieth century changed the way food was grown, shipped, stored, prepared, and eaten. Since the economic emphasis was rerouted from agriculture to industry, even the supply of food became an industry. Food became a commodity, subject to mechanization and automation. This has led to the reduced nutritional quality of foods. As an example, look at grains:

Prior to the industrial revolution, grains were stone ground or hand milled into flour. This unrefined flour would then be used for baked goods or cooked cereals. With the industrial revolution came large mills and better refining processes that created a new food—refined flour. These lighter flours were considered superior, until it was discovered that people were developing nutritional deficiencies because the nutrients inherent to the grain were separated out in the refining process. All that was best in the grain—the germ, the bran, and the fiber—were lost.

Other agricultural and food industry practices have even compromised the nutritional content of the soil itself. And if needed nutrients are not in the soil to begin with, how can they get into the food grown on it? In the agriculture ages, when farming of grains became more commonplace, farmers realized that the land could only be planted for so long before it became depleted and would not produce well. To put nutrients back into the soil, techniques such as crop rotation and soil fertilization were employed. Fertilizers, at the time, were primarily manure, compost, and lime—substances that place organic matter and a full range of nutrients back into the soil. Today, synthetic inorganic fertilizers are used.

The very use of synthetic fertilizers presents a classic problem. The modern need to grow large quantities of food in relatively small areas of land has led to the depletion of soil and the need for commercial fertilizers. Cheaper and more readily available than organic fertilizers, synthetic fertilizers are the popular choice of commercial farmers. Rather than replenishing the soil with all the essential minerals and nutrients, synthetic fertilizers like NPK (a nitrogen, phosphorus, and potassium blend) use fewer nutrients to replenish the soil, eliminating nutrients that are essential for humans but not plants.

It has been demonstrated that poor fertilization of soil can lead to widespread deficiencies in trace minerals. Fertilization of soil is just one issue facing modern farmers; some research reveals that although the nutrients may be present in the soil, soil conditions prevent the plants from absorbing them.

Another problem affecting the nutritional content of foods involves the ripening of foods. In preindustrial times, when foods were grown on the family farm, they were ripened on the tree or vine before being picked or harvested. These vine-ripened foods absorbed more nutrients from the soil. Because these ripe foods would spoil if transported too far, foods were sold locally.

Once again, contrast these farming methods with current practices. Today, food is often grown far from the point of sale. In order to preserve freshness, crops are picked *before* they are ripe or forced to ripen quickly under unnatural conditions. Other crops are sprayed, gassed, and fumigated in order to delay ripening during shipping. Some foods are refrigerated or frozen en route to market. This affects nutritional content in our foods because those last stages of ripening allow for the formation of more vitamins and absorption of more minerals.

There is also the issue of the mineral content of our soil, and how it differs from commercial farm to commercial farm. This issue was best illustrated a few years back when a classic study conducted at Rutgers University revealed the differences in mineral content of vegetables grown in ten different states. The researchers evaluated snap peas, cabbage, lettuce, tomatoes, and spinach for their mineral content. The results demonstrated the staggering variation in the mineral content of foods grown in different soils. It was found that the calcium content of tomatoes, for example ranged from 4.5 millequivalents (mEq) per 100 grams to 23 mEq per 100 grams. Calcium content of lettuce varied from 6 mEq per 100 grams to 71 mEq per 100 grams. The iron content of lettuce ranged from 9 parts per million (ppm) to 516 ppm. Iron in tomatoes ranged from a low of 1 ppm to a high of 1,938 ppm. This variability has a direct effect on our nutritional status as the level of nutrients needed to maintain good, vibrant health may not be consistent in our plant foods.

The use of insecticides, pesticides, and herbicides on most of the crops grown in America has lead to another insidious health dilemma. It is well known that traces of carcinogens in the food and water supply are derived from chemical insecticides. Most of the insecticides sprayed on crops actually land on the soil, killing beneficial bacteria and earthworms in the soil and leaching into ground water. Earthworms are needed to aerate the soil, and the bacteria are important for the uptake of nutrients into the growing roots of the plants.

Another important study compared the nutritional content of organically grown foods (foods grown with no synthetic chemical pesticides or herbicides) with those grown under modern agricultural (non-organic) conditions. Both foods were selected randomly from grocery store bins on the same day. After laboratory analysis for nutritional content, it was revealed that the organically grown produce contained approximately twice the nutritional value of the commercially grown food. Other studies comparing the nutritional content of organic versus non-organic foods find higher levels in a range of nutrients, as well as lower levels of nitrates and heavy metals.

The Effect of New Lifestyle Demands on Nutritional Status

In addition to changing the way food is grown, transported, and processed, modern life has also introduced new lifestyle demands. Lifestyle changes have altered how food is prepared and eaten in the American home, and how the American people spend their leisure time. From the early 1900s through the 1940s, most Americans ate home-cooked meals, which incorporated fruits and vegetables—most of which were still grown in home gardens.

In the early 1950s, convenience foods transformed the lives of millions of American women and men. The TV dinner was wholly embraced as a cultural and lifestyle advantage. And this was just the tip of the processed-food iceberg. As the years passed and more women began working outside the home, less time was available to prepare meals from whole foods. Much more food was purchased in the supermarket rather than grown at home, and the American diet started the shift away from incorporating fresh fruits and vegetables into daily meals.

In the 1960s, the advent of fast food offered a cheap and convenient alternative to home cooking. It also began the American love affair with high-fat, salt-laden meals accompanied by soft drinks. From the 1970s onward, the trend continues. These days, families eat out or order takeout foods more often than they prepare home-cooked meals. Sugar, salt, and fat intakes are at an all-time high. And more than 90 percent of Americans get less than two daily servings of fruits and vegetables.

Oh, and one last thing about the modern American diet—*nonnutritive foods.* These are "foods" that have little or no nutritional value, such as soft drinks, candy, and sugar-free gelatin—just to name a few. Have you looked at the nutrition label on some of the substances you drink or eat? Have you seen how many have little or no complex carbohydrates, no protein, no fat, no vitamins, no minerals—nothing— sometimes not even calories? Somehow, these nonnutritive ("Frankenstein") foods leap off the supermarket shelves into our homes.

It is estimated that, on average, up to one-third of a typical American's daily nutritional intake is from nonnutritive foods. In other words, in today's America, it is entirely possible to be overweight and yet be starving to death. To drive the point home, let's consider again the example of bread:

According to recent surveys, most Americans consume less than 1 serving of whole-grain bread or cereal per day. This means Americans are relying on white bread and other refined breads and cereal products. But white flour, when processed, loses almost all the iron, vitamin B_1 (thiamine), vitamin B_2 (riboflavin), and vitamin B_3 (niacin). This is why these nutrients were required by the Enrichment Act of 1942 to be added back into white flour used for breads, pastas, and cereal. That's why white breads are called "enriched." However, these so-called enriched breads still fall short in nutrients. Compared with whole-grain bread, enriched bread contains 15 percent less iron, 75 percent less magnesium, 60 percent less zinc, 80 percent less vitamin B_6, 35 percent less folate, and 75 percent less fiber. Multiply this effect by all the other refined, processed foods and think about how your nutrition is going to suffer.

And suffer it has. While full-blown clinical nutritional deficiencies such as scurvy (resulting from a lack of vitamin C) and beriberi (resulting from a lack of vitamin B_1) are rare, a new area of concern has emerged: *subclinical* nutrition deficiencies. By this I mean nutritional insufficiencies that, while they do not show themselves on any medical test, are slowly and subtly eroding the state of your health. A subclinical deficiency can take years to show up as a symptom, and yet the changes it creates can be influencing your personal metabolic code over a lifetime.

Due to all the factors influencing the nutritional content of our foods, I honestly do not believe that people can get optimal nutrient intakes simply from eating the food that is available today. And the situation becomes even more difficult for people who are also taking medications that are depleting nutrients from their bodies, or who have a specific disease or condition that may demand more nutrients. (For specific medications, see Appendix 3: "Prescription and Nonprescription Nutrient Depletions" on page 512.) And finally, nutrient needs also increase with the demands placed on our bodies from a toxic environment—a point that many health and nutrition experts fail to include when considering human nutrition needs.

Now, thanks to modern science, we can make up for some of the nutrients not obtained in the diet with multivitamin and mineral supplements. In addition, other nutraceuticals and herbal compounds are available that can help correct a multitude of health problems and can have a profound effect on disease management, performance enhancement, and longevity. But while these nutraceuticals represent a stride toward health, it is indeed sad that we have lost our ability to be well and happy just from the foods we eat.

The Effect of Modern Conveniences on Health

Along with decreased nutritional intake, another huge factor is making us the obese nation that we are: decreased activity levels. Going back again to preindustrial times, men and women worked very hard to keep food on their tables and to do household chores. Walking was the primary mode of transportation. In addition to a whole-foods existence, people worked much harder and engaged more often in physical activity. A good example of this was demonstrated in the Public Broadcasting Service (PBS) series "Frontier House." In this "reality" series, people were chosen to live as settlers did on the frontier in the 1800s. It was not long before the participants realized that more calories were getting burned in a day than they could possibly take in! One settler swore that he was becoming malnourished because of the weight loss he was experiencing. When the army physician examined the modern-day settler, all that was found was that he was dehydrated; he wasn't keeping up with the fluid demands that his body needed. In addition, the army physician stated the man had become a "lean, mean fighting machine."

Today, with modern conveniences such as cars, household appliances, and an abundance of desk jobs, one can get through a day and exert little physical effort doing it. Also, television has contributed to much of our free time being inactive. During the second half of the twentieth century, Americans began developing cardiovascular disease, diabetes, and cancer in epidemic proportions. Hypertension, high cholesterol, and obesity are becoming the norm rather than the exception. Dietary changes along with increasingly sedentary lifestyles are attributed to the declining health of the population. Between 1946 and 1967, the rate of heart disease increased so dramatically that the World Health Organization (WHO) called it the world's most serious epidemic.

In 1948, a thirty-year study began in Framingham, Massachusetts, known as the Framingham Study. It was designed to study predictors of heart disease by following 5,127 people, aged thirty to sixty-two, who had no signs of existing heart disease. Every two years, subjects were given complete physical exams. The outcome of the study was a compilation of risk factors for the development of heart disease. These risk factors were identified as age, blood levels of high-density lipoprotein (HDL) cholesterol, blood pressure, cigarette smoking, and diabetes mellitus. Obesity was later identified as an independent risk factor for the development of diabetes and heart disease, stroke, reduced life expectancy, and increased cost of lifetime medical care. Obesity and diabetes are fast becoming our number-one health problem. In addition, we now have the added disruptors of cellular metabolism from our environment to compound these health problems.

WHAT WE ARE GETTING TOO MUCH OF

The effects of modern-day nutrition on our metabolism and health can be discussed by breaking it down into two categories: first, we must consider what foods we may be getting too much of in our diet, and second, we must consider what foods we may not be getting enough of in our diet. In other words, we have our food priorities backward; we don't eat enough of the healthier foods, like fruits and vegetables, and we eat way too much junk, a term for foods that are high in fat and/or sugar and low in vitamins and minerals. People inherently know that a diet that is based on refined, processed foods simply can't be healthy.

The typical American diet is too high in refined sugars and other refined carbohydrates, food additives, preservatives, saturated fats, and trans-fatty acids. In addition, Americans consume excessive amounts of artificial sweeteners, caffeine, alcohol, and salt, all of which are detrimental to health in large quantities. And finally, pesticide residues on foods are a health concern today. All of these modern health- and metabolism-destroying culprits are discussed below.

Sugar, Artificial Sweeteners, and Refined Carbohydrates

The typical American consumes an average of 150 pounds of sugar every year. In fact, approximately 18 percent of the average American's caloric intake comes from sugar. These figures continue to rise annually and show no sign of slowing. This is one of the most disturbing trends in the American diet today.

The overabundance of sugar in the American diet stems from a number of factors. But first and foremost is the consumption of soft drinks. Secondly, the addition of sugar in processed foods contributes greatly to its consumption. Sugar is everywhere. It can be found in surprising places like tomato sauce, mustard, bread, frozen dinners, canned soup, and coffee creamer. Commercial cereals can pack as much as two tablespoons of sugar into one serving. A 12-ounce bottle of soda contains about nine to eleven teaspoons of refined sugar. Just take the time to spoon out ten teaspoons of sugar onto a plate. Look at it and think about what you're doing with every soda that you drink.

A diet high in sugar has a number of adverse effects on health. Probably of greatest concern is its effect on blood-sugar regulation. Foods cause different insulin responses based on the carbohydrate, fiber, and protein content. The degree of insulin response to a given food is known as the glycemic index. A diet high in sugar stimulates the pancreas to release insulin. Insulin delivers glucose (sugar) to the cells to use as fuel. Sometimes when insulin is released in large quantities, as after eating a food high in sugar, instead of just bringing blood sugar levels back to normal, the blood sugar will drop to below normal levels (hypoglycemia). The hypoglycemic state signals the brain to seek out more food. Many times a person experiencing low blood sugar will resort to eating more high-sugar foods or drinks to quickly get the blood glucose back up to a comfortable level. This cycle can create a sugar "addiction" of sorts and may be one reason sugar intake is so high.

The effect of refined carbohydrates is similar to the effect of plain sugar. Carbohydrates stripped of fiber and nutrients are quickly converted to glucose, resulting in high blood sugar and a release of insulin from the pancreas.

When blood sugar drops in a hypoglycemic reaction, the most common physical symptoms are weakness, shakiness, sweating, and light-headedness. The cycle of high and low blood sugar swings is uncomfortable enough, but other immediately felt effects of low blood sugar are headaches, mood swings, irritability, and lethargy. However, it is the unfelt long-term effects that are of the most concern.

Repeated spikes in blood sugar force the pancreas to overwork. When insulin levels are elevated, the body is in an anabolic state, which means the body is making deposits into cells and building or gaining weight. If a person is exercising a lot or weight training, he or she will burn the calories and gain muscle. However, elevated insulin in a sedentary person means the calories will likely be stored as fat. Another unfelt effect is from the excess workload on the pancreas. The pancreas is an endocrine gland that can simply "wear out" with overuse. This may be one reason why people with hypoglycemia are at an increased risk of becoming diabetic.

Additionally, with weight gain that can result from excess sugar intake, the body's cells can get to a point where they no longer recognize insulin, resulting in insulin resistance. As you have read, insulin resistance leads to impaired glucose delivery to the cells, chronically elevated blood sugar, and can result in diabetes. Insulin resistance is one way sugar can contribute to obesity as chronically high insulin levels cause weight gain.

There are other negative effects of excessive dietary sugar intake. When blood sugar levels remain too high for too long, the body can convert the sugar to fatty acids; this increases blood lipids and can enhance platelet aggregation and encourage atherosclerosis. Excess sugar also causes excretion of vitamins, minerals, and other nutrients, including calcium, chromium, magnesium, zinc, and copper. And any food that causes us to lose nutrients rather than gain them is a problem.

In the case of calcium, this reduction in calcium stimulates the secretion of parathyroid hormone. Parathyroid hormone reestablishes blood calcium levels by drawing from calcium reserves in the bones. Thus, excess sugar can contribute to bone loss and osteoporosis.

Sugar-laden foods that are dense with calories but low in fiber and vitamins and minerals make it easy to eat 1,000 or more calories in one sitting without feeling full. This is another way sugar contributes to obesity. And often, the high-sugar foods are displacing other more nutrient-dense foods. So not only are the high-sugar foods causing excretion of nutrients, they are displacing foods with higher nutrient content.

Another negative effect of sugar is that it weakens the immune system by interfering with the ability of white blood cells to scavenge and destroy bacteria. This means our bodies will have a harder time fighting off infections. Also, sugar can lead to increased oxidative stress by increasing free-radical production in the body. One study reported in the *American Journal of Clinical Nutrition* found that high-glycemic diets significantly increased production of C-reactive protein, a substance known to cause atherosclerosis and to increase risk of stroke and certain cancers.

Although it may be difficult, many Americans need to severely restrict the amount of refined sugar they consume. And like any other addiction, the more difficult the habit is to break, the more it probably needs to be done.

Some people find that allowing themselves occasional sugary "treats" leaves them wanting more. Such people may be better off eliminating sweets entirely. I have always felt that reasonable intake of sweets is not a problem *once your chemistry is in check*. But that is a big caveat. Epidemic numbers of Americans are becoming obese and diabetic. Metabolic syndrome, of which the primary symptom is elevated blood sugar, is also drastically increasing. Most of us need to cut down on sweets! This is especially important for those of you who have already been diagnosed with metabolic syndrome, insulin resistance, or diabetes.

When blood sugar levels are above normal, the effects of consuming sugar are especially harmful. A 2002 study on the effects of glucose load were reported in *Diabetes Care*. In this study, people with type 2 diabetes were given a 75 gram load of glucose. The isoprostane levels in their blood were then measured. Isoprostane is an inflammatory prostaglandin that can cause free-radical damage in cell membranes. An elevation in isoprostanes indicates a direct link to oxidative stress (free-radical damage) to membrane phospholipids. What the researchers found was startling: The level of isoprostanes significantly increased within just ninety minutes. Although this study was conducted in diabetics, there is no reason to believe that the results would be any different in people with insulin resistance or metabolic syndrome.

Another harmful effect of high blood sugar levels is *glycation*. Glycation is the metabolic process of adding a sugar molecule to fat or protein. Glycation can damage enzymes and proteins in the body leading to the formation of advanced glycation end products (AGEs). Researchers feel that AGEs may actually be more damaging to the body on a cellular level than oxidation. Both are thought to be principle factors in accelerated aging and contributors to the onset of disease.

The bottom line is that if you are insulin resistant or have type 2 diabetes, every time you load up on glucose or simple sugars (cakes, pies, sodas, and other highly refined carbohydrate foods), you are slowly destroying your cell membranes and generating tremendous free-radical damage inside your body.

For those who have broken the cycle of insulin resistance and have balanced their body chemistries, eating a small amount of something sweet no more than once or twice a week is acceptable. This approximates to a few bites of very sweet foods such as cakes or candies per week, and a 4-ounce soft drink once or twice a week. Also, read labels of processed foods to ensure you are not getting more sugar than desired. When checking food labels for sugars, look for other sources of sugar, such as corn syrup, high fructose corn syrup, dextrose, sucrose, glucose, and maltose.

Although artificial sweeteners are low in calories or are calorie-free, many health advocates consider it best to use them in extreme moderation or to avoid them completely. Analysis of aspartame studies conducted in the mid-1990s revealed that nearly all independent third-party research showed harmful effects from aspartame, while industry-sponsored research showed no negative effects. However, many people have reported adverse reactions to aspartame, such as headaches, gastrointestinal upset, heart palpitations, and joint and muscular pain.

Other artificial sweeteners such as sucralose and acesulfame K are wrought with similar problems. Not enough research has been done on these sweeteners, and some of the research that has been done is questionable. Saccharin has been proven to cause cancer in animals when consumed in huge amounts, but in modest consumption is safe. The low-calorie sugar alcohols sorbitol, maltitol, xylitol, and mannitol can cause intestinal disturbances, such as cramping, gas, and diarrhea in some people.

Contrary to popular perception, artificial sweeteners do not help people to lose weight. One theory to explain why people have not lost weight with the use of artificial sweeteners is that by eating products that contain these sweeteners, people get a false sense that they are reducing their overall calorie intake when, in reality, they are not. Another theory is that artificial sweeteners, which are hundreds of times sweeter tasting than sugar, perpetuate our sweet tooth rather than taming it.

Many of my patients report that they experience bouts of low blood sugar after drinking diet soft drinks, especially those containing aspartame. Although technically there should be no rise in blood sugar to stimulate an insulin response since there are no carbohydrates in diet soft drinks, it is theorized that their sweet taste may trick the brain into responding as if carbohydrates had been consumed, thereby triggering an insulin response. Although this has yet to be proven, if diet soft drinks do induce an insulin response in some people, then they are no better to consume than regular soft drinks. Nevertheless, due to the amount of artificial sweeteners in diet soft drinks, I recommend avoiding them all together. If one of my patients is accustomed to drinking numerous cans of diet soft drinks daily, I recommend cutting it down to one or two daily, and then eventually recommend eliminating even those, other than on occasion.

If you are going to use any artificial sweeteners or sugar alcohols, do so in moderation. Good alternatives to refined sugar and artificial sweeteners are honey, molasses, rice syrup, barley malt, fruit juices, and maple syrup. However, even these alternatives should be used sparingly, as they feed the taste for sweets and elevate blood glucose.

Harmful Fats

The body needs some fat. The problem is that most Americans eat excessive amounts of the wrong types of fat. An excess intake of fats—saturated, hydrogenated, and trans-fatty acids—is a major contributing factor to the development of obesity and cardiovascular disease, among many other disorders. To understand how fat affects your health, it is necessary to briefly explain the different types of fats. The type of fats you eat or don't eat can affect everything from pain management and arthritis to memory and depression.

Fats are the structural components of cell walls and hormones. They provide insulation for the body, store energy, and supply the precursors for important regulatory molecules called *prostaglandins*. Fats are part of a class of nutrients known as *lipids*. Like carbohydrates and protein, lipids contain carbon, hydrogen, and oxygen, but they are attached to a glycerol backbone.

Lipids that are transported through the circulatory system encased in a protein coat are referred to as *lipoproteins*. The amount and density of lipoproteins in the blood are considered important determinants of health. High-density lipoproteins (HDL) are dense because of their high protein content relative to cholesterol. Low-density lipoproteins (LDL) contain less protein and more cholesterol. Very low-density lipoproteins (VLDL) are extremely low in protein, and high in triglycerides, the most common form of dietary fat. The lower the density, the more fat contained within the lipoprotein, and the more damaging it is to the cardiovascular system. These lipoproteins contribute to fatty deposits and plaque formation in the arteries.

Triglycerides are created when three fatty-acid chains attach to a glycerol molecule. While all glycerol molecules are the same, fatty-acid chains vary in their length and degree of saturation. Some fatty-acid chains contain just two carbon atoms, while others contain as many as eighteen.

The "degree of saturation" refers to the number of carbon atoms in a chain that have bonded with hydrogen. A *saturated fatty acid* is one in which all the carbon atoms are bonded with hydrogen. Long chain, saturated fatty acids are considered the most detrimental to cardiovascular health. Too much saturated fat in the diet can significantly raise blood cholesterol levels and therefore, the levels of LDL, or harmful cholesterol. Saturated fats are found primarily in animal products, including high-fat meats such as beef, ham, lamb, and pork, and in dairy products, such as whole milk, cream, and cheese.

An *unsaturated fatty acid* describes a chain in which at least one carbon atom is free of hydrogen (monounsaturated). Monounsaturated fatty acids are most abundant in canola, olive, and peanut oils. These fats tend to lower LDL cholesterol while having no effect on HDL, or good cholesterol, levels.

If more than one carbon is unsaturated, it is called a *polyunsaturated fatty acid.* Polyunsaturated fatty acids are found mostly in corn, safflower, soybean, and sunflower oils, and in some fish oils. These fats, unlike saturated fats, actually lower levels of both LDL and HDL cholesterol. For this reason, these fats can be eaten, but in moderation.

The carbon atoms that do not bond with hydrogen form double bonds with other carbons in the fatty-acid chain. The location of these double bonds distinguishes one fatty acid from another. For example, the unsaturated fatty acid linoleic acid is double-bonded at the sixth carbon, making it an omega-6 fatty acid, an essential fatty acid.

Essential fatty acids (EFAs) are unsaturated fatty acids that the body is unable to synthesize and must, therefore, be supplied through the diet. Every living cell needs EFAs. The two most important are *linoleic acid* (an omega-6 fatty acid) and *alpha-linolenic acid* (an omega-3 fatty acid). Omega-6 fatty acids are found primarily in raw nuts, seeds, and legumes, and in many vegetable oils, including corn and safflower oil. Omega-3 fatty acids are found in fish, fish oil, and certain vegetable oils.

The body uses EFAs for rebuilding and producing new cells, and for the production of *eicosanoids,* which regulate a number of bodily functions. Subsets of eicosanoids, known as *prostaglandins* and *thromboxanes,* have a profound influence over the immune response, inflammation, clot formation, blood lipid concentrations, and response to injury.

The importance of the *eicosanoids* is, sadly, one of the least noted and least understood aspects of health. EFA deficiency disrupts the important balance of eicosanoids and their health-protective benefits. Furthermore, certain dietary, environmental, and lifestyle influences can alter the conversion of EFAs to health-promoting eicosanoids. (To help you further understand the role of prostaglandins, see the inset "How Balanced EFAs Make Us Healthier"" on page 286.)

Hydrogenated oils were developed partially in response to the recommendation to avoid saturated fats. These supposedly "healthy" and convenient alternatives to lard and butter were created from polyunsaturated oils. The process of hydrogenation involves artificially saturating the carbon molecules of a fatty-acid chain with hydrogen. This is done under extremely high heat and pressure, with the aid of a metal catalyst such as copper, nickel, or platinum.

The degree of hydrogenation determines the solidity of the oil. If a fat is hydrogenated, it is completely solid at room temperature. *Partially hydrogenated oils* are semisolid at room temperature. This makes partially hydrogenated products such as margarine easy to work with. Hydrogenation also retards spoilage, and hydrogenated oils can be heated to high temperatures without becoming rancid like unsaturated oils. But all this convenience comes at a high price to our health.

During the chemical process of hydrogenation, chemically unstable molecules called *trans-fatty* acids are produced. Trans-fatty acids are altered forms of essential

How Balanced EFAs Make Us Healthier

Prostaglandins are hormones, distinct from the type of hormones secreted by endocrine glands. Prostaglandins are manufactured, secreted, and used at the cellular level. The body uses them instantaneously. More than thirty different prostaglandins have been identified and classified into three categories. Prostaglandins that have general health-promoting activities are classified as prostaglandin E-1 (PGE-1) and prostaglandin E-3 (PGE-3). Prostaglandins that are considered detrimental to health if overproduced are prostaglandin E-2 (PGE-2),

PGE-1 and PGE-3 strengthen the immune system, prevent platelets from becoming sticky (and therefore prevent clots, strokes, and heart attacks), dilate arteries, and fight inflammation. PGE-2 can increase inflammatory substances known as eicosanoids and free-radical activity. They also promote constriction of the blood vessels and clotting of the blood. This is good if your blood pressure has fallen, but very detrimental of you have high blood pressure. In reality, all prostaglandins serve a purpose and are not exclusively "healthy" or "unhealthy." The health effects of prostaglandins are found in their over- or underproduction, which is determined by several factors in the diet. An overabundance of PGE-2 will override the healthy benefits of PGE-1 and PGE-3.

Dietary intake of fats and oils is the single most influential factor in the healthy balance of prostaglandin production. Overproduction of PGE-2 and other inflammatory substances is primarily caused by the overconsumption of two types of fatty acids: arachidonic acid and linoleic acid. Arachidonic acid is abundant in animal proteins, especially red meat, and linoleic acid, an omega-6 fat, is the primary fatty acid in corn oil, sunflower oil, and safflower oil. Linoleic acid can be converted both to PGE-1, a health-promoting prostaglandin, as well as to arachidonic acid, which then forms PGE-2, a pro-inflammatory prostaglandin. To limit your intake of arachidonic acid, eat lean meats such as fish, chicken, and turkey and make sure to have very lean cuts of beef and pork.

PGE-3 is derived from substances in omega-3 fats called EPA (eicosapentaenoic acid) and DHA (docosahexaenoic acid), which are found primarily in fish oils. A diet excessively high in saturated, hydrogenated, or trans-fatty acids will divert the synthesis of EFAs from production of healthy prostaglandins to unhealthy prostaglandins. EFA deficiency, especially a lack of omega-3 fatty acids, fails to supply the ingredients needed to form healthy prostaglandins. A diet that is lacking in certain vitamins and minerals will also slow the synthesis of PGE-1 and PGE-3. Omega-3 fatty acids are also needed for healthy brain and nerve cell development, for healthy cell membranes, and to positively affect the genetic expression of certain proteins that can control cancer cell development.

The conversion of dietary omega-6 EFAs to healthy prostaglandins is regulated by two important enzymes: delta-6 and delta-5 desaturase. Delta-6 desaturase converts linoleic acid to the metabolically active gamma-linolenic acid, which can then be converted to either PGE-1 or PGE-2. It also converts alpha-linolenic acid (an omega-3 fat) to EPA. In general, allowing delta-6 desaturase activity and inhibiting delta-5 desaturase activity is what will lead to a more favorable balance of prostaglandin production.

Delta-6 desaturase is inhibited by several conditions. One is age. The body's ability to convert EFAs to prostaglandins diminishes after age thirty. Obviously, we can't stop time, but delta-6 desaturase can also be inhibited by diet—a factor we can control. Anything that elevates blood sugar such as a diet high in refined carbohydrates slows delta-6-desaturase activity and decreases production of healthy prostaglandins. A diet high in trans-fatty acids from hydrogenated oils, as well as stress, alcohol consumption, or a genetic weakness of the enzyme, will inhibit the activity of delta-6-desaturase.

In the presence of delta-5 desaturase, gamma-linolenic acid can become arachidonic acid, which is ultimately converted to inflammatory prostaglandins. This enzyme is actually the gatekeeper of the critical balance in prostaglandin synthesis and is an enzyme you generally want to control. Elevated insulin levels increase delta-5 desaturase activity, which is an unfavorable condition. Controlling blood sugar levels is an important factor in slowing delta-5 desaturase. The other way to inhibit delta-5 desaturase is by making sure there is enough eicosapentaenoic acid (EPA) in the diet. EPA is an important inhibitor of delta-5 desaturase and is found in cold-water fish oils.

If the body has insufficient delta-6 desaturase activity, it will not adequately produce PGE-1 and PGE-3, which strengthen the immune system and fight inflammation. (There is one caveat: omega-6 fatty acids can also be converted to PGE-2. It is important not to overconsume omega-6s but to find the healthy balance between omega-6s and omega-3s. Overactive delta-5 desaturase will increase PGE-2s.)

So, to encourage production of PGE-1 and PGE-3s and discourage production of PGE-2s, limit your intake of saturated fat, trans-fatty acids, and arachidonic acid; control your blood sugar levels; and consume healthy omega-3 fatty acids, especially fish oils. Adequate vitamin and mineral intake is also important.

fatty acids that are actually more damaging to health than saturated fats. For one, trans-fatty acids block an important enzyme that is responsible for the conversion of linoleic acid to its metabolically active form, gamma-linolenic acid (GLA), which interferes with the synthesis of prostaglandins.

Trans-fatty acids are nutritionally inert, replacing potential sources of essential fatty acids with fatty acids that do not function properly in the body. They have been associated with serious health problems, including cardiovascular disease and cancer. The Harvard School of Public Health estimates that 30,000 premature deaths per year in the United States are attributable to the consumption of trans-fatty acids. The

National Academy of Sciences (NAS) is currently reviewing trans-fatty acid research to determine a safe limit of intake. The research thus far shows negative effects in even small amounts. These findings have led to an initiative sponsored by the FDA requiring food manufacturers to declare trans-fatty acid content on food labels by the year 2006.

It is thought that trans-fatty acids contribute to cardiovascular disease in a number of ways. Although hydrogenated oils may not contain cholesterol, they do influence cholesterol production. Until recently, it was believed that eating foods that contain cholesterol was one of the main contributors to increased blood cholesterol levels, which is a risk factor for cardiovascular disease. Now it is known that trans-fats and other dietary habits may be influencing cholesterol levels as much or more than eating foods high in cholesterol.

While saturated fats increase LDL ("bad") cholesterol, they also increase HDL ("good") cholesterol. Trans-fatty acids raise LDL cholesterol *and* decrease HDL cholesterol. One way trans-fatty acids increase cholesterol is by blocking the synthesis of healthy *prostaglandins*. Healthy prostaglandins (PGE-1 and PGE-3) help control the production of cholesterol in the liver. Without them, cholesterol synthesis is increased. (Ironically, margarine—a common source of hydrogenated oil—which many people use to help control cholesterol in the diet, can actually *increase* cholesterol depending on the trans-fatty acid content.)

Secondly, because trans-fatty acids block the synthesis of healthy prostaglandins, unhealthy prostaglandins (PGE-2) are left to exert their cardiovascular-damaging effects. And finally, trans-fatty acids are highly unstable molecules that generate a lot of free radicals in the body. Free radicals and free-radical damage to tissues (oxidation) contribute to atherosclerosis, ischemia (decreased blood flow), premature aging, cancer, and inflammatory and degenerative diseases. (Polyunsaturated fats and oils that become rancid from exposure to high heat or damaged by exposure to light and air also promote the generation of free radicals—another reason why they should be consumed in moderation.)

Foods highest in trans-fatty acids are foods that are made with, or are fried in, hydrogenated or partially hydrogenated oils. Fast foods or any fried restaurant foods are typically loaded with trans-fatty acids because the oils used in frying machines are usually partially hydrogenated oils. This includes any deep-fried foods such as French fries, hash brown potatoes, fish or chicken patties or nuggets, doughnuts, as well as deep-fried dessert items like apple or cherry pies. Snack chips are a primary source of trans-fatty acids, although some manufacturers are no longer using hydrogenated oils—be sure to read labels. Commercially prepared crackers and baked goods such as cookies and snack cakes are also loaded with partially hydrogenated oils and therefore with trans-fatty acids.

No limit for trans-fatty acid intake has been established, but some experts suggest the daily intake should not exceed 5 percent of total daily calories. On an 1,800-

calorie diet, for example, the intake of trans-fatty acids should be less than 10 grams a day. It is estimated that 25 to 45 percent of the fat in foods containing hydrogenated or partially hydrogenated can be trans-fatty acids. This is why it is wise to avoid hydrogenated or partially hydrogenated oils all together.

When you consider the trans-fatty acid content in one Danish pastry (3 g), one doughnut (13 g), one 4-ounce order of French fries (4–8 g), one tablespoon of margarine (2 g), six crackers (approximately 1 g), 1 ounce of corn chips (1.4 g), and one deep-fried fish filet (8 g), you can see how one fast-food meal, or a meal made up of highly processed foods, could easily exceed the 10-gram daily limit.

Pesticides

Pesticides, by nature, are killers. They are compounds designed to destroy living, organic substances. (That fact alone should raise some concern about the safety of their residue in the food supply.) Pesticides are difficult to identify because they are invisible and tasteless, and do not appear on food labels. The food and agricultural industries use more than 3,000 different chemicals for the growth, appearance, and preservation of food. In the 1980s, an NAS study found that 78 percent of the most widely used commercial chemicals had not undergone "minimal toxicity testing."

To date, the Environmental Protection Agency (EPA) has identified sixty-six different carcinogenic pesticides, and has restricted the use of none. The EPA has an established criteria of "acceptable cancer risk," which serves as a benchmark for the allowance of pesticide use. However, it may not be so cut and dried. In 1997, the EPA identified the pesticides thought to pose the greatest health risk to both adults and children, including nerve poisons, carcinogens, and endocrine disrupters. The EPA named *organophosphates* (OPs) and *carbamate* as the insecticides (a type of pesticide used to kill insects) most threatening to public health. Both compounds are known to be toxic to the nervous system.

Although the EPA is developing screening protocols to determine the effects of pesticides on endocrine function, these tests are not currently in place. However, there is no doubt that there is concern regarding the effects these endocrine disrupters will have in the human body. (The role of pesticides as disruptors of the endocrine system by mimicking or antagonizing endocrine hormones is discussed in Chapter 10.) Many pesticides are known endocrine disruptors, and because of the risk of cancer and other health risks from their consumption, it is wise the limit the intake of pesticides whenever possible.

Antibiotics

Meats and dairy products are tainted with antibiotics, growth hormones, and other chemicals. There is a significant correlation between consumption of animal products, and the subsequent ingestion of antibiotics and other chemical residues, and the incidence of certain cancers.

Consider the following facts about the use of antibiotics in animals: Small doses of antibiotics have been used as agents to increase growth and maturity and to prevent infection of animals raised for food. Antibiotics given to these animals causes an increase in antibiotic resistance in humans, a common problem that has many scientists worried about the possibility of creating "super-resistant" bacterium that conventional antibiotics will not destroy. It has been reported that antibiotic-resistant bacteria, which are present in many retail meats, may survive the gastric passage in our bodies and be present in human stools. Once in the gastrointestinal tract, the bacteria may multiply and cause illness. In response to the growing concern about the use of antibiotics in meat, even the McDonald's corporation is considering mandating that their meat suppliers not use antibiotics in their animals.

Hormones

The recent spread of a Western-type, meat-based diet is now associated with breast and prostate cancer throughout the world. It is believed that exposure to and metabolism of estrogens and other hormones in meats may cause the appearance of secondary sex characteristics in girls before age eight (or menstruation before age nine) and in boys before age nine. Further, it may potentially contribute to various gender-related cancers and infertility in both males and females in their later years.

In the United States steroid hormones are used to increase the growth of beef cattle and poultry. Such use has been banned in the European Union. The Union's concern over the health effects of certain growth hormones has also resulted in a ban on the importation of meat from the United States.

Food Additives and Preservatives

A food additive is any substance that a food manufacturer intentionally puts into a food product in order to achieve a specific desired effect during production or processing. While many additives, such as added nutritional supplements (discussed below), are helpful and have no known side effects, others can be harmful. Francis Moore Lappé, author of *Diet for a Small Planet* (Ballantine Books, 1992), gives a comprehensive discussion of the scope of the food-additive problem. She points out that there are 3,000 types of additives currently being used in this country, and that the average American consumes approximately 150 pounds of them a year. Some people have developed chemical sensitivities to certain additives, causing allergies, asthma, and a host of other health problems. Some additives are thought to negatively impact behavior, particularly in small children. Others can cause allergic reactions severe enough to warrant hospitalization. The safety of long-term ingestion of harmful additives is unknown.

Many food additives that have been outlawed in other countries are still widely used in the United States. Many food colorings, for example, have been banned in different European countries. Red No. 40 is banned in Austria, Belgium, Denmark,

France, Germany, Norway, Sweden, and Switzerland, but is still not banned in the United States. Blue Dye No. 1 is also banned in many European countries, but not in our country. Among the food colorings, Yellow #5 (tartrazine) has the strongest association with allergic and behavioral reactions in children. Yellow #5 is presently banned in Norway and Austria.

Processed, packaged, frozen, ready-to-heat and "microwaveable" foods are the most abundant in artificial preservatives, flavoring, and coloring. Emulsifiers, binders, and anticaking agents are added to most processed foods to improve appearance and texture. Some commonly used food additives include nutritional supplements, flavoring and coloring agents, and preservatives.

Nutritional supplements are an example of an obviously helpful food additive. Many foods are fortified with vitamins and minerals primarily to replace nutrients lost during processing and, therefore, to prevent deficiency diseases. Some of the common fortifications include vitamin D in milk, vitamin A in margarine, iron and vitamin B_1 (thiamine) in breads, and iodine in table salt.

Artificial flavoring agents are the most commonly used additives. Some, such as monosodium glutamate (MSG), are used to enhance flavor. MSG can cause severe headaches and nausea, among other problems. Others flavoring agents, such as chemical concentrates of an artificial flavor such as strawberry, are used to boost flavor. Artificial flavorings are often used when a natural flavoring is unavailable or too expensive to use in a particular commercial product. The proliferation of artificial flavoring agents has so saturated our taste buds that many of us can no longer appreciate the natural flavors in fruits and vegetables, especially when flavoring agents are combined with other flavor enhances such as salt and sugar. By cutting down on processed foods that are high in salt, sugar, and/or flavor enhancers, we can once again begin to eat and enjoy healthier foods.

Coloring agents are used to make foods more attractive. Even the color of some fresh fruits, such as oranges, has been enhanced with coloring agents to meet consumers' expectations. Coloring agents are especially prominent in foods targeted for children. Some allergists feel that coloring agents and other additives are problematic for some kids and that they can cause behavioral disturbances (especially ADHD), headaches, and many other symptoms in children. Ben Feingold, M.D., raised awareness on the relationship between food coloring, additives, sugar and highly allergenic foods to ADD/ADHD and other behavioral disturbances in the 1980s. This is such a large problem as evidence by the record number of children diagnosed with ADD/ADHD that in 1999 a group of scientists urged the National Institutes of Health (NIH) to begin allocating dollars for research in this area. They are urging action in this area, because rather than dietary changes being the first course of action, children are being placed on methylphenidate (Ritalin), a drug with very serious side effects.

Preservatives, such as nitrites and sulfites, retard spoilage, preserve flavor and color, and keep oils from turning rancid, thereby greatly extending the safe-use period of many foods. Preservatives protect foods, such as cured meats, from developing dangerous toxins, including botulism (a type of food poisoning). Nitrites are used in cured meats to delay rancidity, inhibit microbial growth, and improve color. Nitrites may combine under certain conditions with protein to form nitrosamines, compounds that have been shown in studies to cause cancer in animals and increase the risk of cancer in humans. When nitrites are used in a product, the USDA requires the manufacturer to also add sodium ascorbate or sodium erythorbate, substances that prevent nitrites from converting to nitrosamines. Fortunately, nitrite-free cured meats are also available. Sulfites are used to preserve color in dried fruits, frozen French fries, and sauerkraut. They can trigger asthmatic attacks in susceptible people.

Genetically Engineered Foods

The technology that has allowed scientists to alter the genetic code of living organisms is relatively new. From a scientific standpoint, it is exciting technology. However, genetically engineered food crops introduces a realm of technology that may have grown too far, too fast.

The purpose of altering the genetic makeup of a food, in theory, is to improve its resistance to disease, decrease its ripening time (so food stays fresher longer), and, in some cases, allow it to withstand stronger herbicides. The process involves introducing strands of DNA from one organism (known as the *gene source*) into the DNA of a particular food (known as the *unmodified organism* or UMO). This process is known as *gene splicing*. Splicing the genetic code for a "desirable" trait, such as resistance to bacteria or fungus, from the gene source changes the trait in the UMO, thereby transforming it into a genetically engineered food.

For a number of reasons, the safety of genetically engineered foods is questionable and has created an enormous debate. The hazards that can be introduced into foods from gene splicing include the increased chance for allergic reactions, the introduction of potential toxins, and the reduction of nutritional quality.

John B. Fagan, Ph.D., is a molecular biologist and biochemist who has devoted his career to genetic research. Since 1994, he has been speaking out about the dangers of genetically engineered foods, the environmental hazards of releasing genetically engineered organisms into the environment, and the risks of germ-line genetic engineering in humans. According to Dr. Fagan, current recombinant DNA methods are capable of introducing unwanted changes in the function and structure of the food-producing organisms. He states that genetically altered food may have characteristics unintended by the genetic engineer, which cannot be foreseen. Currently, safety tests conducted on genetically engineered foods are based on the known health hazards of the gene source and the UMO, not on the final product.

Since a gene is the blueprint for protein, the food produced by the genetically engineered organism will contain new proteins. These proteins can come from viruses, pigs, bacteria, plants, or any other living organism. The new proteins can produce toxins or act as allergens. They may cause changes in the metabolism of the food-producing organism that alters its nutritional content. Altering genetic information can also produce mutations in the organism, resulting in changes in enzymes or protein levels. These changes, according to Dr. Fagan, can render the organism allergenic or toxic.

Supporters of genetically engineered foods state that the risk associated with these foods is minimal. However, there is little scientific evidence to substantiate the long-term safety of consumption by humans. There are currently no laws requiring that genetically engineered food be labeled as such. There are now tomatoes, corn, and potatoes sold in the grocery stores that have been genetically altered. Until legislation is enacted that requires labeling, the only way to assure unaltered food is to buy organically grown products that specifically state "non-genetically modified," (often abbreviated as "non-GMO") or "non-genetically engineered."

Alcohol

According to the National Institute of Alcohol Abuse and Alcoholism, approximately 14 million Americans either abuse alcohol or are alcoholic. Clearly, for many Americans, alcohol qualifies as a substance that we are getting too much of. Aside from its addicting qualities, alcohol has potential negative effects on nutritional status when consumed in excess. Alcohol metabolism creates a need for more vitamin B_3 (niacin) and vitamin B_6 (pyridoxine); it causes the excretion of magnesium, calcium, potassium, and zinc in the urine and a decreased absorption of vitamin B_1 (thiamine) folate, and vitamin B_{12} (cyanocobalamin). It is associated with many problems, including high blood pressure, stroke, birth defects, cirrhosis, and cancer.

There appears to be a heart-protective effect from moderate consumption of all forms of alcohol, including beer, wine, and hard liquor. At one or two drinks a day (equivalent to 12-ounces of beer, 4 to 5 ounces of wine, and 1 ounce of 80-proof alcohol) alcohol lowers the risk of having a heart attack. Alcohol prevents blood clots and increases HDL. Moderate intake is considered one or two drinks per day (no more than five out of seven days per week) for women, and two drinks for men. This is truly a case where moderation is key—more than two drinks a day is associated with an increased risk of cancer, especially in women.

WHAT WE ARE NOT GETTING ENOUGH OF

Americans consume too many hazardous food products and not enough of the nutrients needed to support good health. Processing and refining foods strips them of valuable vitamins and minerals. This is evident in refined flour and rice products, which must be enriched to meet even minimal standards of nutrition. In addition, the decreased intake of healthier foods means Americans are not getting enough fiber and beneficial phytochemicals, among other important nutrients.

Essential Vitamins and Minerals

While many refined foods provide calories, they do not supply essential nutrients. Eating these foods supplants the appetite for nutrient-dense foods, leaving wide gaps in nutrient intake. In one study conducted by the United States Department of Agriculture (USDA), it was reported that most Americans are deficient in one or more essential nutrients. It was found that:

- 80 percent consumed less than the RDA* for vitamin B_6

- 75 percent consumed less than the RDA for magnesium

- 68 percent consumed less than the RDA for calcium

- 50 percent consumed less than the RDA for vitamin A

- 45 percent consumed less than the RDA for vitamin B_1

- 45 percent consumed less than the RDA for vitamin C

- 34 percent consumed less than the RDA for vitamins B_2, B_3, and B_{12}.

* Recommended Daily Allowance

Another study at the Boston University School of Public Health examined dietary intake of men and women from the Framingham Study (1984–1988 Cycle III, Framingham Offspring-Spouse Cohort). The dietary data indicated that 30 to 50 percent of subjects exceeded cholesterol intake objectives (less than 300 milligrams [mg] daily); and 6 to 45 percent exceeded the recommended intake of sodium (less than 3 grams daily). The mean total fat intakes were 38 percent of caloric intake, and more than 90 percent of subjects exceeded recommended daily fat intake. Fewer than 3 percent of subjects met the dietary fiber guidelines.

The National Health and Nutrition Examination Survey II (NHANES II) concluded that 91 percent of Americans do not eat the suggested three daily servings of vegetables and two daily servings of fruits. In the same survey, it was found that 50 percent of Americans consume less than the RDA for vitamins A and C, and the minerals calcium and iron.

Educating yourself about what each nutrient does in the body can be a great motivator for improving your diet. When you understand the role of each nutrient, you will want to make sure you are getting enough of them.

In addition to essential vitamin and minerals, macronutrients are required in large amounts by the body. These include carbohydrates, fats, and protein. An average 1,800-calorie diet contains approximately 250 grams of carbohydrates, 100 grams of protein, and 50 grams of fat. Americans are not consuming enough of whole foods as their source of carbohydrates (whole grains, vegetables, and fruits). In general, we consume plenty of protein, but many of the proteins eaten are poor-quality high-fat meats, such as hot dogs and luncheon meats. As for fats, again Americans consume too many poor-quality harmful fats, such as partially hydrogenated oils, and do not get nearly enough of the healthy omega-3 fats.

Complex Carbohydrates

Although carbohydrates have taken a significant amount of criticism, not all carbohydrates are bad for you—the same way not all fats are bad for you. Carbohydrates are the preferred fuel source for the human body. Carbohydrates are made up of carbon, hydrogen, and oxygen. They are found mostly in foods of plant origin.

Carbohydrates are composed of single sugars (monosaccharides), double sugars (disaccharides), and multiple chains of sugars (polysaccharides). The monosaccharides are glucose, fructose, and galactose. An example of a disaccharide is table sugar (a combination of glucose and fructose). *Complex carbohydrates* and fiber are made up of polysaccharides, chains created by thousands of monosaccharides. Complex carbohydrates are broken down during digestion to form glucose. Cellulose, the polysaccharide abundant in plant foods cannot be broken down. Cellulose passes through the digestive tract undigested, providing bulk and helping to move foods through the intestines. Cellulose is the principle component of fiber.

The best sources of carbohydrates are complex carbohydrates. This is because the break down of complex carbohydrates into simple sugars is slower, allowing a more gradual release of glucose into the blood. This is especially true if the carbohydrate-containing food is also high in fiber. Complex carbohydrates that contain fiber have a number of important health benefits, including a decreased risk of cancer and cardiovascular disease. Vegetables are a wonderful low-calorie, nutrient-rich source of complex carbohydrates. Fruits contain a lot of natural simple sugars, but these sugars are balanced by fiber and water in the fruit; fruits, therefore, can also be consumed in moderation. Two servings of fruit a day is best.

Americans simply take in too many refined simple carbohydrates, such as bread, pasta, and sugar. This is sometimes the most difficult food group to moderate, especially with the effects of stress driving us to crave these foods.

Fiber

For years, we have known about the many health benefits of adequate dietary fiber, and even more benefits are being discovered almost daily. Fiber may be classified as *soluble* or *insoluble.* Soluble fiber dissolves in water. An example of soluble fiber is pectin, a gelatinous substance found in fruit. Pectin stimulates the secretion of pancreatic and intestinal enzymes, and relieves constipation. Soluble fiber binds with bile acids and helps reduce cholesterol.

Insoluble fiber does not dissolve in water. Cellulose and hemicellulose, the roughage portions of plants, are considered insoluble. Insoluble fiber binds with water, creating bulk in the stools. It decreases the transit time of digestible material in the digestive tract and prevents the accumulation of toxins in the small and large intestines. Insoluble fiber decreases the occurrence of constipation, hemorrhoids, and diverticulitis.

While study findings have both confirmed and denied the ability of a high-fiber diet to cut risk of colon cancer, a recent article in the *Lancet* reported on the results from two large studies, which showed that diets containing at least 30 grams of fiber a day reduced the risk of developing colon polyps and colon cancer when compared with low-fiber intakes of approximately 15 grams or less.

Fibers increase the sensation of fullness, helping to reduce appetite. It also helps to regulate blood sugar and insulin response. The higher the fiber content of a food, the more slowly glucose will be released into the blood. A high-fiber diet is also important for the regulation of healthy intestinal flora. Bacteria in the digestive tract use fiber to form some of the B vitamins. The recommended daily fiber intake is a minimum of 25 grams.

Whole-grain cereals and flours, as well as whole grains themselves, are excellent sources of complex carbohydrates and fiber. The fiber content in a slice of whole-grain bread is approximately 2 grams and in one cup of whole-grain cereal is about 5 grams. On average, there is about 2 grams of fiber per cup of vegetable or fruit. Beans, a wonderful source of fiber, average about 5 grams per one-half cup serving.

Using flaxseed meal can increase the daily intake of dietary fiber. I recommend adding 1–2 tablespoons of flaxseed meal to a morning protein drink or on cereal daily.

Quality Proteins

Proteins are compounds formed from carbon, hydrogen, oxygen, and nitrogen. The nitrogen component separates proteins from carbohydrates. Proteins are made up of chains of amino acids. There are twenty amino acids, half of which the body can synthesize. Ten amino acids are considered essential, which means they must be obtained through the diet. The essential amino acids include *arginine* (essential in children), *histidine* (essential in children), *isoleucine, leucine, lysine, methionine, phenylalanine, threonine, tryptophan,* and *valine.*

Muscle, skin, hair, nails, blood cells, enzymes, hormones, neurotransmitters, and antibodies are all made up of protein. In fact, all of the tissues in the body are made up of proteins. Protein is a vital component of life. It needs to be consumed in adequate amounts to maintain health and optimal metabolism.

There is some debate over how much protein is adequate, but most experts agree that between 0.8 and 1.0 grams per kilogram of body weight is a good daily intake of protein. (1 kilogram equals 2.2 pounds.) According to this guideline, a woman who weighs 57 kilograms (approximately 125 pounds) should consume about 45 grams of protein daily. Others recommend calculating protein requirements based on *lean body mass,* making adjustments for levels of activity. Diets high in protein are required during early childhood, pregnancy, and during recovery from injury, surgery, illness, or disease.

Americans generally consume large amounts of protein—as much as two to three times the recommended amount. However, when I perform an amino acid panel on my clients, I generally find that they are low in several important amino acids. While this can be due to an inadequate intake of protein, it can also be caused by poor digestion and/or absorption. Poor digestion and/or absorption can be caused by dysbiosis or as a result of disease states and/or conditions such as high levels of stress. High levels of stress cause an increased utilization of certain amino acids. The balance between protein intake and other vitamins and minerals may also affect protein absorption and utilization. When a person has low levels of amino acids, it is most likely due to a combination of these and other factors, which, of course, may differ from person to person.

Because protein is needed for the maintenance of almost every cell in the body, it is extremely important to ensure adequate intakes and proper utilization of the amino acids. Working to improve the overall quality of your diet by increasing fiber intake, phytochemical intake, balancing gut terrain (see Chapter 11), and controlling stress will ensure better utilization of proteins by the body.

One of the important roles of protein with regard to metabolic syndrome is its role in controlling glycemic response. Eating high-protein foods with carbohydrates will help slow the release of glucose into the bloodstream. Any high-protein food will perform this function; however, it is still important to consider the quality of your protein.

Some foods that are highest in saturated fats are animal proteins, one of the best sources of protein for humans. However, foods high in saturated fat are known to increase arachidonic acid levels and thereby increase inflammatory processes in the body associated with the development of cardiovascular disease, cancer, and autoimmune diseases, among others. Also, as you've learned, beef and poultry are raised with antibiotics and growth hormones or are fed pesticide-laden feed. Some meats are also processed and treated with chemicals such as nitrates (for example, luncheon meats and hot dogs).

To avoid the possible metabolic interferences of hormone- and pesticide-containing meats, I recommend free-range poultry, antibiotic- and hormone-free beef, free-range chicken eggs, and buffalo meat. Not only is meat from animals that were allowed to grass feed or feed on a free-range hormone and antibiotic free, but they are also lower in saturated fat and higher in omega-3 fats than their unhealthy counterparts. Eggs are a highly biologically available protein source. Eggs that come from free-range chickens contain twenty times more omega-3 fats than typical eggs. Although fish is a wonderful source of protein and healthy fats, care must be taken to eat it no more often than one to two times per week due to contamination from polluted waters.

Strict vegetarians, known as vegans, do not eat any animal protein or animal products, and must therefore get their protein from plant sources. Studies suggest that all types of vegetarian diets—even those that include eggs, dairy, or fish—lead to lower risks of many diseases, including heart disease, cancer, and high blood pressure. Beans, legumes, and grains are often used as vegetarian sources of protein; however, plant proteins typically lack one or more essential amino acids. Fortunately, these can be provided by complementary plant proteins. For example, beans lack the essential amino acid *methionine* and rice lacks *lysine.* If eaten together, the beans provide the lysine, the rice provides methionine, and thus a *complete protein* is obtained.

Soy is a plant source of protein that is a complete protein and has many health benefits; however, some people have allergies to soy; so care must be taken to screen for any possible allergies.

In addition to eating high-quality protein, I strongly support the use of predigested protein meal replacements. These are proteins that are already broken down into smaller units of amino acids or peptides, making them easier to absorb and utilize in the body. Whey protein, rice protein, split-pea protein, and egg white protein are forms of predigested protein. Predigested protein is a great way to insure intake of all amino acids.

Healthy Fats

Although Americans get an overabundance of unhealthy saturated, hydrogenated, and trans-fatty acids, our diets are lacking in the right kinds of fats. *Essential fatty acids* (EFAs) have many important disease-controlling roles in the body. Our bodies could not function without fat. As you've learned, fats are the structural components of cell walls and hormones, provide insulation for the body, store energy, and supply the precursors for important regulatory molecules called prostaglandins. (See the inset "How Balanced EFAs Make Us Healthier" on page 286.)

EFAs are unsaturated fatty acids that the body is unable to synthesize and therefore must be obtained from the diet. There are eight essential fatty acids. The two most important are *linoleic acid* (an omega-6 fatty acid) and *alpha-linolenic acid* (an omega-3 fatty acid). Americans get an overabundance of omega-6 fatty acids in their diet from poor sources, such as margarine, salad dressing, chips, crackers, and ready-made baked goods. Care should be taken to limit your intake of omega-6 fatty acids and to get them from quality sources. Avoid or severely limit your intake of margarine, packaged foods containing partially hydrogenated or hydrogenated oils, and fried food. Limit saturated fats from meat.

Table 12.1 on page 299 lists the best food sources of omega-3 and omega-6 fatty acids.

While total fat intake should be limited to 20 to 30 percent of daily caloric intake, the emphasis should be on selecting fats that provide EFAs. Cold pressed oils,

Table 12.1. Sources of Omega-3 and Omega-6 Essential Fatty Acids

OMEGA-3 FATTY ACIDS		OMEGA-6 FATTY ACIDS	
Cod liver oil	Salmon	Borage oil	Peanut oil
Egg	Sardines	Canola oil	Pork
Flax oil	Trout	Chicken	Safflower oil
Haddock	Tuna	Egg	Sesame oil
Leafy green vegetables	Wild game	Evening primrose oil	Turkey
Mackerel			

including olive and safflower oils, are recommended for cooking. Sesame, walnut, flaxseed, and avocado oil should not be heated, but can be used for flavoring and salad dressings. Lean meat, poultry, fish (see the inset "Safe Sources of Fish and Fish Oil" below), and game provide EFAs. Butter and ghee (clarified butter) in moderation are also quality sources of fat.

Phytochemicals

Phytochemicals are active chemicals in plant foods. Because the chemical compounds are neither vitamins nor minerals, phytochemicals have a unique classifica-

Safe Sources of Fish and Fish Oil

Fish is one of the best sources omega-3 fats because it is high in EPA and DHA. Although ocean fish can be contaminated by mercury, which is toxic to humans, studies still support the cardioprotective benefit from eating fish. The fish with the highest levels of mercury are swordfish, king mackerel, tilefish, and shark, and should therefore be avoided. Current EPA guidelines recommend eating no more than one or two servings of fish per week. Pregnant women and children should eat even less. Check the EPA website and local extension agents for updates on warnings for fish consumption. All fish have some level of mercury, even farm-raised salmon. Many people have turned to farm-raised fish under the assumption that their contamination levels are lower. While their mercury levels may be lower, they contain high levels of PCBs, cancer-causing chemicals from hydraulic fluids, oils, and electrical transformers. Moreover, farm-raised fish are not high in omega-3 fats, which is the primary reason for eating them. Instead, farm-raised fish are high in omega-6 fats due to their diet of cornmeal. For all of these reasons, eat only wild fish occasionally and take purified fish-oil supplements to ensure adequate omega-3 intake. Make sure these supplements are purified of mercury and other pollutants. Smaller fish such as anchovies and sardines pose less risk of contamination.

tion. These naturally occurring substances have protective, disease-preventing properties from which many pharmaceutical drugs are derived.

Bioflavonoids are a class of phytochemicals found in citrus fruits, garlic, onions, and in all other vegetables. Bioflavonoids are potent antioxidants (substances that neutralize free radicals). The many known health benefits of bioflavonoids' include strengthening blood vessel walls, inhibiting LDL oxidation, and immune enhancement.

Other phytochemicals found in fruits and vegetables known to have protective benefits include the following:

- *Indoles* and *dithiolthiones,* found in broccoli, cabbage, cauliflower, and other members of the cruciferous family—activate cancer-fighting liver enzymes.

- *allicin,* found in garlic, onions, scallions, and other members of the allium family—can reduce the risk of blood clots and lower cholesterol.

- *curcumin,* found in the spice turmeric—exhibits very potent antioxidant, anti-inflammatory, and anticancer activity.

- *lycopene,* found in tomatoes—protects against prostate cancer.

- *lutein,* found in dark-green leafy vegetables—protects against the oxidation in the eyes that can lead to macular degeneration (a common cause of blindness in older people).

- *genistein,* found primarily in soybeans—belongs to a class of phytochemicals called *isoflavones,* which reduce cholesterol and fight cancer cells.

- *anthocyanidins,* abundant in wine and grape juice—strong antioxidants that fight cancer and cardiovascular disease.

Virtually every day, researchers discover even more health benefits of the various phytochemicals. One 2003 study reported in *The American Society for Nutritional Sciences Journal of Nutrition* found that women with the highest phytochemical intakes had the lowest risk of developing ovarian cancer.

If you are like the average American, your intake of fruits and vegetables is very low (less than five servings per day), and consequently so is your intake of phytochemicals. The best way to increase your intake of phytochemicals is to eat at least two servings of fresh fruits and five servings of vegetables daily, to use spices such as turmeric, rosemary, and oregano in your cooking, and to drink black and green teas.

HOW FOOD BECOMES ENERGY

Carbohydrates are the main source of energy used to fuel the body. When carbohydrates enter the digestive system, complex sugar molecules are broken down into single sugar molecules such as sucrose (table sugar), fructose (fruit sugar), and lactose (milk sugar), and are converted into glucose and absorbed into the bloodstream. Digestive enzymes perform this function in the small intestine before the monosaccharides are absorbed into the capillaries.

From there, the circulating glucose is transported by insulin to cells with insulin receptors. Some cells, like the neurons in the brain, absorb glucose directly from the bloodstream without the help of insulin. Skeletal muscle cells and adipose (fat) cells are the most receptive to the insulin-glucose compounds. Once inside the cell, glucose enters metabolic pathways, where it is broken down further.

The process of splitting glucose into smaller compounds is called *glycolysis.* During glycolysis, the 6-carbon glucose molecule undergoes a series of chemical changes that uses enzymes, coenzymes, and oxygen to eventually convert the glucose into energy. Carbon dioxide is formed as waste product by way of this process. The series of chemical reactions in cellular metabolism are known as the *citric acid cycle.* The citric acid cycle provides the fuel (energy) for most cellular activities.

Glucose can be broken down into 3-carbon molecules, which can either enter the citric acid cycle or go back and be made into glucose, when needed. Glycerol, a breakdown product from fat, can also be used in this metabolic pathway known as *glucogenesis.*

Fatty acids (another breakdown product of fat metabolism) and a few amino acids (the products of protein metabolism) are 2-carbon molecules. Two-carbon molecules cannot be converted into glucose for cellular energy. This is why fat is a poor source of quick energy. Only about 5 percent of fat can be used to form glucose.

Fat enters the digestive system and, like glucose, is broken down into smaller compounds by enzymes from the pancreas and small intestine. The breakdown of a triglyceride produces one glycerol and three fatty acid molecules. The glycerol, a 3-carbon molecule, can be used to make glucose. The fatty acid molecules cannot. Instead, the fatty-acid chain enters the citric acid cycle at a later point, helping to fuel cellular activity. When fat is consumed in excess of energy demands, the extra fatty acid molecules are transported to the liver where cholesterol is formed and fat is reformed to be stored in fat cells.

Proteins are broken down into separate amino acids during digestion. Essential amino acids are derived from food, and the body can produce the rest if it is not under any extra metabolic demands. The amino acids are used to synthesize the structural proteins, enzymes, and hormones needed by the body. The amino acids that are not used to make other proteins are used for cellular energy. In the absence of adequate glucose from carbohydrates, amino acids can be converted to glucose and fat.

When amino acids enter the citric acid cycle, they lose nitrogen (termed *deamination*) and produce ammonia. Ammonia is then detoxified by the liver and excreted by the kidneys as urea. Relying on protein to fuel cellular energy places inordinate stress on the liver and kidneys. The excretion of urea in urine demands large quantities of water, which can result in dehydration.

Obviously, the process of how macronutrients become energy for the body is another complicated biochemistry lesson. However, the important fact here is that during all of these steps, or *biochemical pathways,* many enzymes and coenzymes act as catalysts to make all of these reactions occur. Vitamins and minerals act as coenzymes; their ability to function as coenzymes is one of the largest jobs vitamins and minerals perform in our bodies. The body needs vitamins and minerals to break down carbohydrates, proteins, and fats in foods in order to rebuild them into body tissues. While vitamins and minerals do not provide glucose, they act as coenzymes to make energy-producing metabolic pathways possible. Without adequate intake of vitamins and minerals, our vitality is negatively affected because the metabolic pathways are not properly carried out. Moreover, if the body does not have adequate supplies of vitamins and minerals for the metabolic process of burning glucose, the glucose will be stored as fat. Therefore, poor nutritional status may also lead to weight gain.

KEY INFLUENCES ON NUTRITIONAL INTAKE

Before closing this chapter, it is important to consider how nutritional intake is influenced by several other key metabolic factors.

Insulin and Pancreatic Function

Before nutrients can be absorbed from the digestive tract, they must be split into small molecules. Pancreatic enzymes perform some of this work. Pancreatic enzymes are secreted into the small intestine, where they split large protein, carbohydrate, and fat molecules into smaller compounds. From there, intestinal enzymes and bile from the liver complete the process before the food is absorbed into the blood and lymph. Without these enzymes, digestion and absorption of critical nutrients is incomplete. Pancreatic enzyme deficiency can lead to malabsorption syndromes and EFA deficiency.

The catalysts for every activity in the digestive process—from start to finish—is dependent upon enzymes. Digestive enzymes are involved in the breakdown of ingested proteins, carbohydrates, and lipids (fats). Proper breakdown of these ingested foods is necessary to allow proper absorption of the nutrients to occur. Digestive enzymes can be depleted, either by genetic predisposition, prescription medications, or various diseases. Including raw foods such as fruits, vegetables, and lots of salad greens in your diet provides tremendous support to the pancreas because uncooked foods are rich in enzymes that aid digestion. These enzymes take some of the burden off the pancreas by reducing the amount of digestive enzymes needed from it and, in the long run, helps save the pancreatic cells from overuse.

The pancreas also secretes insulin in response to fluctuations in blood sugar. After a high-sugar or high-carbohydrate meal, insulin is secreted quickly in response to the rapid rise in blood sugar. The result is a subsequent dip in blood sugar, which triggers a rebound hunger. Typically, the urge is to eat more quick sources of sugar and the cycle continues. Rising and falling insulin influences nutrition in two ways. First, insulin increases hunger. Second, because the need to replenish blood sugar is the first order, dietary choices are affected. People tend to choose the first sugary or starchy food they can get their hands on because these foods raise blood sugar quickly.

Age, a diet high in sugar, and other factors can result in insulin resistance and impaired glucose tolerance, in which the cells lose their ability to utilize glucose for energy. The first consequence of impaired glucose uptake is a decrease in energy. Fatigue results from a decline in cellular respiration and ATP (energy) production. Since blood sugar remains elevated, there is a simultaneous increase in insulin output from the pancreas. This is known as hyperinsulinemia, characterized by abnormally high levels of circulating insulin. Hyperinsulinemia can ultimately lead to insulin resistance, type 2 diabetes, and cardiovascular disease.

Hyperinsulinemia promotes the storage of belly fat, and belly fat is known to increase the production of certain inflammatory substances in the body. Hyperinsulinemia also increases the synthesis of triglycerides in the liver. Insulin decreases HDL cholesterol and dangerously alters LDL cholesterol. Insulin promotes free-radical damage in the arteries and contributes to cardiovascular disease and chronic conditions associated with aging. Hyperinsulinemia increases the need for antioxidant nutrients, including vitamins A, C, E and the mineral selenium. Chromium, zinc, and magnesium are needed in greater quantities by those with elevated insulin and blood glucose.

Hyperinsulinemia can also result in a deficiency of essential fatty acids (EFAs) in two ways. First, the free radicals generated by excess insulin are most attracted to polyunsaturated fatty acids. Most polyunsaturated fatty acids in the body are omega-3 and omega-6 EFAs. Once oxidized, EFAs are unable to become healthy prostaglandins. Second, insulin blocks delta-6 desaturase, the enzyme necessary for the conversion of EFAs to their metabolically active state.

Thyroid and Pituitary Function

The thyroid gland controls the rate at which nutrients are utilized. The thyroid is the metabolic regulator of the body; it determines how quickly carbohydrates, protein, and fats are utilized. When metabolism increases, more of these macronutrients are required to fuel energy. If metabolism slows, fewer macronutrients are needed. Typically, if metabolism increases or decreases, the appetite follows. The thyroid gland affects food absorption, gastric emptying, secretion of digestive enzymes, and motility of the gastrointestinal tract.

As we've discussed, hypothyroidism lowers your metabolism; therefore, weight gain is common, even if activity level remains the same. Hyperthyroidism speeds up the metabolism of both macro- and micronutrients. Vitamin deficiency is common in hyperthyroid states. Hyperthyroidism increases the demand for calories by as much as 200 percent, simply to stay at a constant weight. Weight loss is a typical sign of hyperthyroidism, as the increased consumption of calories fails to match the increase in basal metabolic rate.

Hyperthyroidism also increases the blood levels of the thyroid hormone calcitonin, which stimulates calcium loss from the bones. Extra calcium is needed in the diet to offset this effect. Those with hyperthyroidism can develop lactose intolerance, limiting tolerable dietary sources of calcium.

Stress and Adrenal Function

Under acute stress conditions, the adrenals work to secrete hormones needed for the "fight-or-flight" response. These hormones, including epinephrine and cortisol, require nutrients for their synthesis. Under chronic stress, the adrenals must work to maintain consistently high levels of epinephrine and cortisol, and the body must adapt to physiological changes in the presence of these hormones. While acute stress is an adaptive response from which the body quickly returns to normal, chronic stress is maladaptive and depletes the body of vital energy and nutrients.

The adrenal glands have the highest content of vitamin C than any other tissue or gland in the body. It is thought that vitamin C plays an important role in the synthesis of cortisol, as well as of other endocrine hormones. Overproduction of cortisol can deplete the body of vitamin C, which is an important antioxidant. This, in turn, can increase oxidative stress and free-radical damage, which are forms of stress. In other words, depletion of vitamin C can actually increase stress and result in its further depletion. Other antioxidants, including vitamins A and E and the mineral selenium, are also consumed by stress.

Stress often increases the use of caffeine, prescription drugs, nicotine, and alcohol. All of these substances exhaust nutrient stores. Another vital nutrient depleted by stress is vitamin B_5 (pantothenic acid). Vitamin B_5 is needed for the production of adrenal hormones, and deficiency is associated with a decline in cortisol output. Stress is linked to a reduction of iron absorption due to insufficient hydrochloric acid secretion by the stomach. Chronic stress increases the need for zinc, calcium, and magnesium. Zinc supports the immune system and neutralizes free radicals, which are abundant during times of stress. Magnesium and calcium are required for healthy nervous system function.

Gastrointestinal problems are common during stress. Stress initially increases the secretion of hydrochloric acid (HCL, a strong stomach acid necessary for the breakdown and digestion of many foods). This is a time when peptic ulcers can be initiated or aggravated. Eventually HCL secretion diminishes, and certain digestive enzymes are rendered ineffective. During stress, blood flow to the gastrointestinal tract is diverted, and autonomic nervous impulses are reduced. Constipation and diarrhea are both common signs of stress. Stress can deplete probiotic bacteria in the intestine, resulting in reduced nutrient absorption.

Cortisol stimulates glucose production by the liver, promotes protein breakdown, and increases the mobilization of fatty acids. These actions increase blood sugar (and therefore insulin release from the pancreas) and LDL cholesterol. The need for protein increases under the effects of cortisol. Proteins are split into amino acids and utilized for the production of glucose. This can result in muscle wasting and protein deficiency. Fatty acid deficiency is a concern for several reasons. As fats are mobilized and converted to glucose, fat stores are depleted (along with fat-soluble vitamins). Cortisol and other stress-related factors interfere with the conversion of EFAs to healthy prostaglandins.

Bowel Terrain

The large intestine, or bowel, is critical for the final phases of digestion. In the large intestine, some vitamins are synthesized, toxins are neutralized and eliminated in the stool, and nutrients, water, and electrolytes are absorbed into the blood. The health of the large intestine is so critical to overall well-being that many experts suggest that many illnesses, in part, can be traced to poor bowel function. Bowel imbalance, known as dysbiosis, is a factor in nutritional deficiencies.

The primary causes of dysbiosis are overgrowth of pathogenic microorganisms; lack of dietary fiber; excessive intake of sugar and animal protein; alcohol and drug use; poor thyroid, liver, or gallbladder function; food allergies; and inadequate upper gastrointestinal digestion. Inadequate digestion of food interferes with the absorption of protein and trace minerals, more than the absorption of carbohydrates and fat. This can result in weight gain despite inadequate absorption of nutrients. When upper intestinal digestion is poor, large food particles enter the bowel and ferment pathogenic bacteria. The byproducts of fermentation, known as bacterial endotoxins, are toxic to the bowel and can be absorbed systemically through the bloodstream. Endotoxins can damage cell membranes and disturb intracellular activity.

Healthy intestinal flora contributes to the synthesis of some B vitamins (B_1, B_2, and B_{12}) and vitamin K. Healthy intestinal bacteria feed on cellulose from fiber. A diet low in fiber, or any condition that feeds the overgrowth of unhealthy bacteria, can lead to deficiencies of those vitamins synthesized in the bowel.

Water

Quality water is essential for digestion and metabolism. Numerous enzymatic and chemical reactions required for the breakdown of food need water. Water is also responsible for transporting nutrients via blood to cells throughout the body. Water is involved in every bodily function, not only for digestion, but also for circulation, elimination/detoxification, and the total "balance" of health. An inadequate intake of water, therefore, results in digestive problems, dehydration, constipation, and a buildup of toxic waste.

Darlene's Story

I was forty-nine years old and rarely perspired. I had been to many doctors, but none could diagnose my problem. Because my body retained so much water, I needed to take diuretics (water pills), and had been taking them for thirty years. It was not unusual for me to retain twenty to sixty pounds of water weight. I was always uncomfortably hot and my whole body was achy. I felt like I was sick with the flu all of the time. Because of the variation in my water weight, I had to keep five different sizes of clothing in my closet. If we were having hot weather, I'd wear the largest size because I knew I'd "grow" into it in several hours. The problem progressively worsened as I got older. I couldn't sleep at night because my body heat was unbearable. I slept with the window opened all winter and the heat turned off. I couldn't go outside during hot days except for short amounts of time. I was miserable. I could honestly say, "No sweat."

After Dr. LaValle's evaluation of my case, he felt that I needed nutritional support for my pituitary gland. He gave me supplement recommendations along with his Healthy Living Guidelines. Within a few weeks of following the guidelines and taking the supplements, my body began to sweat. Other changes I have noticed are that my skin is softer, my joints don't ache, and at fifty years old, I grew an inch! I'm more energetic, and I can stay outside on hot days. I wore a size five all summer. People tell me I look younger, and I feel great! Dr. LaValle's knowledge, and the supplements have been a miracle for me. My sister says I have a smile that says, "You ain't seen nothin' yet!"

Darlene contracted a virus at age six that most likely affected her pituitary gland. She was fatigued, and it was obvious from our initial interview that she needed to rejuvenate her chemistry. Now in her fifties, Darlene has a new lease on life and is enthusiastically charge in other areas of her life. When the functioning of the pituitary gland is disturbed, many times problems involving adrenal and thyroid function follow. By correcting her imbalances, we realigned her endocrine hormones and awakened her metabolism.

TIME FOR A CHANGE

Our health is directly affected by the foods we eat, or don't eat enough of. Our metabolism, our very lives, depend upon the elements we allow to enter our bodies. We have all read the statistics that tell us that Americans are in real trouble when it comes to chronic diseases, such as cardiovascular disease, diabetes, and obesity—the end products of metabolic syndrome. But, for many people, statistics aren't enough. They would rather point to the one person in their family—some great aunt or uncle—who lived to beat the odds until they were in their eighties despite drinking coffee, eating donuts, and smoking. They would rather live in this dream state than open their eyes to the many, many people around them who are living lives of chronic illness, or dying young, just because they will not alter their eating habits.

I try to remind these folks that their aunt or uncle was the exception. I try to explain to them that the human body is a miraculous thing. The human body has all kinds of ways in which it can compensate for nutritional deficiencies and inadequacies, for a while, but only for a while. Eventually these deficiencies and inadequacies will begin to show themselves in your health. They will begin to wear down that wonderful, miraculous body of yours.

Believe me, and I speak from twenty years of clinical experience, as well as from the experiences of hundreds of my patients, good nutrition makes a difference. I readily admit that it can be hard to change your diet. After all, here in America we are surrounded by nutritionally inadequate food choices. Not only are we surrounded by these foods, but we are always getting them thrust at us by every type of media. You rarely get reinforcing media. When is the last time you saw a broccoli commercial on television? Yet, the time has come for us to take responsibility for our own health, and not expect a doctor to fix us without at least offering to help him or her do so.

The effort to make the change is worth it. It doesn't have to be difficult or complex, but I have found that the ease with which people make dietary changes depends on a person's true readiness for change. If you are really ready, you will be able to make the changes and make them stick. There is no trick or gimmick that is going to change that. If you are ready to make the change to improve your diet, let me help you with a few simple guidelines that have worked for many of my patients over the years.

Now, onward for Key Seven . . .

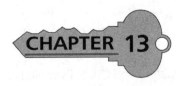

CHAPTER 13

KEY SEVEN:
Understanding Diet and How to Get the Most from What You Eat

A re you unsure of what you should or should not be eating? Do you know how to eat healthier, but you just can't seem to do it? The reason most eating plans fail over time is that they work against human nature. Human beings seek pleasure. And while food is pleasurable, scrutinizing what we eat is not.

In general, diet plans leave people feeling exhausted—either physically or psychologically, or both. Some argue that many of the foods and substances we eat these days are really more like addictive drugs (for example, chocolate, caffeine, and added flavorings, which evoke certain responses in the brain). This may be one reason why it is so challenging for people to make healthy dietary changes. Another problem is that most people look at eating healthier as something they do temporarily until they lose some weight, and then they go back to the old way of eating. Our main challenge is to find ways to enjoy a new way of eating so that we don't want to go back to the old way.

The basis of my "Healthy Living Guidelines" is to help you learn to eat the foods that support health, not foods that destroy health like most people eat today. Food choices are the most simple and powerful ways in which you can take control over your own state of health. Eating foods that promote health, and avoiding foods that deplete health, are the building blocks of wellness. If you ever hope to be healthy, you must find a way to like the foods that support your health.

As you'll learn in this chapter, when chosen from quality sources and eaten wisely, the four basic components of the diet—carbohydrate, protein, fat, and water—supply the calories, vitamins, minerals, essential nutrients, fiber, and enzymes our bodies need to run efficiently. The quantities and portions of each of these classifications of foods have been manipulated in an infinite number of ways over the years, resulting in a confusing mix of information and misinformation when it comes to diet and nutrition, and about what it means to "eat right."

CONTROVERSIES OVER WHAT MAKES UP
A HEALTHFUL DIET

In the United States, the USDA's Food Guide Pyramid is the most widely accepted set of dietary recommendations for what constitutes a "balanced daily diet." The base of the pyramid contains bread, cereal, rice, pasta, and other grains as the foundation of a healthful diet. The second level of the pyramid is shared by fruits and vegetables. The next level higher contains the milk, yogurt, and cheese group. This level of the pyramid also contains the meat, poultry, fish, dry beans, eggs, and nut group. At the top of the pyramid, representing the smallest category, is fats, oils, and sweets.

The pyramid has come under criticism from many health professionals who feel that—among its many shortfalls—it encourages too high a carbohydrate intake, especially in light of the growing numbers of people with insulin resistance and diabetes. The government-issued pyramid recommends that approximately 50 to 60 percent of your daily caloric intake consist of carbohydrates, with the majority coming from breads and cereal (grains). The recommendation is based on a 1,600 to 2,800 calorie diet and, if followed, would provide anywhere from 200 to 350 grams of carbohydrate a day. The USDA pyramid has also been criticized for not emphasizing the importance of choosing whole grain versions of the breads, cereals, rice, or pastas eaten and for recommending a low-fat diet without emphasizing the importance of the quality of the fats consumed. The pyramid makes no mention of trans fatty acid intake, and nuts are to be eaten sparingly because of their high fat content, as are sweets, which the guidelines simply state can contribute to dental caries.

Americans clearly adopted the higher-carbohydrate and lower-fat dietary pattern suggested by the USDA's food pyramid, but did not take to heart the recommendations to increase fiber intake, to increase fruit and vegetable intake, or to curb their intake of sweets. The result is evident in the disastrous levels of obesity and diabetes that we are experiencing today.

The controversies that have developed over the last few years concerning the appropriate levels of carbohydrate, fat, and even protein in our diets is based on new research that continues to change our understanding of the effects of diet on health. For example, there is a body of research now that shows that a high-carbohydrate intake, which the USDA pyramid encourages, contributes to several factors that increase risk of cardiovascular disease such as increased VLDL and triglyceride levels, and decreased HDL levels. Diets high in carbohydrates have also been proven to contribute to increased circulating insulin levels, which cause weight gain (belly fat in particular), inflammation, and eventual insulin resistance. (Unfortunately, such findings have repopularized high-protein, low-carbohydrate diets.) There is also now plenty of evidence on the harmful effects of trans-fatty acids, and the helpful roles of omega-3 fatty acids found in foods such as nuts.

Since the USDA issued its food pyramid and subsequent nutrition campaigns, such as the slogan "Five a Day," which was used to encourage people to eat at least a minimum of five servings of fruits and vegetables, the DASH (Dietary Approaches to Stop Hypertension) study found that people should eat a minimum of nine servings of fruits and vegetables daily. Participants of the study who were on the DASH diet versus control subjects were able to lower blood pressure with diet alone. In addition to fruits and vegetables, a small handful of nuts and seeds were eaten daily on this diet, and were also felt to play a helpful role in the results participants were able to achieve. Since this study, many health organizations have increased their recommendations from five servings of fruits and vegetables daily to at least nine servings daily. Continued study on the health effects of nuts and seeds have also led to a universal standard of recommending a daily serving of them.

To add to the confusion, many studies now show that vegetarian diets (those that include very little or no animal protein) greatly reduce risk of developing heart disease, cancer, and high blood pressure. Vegetarian diets are by nature higher in carbohydrates because they typically include lots of whole grains, fruits, and vegetables. On the other hand, research indicates that eating a high-protein/low-carbohydrate diet can lead to improved control of blood sugar and, therefore, can reduce risk for cardiovascular disease. There are compelling arguments on both sides of the animal protein issue.

Protein intake in the form of dairy products is also amazingly controversial. There are numerous studies on the effects of dairy products on human health. Recent studies have proven a moderate intake of dairy products to be beneficial in lowering high blood pressure and helping to regulate weight, while earlier studies link dairy products to an increased risk of prostate and breast cancers. Studies conducted in the early 1990s also correlated a high cow's milk intake in early childhood with a greatly increased risk of developing type 1 diabetes. And, despite the U.S. Dairy Council advisory to drink milk to prevent osteoporosis, an increase intake in dairy has not been proven to decrease risk of bone fractures in older adults. In fact, the latest studies show that vitamin D intake may be more important than milk intake for reducing hip fracture.

Emerging theories also suggest that genetics may play a role in what foods different individuals can tolerate. In addition, a person's activity level will have an influence over the amount of carbohydrates, protein, and fats a person can eat without ill effects.

It is findings such as these that have lead many health professionals, including the American Dietetics Association (ADA), to the conclusion that no one diet fits all. While there are certain components of a healthy eating plan that virtually everyone should incorporate, such as eating more fruits and vegetables and greatly reducing sugar intake, the truth is that there is no single eating plan that is right for everyone. However, there is a way to customize your diet to your metabolism—discover which foods you may be sensitive to and determine the quantity of carbohydrates your body can tolerate.

That's what I invite you to do here and now. In this chapter, you will be presented with information that will allow you to create an eating plan specific to you. The Healthy Living Guidelines will serve as a road map for you to follow in achieving your long-term goals of health and vitality, and for many, a lifetime of weight control.

How stringently you follow the Healthy Living Guidelines revolves around one factor: your desire to crack your metabolic code—your desire to, once and for all, understand your own body, your own metabolic system, and how you can best keep it healthy. Eating is a *lifestyle* choice not just part of a diet plan. If you want to be well, you must make permanent changes concerning food and exercise, and other lifestyle issues. This is what will put you on the path to optimal health. It may not be an easy journey. The Healthy Living Guidelines require some commitment and willingness to change. The first few days may prove challenging as you give up some of the high-fat and/or high-sugar foods you enjoy, but don't quit, the rewards of good nutrition and a healthier lifestyle are well worth it.

THE HEALTHY LIVING GUIDELINES

To begin with, the word "diet" stems from the Greek word *diaita,* meaning "a manner of living" or "way of life." This is not the same thing as a desperate scheme to shed extra pounds or add bulk to muscle. Dieting as a manner of living implies that your intention, in choosing to eat the foods that you do, is the creation of health and vitality. One thing is for sure—we must give up the notion that we can somehow get by without eating whole foods. We must "stop the madness" of the typical American diet that relies on desperately poor quality foods and that does not include fruits and vegetables.

I developed and began using the Healthy Living Guidelines in my clinical practice nearly twenty years ago. The guidelines are based on nutrition principles that use wholesome foods and nutrients to correct imbalances of metabolism and to promote optimal metabolic function. The diet relies on vegetables and legumes/beans to constitute most of your carbohydrate requirements, with grains and cereals supplying only a small portion of your carbohydrate intake, followed by protein, fat, and fruit, which provide the remainder of your nutritional needs. Figure 13.1 on page 313 illustrates the guideline's recommendations for optimum intakes of carbohydrate, protein, and fat.

This pyramid differs from the current USDA Food Guide Pyramid, which recommends eating six to eleven servings from the carbohydrate group (bread and cereal), two to three servings each from the protein groups (meat and milk), three to five servings of vegetables, two to four servings of fruits, and to eat sparingly from the fats, oil, and sweets group.

The Healthy Living Guidelines de-emphasize simple carbohydrates, especially carbohydrates from sugar and grains. Limiting the intake of simple carbohydrates coun-

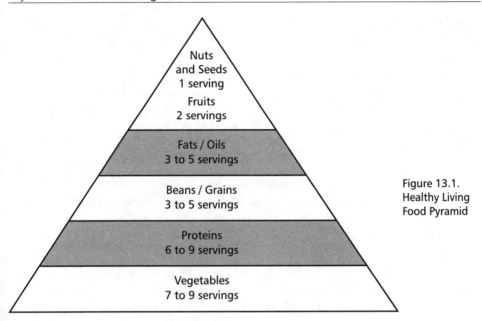

Figure 13.1.
Healthy Living
Food Pyramid

ters the glycemic effects, which lead to weight gain and the health problems associated with metabolic syndrome. While most people do better (controlling weight, blood sugar, and total health) with a lower-carbohydrate diet, others can consume more carbohydrates without ill effects. However, I haven't found anyone who does well consuming large amounts of refined carbohydrates. The guidelines will help you discover your own personal optimal intake of carbohydrates—the highest amount you can consume without gaining weight or negatively affecting blood sugar.

Although the guidelines de-emphasize carbohydrates, they do not exclude them entirely. Carbohydrates are an abundant source of energy. Carbohydrates provide the body with glucose, a preferred unit of fuel. Without carbohydrates, the body becomes easily fatigued, tissue and muscle are broken down for energy, and minerals are depleted. In comparison to the Atkins diet, which recommends eating less than 40 grams of carbohydrate per day, the guidelines provide 100 to 125 grams of carbohydrate daily. The additional carbohydrates are encouraged because people generally find it difficult to comply long term with a diet that only allows for an extremely low carbohydrate intake. When people who are on an extremely low-carbohydrate diet finally "crack" and begin to reincorporate more carbohydrates into their daily diets, the weight often returns with a vengeance.

The primary reason most people cannot adhere to very low-carbohydrate diets involves the neurotransmitter serotonin. As you may recall from Chapter 5, serotonin production is depleted during times of stress and during chronic stress. Serotonin is the neurotransmitter that helps regulate our sleep, mood, and even tolerance to pain. When this neurotransmitter is depleted, we become depressed, have difficulty sleeping, experience an increased sensitivity to pain, and most significantly, develop food cravings.

Serotonin is made from the amino acid tryptophan. Tryptophan is made from protein. Eating a high-protein diet will not lead to increased serotonin production. There are many other amino acids in the body that compete for absorption and lower the uptake of tryptophan. It is actually a higher-carbohydrate meal that leads to increased tryptophan absorption and serotonin production. The carbohydrate triggers insulin. Insulin reduces amino acid levels in the blood, all except tryptophan, which can then easily cross the blood-brain barrier (a semipermeable membrane that controls entry of substances into the brain) due to lack of competition from other amino acids.

Another reason the guidelines encourage you to incorporate adequate amounts of carbohydrate into your diet is that the muscles need carbohydrate to provide glycogen stores for fuel during exercise. If you are going to try to exercise more—as you should—you will find you do better with a little more carbohydrate intake. As long as whole foods and not refined foods are used as the source of carbohydrate, the effect on blood sugar is moderated. The guidelines provide more carbohydrate to allow for improved serotonin production and to provide more fuel for muscles during exercise, but not so much that blood sugar and insulin levels are continually elevated.

The guidelines also recommend increasing your daily intake of vegetables (seven servings) and fruits (two servings). This will provide optimum intakes of fiber and other nutrients responsible not only for fueling biochemical pathways in the body, but also for maintaining alkalinity and for the cancer protection provided by their phytonutrients.

As for what constitutes an optimum intake of protein, well, in my opinion, the incisors and flat crushing molars in humans suit us to eat plant foods *and* some animal foods. Proteins are the building blocks of all cells, tissue, and organs. Protein is required for the maintenance and repair of all systems. Protein deficiency leads to poor wound healing, weakened immunity, poor appetite, and muscle wasting. Protein is essential to maintaining anabolic metabolism and providing the building blocks need to make neurotransmitters and enzymes. However, excess animal protein puts undue stress on the body, especially on the liver and kidneys, which are responsible for processing the waste products of protein metabolism. In addition, medical literature shows that a diet too high in saturated fats (found in animal meats and dairy) increases risk factors for cardiovascular disease and cancer, especially when not accompanied by lots of the phytochemicals and antioxidants found in vegetables and greens. Therefore, the guidelines encourage eating both plant and animal sources of proteins, but making sure that animal proteins are of very high quality, meaning organic and free range. Following the guidelines will provide an average of 30–35 grams of protein a day from non-animal proteins and 50 grams from animal proteins.

In my clinical experience, I observe that most people feel better and are able to maintain good health when they eat at least some animal proteins. (I am not against vegan diets—a diet containing no meat, eggs, or dairy—as long you can maintain good health and vitality. I have found that only a minority of people are able to feel energetic after following a vegan diet long term.) An important benefit of including at least occasional animal proteins in the diet is that they are the only source of vitamin B_{12}. The guidelines recommend between 1 and 1.5 grams of protein per kilogram (kg) of body weight, which is slightly higher than the minimum .8 grams per kg recommended by medical guidelines. However, it is still less than the two to three times their daily protein needs most Americans consume.

As for fat, the guidelines emphasize moderating total fat intake but making sure that the fat consumed is from healthier sources. The guidelines replace saturated fats and trans-fatty acids with essential fatty acids (EFAs). EFAs are needed to maintain integrity of cellular membranes and to regulate cholesterol. EFAs produce prostaglandins that have regulatory effects over inflammation, immune function, cardiovascular function, and the nervous system. EFA deficiency is also associated with poor skin integrity and depletion of fat-soluble vitamins. So, fat intake has to do more with quality than quantity. Eating nuts and seeds daily is encouraged as a source of healthy omega-3 essential fatty acids and several important minerals.

Keep in mind when evaluating a fat or oil that there are three factors that determine its health-giving qualities: The type of fat (no hydrogenated or trans-fatty acids), the way the fat is extracted, and how the fat is used. Polyunsaturated oils have a tendency to oxidize easily. When oxidized, they become a source of free radicals to the body. Oils that are pressed or extracted at high temperatures, therefore, have a higher free-radical content. This is why I recommend cold-pressed oils. Monounsaturated and saturated fats are the best cooking oils.

Lastly, the guidelines are designed to help you discover food intolerances or allergies that may be compromising your immune system and your metabolism. In particular, it excludes wheat and dairy products from the diet at first, because so many people have sensitivities to them. This is consistent with the recent findings by the University of Maryland Center for Celiac Research, which found that as many as 1.5 million Americans are suffering from celiac disease (also called celiac sprue), a chronic digestive condition in which people develop an autoimmune reaction to gluten, a protein fragment in a number of grains—most notably wheat, rye, barley, and oats. According to their research, even in those groups at low risk for developing celiac disease, 1 out of every 133 Americans is gluten intolerant. If a person knows he or she had celiac disease, gluten must be eliminated from the diet. For people who do not have gluten intolerance, the guidelines attempt to reincorporate some wheat into the diet.

Milk products are also restricted from the diet at first. Research shows that up to 25 percent of people of northern European descent and between 50 to 95 percent of people from other ethnic backgrounds may be lactose intolerant. Lactose is the natural sugar in milk and milk products. The widespread problems associated with milk consumption may also be from the contaminants in milk (antibiotics, hormones, and pesticides) or it may due to an inability in many individuals to properly digest the proteins in milk. Because of the high risk of contamination from antibiotics, hormones, and pesticides, the guidelines recommend only moderate intake of organic milk and milk products when they are reincorporated into the diet.

In addition, yeast and fermented foods are excluded from the diet initially in order to minimize the further proliferation of yeast and other dysbiotic organisms in people with an overgrowth of *Candida albicans,* known as candidiasis. Candidiasis contributes to the breakdown of the gastrointestinal linings and wall, which, in turn, can contribute to a wheat, gluten, dairy, and other sensitivities. As the digestive tract is rebuilt with key supplements and a better quality diet, an attempt at reincorporating these foods can be made, if possible.

CHALLENGES TO EXPECT AT THE START

I think many people want to eat a healthier diet, but too often find themselves returning to a less healthy diet for one reason: many unhealthy foods taste good. Sweet desserts and fast foods saturate the taste buds, as do salty foods such as snack chips. In comparison, salad greens and an apple don't have the high-fat, high-sugar, or high-salt content and may not taste as appealing. However, with time, as you gradually eat fewer desserts, fast foods, and other junk food, your taste buds will regain the ability to recognize the natural flavors in fruits and vegetables. If you keep away from junk foods long enough, you will notice negative physical effects, such as headaches and hypoglycemia, when you do try to eat them again; this becomes a disincentive for eating them. And in time, believe it or not, the junk foods will not taste as good as they used to.

The way to overcome these challenges is twofold: The first survival technique is to retrain your taste buds; the second technique is to surround yourself with healthy foods. This means getting the unhealthy foods out of the house and out of your reach. It also means experimenting with healthier food choices until you find recipes and foods that you like. Finding healthier options that taste good to you is critical, because the only way you will continue to eat foods is if you like how they taste. Of course, you'll need to exert some willpower at the start, because no matter how hard you try, a lunch consisting of a salad and whole-grain crackers isn't going to taste as good as a hot-fudge sundae. However, after time, your taste buds will begin to adapt to the lower levels of fat, sugar, and salt, and you will find that you are actually enjoying many of the healthier foods. This may sound simplistic, but I have found that too often people use their grit and willpower to keep eating foods that don't taste good to them. And this just won't last long term. Usually willpower will eventually lose out because eating must be pleasurable.

Another challenge to successfully switching over to a healthy eating plan is that healthy foods take a little extra time to prepare. If you don't know how to cook or prepare foods, take cooking classes at a local culinary school or even at a high school. Learning to prepare home-cooked meals is a great way to solve the problem of finding foods you like. Also, more restaurants and delis are offering healthy take home meals these days, so if you simply cannot cook, this might be an option. Even if they only provide a healthy main entrée, it's easy enough to prepare a salad and vegetables to go with it.

Maintaining a healthy diet may also be a challenge for people who do not like fruits and vegetables. Unfortunately, I have no magic for you folks, but I do have some suggestions that have helped many people learn to like them.

- Learn how to choose ripe and good-quality fruits and vegetables. Many people think they do not like fruits and vegetables when the real problem is that they are choosing unripe or nearly spoiled produce. There are some informative fruit- and vegetable-buying guides available that can teach you how to select ripe fruits and to recognize freshness in produce. Also, ask your supermarket's produce manager to give you some pointers.

- Retry fruits and vegetables that you think you don't like. Often as we age and mature, we start liking the very foods we refused to eat when we were young. You may suddenly discover, for example, that you do like grapefruits after all. Also, try foods in different forms. For example, if you don't like cooked broccoli, try eating it raw or vice versa. Experiment to find your preference.

- Buy organic produce. Organically grown fruits are generally sweeter and organically grown vegetables are generally more flavorful and less bitter. In addition, organically grown foods are free of pesticides and fungicides, so eating them lightens the chemical load in the body. This is important since one of the advantages of this diet is that it can help the body to detoxify.

- Try at least one new fruit, vegetable, or healthy recipe each week. (It helps to try new foods after several hours of not eating, since foods tend to taste better when we're very hungry.) By the end of a year, even if you only like half of the new foods you've tried, you will have added twenty-six new foods to your repertoire!

Going out to eat also challenges our ability to stick to a healthy-eating meal plan. There are a number of helpful booklets available that provide nutrition information on the foods served at chain restaurants and fast-food restaurants. Such information can help you become skilled in finding healthy food choices or foods that are a lesser of the evils when eating out. For additional pointers, see the inset "How to Dine Out and Stay Healthy" on page 340.

IMPLEMENTING THE HEALTHY LIVING GUIDELINES

Implementation of the Healthy Living Guidelines occurs in two phases. *Phase one* involves relearning how to eat from each of the five food groups and how to reintegrate whole foods into your life. This phase lasts approximately four to eight weeks. These foods will remain the staples of your diet. During this phase, common allergy-producing foods are eliminated, as well as foods that can contribute to insulin resistance, dysbiosis, an overgrowth of *Candida albicans,* and other conditions that disrupt metabolism. Phase one encourages the detoxification process. However, if a more intensive diet for detoxification is desired, then follow the additional guidelines in Chapter 11.

Once your health has improved, *phase two* can be implemented. In this phase, the process of reintroducing some of the restricted or eliminated foods begins. This phase involves detective work to uncover food sensitivities. Once you accomplish phase two, you will have composed an eating plan for life.

By now, I hope you have come to the conclusion that by changing the foods you eat, you can change the pathway of your health. You can stop the downward spiral that leads to metabolic syndrome and an out-of-control metabolism. You can, instead, restore yourself to optimal health. Read on to begin phase one.

PHASE ONE

Your reeducation begins by learning how to select foods and eat the recommended servings from each of the following five food groups.

The number of servings from each food category total approximately 1,300 calories a day during phase one. Some larger men or very active people may need to increase this number of calories up to 1,800 calories a day. If your goal is not only to feel better, but also to lose weight, and you have not begun to lose pounds after four weeks on phase one, it is better not to reduce calories much further. A shorter person could reduce their calorie intake to 1,200 calories, however, it is not healthy for anyone to go below 1,000 to 1,200 calories a day. Occasionally, obese individuals will undertake very low-calorie diets of less than 1,000 calories a day to achieve weight loss, however, such diets should be supervised by a physician. It is much better to increase your activity level rather than risk taking in too few calories. (Interferences to weight loss can sometimes occur from environmental endocrine disrupters. You may want to consider getting one of the tests described on page 235 to determine the levels of heavy metals in your body.)

To calculate serving sizes, I use the exchange list system developed by the American Diabetes Association (ADA) and the American Dietetics Association. In the exchange system, foods are grouped into starches, vegetables, fruits, meats, milk products, and fats. The foods are proportioned to measure and control calories, carbohydrates, and other nutrients. An exchange is basically one portion of a food type.

You can exchange or trade foods within a group because they are similar in nutrient content and in the way they affect blood sugar. The complete list of exchanges for each food group is available in *The Exchange Lists for Meal Planning* through most hospital dietetic departments, or you can buy *The Official Pocket Guide to Diabetic Exchanges* (McGraw-Hill/Contemporary Books, 1998). You may also download and print the list for free from the following websites: www.webmd.com or www.nhlbi. nih.gov. Type in the web address and use the site search to look for the food exchange list.

Vegetables

Vegetables should make up the bulk of your diet with seven to nine servings a day. Even though you will be eating the greatest number of servings from this group, it will only make up a small percentage—about 20 percent—of your total caloric intake. Seven to nine servings may seem like a lot at first, but you will eventually find this is a comfortable level that is easy to achieve. It usually means having a large salad every day, in addition to some steamed, roasted, or stir-fried vegetables, as well as some raw vegetables.

Vegetables are fiber rich and nutrient dense. Studies have shown that people who eat at least five to nine servings of vegetables a day have a much lower risk of cancer, diabetes, heart disease, and high blood pressure. The disease-preventing effects are due to antioxidants and phytochemicals so abundant in vegetables.

Vegetables can be grouped by carbohydrate content as shown in Table 13.1 on page 320. Choose vegetables primarily from groups 1 and 2, and occasionally from group 3. Vegetables with lower carbohydrate content have a lower glycemic index and therefore do not exert as great an effect on blood sugar. Groups 4 and 5 list the higher-carbohydrate vegetables. High-carbohydrate vegetables such as potatoes and corn should be grouped with grains and legumes, and because of their high-glycemic index, they should be limited from phase one. If you would like to eat a serving of either potatoes or corn, count it as one of your servings from the grain/legume group below. You can substitute one of the foods from group 4 or 5 vegetable group for a grain/legume serving.

There are many low-carbohydrate vegetables to choose from. Variety is important. If you are not presently eating much variety from this group, it will be important to follow some of my earlier suggestions for learning to like vegetables. If you are eating only two or three different kinds, it will be difficult to get the quantity of vegetables you need and you will soon grow tired of those you are eating.

Try to avoid iceberg lettuce, which has a low nutritional value when compared with other darker-green lettuces. If you are not accustomed to eating the darker-green lettuces, begin by mixing iceberg lettuce with a little bit of a darker-green lettuce or with romaine lettuce. Do this until your taste buds have become accustomed

Table 13.1. Vegetables Grouped by Carbohydrate Content

GROUP 1 LOWEST	GROUP 2	GROUP 3 MODERATE	GROUP 4	GROUP 5 HIGHEST
Asparagus	Beans, string	Artichokes	Lima beans	Potato, sweet
Bean sprouts	Beets	Hominy	Corn	Yams
Beet greens	Brussels sprouts	Oyster plant	Potato, white	
Broccoli	Carrots	Parsnips		
Cabbage	Chives	Peas, green		
Cauliflower	Collards			
Celery	Dandelion greens			
Chard, Swiss	Eggplant			
Cucumber	Kale			
Endive	Kohlrabi			
Lettuce	Leeks			
Mustard greens	Okra			
Radishes	Onions			
Spinach	Parsley			
Turnip greens	Peppers			
Watercress	Pimento			
	Pumpkin			
	Rutabagas			
	Tomatoes			
	Turnips			
	Zucchini			

to the taste, and then increase the amount of dark-green lettuces until you have eliminated iceberg lettuce entirely.

To avoid getting tired of salad, top your lettuce greens with a variety of cut up vegetables, nuts, or seeds, and soy or rice cheeses (alternatives to cow's milk cheese to be used while eliminating dairy during phase one), and seasonings such as sea salt, pepper, onion powder, and other spices, and toss with your dressing. Experiment with different types of dark-green lettuce and combinations of toppings and dressings. Many bottled salad dressings contain vinegar, a substance avoided during phase one. Look for dressings that are vinegar- and dairy-free, or make your own by blending lemon juice with an oil such as olive, flaxseed, or walnut.

Proteins

Your total caloric intake should be made up of 20 to 30 percent proteins. This is approximately 80 grams of protein on a 1,300-calorie diet and 100 grams on a 1,800-calorie diet. Proteins are important for rebuilding tissues. They also help regulate blood sugar. Organic, grass-fed, and hormone-free meat products are preferable, whenever an option, because they have a better fatty-acid content. Chicken, turkey, fish, and game meats (venison, buffalo, and even ostrich) are best. The top twelve foods highest in quality protein are:

- Beef, Lean
- Orange roughy
- Buffalo
- Pork, Lean (no ham or cured pork)
- Chicken
- Scallops
- Cod
- Tilapia
- Eggs
- Turkey
- Halibut
- White Fish
- Lamb

Protein needs for healthy individuals can be calculated by first dividing desired or ideal body weight by 2.2. This figure converts your body weight into kilograms (kg). Multiply the number of kg by 1.0 gram/kg and this figure represents an estimate of protein needs in grams.

Some of your protein needs will be met with vegetables, beans/legumes, and nuts. There is an average of 2 grams of protein per vegetable serving, so eating nine servings a day will provide 18 grams. Beans and legumes provide about 7 grams per serving, starchy foods such as potatoes or corn about 3 grams per serving, and nuts about 7 grams per serving. There are approximately 7 grams of protein per ounce of meat.

For example, 150 pounds divided by 2.2 equals 68 kg. Sixty-eight kilograms multiplied by 1.0 gram equals 68 grams of protein. Sixty-eight grams of protein minus approximately 30 grams from starch, vegetables, and nuts equals 38 grams that is needed from meat. Thirty-eight divided by 7 grams per ounce of meat equals 5–6 ounces of meat. If you eat a little under your daily amount of protein one day, or a little over the next, it's not that critical; it all averages out. This is simply a way to determine a guideline. Many people determine their needs by seeing how they feel after eating higher or lower amounts. As long as you are feeling well and energetic, your body usually knows best.

Note: This protein requirement has been established for those in good health, who exercise moderately, and who have no existing renal (kidney) failure. It has not been established for those with special needs, such as an athlete or someone recovering from an illness. Your individual protein needs may vary.

Grains and Beans/Legumes

Grains, combined with beans and legumes, should make up about 15 percent of your daily calories. This translates to three servings a day with a serving being equal to 15 grams of carbohydrate. Examples of one serving include one slice of whole-grain bread, one-third cup of cooked millet or rice, one-third cup of cooked beans, three-fourths cup unsweetened ready-to-eat cereals, and one-third to one-half cup cooked pasta. While these amounts indicate the precise servings that equate to 15 grams of carbohydrate, it is safe to use a half-cup serving of any type of grain or bean such as cooked cereals, corn, pasta, beans, or potatoes as the single serving size. For some foods, this may put you slightly over the 15 grams of carbohydrates, but the difference will be negligible. Most people overindulge in this food category, so be sure to carefully measure your servings.

Some people are very sensitive to carbohydrates. If you are insulin resistant and overweight and find that you have not lost weight or inches after four to eight weeks on phase one, reduce the number of servings from this group until you begin to see weight loss. (Measure blood levels with a home-monitoring device.) Follow the reduced level for two to three weeks, then begin adding in one serving a day. Do this for several days and monitor your weight again. If you continue to lose weight, increase by another serving per day, and follow this same procedure until you have determined your level of tolerance.

Included in this category are wheat-free, whole-grain flours, breads, cereals, pasta, crackers, and snacks. Choose whole grains in the form of yeast-free flat bread, crackers, rice, or pasta. Whole-grain rye or rice crackers are a good substitute for bread. Other wheat-free choices are amaranth, barley, brown rice, buckwheat, cornmeal, kamut, millet, oats, quinoa, rye, and spelt.

Do not overcook grains. Cook grains until they retain some firmness, but are not chewy or soggy. Overcooking grains increases their glycemic index.

Spelt and kamut are in the wheat family; therefore, anyone with wheat allergies or known gluten intolerance may find these grains intolerable. Those on gluten-restricted diets should avoid oats, rye, barley, spelt, kamut, couscous, and triticale (a hybrid of rye and wheat), as well as whole wheat. Acceptable grains for those on gluten-restricted diets are corn flour, corn meal, cornstarch, potato flour, brown rice, soy flour, and millet, quinoa, and buckwheat. (Buckwheat, in spite of its name, is not wheat, but a seed and is gluten-free.) Other available flours include bean flours and hazelnut flour.

Note: Some people find that the starch, or complex carbohydrate, in grains can cause gas when eaten with meats. If this is the case, it can be easily remedied by avoiding eating complex carbohydrates and meats together. Instead, have your grains with vegetables at one meal, and your meats and vegetables at another meal. Also, if the beans and legumes cause gas when eaten, digestive aids such as Beano can be used to eliminate this problem.

Legumes are an excellent source of water-soluble fiber and can aid in controlling blood sugar and constipation. Legumes are an important source of protein for vegetarians when eaten with grains. Most legume and grain combinations provide all of the essential amino acids.

Try lentils, split peas, and any of the following beans: adzuki, anasazi, black, fava, garbanzo, kidney, lima, mung, or navy, or any of the other quality grains and beans listed in Table 13.2 below.

Table 13.2. Sources of Quality Grains and Beans/Legumes

GRAINS	BEANS/LEGUMES
Amaranth	Adzuki
Barley*	Anasazi
Bran* (Oat)	Black
Buckwheat*	Fava
Cornmeal (high lysine, limit to twice per week)	Garbanzo
Grits	Kidney
Job's tears	Lentil
Kamut	Lima
Millet	Mung
Quinoa	Navy
Rice, Basmati	Split Pea
Rice, brown and wild	
Rye*	
Spelt	
Teff grain	

Do not use these grains if you are on a gluten-restricted diet.

Added Fats and Oils

Added fats and oils make up 10 to 15 percent of your total caloric intake. When the fat from added fats and the fat content of meats are added together, the amount should not exceed 30 percent of calories from fat. On a 1,300-calorie diet, this would mean eating no more than 43 grams of fat a day, and about 60 grams of fat on a 1,800 calorie a day diet.

If you eat 7 ounces of lean or very lean meat a day, you will obtain 14–21 grams of fat. One small handful of nuts or seeds a day provides roughly 7 grams of fat. This leaves the remainder for added fats. An added fat serving is the equivalent of 5 grams of fat; for example, 1 teaspoon of butter or oil, 2 teaspoons of tahini (sesame seed paste), or 1 tablespoon of mayonnaise or salad dressing.

Fats are essential for the production of hormones, the health of skin and cell membranes, and for body temperature regulation. The importance of choosing the right fats cannot be overstated. Quality fat sources will contribute to health and vitality.

Poor-quality, hydrogenated fats such as shortening, and trans-fatty acids (from hydrogenated fats and oils, margarines, and fried foods) will contribute to cardio-vascular disease, inflammation, suppressed immune function, and other conditions.

Good fats to incorporate into the diet include those contained in nuts and seeds, cold-pressed olive and canola oils, flaxseed oil, sesame oil, avocado oil, and ghee (clarified butter).

Some fats are less stable when heated, meaning they lose their double carbon bond when heated, forming trans-fatty acids. Polyunsaturated or monounsaturated oils, including canola, corn, flaxseed, safflower, and sunflower oils tend to be unstable when heated. Canola and flaxseed oil are very unstable and should never be heated; they are great to use for salad dressings, however.

High-oleic monounsaturated oils such as olive oil and high-oleic sunflower and sesame seed oils, on the other hand, are more heat-stable oils. Butter, while high in saturated fat, is stable when heated. Use butter sparingly, but a little bit here and there adds a lot of flavor to your foods. *Note:* As a healthier alternative to butter or margarine, soften one pound of butter. Mix with 16 ounces of a cold-pressed oil. Let stand in the refrigerator until firm. This has the spreadability of margarine, but provides a quality source of fats.

In addition to the healthy fats and oils listed below, sesame, avocado, rice bran, and walnut oils can be used in limited amounts for flavoring.

Sources of healthy fats and oils include:

- Butter
- Olive*
- Canola
- Organic peanut oil*
- Flax seed oil

- Coconut oil**
- Ghee (clarified butter)
- Safflower
- Macadamia nuts

*Highly recommended for cooking.

** Very good for cooking. In its non-hydrogenated form, coconut oil is very heat stable. Although it contains some saturated fat, the fatty-acid chains are medium in length and have some health benefits. Evidence suggests that coconut oil supports thyroid health and may be beneficial for promoting weight loss.

Nuts, Seeds, and Fruit

Nuts and seeds, combined with fruit, should make up the remainder of the diet—about 5 to 10 percent of your daily calories. Nuts and seeds are a good source of minerals, especially magnesium, and healthy fatty acids. Nuts and seeds have some protein, but are highest in fat content. Incorporate them into your diet by eating a small handful a day, either plain or mixed into other foods. One handful of nuts or seeds—the equivalent of approximately twelve to fifteen almonds, or one-half ounce of nuts or seeds, or 1 tablespoon of nut or seed butter—contains approximately 90 calories.

If you find that you are not losing weight during phase one, cut out one fat serving a day, but be sure to keep nuts and seeds in your diet. Nuts, seeds, and nut butters are a convenient and tasty way to incorporate many nutrients into the diet. *Note:* Nuts and seeds should always be dry-roasted or raw. Roasted nuts are coated in low-quality unsaturated fats before they are roasted.

Recommended high-quality nuts and seeds, which are also free of allergenic molds include:

- almonds
- filberts
- pumpkin seeds
- pistachio nuts
- sesame seeds
- sunflower seeds

Some nuts should be avoided altogether, particularly peanuts. Peanuts contain dietary lectin, which binds with *glycoproteins* (proteins with glucose attached) on arterial smooth muscle cells, and may contribute to atherosclerosis. Peanuts are often contaminated with a mold called *aflatoxin,* which is thought to be highly carcinogenic. Peanut ingestion in pregnant women has been shown to increase peanut, wheat, and soy sensitivity in their children. Peanut allergies in children can induce anaphylactic shock and death. There is often a cross-sensitivity to Brazil nuts and hazelnuts among those allergic to peanuts.

Warning: If you have diverticulosis, you may be unable to tolerate whole or pieces of nuts or seeds; however, nut and seed butters (smooth-style, not chunky) are acceptable. To obtain magnesium and fatty acids, the two most important nutrients found in nuts, try alternative sources such as nut or seed butters, supplements, or other food sources. Magnesium is abundant in dark-green leafy vegetables, whole grains, legumes, squash, broccoli, and figs, for example. Sesame and walnut oils are especially rich in fatty acids.

Including fruits as part of your 5 to 10 percent of your daily calories in this category translates to two servings a day. One serving is roughly equivalent to 15 grams of carbohydrate. One-half of a large grapefruit, three-fourths cup of blackberries or blueberries, two small plums, one medium peach, one small banana, and one small apple, for example, are equal to one serving.

Like vegetables, fruits are a valuable source of soluble fiber, phytochemicals, vitamins, and minerals. Table 13.3 on page 326 breaks down fruits according to their carbohydrate content. Balance your intake of higher-carbohydrate fruits with lower-carbohydrate fruits. Choose two fruits from Groups 1, 2, and 3, or choose one fruit from either Group 1, 2, or 3 and one from Group 4. Dried fruit and bananas have the

Table 13.3. Fruits Grouped by Carbohydrate Content

GROUP 1 LOWEST CONTENT	GROUP 2	GROUP 3	GROUP 4 HIGHEST CONTENT
Rhubarb	Apricots	Apples	Bananas
Strawberries	Blackberries	Blueberries	Figs
	Cranberries	Cherries	Prunes
	Currants	Kumquats	
	Gooseberries	Loganberries	
	Grapefruit	Mangoes	
	Guava	Mulberries	
	Lemons	Pears	
	Limes	Pomegranates	
	Papayas		
	Peaches		
	Plums		
	Raspberries		
	Kiwi		

highest sugar content of all fruit, and should be eaten sparingly. Also, berries are susceptible to mold, so make sure they are very fresh and well washed.

Some people do not tolerate fruit well. It may create gas. If that is the case, you may need to avoid fruit altogether in the first four weeks of phase one. To reduce gas, eat fruits alone, separate from other foods. It also often helps to eat your fruit first thing in the morning. If gas production persists, eliminate fruit entirely and then try reintroducing it a few weeks later during phase two.

Foods to Avoid During Phase One

Some foods have a tendency to contribute to overgrowth of the yeast *Candida albicans* (like sugar, yeast, or fermented foods), or to the deterioration of health either because they are high in harmful food additives or because they are allergenic foods. Table 13.4 on page 327 lists these most common foods. Avoid these foods during phase one. Some of these foods will be reintroduced back into your diet during phase two. (An occasional indulgence is fine for most people, but some find it easier to eliminate these foods altogether feeling that it is sometimes easier to make a clean break from bad habits.)

Table 13.4. Foods to Avoid During Phase One

FOOD TO AVOID	COMMENTS
Alcoholic beverages, including beer, brandy, gin, rum, whiskey, wine, or any other fermented or aged liquors or liqueurs	If you wish, you may drink a small amount of vodka, but limit it to no more than two drinks per week. Alcohol is difficult for the body to metabolize, and stresses the liver, kidneys, pancreas, and intestines—the very organs you are trying to rejuvenate.
Baked goods, including rolls, bread, coffee cakes, and pastries	Avoid all raised baked goods that contain yeast, wheat, enriched flour, and/or hydrogenated fats.
Dairy products, including milk, yogurt, cheese, and cottage cheese	Avoid all dairy products, including cheeses.
Fruits, including oranges, tangerines, pineapples, grapes, and all melons (including watermelon, cantaloupe, and honey-dew), as well as all fruit juice	The fruits listed here tend to contain molds or yeast and/or have a high-sugar content.
Dried and canned fruit	These are generally too high in simple sugars and may contain sulfites.
Fungi	This category includes all types of edible mushrooms and truffles.
Hydrogenated oils and saturated fats, including margarine, shortening, palm oil, lard, animal fat, and any other oil that is hydrogenated or partially hydrogenated	These are undesirable fats that have been associated with elevated cholesterol and increased cancer risk. These fats will not build healthy cells. (Read ingredient labels carefully.)
Malt Products, including cereals and candies and malt beverages	Malt is a kiln-dried, sprouted grain. It is used in many beverages and processed foods.
Some meats and fish, including ham, all pickled meats, smoked meats, smoked fish, sausages, hot dogs, luncheon meats, corned beef, pastrami, pickled tongue, and pickled herring	Some meats and fish are cured or pickled with nitrates and nitrites. Other foods listed here may be difficult for the body to digest when detoxifying.
Nuts, including peanuts, cashews, chestnuts, hazelnuts, pecans, pine nuts, and walnuts	Avoid all nuts and seeds that are roasted in oil or that have high mold content.
Refined sugar and sugar-containing foods, including all desserts, ice cream, candy, and soda, that contains any of the following sugars: sucrose, dextrose, fructose, maltose, lactose, glucose, mannitol, sorbitol, honey, molasses, maple syrup, date sugar, brown sugar, and turbinado sugar	Simple sugars release glucose too quickly into the bloodstream and when overeaten cause a host of health problems described in this book.
Wheat, including all wheat breads, rolls, pastas, and cereals	Avoid all wheat, whether refined or whole grains.
Yeast, including baker's yeast and brewer's yeast	Avoid all foods whose preparation includes yeast.

A Sample Seven-Day Eating Plan for Phase-One

There are many ways to approach the phase-one eating program. The best approach is to rotate foods, eating no one food more often than every four days. Many people eat the same foods over and over, which results in anxiety, boredom, and viewing this eating plan as a diet, instead of as an interim way of life. More important, rotating foods helps prevent the possible development of food allergies. And of course, the variety also naturally provides a wider range of nutrients.

To help get you started, I have put together the following seven-day sample menu. It rotates your foods and follows the recommended number of servings from each food group. Feel free to mix and match foods as you like during phase one as long as you avoid the foods listed in Table 13.4 and follow the serving sizes from the five food groups. If you have trouble with weight loss or sustaining energy, shift to using a protein shake with flaxseed meal for breakfast (see page 332 for recipes).

DAY 1

Breakfast: 1 poached egg, and 1 slice yeast-free bread with 1 teaspoon of olive oil and butter mixture spread

Lunch: 4 cups salad greens topped with a half cup of garbanzo beans, a small handful of nuts or seeds, and 1 tablespoon of salad dressing

Snack: Two fruit servings, such as three-quarters cup of blueberries and three-quarters cup cherries, anytime during the day.

Dinner: 6-ounces of baked, grilled, or pan-fried chicken with light spray of olive oil and seasonings, 1 small or a half of a large baked potato with 1 teaspoon of butter, 2 cups of steamed broccoli, and 1 cup of raw celery and carrots

> ***Nutritional content:*** *1,235 calories; 125 grams carbohydrate; 87 grams protein, (49 grams from animal protein); and 43 grams fat*

DAY 2

Breakfast: A half cup of oat bran or other whole grain, wheat-free, low-sugar cereal or 1 small oat-bran muffin sweetened with unrefined sugar, with a hard-boiled egg and a cup of hot tea

Lunch: 3 cups of vegetables, stir-fried with 2 ounces of lean beef (use 1 teaspoon of oil for stir-fry), two small kiwis, sliced

Snack: 1 small apple

Dinner: 4-ounces of roasted turkey breast, 1 cup of sweet potato with 4 cups of salad greens (2 tablespoons of salad dressing), and 1 cup of green beans (cooked to taste) sprinkled with a half ounce of slivered almonds

> ***Nutritional content:*** *1,210 calories; 122 grams carbohydrate; 79 grams protein (49 grams from animal protein); and 45 grams fat*

DAY 3

Breakfast: Mixed fruit bowl ($^3/_4$ cup of blueberries and 1 cup of strawberries or $^3/_4$ cup of blackberries), sprinkled with a half ounce of sunflower seeds, and 1 cup coffee or tea (use a coffee substitute such as chicory if drinking more than one cup of coffee daily)

Lunch: 3 cups of mixed steamed vegetables with 1 teaspoon of butter and $^1/_2$ cup of adzuki beans

Snack: 10 cherries

Dinner: 1 cup of couscous, 7 ounces of buffalo meat seasoned to taste, 1 cup of cooked carrots, 3 cups of salad greens with 1 cup of sliced radishes and celery and 2 tablespoons of salad dressing

> **Nutritional content:** *1,271 Calories; 137 grams carbohydrate; 84 grams protein, (49 grams from animal protein); and 43 grams fat*

DAY 4

Breakfast: Three-quarters cup of millet flake cereal with 4 ounces of soymilk and 1 cup of strawberries

Lunch: 1 large bowl of beef vegetable soup and 3 cups of salad with 1 tablespoon of salad dressing and three yeast-free sesame-rye crackers

Snack: 1 medium pear

Dinner: 2 cups of steamed vegetables, and 5 ounces of baked orange roughy dotted with a half teaspoon of clarified butter, seasoned and baked, 2 cups of salad greens topped with a half ounce of nuts or seeds and 2 tablespoons of salad dressing

> **Nutritional content:** *1,285 calories; 141 grams carbohydrate; 90 grams protein (52 grams from animal protein); and 40 grams fat*

DAY 5

Breakfast: 1 celery stalk cut into sections stuffed with 1 ounce of almond butter and a fresh fruit and vegetable drink prepared with a juicer. (For recipe, see "Option 2 Morning Drink" below.)

Lunch: Bowl of chili made with 3 ounces of ground beef with 2 to 3 cups of romaine or spring-mix greens and 2 tablespoons of salad dressing

Snack: 1 medium peach

Dinner: 4 ounces of baked cod, seasoned to taste, with 1 cup of rice salad made with chopped tomatoes, green onions, basil, lemon juice, and seasonings, and 1 cup of cole slaw made with 1 tablespoon of low-fat mayonnaise, salt, and pepper.

> **Nutritional content:** *1,300 calories; 121 grams carbohydrate; 86 grams protein (49 grams from animal protein); 55 grams fat*

DAY 6

Breakfast: Half a large grapefruit, 2 ounces of tuna with 1 tablespoon of low-fat mayonnaise, chopped celery, and onions on 2 yeast-free rye crackers

Lunch: Caesar salad or a large salad with 3 to 4 cups salad greens with one grilled chicken breast and 2 tablespoons of low-fat salad dressing

Snack: 2 small plums and a small handful of pistachio nuts

Dinner: 5 ounces of grilled steak with 1 cup of lima beans, 2 cups of sautéed zucchini with stewed tomatoes, and 1 cup of salad with 1 tablespoon of salad dressing

Nutritional content: 1,400 calories; 122 grams carbohydrate; 111 grams protein (70 grams from animal protein); and 52 grams fat

DAY 7

Breakfast: 1 egg topped with 1 cup of fresh spinach and $\frac{1}{4}$ cup chopped onion sautéed in 1 teaspoon of ghee, and $\frac{1}{2}$ cup cranberry juice diluted with water

Snack: One-half to one ounce of sunflower seeds

Lunch: Chef's salad made with 4 cups of lettuce greens, 1 ounce of turkey, 1 ounce roast beef, including cut-up vegetables, such as celery, cucumber, and carrots with 2 tablespoons of low-fat salad dressing, and 1 cup of potato salad

Dinner: Lamb kabobs made with 4 ounces of lamb, tomato, onion, and green peppers with 2 cups of Bibb lettuce salad and 2 tablespoons fat-free salad dressing and 1 pear, sliced

Nutritional content: 1,200 calories; 123 grams carbohydrate; 79 grams protein (49 grams from animal protein); 41 grams fat

An additional serving of a half cup of complex carbohydrates, two ounces of meat, and 5 grams of fat adds 235 calories to each of the suggested phase-one menus. An additional serving of fruit adds another 60 calories.

It is extremely important to make sure that the added fats in these menus are from sources that provide plenty of omega-3 fatty acids in the proper balance with omega-6 fatty acids. Omega-6 fats are usually abundant in the diet because they are found in commonly used vegetable oils such as corn oil, safflower oil, sunflower oil, soybean oil, and in animal proteins, especially those that are grain fed (beef, chicken, and fish). Canola oil and flaxseed oil are sources of omega-3 fatty acids; however, neither of these oils should be used for cooking as heat causes rancidity in these oils. (Flaxseed oil is particularly prone to rancidity from heat and light, and should be stored in the refrigerator.) Although using canola or flaxseed oils in homemade salad dressings helps to increase your omega-3 fatty acid intake, it does not appreciably contribute to EPA and DHA levels.

Unsaturated oils do not tolerate high temperatures well because they are easily oxidized at high temperatures. Olive oil is the best oil to use when cooking with oil.

Saturated fats do not oxidize when heated in cooking, so they are a good choice for cooking. While the milk solids in butter will scorch at high temperatures, clarified butter, also called ghee, is an excellent choice for cooking because the milk solids have been removed. You can purchase clarified butter, or follow the directions below to make it yourself at home:

1. Melt 2 pounds of organic butter in a pan over low heat. Do not let it burn. Decrease the heat slightly if the liquid starts to smoke or show signs of scorching.

2. Cook over low heat for approximately one hour. You will notice milk solids sinking and foam at the top. Avoid stirring while the solids are separating.

3. Remove pan from heat and leave the liquid to cool for approximately 15 minutes.

4. Carefully skim foam or floating substances off the top. Filter the remaining clear liquid into a clean white jar, using cheesecloth or a coffee filter. Your finished product will have a rich golden color and buttery aroma. It will solidify somewhat, but will not be hard.

5. Covered and stored in a refrigerator, it will keep indefinitely.

Remember, it is still considered best to moderate your intake of saturated fats, so use butter and ghee in moderation.

It is important to eat three meals a day. Eating in the morning is extremely important as it breaks your night-long fast—thus the word "breakfast." Studies show that eating breakfast jump-starts your metabolism for the day. When you skip the morning meal, your metabolism stays at its lower morning rate all day. Taking time to eat a small morning meal gets your metabolism going and helps you burn more calories throughout the day.

Non-breakfast eaters also tend to be overweight. If you are not a breakfast eater, you are probably like the many people I see who feel that they "just don't have an appetite in the morning" or they "just can't eat." You don't have to accept this as your natural state. There are ways you can build up an appetite in the morning. Start by eating just a few nibbles of food—for example, a few nuts, a half a piece of fruit, or even some tuna salad on a cracker. At first you may not feel like eating even this, but force yourself. As your stomach gets used to having food in it at this time of day, your appetite in the morning will increase. Also, reducing late-night snacks increases your fasting time and will usually cause you to wake up hungrier.

For people on the run, protein drinks are a good breakfast option. I am a big advocate for starting the day with a protein drink. Protein drinks made from whey, rice, or pea protein are satisfying and prevent carbohydrate cravings throughout the day. Here are two options for morning drinks. They can also be used during phase one.

OPTION 1 MORNING DRINK

20–30 grams protein from a low-carbohydrate protein powder
Strawberries or other berries equal to 1 fruit serving
4–6 ounces soy, rice, or almond milk (organic cow's milk may be substituted in phase two, if well tolerated)
1–2 tablespoons flaxseed meal

Combine all of the ingredients in a blender. Blend for approximately one minute or until the powder is well mixed.

OPTION 2 MORNING DRINK

2 carrots
One-half beet
2 celery stalks
1 apple or 10 strawberries
One-half parsnip or small zucchini

Wash your fruits and vegetables well. Leave on peel, but remove any bad spots. Cut off stems, slice fruits and vegetables, and put into juicer.

Cookbooks for Inspiration

Bookstores stock a variety of whole-food cookbooks that you can put to good use in your kitchen. When preparing a dish, be sure to substitute acceptable ingredients if necessary, especially during phase one. Look for cookbooks with key words such as "no refined sugars," "dairy-free," "gluten-free," "low carbohydrate," and "low fat" on their covers. The cookbooks listed below are highly recommended and can help ease the challenge of giving up tastes to which you are accustomed.

• *A Celebration of Wellness: A Cookbook for Vibrant Living—Over 300 Heart Healthy, No Dairy, No Cholesterol, Nonfat and Lowfat Inspired Recipes* by Natalie Cederquist and James Levin, M.D. (Avery Penguin Putnam, 1998)

• *Guilt-Free Indulgence: A Cookbook with a Conscience* by Cheri Percival, Mark Percival D.C., N.D., and Eric Blais, N.D. (Health Coach System International, 6th Ed., 1995)

• *Sweet and Natural: Desserts without Sugar, Honey, Molasses, or Artificial Sweeteners* by Janet Warrington (Crossing Press, 1985)

• *The Yeast Connection Cookbook: A Guide to Good Nutrition and Better Health* by William G. Crook, M.D. and Marjorie Hurt Jones, R.N. (Professional Books, Rev., 1989)

Freshly made juices provide a wide range of healthful nutrients. There are many different combinations of fruits and vegetables that taste great. Check out some of the available juicing books and try different recipes to find something that is right for you.

PHASE TWO

Once you begin to notice that your health is improving (typically in four to six weeks on phase one) and that you are losing weight, regaining control of your blood sugar, and getting rid of gastrointestinal problems, you may start reintroducing some of the restricted foods you eliminated during phase one. However, any foods to which you are intolerant will trigger an immune response and will tend to have an inflammatory effect in your body. Eating these foods will keep your metabolism out of balance, so continue to avoid them. Also, there are some foods that you should continue to avoid as much as possible all through life even if you're not allergic to them, including the following:

- **Hydrogenated and partially hydrogenated oils**—Foods with hydrogenated or partially hydrogenated oils will never support good health. It is not a matter of whether you as an individual can tolerate them; these foods are very bad for health.

- **Refined sugars from cakes, cookies, sodas, ice cream, and candies and other sweetened packaged foods such as breakfast cereals**—Refined sugars and foods containing them will only throw metabolism out of balance if eaten too often. They should never be eaten more than occasionally, and only by those who have corrected blood sugar imbalances and realkalinized their body with minerals. We'll discuss the importance of alkalinity in the body later in this chapter.

- **Excessive intake of carbohydrates**—Carbohydrate foods, especially those from the bread and cereal group like bread, rolls, and pasta should be eaten in moderation. Like sugar, an excess intake of carbohydrates contributes to chronically raised blood sugar levels. If carbohydrates are from whole-food sources, the fiber and mineral content will moderate that effect. However, there are some people who will probably never tolerate even whole grains in anything other than small amounts. Implementing phase two will help you establish what your optimum intake level will be.

Although both fruits and vegetables contain carbohydrates, the carbohydrate content of vegetables is very low and is well balanced by fiber and vitamins and minerals, which will moderate their effects. Fruits, on the other hand, have much higher carbohydrate content than vegetables, and even though they contain fiber and vitamins and minerals as well, they should be eaten moderately. The guideline I use is one fruit for every three vegetables. If you are eating nine servings of vegetables a day, eat no more than three servings of fruit.

- **Meats and fish with added nitrates/nitrites**—Most lunch meats, hot dogs, and smoked fish have nitrates or nitrites added. In the body, nitrates and nitrites are converted to nitrosamines, which are known to be carcinogenic. Also, nitrates and nitrites can bond with hemoglobin, rendering it unable to carry oxygen. Smoked and cured foods also contain nitrosamines, and should be avoided.

- **Undiluted fruit juices**—Fruit juices should be consumed minimally, and only if diluted with equal parts of water. Juices have almost no fiber content, but have a very high carbohydrate content, and their effect on blood sugar is substantial. Use them to flavor water as a treat.

Reintroducing Foods During Phase Two

There is no particular order to follow when deciding which foods to reintroduce into your diet. You can start by reintroducing the food you have missed the most. (Be aware, however, that foods that you ate most often are usually the foods to which you had a food sensitivity; therefore, you may not tolerate the food very well on the first try.)

It is best to reintroduce only one food every two to three days. Introducing more than one food every two to three days will make it virtually impossible to determine which food may have caused a reaction, if any. Keep a daily log of every food you eat. Observe your body carefully and pay attention to any reaction and how you feel.

Begin by eating a serving of food from one of the categories of foods that are eliminated in phase one, for example, a slice of whole-wheat bread. (See Table 13.4 for foods to avoid during phase one.) Then, for the next forty-eight to seventy-two hours observe your body for any symptoms of intolerance, such as abdominal cramping, gas, diarrhea, headaches, or even a runny nose. If you display any symptoms, you should eliminate the food once again, in this case wheat, for another two to four weeks. If you try this cycle a number of times, and eating wheat still causes symptoms, you know that this is a food you may need to eliminate completely or cut back on significantly. Repeat this process for each of the following foods you eliminated during phase one to find out your level of tolerance to them.

- *Whole grains.* Make sure the product you choose for reintroduction is truly made from whole grains. The label of a whole-grain bread will usually state "100 percent whole grain." If wheat flour is listed as an ingredient, but the label does not say "whole-wheat" flour, the bread contains refined white flour, not whole-wheat flour. (Manufacturers may call refined flour "wheat flour" because it does come from wheat.) Normally, white flour is listed in the ingredients as "enriched wheat flour." Sometimes companies use unbleached wheat flour, which is a little better than regular flour because it is not chemically bleached, but neither is it whole grain. You will be able to tell the difference in a "true" whole-grain bread, because the loaves feel heavy compared with other breads. Some people find it easier to eat whole-grain breads toasted.

To determine wheat sensitivity, however, it is best to eat 100 percent whole-wheat crackers or flat bread rather than a mixed-grain bread or whole-wheat bread with yeast. This way, if you get symptoms from eating it, you know for certain the reaction is to wheat and not to the yeast or another grain. If bloating or allergic symptoms occur, you may also be sensitive to gluten, in which case you may always have to avoid this family of grains. Natural food stores carry a large selection of wheat-free and gluten-free breads, crackers, and cookies. There are also many Internet resources for these foods.

If after several tries, you can once again tolerate whole wheat, it is still best not to overeat it. Try not to rely on wheat as your primary source of bread and pasta. Continue to select alternative grain products and pasta made from artichoke, rice, soy, corn, spelt, and quinoa flour and to rotate these and other grains throughout your diet regularly to avoid developing or redeveloping a sensitivity to wheat. It is also acceptable to occasionally have regular (non-whole-grain) pasta.

Again, be careful not to revert back to excessive carbohydrate use. One or two pieces of bread a day for five out of seven days is a good guideline, especially if you are not trying to lose weight. You might find that you need to increase your carbohydrate intake as you begin to incorporate exercise into your lifestyle. Contracting muscles use carbohydrates as their source of fuel—one incentive to begin an exercise program! As you use the nine keys and overcome insulin resistance, you may be able to increase the number of servings of high-carbohydrate foods.

- *Dairy.* When reintroducing dairy, begin with plain yogurt, cottage cheese, goat cheese, or sheep's milk cheese in limited quantities, as long as bloating, gastrointestinal upset, sinus congestion, or increased mucus production does not occur. Hard and soft whole-milk cheeses such as cheddar cheese, Colby cheese, Swiss cheese, and mozzarella should never be consumed in large amounts. They are very high in fat, are acid-forming, and can be constipating. Some people may never be able to tolerate dairy products well, especially plain cow's milk. Be conservative in your milk intake—especially if the above symptoms start to occur.

  Here is an example of how dairy products count in your daily servings: 1 ounce of cheese counts as one protein serving and one fat serving; an 8-ounce glass of 2 percent milk counts as one carbohydrate serving, one protein serving, and one fat serving; 1 percent milk or skim (fat-free) milk counts as one carbohydrate serving and one protein serving. Use organic sources when possible.

- *Sweeteners.* Natural sweeteners such as agave nectar, brown rice syrup, date sugar, honey, maple syrup, molasses, and granulated sugar cane (Sucanat) and cane juice may be introduced sparingly from 1 to 4 teaspoons weekly. Watch closely for effects on blood sugar. Stevia and xylitol are other natural sweeteners that are a good alternative and which have very minimal effect on blood sugar, if any.

- **Condiments.** The following pickled and vinegar-containing condiments can be used in moderation: ketchup, mustard, mayonnaise, soy, tamari, vinegar, olives, pickles, and similar foods. Since condiments are usually used in smaller amounts, they are often well tolerated when reintroduced. However, some people may be especially sensitive to substances in these foods. For instance, people who have an overgrowth of *Candida* may have an increased sensitivity to vinegar and vinegar-containing foods. Also, up to 30 percent of the population is especially sensitive to glutamates, metal compounds found in the amino acid glutamic acid. Glutamates are formed during the fermentation process that is used to make bouillons, miso, and soy sauce. They cause headaches and are neural toxins.

- **Fungi.** Mushrooms, including maitake and shiitake, truffles, and medicinal mushrooms can now be added back to the diet, but watch closely for any signs of sensitivity. If you have no signs of reaction, fungi can be included regularly in your diet.

Follow the phase-two program with the reincorporated foods mentioned above—wheat and dairy (to tolerance), condiments, mushrooms, and healthy sweeteners (in moderation)—until your health has improved quite a bit and has stabilized. Once this has occurred, you can begin to reincorporate the fruits and nuts listed on page 327. As always, add foods one at a time (one food every two or three days) and watch for any reactions. If a food tends to cause symptoms, eat it occasionally or not at all.

During phase two, you can also begin to increase your calorie intake, but only if you have accomplished your weight goal. Experiment by gradually increasing calories from high-carbohydrate foods such as potatoes, whole grains, and cereals, to find the maximum amount of calories you can consume while still feeling energetic and maintaining your ideal weight and without triggering blood-sugar disturbances.

Follow your customized phase-two program for several weeks. If you start to regain weight, you may have added too many carbohydrates back into your diet or you may be eating too many foods to which you were sensitive. Cutting back on these foods should help stabilize your weight. Also, cut back or eliminate added sweeteners, which should only be unrefined at this point anyway. At any time, if you need to lose extra weight, go back to following the phase-one guidelines.

Let's be honest, people want an occasional dessert. When you have followed phase two for several weeks and feel you have attained equilibrium with the reincorporated foods, you can begin to add in an occasional dessert or sweet—a small piece of cake or pie. As long as you eat desserts and candy only occasionally, you should not gain weight or become insulin resistant. What is occasionally? Well, that depends on portion size. You can eat small portions one time a week—for example, one scoop of ice cream, a small piece of cake or pie, or a cookie. If you want to eat a whole ice cream sundae or a normal-size piece of pie à la mode, do not eat more than one serving each month. Strive to choose healthy versions of these foods, that is, desserts and sweets made with natural ingredients rather than processed products containing refined sugars and partially hydrogenated oils.

The Healthy Living Guidelines present a way of eating that supports good health, energy, and vitality into old age. However, for most people, this will be a very different way of eating. Because you were probably not raised on an eating plan such as this one, you will tend to get hungry for the foods that you grew up on or that you'd become accustomed to eating, such as mashed potatoes and gravy, chicken pot pie, or snacks chips, sometimes called "comfort foods." For almost any food, there is a healthier version available. You can modify recipes by substituting healthier ingredients, and you can find premade healthier versions of many foods, such as pizza or chicken pot pie, in the natural foods section of your supermarket.

For those of you who have a very hard time adjusting to this new way of eating, a popular survival technique is to eat according to the Healthy Living Guidelines six days a week, and on the seventh day, eat whatever you want for one meal. Eventually, cravings for "cheating" meals will begin to dwindle, simply because you will feel worse after eating them. If you know you can eat whatever you want for that one meal, it can help you get through the healthy days until you begin to enjoy them more than the unhealthy foods. Continue to strive to incorporate whole-food alternatives into your diet and lifestyle so that you can benefit from the nutrition these foods provide.

Some people will not be able to tolerate a "cheating" meal until they have followed the phase-two guidelines for several months. These are people who had a severely imbalanced intestinal terrain. You will know if you are one of these people if you develop a lot of symptoms after eating restricted foods. For those of you who fall into this category, I encourage you to hang in there. Sticking to the Healthier Living Guidelines is better than going back to your old eating habits and feeling miserable every day. Although it may take a while, you should eventually progress enough to occasionally enjoy some restricted foods. Your "occasionally" may be different from the next person's "occasionally." It may be as often as once every two weeks or as seldom as once a month. That is the point of following the phase-one and phase-two programs—to help you determine your level of tolerance with each food and with how often you can eat it, if at all.

You may find that you feel so well with your new way of eating that you won't ever want to eat sweets, snack chips, or other restricted foods again. You may not even understand other people's needs to eat these foods even occasionally. To you, I say congratulations and keep up the good work!

COMBINING THE HEALTHY LIVING GUIDELINES
WITH SENSIBLE EATING HABITS

The following suggestions will help improve your digestion and nutrient absorption, as well as make eating a more pleasurable experience overall.

Do not use refrigerated leftovers after two days. Mold begins to grow on most foods after a couple of days. Freezing preserves most foods up to a month.

Eat a variety of foods. Variety ensures a broad intake of nutrients and phytochemicals, helps prevent food allergies, and staves off boredom.

Rotate the foods you eat. Too many people eat the same foods over and over. Food rotation helps prevent food allergies that can develop, and again, variety also provides more sources of nutrients. Expand your taste for new foods. Be open to change. For example, experimenting with different oils and spices is a great way to change and enhance the flavor of your foods.

Avoid prepackaged foods. Try to eat fresh foods whenever possible. Many times, prepackaged foods contain additives, preservatives, hidden sugars, and low-quality fats. Most prepackaged foods are cooked until sterile. Because of this, most of the enzymes that were present in the food are destroyed. My mentor, Dr. Alexander Wood, always said, "Eat foods that spoil, just eat them before they do." It is so true. Foods that spoil are foods that support life. However, there are some quality prepackaged foods that you can buy at food stores that can help your busy schedule. Also, some restaurants are now providing fresh or frozen, healthy take-home entrees (low salt, low fat, low sugar) that are also preservative free.

Wash fruits and vegetables before eating. To remove pesticide residue, fill a sink with water, add a tablespoon of apple cider vinegar, a small amount of dish soap, or a special fruit and vegetable wash, and fill with produce. Soak for twenty minutes, then rinse well. Also, there are a variety of produce washes on the market. Whenever possible, buy produce that has been grown organically without the use of insecticides, herbicides, artificial fertilizers, or genetically engineered organisms. However, it is still a good idea to wash even organic fruits and vegetables because of other possible pathogens from soil or human hands that have handled them.

Opt for natural sweeteners. Sweeteners that are acceptable include agave nectar, brown rice syrup, date sugar, honey, maple syrup, molasses, and granulated sugar cane (Sucanat) and cane juice, stevia, and xylitol, but use them sparingly. They can be used in baking. You can also use fruits such as apples and raisins to help sweeten baked goods. Stevia is a natural flavoring agent that adds a sweet taste. Xylitol is a natural sweetener that tastes very much like sugar and also bakes well. I have found it to be much more appealing than stevia, and it actually helps with blood sugar and fights dental caries. It does not induce a spike in blood sugar and has been used in foods commercially for years. It recently became available for purchase by consumers in natural foods stores.

Limit portion size. The issue of portion size is one of the most important factors in diet. "Biggie" sizing has become epidemic in America. It may be of benefit to the businesses that offer this option, but all it does for the average person is cause weight gain. People are also increasing portions at home. By following the Healthy Living Guidelines, you will be eating a diet higher in fiber and nutrient content. Most people will naturally begin to reduce portion size when they eat this way.

Chew your food. Chew food thoroughly before swallowing. This is the most important part of digestion. If you do not chew your food well, your body cannot extract the nutrients it needs from the food. You also will find that you will eat less if you take your time.

Drink a wide range of healthful beverages. Good beverage choices include vegetable juices, water, carbonated water (in moderation), diluted fruit juices, tea, herbal teas, soymilk, rice milk, and almond milk. One or two cups of coffee per day is acceptable, if tolerated and desired.

Drink water. Water is your most valuable drink. You should drink six to eight 8-ounce glasses per day. Our bodies are made up mostly of water. It is needed for cleansing all tissues. A purifying system that uses reverse osmosis water is best, but some kind of filtered water is a must. If you are interested in water systems for your home and don't know where to start, look to our reference guide in the appendix. When you are hungry, try drinking a glass of water. Many times, the body's signals of thirst are felt as hunger. Drinking water can often alleviate a feeling of hunger and prevent unnecessary snacking.

Drink most fluids alone. Drink the majority of your fluids without food. Try to drink less with meals and more between meals. You may dilute the acids and enzymes needed for proper food digestion.

Limit snacks. Snacks may be eaten as needed, but avoid overindulging in high-carbohydrate foods. Look for the healthier alternatives to many snack foods (no hydrogenated oils or refined sugars) such as potato chips, tortilla chips, and cookies. Snacks can be substituted for one of your grain servings to keep your calorie level constant or can be eaten occasionally in addition to your grain servings. Limiting snacks is one way to avoid weight gain from excessive calorie intake.

Consider your individual needs. Remember that activity level, individual metabolism, and specific problems, such as diabetes, may alter your need for food consumption. For instance, an athlete or a person who is exercising heavily will need more calories. A person with diabetes may have been given a prescription diet (for example, the

How to Dine Out and Stay Healthy

Dining out can be a challenge. Not because it is difficult to find acceptable foods, but more so because of the demands on your willpower. Foods that you will have to pass up when eating out include anything fried, most breads, and desserts. Other than these foods, eating at a sit-down restaurant can be accommodated.

Always order a large salad. Ask for the salad without cheese or ask for the cheese on the side (only if you have completed phase two and are tolerating dairy). Order the salad dressing on the side and lightly dip each bite of salad before eating. Using this method you usually won't exceed 1 or 2 tablespoons of salad dressing.

Broth-based soups are acceptable; skip cream soups because of the milk content.

Order an entrée of fish, chicken, turkey, or beef. Roasted, broiled, baked, or steamed is best. Usually gravies and sauces are not made with quality fats, so avoid them. It's okay if the fish was sautéed in butter.

Rice, beans, or potato can be a side dish. Think small, limit your portion size of the starchy foods to a half cup (take the rest home for another meal). And always order at least another steamed or cooked vegetable if possible—green beans, carrots, asparagus, broccoli, and cauliflower blends are usually available.

1,800-calorie ADA diet) from their doctor. A person who is following a specific diet for medical reasons should not change their diet without consulting their doctor.

De-stress. Spend fifteen minutes each day doing something that you enjoy and that helps to reduce stress in your life.

Enjoy and give thanks. Take pleasure in food and give thanks for each meal. Eat in a pleasant state of mind. Digestion will improve, and the meal will be relaxing.

THE IMPORTANCE OF ALKALINE FOODS

The Healthy Living Guidelines are designed to address several important dietary considerations. One extremely important issue that has not yet been discussed is that the human body is greatly affected by the pH levels our food choices have on our blood and interstitial fluids (lymph and other fluid that bathes our cells). The body's pH, or acid-alkaline balance, must be kept within a limited range to maintain the body's delicate balance.

Many organs and systems, especially the kidneys, adrenals, and lungs, play important roles in maintaining proper pH. In fact, the pH of the blood must be maintained at 7.4. If not maintained at that level, it can be fatal. Our cells just don't function well in an acidic environment. Energy production is affected, and therefore, so is every cellular function. Fluid balance is also greatly affected by the body's acid-alkaline balance. So, the body will go to great lengths to maintain the proper pH level.

Do not order pasta (unless it is non-wheat) until you have completed phase two, are at your ideal weight, and have successfully reincorporated occasional wheat foods. Sandwiches will not generally be an option because of the bun or bread.

If you are eating out with friends who choose an Italian restaurant, stick to soup and salad along with protein if you don't like the non-pasta choices. Chinese or other Asian restaurants are generally good choices because of the wide variety of vegetables they offer. Avoid the white rice, sweet and sour sauces, which are high in sugar, and any fried foods, however. Mexican restaurants are another option if you limit the portion of the beans and rice, and if they have corn tortilla shells available. Again, no wheat-flour tortillas. Taco salads are generally loaded with very high-fat meat and cheeses, so avoid them.

It is virtually impossible to find healthy foods at fast-food restaurants. If you do choose to eat at a fast-food restaurant, order a salad if one is offered. A grilled chicken breast sandwich is also acceptable. Remove the bun, and eat the plain chicken along with your salad.

When dining out, it's perfectly acceptable to partake in an occasional glass of red wine, if you wish.

The pH scale goes from 0 to 14, with 0 being the most acidic and 14 being the most alkaline (or basic). An element with a pH of 7, water for example, is neutral. The cells of the body in a state of health are slightly alkaline and vary between 7 to 7.4. In a disease state, the pH moves below 7.0, resulting in a more acidic environment.

Although our body fluids must be alkaline, the metabolic processes of the body produce a great deal of acid. As such, the body's buffering systems are called upon to neutralize the acids to maintain an alkaline pH. Alkaline minerals in their salt forms are used to neutralize the acids of metabolism. If the body fluids begin to run low on these minerals, they can be pulled from tissues where they are stored in the cells. Potassium salts are extracted from the muscles, leaving them in what is sometimes called an acid-contracted state. Sodium salts are used up, weakening digestive processes. Calcium salts are extracted from bones and teeth. In fact, chronic low-grade metabolic acidity is thought by many health professionals to be a major contributor to osteoporosis, and urologists have long known the connection between metabolic acidity and kidney stones. Yet, even though many doctors are aware of this problem, which is called *metabolic acidosis,* most practitioners do not usually acknowledge it until it is in an advanced stage. Most of these practitioners are also unaware of the many effects of chronic low-grade acidosis.

What are the major contributors to a chronic low-grade acidosis? Diet and dysbiosis. The American diet consists mostly of acid-forming foods and is low in alkaline-forming foods. The primary acid-forming foods are meats, dairy foods, grains, sugar, and refined foods. Fruits and vegetables, which contain an abundance of mineral salts necessary to help neutralize metabolic acids, are the primary alkaline-forming foods. The average American diet consists of 20 to 30 percent alkaline foods.

A diet high in animal protein, sugar, caffeine, and processed foods disrupts healthy pH balance. This unbalanced diet pushes the body toward an acid state and depletion of calcium and other alkalinizing minerals from the blood and tissues.

Ideally, the diet should contain moderate amounts of acid-forming foods with enough alkaline-forming foods to supply the minerals needed to prevent metabolic acidosis. Estimates vary regarding how much acid-forming food can be tolerated by the body. Conservative estimates say the diet should be composed of about 35 percent acid-forming foods and 65 percent alkaline-forming foods.

Phases one and two of the Healthy Living Guidelines contain more than adequate levels of fruit and vegetable servings to preserve the alkalinity of the body. Most people are surprised to find the return of energy while following the guidelines. Returning your body to the alkaline state it was intended to operate in is one of the primary reasons why such energy and vitality is regained. If you are finding it difficult to eat the recommended amount of vegetables in the guidelines, I urge you to research the importance of an alkaline diet to health.

You can also monitor the pH of your body with pH test strips that can be purchased at most pharmacies. Put the strip in your mouth and soak it with some saliva, and compare the color of it to the chart on the test-strip packaging. It is best to check pH first thing in the morning after drinking a small amount of water (two or three small sips), but before drinking any other beverage. The pH of saliva in the morning should be between 7.0 and 7.4.

You can also check urinary pH. Urine pH will be slightly acidic in the morning due to the clearing of acids that occurs during sleep. However, a urinary pH between 6.0 and 7.0 will indicate that the body is adequately alkaline.

A food is considered acid or alkaline not based on the pH of the food, but on the effect it produces in the body. This is referred to as the ash value of a food—meaning the type of residue that occurs in the body after the food is digested and processed. For example, oranges and other citrus fruits are acidic in pH themselves, but they produce an alkaline effect in the body. Because the body is an alkaline entity, in order to maintain health, the majority of our diet must consist of alkaline ash foods.

If we become too alkaline by eating a majority of alkaline foods, a loss of appetite will result. Fasting will cause an eventual buildup of the normal acid metabolic byproducts and will return the body' s pH back to normal.

Considering the acid to alkaline imbalance inherent in the American diet, it is no wonder that so many of us are unable to maintain good health and vitality. In fact, it is not uncommon for a person in this country to go several days without eating *any* fruits and vegetables, the alkaline foods. Table 13.5 provides a list of the most common foods that help to maintain an alkaline pH.

Table 13.5. Acid and Alkaline Food Chart

ALKALINE FRUITS		ACID FRUITS	
Apples/cider	Loquats	Blueberries	Olives (pickled)
Apricots	Mangoes	Canned fruit with sugar (all)	Plums
Avocados	Melons (all)	Cranberries	Pomegranates
Bananas	Nectarines*	Dried-sulphured fruit (all)	Preserves (all)
Berries (most)	Olives (ripe)	Glazed fruit (all)	Prunes
Cantaloupe	Oranges		
Carob (pod only)	Papayas		
Cherries	Passion Fruit		
Citron	Peaches		
Currants	Pears		
Dates	Persimmons*		
Figs	Pineapple* (fresh)		
Grapes	Raisins		
Grapefruit	Raspberries*		
Guavas	Tamarind		
Kumquats	Tangerines*		
Lemons (ripe)	Tomatoes		
Limes**	(fully ripened)		
ALKALINE VEGETABLES		**ACID VEGETABLES**	
Alfalfa sprouts	Jerusalem artichokes	Asparagus (white only) tips	Lentils (legume)
Artichokes	Kale	Beans (all dried)	Peanuts (legume)
Asparagus (green only)	Leeks	Corn	Peas
Bamboo shoots	Lettuce	Garbanzos (legume)	Soybeans**
Beans (green, lima, wax, string)	Mushrooms		
	Okra		
Beets	Onions*		
Broccoli	Oyster plant		
Brussels sprouts	Parsley		
Cabbages	Parsnips		
Carrots	Peppers (bell)		
Cauliflower	Potatoes (skin is		
Celery	best part)		
Chives	Pumpkin		
Cilantro	Radish		
Cucumber	Romaine lettuce		
Dill	Rutabagas		
Dock	Sauerkraut		
Dulse*	Spinach		
Eggplant	Sprouts		
Endive	Squash		
Escarole	Turnips		
Garlic	Watercress		
Horseradish	Yams, sweet potatoes**		

ALKALINE DAIRY		ACID DAIRY	
Acidophilus milk	Raw milk	Butter	Ice cream**
Almond milk	Whey	Cheese (all)	Margarine
Ghee	Yogurt	Cottage cheese	Milk (all, boiled,
		Cream	cooked, malted,
		Custards	dried, canned)
			Processed cheese**
ALKALINE GRAINS		**ACID GRAINS**	
Lentils (a legume)**	Wild rice	Grains and grain products (all) except quinoa	
Quinoa		and wild rice	
ALKALINE FLESH FOOD		**ACID FLESH FOOD**	
Beef juice	Bonemeal	Beef**	Lobster**
		Gelatin	Meats (all)
		Fish	Pheasant**
		Fowl	Shellfish
ALKALINE NUTS		**ACID NUTS**	
Almonds	Coconut (fresh)	Brazil nuts**	Pine nuts
Cashews	Pumpkin	Coconut (dried)	Pistachios (roasted)
Chestnuts	Sunflower seeds	Hazelnuts**	Walnuts**
		Pecans seeds*	
ALKALINE MISC.		**ACID MISC.**	
Agar	Quail eggs	Alcohol	Honey
Apple cider vinegar	Mineral water*	Aspartame	Maple syrup
Baking soda*	Molasses	Balsamic vinegar	Mayonnaise
Coffee substitutes	Most herbs	Beer**	Rice vinegar
(chicory)	Ricesyrup	Black Tea	Saccharin
Duck eggs	Sea salt*	Chicken eggs	Sugar*
Green tea	Spices	Cocoa	Tapioca
Kelp (edible)		Coffee	Tobacco
		Condiments (all)	White vinegar**
		Dressings	Wine
		Fried foods**	Yeast**

* Most alkaline producing   *** Most acid producing*

THE IMPORTANCE OF ENZYMES

No matter how well balanced and nutrient dense your whole-food diet is, it can do nothing to influence your metabolism without enzymes. Without enzymes, we would not be able to digest our foods. Without proper digestive enzyme function, nutrients cannot reach our cells.

Enzymes are catalysts for every chemical reaction that occurs in the body. A catalyst is defined as anything that lowers the metabolic energy required for a particular reaction to take place. This energy is known as the "activation energy." In living organisms, activation energy is measured in the form of heat. Without enzymes, most reactions needed to sustain a living organism could not take place at temperatures below 200°F.

Through the research of the Human Genome Project, an ongoing international collaborative project among scientists which is focused on "decoding" the genetic information within the 23 pairs of chromosomes called our *genome,* we now know that genetic expression guides the manufacturing of proteins that control enzyme functions. And enzymes literally control how the body functions.

There are three classifications of enzymes: *metabolic, digestive,* and *food-based:*

- *Metabolic enzymes* catalyze the reactions that enable life. They activate cellular processes, break down chemical byproducts, and convert food to energy among other functions.

- *Digestive enzymes* break down large food molecules, like protein, carbohydrates, and fats into smaller units that can be absorbed and utilized by the body, and are grouped into several categories. *Proteases* (or proteolytic enzymes) specifically *catabolize* (or break down) proteins, *lipases* aid in breaking down fat, and *amylases* break down carbohydrates. Without these enzymes, which are secreted by the salivary glands and pancreas, digestion of food and absorption of nutrients would be impossible. In fact, burping, bloating, constipation, and general feelings of discomfort after eating are all generally considered to be caused by digestive enzyme dysfunction.

  The digestive organs each secrete different types of enzymes, and operate under their own optimal pH. In general, they require a more acidic environment. For example, the salivary glands secrete salivary amylase, which breaks down carbohydrates. The optimal pH for this enzyme is neutral at 6.0 to 7.0. Pepsin, a protease secreted in the stomach, requires an acidic pH in the range of 1.0 to 2.0.

- *Food enzymes* are those that occur naturally in raw foods. They support the digestive process and relieve some of the burden on digestive enzymes. Food enzymes are found in all raw foods, from both plant and animal sources. Examples are papaya enzymes (papain) and *bromelain* (from the pineapple) among others. These naturally occurring enzymes are destroyed by heat and processing.

Since the modern Western diet is composed primarily of cooked foods, most of us lack a healthy intake of food enzymes. This places the burden of digestion on the digestive organs, primarily on the pancreas, which must produce the enzymes needed to digest the food we eat. In fact, studies show animals that are fed primarily cooked foods versus raw foods greatly increases the size of the animal's pancreas. According to Edward Howell, M.D., a leading authority on food enzymes, a diet that includes raw foods allows the body to dramatically improve digestion and nutrient absorption, and to concentrate on synthesizing the metabolic enzymes needed for health and healing.

Eating a diet plentiful in raw foods, as the Healthy Living Guidelines recommends, will help to take the burden off the pancreas, thereby saving the nutrients and cellular energy needed for the production of digestive enzymes for other body functions. Be sure to include some raw foods into your diet primarily in the form of fruits and vegetables. Raw fruits, salad greens, and sprouts are great sources of enzymes. (If you have a leaky gut, you may need to cook all vegetables and fruits slightly.)

LAB TESTS FOR CHECKING YOUR NUTRITIONAL STATUS

Taking supplements is a great insurance policy for your health, but many times it is helpful to first evaluate if you are low in any of the essential vitamins, minerals, or essential fatty acids, and more important, to determine how your body is using these nutrients. There are an increasing number of lab tests available to test your vitamin and mineral status. While an experienced practitioner may be able to gain some insight from a traditional panel of blood tests, blood levels are not always a good indicator of nutritional status because the body will keep blood levels of some nutrients constant at the expense of other tissues. Different practitioners will have different preferences for which tests they like to use.

There are a few cutting-edge tests that can provide insight into where you may stand in relation to your body's needs for vitamins and minerals, and amino acids. The following tests are especially valuable for gaining insight into nutritional status and the effects it may be having on the body.

SpectraCell Test

The SpectraCell test measures and assesses long-term intracellular levels and requirements of a wide range of vitamins and minerals. Unlike blood levels, which reflect only the body's present nutritional status, cellular levels reflect the body's nutritional intake over time and are able to determine the amount needed to replenish a vitamin and mineral. Identifying these deficiencies is an essential part of prevention because they influence genetics, metabolism, aging, and symptoms that may be present. Likewise, the SpectraCell test identifies the nutrients that the body is not deficient in and, therefore, that will not need to be taken in supplement form.

Organic Acid Urine Test (OAT)

The OAT test is used to assess how well your metabolism is functioning. It examines various chemicals that are produced during normal metabolism in the body and are then excreted in urine. When these chemicals are out of normal range, it is a sign that certain metabolic processes such as cellular energy production, liver detoxification, or bowel terrain may be out of balance. More than sixty metabolic intermediates are present in urine. Their levels can also provide clues as to the functioning of vitamins, minerals, amino acids, and other cofactors such as CoQ_{10}, which have a direct impact on the efficiency of cellular metabolism.

Amino Acid Profiles

Amino acid profiles indicate how well an individual utilizes their proteins. Amino acids are the building blocks of all proteins, and when certain ones are deficient it can give us clues as to where the body is using up its pool of amino acids. If you don't have a good pool of amino acids to draw from, you can't make serotonin, melatonin, dopamine, and a host of other chemical messengers that regulate your metabolism.

A WHOLESOME DIET AND LIFESTYLE ARE KEY

Now that you're well on your way to cracking your body's metabolic code, these simple food guidelines will help ensure that your nutrition requirements are met and that your cells can receive the energy they need to support your metabolism.

It takes time to retrain old habits and restructure tastes and food preferences. However, once you have completed phases one and two of the Healthy Living Guidelines, you will have already begun to reprogram your taste and food selection habits to include less fat and sugar, and more whole-food carbohydrates and lean protein. The payoff is in the way you feel.

If you find yourself slipping back into unhealthy eating or lifestyle pattern in the future, or if you feel some of your old symptoms of metabolic dysfunction returning, you may want to go back to phase one to help realign your metabolism.

Although the core of these guidelines is nutrition-oriented, you should not overlook the importance of exercise in achieving full benefit from the program. Besides the strengthening of the heart muscle and other aerobic benefits, exercising has a tremendous effect on lowering blood sugar. Many type 2 diabetics, for instance, can stop their medication simply by increasing their level of activity and watching their diet. Exercise and diet together are key to reversing insulin resistance and metabolic syndrome. Exercise has also been found to be the most important lifestyle factor in improving quality of life in old age and increasing life span. But don't underestimate the effect of the other keys on your health.

If you have any doubt as to the importance of exercise, consider these study results: In a recent study conducted at Duke University, researchers found that adults who did not exercise for eight months had an increase in visceral fat (the fat is tucked in and around our organs, in other words, abdominal or belly fat) of 8.6 percent. In contrast, the study participants who exercised the most lost 8.1 percent of their belly fat. Even the researchers were surprised at just how quickly the effects of being sedentary were seen.

While this study shows that only more vigorous exercise was effective, previous studies have shown benefits from even moderate exercise. Imagine what years of

Deanna's Story

Prior to becoming a patient of Dr. LaValle's, life was very difficult for me. I became lightheaded if I ate anything more than a very small meal, and I was extremely tired at the end of the day. Despite these problems, my husband and I decided to try and start a family. My menstrual cycles were very sporadic, which I found out was due to a small tumor in my pituitary gland that was elevating my prolactin levels (elevated prolactin increases the chances of miscarriage). I endured three miscarriages in that year. My doctor put me on a prescription drug to lower my prolactin levels, but the side effects were horrendous. I was tired from morning to night and would some-times get dizzy. I was gaining weight, and I felt moody and depressed. After moni-toring my prolactin levels, the doctor determined that my dosage was too low and would need to be increased to lower the prolactin before I could try to get pregnant again. The increased dosage would mean that I would have difficulty working due to the side effects. So, I had to start looking for other alternatives.

I called our local natural foods store to find out whether there were vitamins I could take that might help with the side effects caused by the drug if I decided to take it again. The staff recommended I call Dr. LaValle, which I did. He evaluated my entire medical history, made nutritional recommendations to support my endocrine system, detoxify my body, and rebuild my health. He recommended the appropriate supplements, including the herb Chaste berry (*Vitex agnus-castus*) which lowers pro-lactin levels, and the Healthy Living Guidelines. Almost immediately, my body began to respond. My energy levels increased. The lightheadedness at mealtimes went away. I lost weight. My menstrual cycles started becoming regular. Friends remarked that my color was improving and how healthy I was looking. The best news of all came when I found out I was pregnant. I had a very easy pregnancy, labor, and deliv-ery, and gave birth to a healthy little girl. I am extremely grateful to Dr. LaValle for his help. I have confidence that with his help I can maintain my health, continue to feel energetic, and have another healthy child!

In the past several years, I have treated at least twenty women who were having difficulty conceiving, but once they were evaluated according to the nine key metabolic principles and began to apply the Healthy Living Guidelines, they became pregnant. By balancing intestinal flora with thyroid and adrenal function, many times hormonal regulation is achieved.

inactivity have done to your body. Getting back into an exercise routine is not only good for your physical health, by leading to improved blood sugar control and weight loss for starters, but it also improves mental health. Exercising regularly helps to control stress hormones and to decrease feelings of depression, tension, and anger.

There is no best form of exercise. However, some exercises can be hard on the body. Running and step aerobics, for example, can be hard on the knees and joints. The key to exercise is finding a form that you like and can easily incorporate into your day. Choose an activity you enjoy and do it at least three times per week. If you have been very inactive, go slowly when you start to exercise. While almost everyone can tolerate walking, it is wise to consult you're a doctor before beginning an exercise program.

And remember throughout the day to always drink plenty of a quality source of water, one of the four basic building blocks of a good diet.

Now, onward for Key Eight . . .

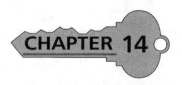

CHAPTER 14

KEY EIGHT:
Understanding the Need for Water—The Body's Most Essential Nutrient

Water. We take it for granted. It's colorless, odorless, and, hopefully, tasteless, and it's readily available to most people in this country at the nearest turn of a faucet. And yet, many people do not realize how absolutely essential water is to optimal health and how drinking impure water can negatively affect our well-being. It is for this reason that this chapter is devoted entirely to a discussion of water. Although water is responsible for and involved in nearly every body function, it can also be a primary source of heavy metals and other contaminants, which can disrupt metabolism. It is important not only that we drink a sufficient quantity of water every day, but also that the water we drink is free of contaminants.

There are three properties of water that enable it to perform such a vast array of processes in our bodies: Water is a solvent, meaning that it can keep many substances suspended in a solution; it is incompressible, meaning it cannot be compressed, and it can hold heat. These three qualities allow the watery fluids of the body to transport tremendous volumes of vitamins, minerals, and other nutrients, as well as oxygen and waste products, in and out of our cells, to cushion and lubricate our organs and tissues, and to help regulate normal body temperature.

Here are some specific examples of water's roles in the body:

- Water releases heat through perspiration, thereby lowering body temperature.

- Water-retaining membranes lubricate the joints, thereby allowing for easy movement.

- Water in the mucous lining of the lungs allows the lungs to expand and contract without drying out, thereby aiding in respiration.

- Water fluids bathe our cells and contain minerals that buffer cellular acids, thereby helping to maintain the body's acid-alkaline balance.

- Water in the blood maintains blood volume, thereby regulating blood pressure.

- Water is needed for certain enzymatic and chemical reactions, thereby facilitating digestion and metabolism.

It's not surprising then that most of the body's tissues contain a large percentage of water. Blood, of course, is nearly all water, and muscles, which are responsible for 40 to 50 percent of the body's weight, are estimated to be 75 percent water. In total, the average person's body is approximately 60 to 70 percent water.

WATER METABOLISM IN THE BODY

Next to the air we breathe, water is the most important substance we will ever put into our bodies. Fereydoon Batmanghelidj, M.D., of St. Mary's Hospital Medical School in London, wrote an enlightening book on the essentials of water. In his book, *Your Body's Many Cries for Water* (Global Health Solutions, 2nd edition, 1995), he shares the results of his research and conclusions he has drawn from his clinical experience on water metabolism in the body. He provides not only compelling case studies and testimonials, but also presents the physiological roles of water based on anatomy and physiology. This book is recommended reading for all my patients.

Batmanghelidj's opinion is that humans tend to lose their sensation of thirst even when the body is giving clear signals that it is not receiving enough water. He believes that much of the illness we see today can be traced back to dehydration of the bodies' cells and tissues from inadequate intake of water. In other words, due to chronic dehydration, the body will begin to lose function and will therefore begin to show signs and symptoms with different illnesses.

Batmanghelidj believes that some of the body's dehydration signals include the following:

- Allergies
- Anginal pain (cardiovascular distress)
- Asthma
- Chronic fatigue syndrome
- Constipation
- Depression
- Diabetes in the elderly
- Dyspeptic pain (gastrointestinal disturbances, such as ulcers)
- Fibromyalgia
- Hypertension (high blood pressure)
- Increased cholesterol levels

- Osteoarthritis and rheumatoid arthritis

- Ulcers

To illustrate the role of water in illness, let's examine Batmanghelidj's theories on the role of water in asthma. Asthma is caused by a histamine-induced constriction of the bronchioles in the lungs, leading to wheezing and difficulty breathing. Histamine is overproduced in the lungs of people with asthma. While there are different theories as to the cause of excessive histamine production, Batmanghelidj claims that one very simple reason may be a lack of water in the lung tissue. You see, histamine is produced in the lungs in response to dehydration. The body loses a good deal of its daily water intake in the simple act of breathing. (You can see the water in your breath when you breathe against a piece of glass). By constricting the bronchioles of the lungs, histamine conserves water for the body. Therefore, asthma is a condition that could be greatly helped by making sure you have adequate water intake. It could be as simple as that.

Asthma and asthma-related illnesses cost individuals, employers, and the health-care system billions of dollars annually. Batmanghelidj's point is, wouldn't it be worthwhile to recommend increasing one's water intake before prescribing expensive treatments?

There are many conditions in which there is an undeniable link with water, based on the established roles of water in the body. Consider water's role in ulcers or other gastrointestinal disorders, for example. The mucus that lines the stomach is composed of 98 percent water. Within this mucous material, sodium bicarbonate neutralizes hydrochloric acid, a powerful digestive acid needed to break down protein, before it reaches the stomach wall. When your body has too little water, the mucous barrier is lost, the sodium bicarbonate is then unable to work, and the unbuffered stomach acid eats away at the stomach lining. When water is taken in, it immediately goes into the stomach where it restores the mucous membranes, potentially decreasing chronic ulcer problems.

Mucus, again made mostly of water, serves other functions in the gastrointestinal tract, such as providing protection for the glands that secrete various chemicals into the gut, allowing for the proper function of digestion. Dehydration can, therefore, cause an imbalance in digestion, in absorbed nutrients (amino acids, carbohydrates, and fats), and can ultimately lead to an imbalance in your most basic biochemistry.

One of the large intestine's functions is to absorb most of the water contained in the stools, which it then reuses in the process of digestion. When the body is dehydrated, the stools will lack the normal amount of water necessary for easy movement of the bowels. The intestines will recycle even the small amount of water contained in these stools, leading to constipation, a condition in which the stools become so hard they are difficult for the intestines to move out of the body. According to the

National Digestive Disease Information Clearinghouse, constipation is responsible for as many as 2 million doctor visits per year.

Batmanghelidj is not the only medical authority to recognize the role of water in preventing constipation. This condition is widely known to be associated with inadequate water intake. In fact, the two most common recommendations for improving constipation are to drink more water and to exercise. Drinking plenty of water allows for proper hydration of fecal material. And because constipation is also associated with colitis and diverticulitis, maintaining hydration could help prevent these conditions.

Common sense tells us that maintaining adequate levels of all the water-containing fluids in the body (cells, serum, blood, mucous linings) will lead to more efficient and optimal functioning of the body. This is why I always recommend that my patients—most of whom report they don't drink more than one or two glasses a day—increase their water intake. Clinically, I have found increased water intake to be particularly valuable for improving bowel function, increasing energy and mental alertness, and improving stamina during exercise. It is also extremely important for improving weight loss. For these reasons, and because adequate water is critical for the delivery of nutrients and the removal of waste products, make sure that you are consuming plenty of quality water daily.

WATER SAFETY AND QUALITY

As water flows through layers of soil and rock in the ground, it dissolves or absorbs the substances that it comes in contact with. While some of these substances are harmless, many are not. This water empties into our ponds, streams, rivers, and lakes, into which industrial waste is being dumped and agricultural runoff from chemically treated soil is leaching. Pesticides, heavy metals, and other environmental pollutants are contaminating our sources of drinking water.

The United States has one of the safest water supplies in the world, but continued contamination from environmental pollutants is quickly changing that. While tap water in our country is required by law to meet certain safety standards, the quality of your drinking water is not guaranteed. That's because drinking water quality varies from place to place, depending on the condition of the source water from which it is drawn and the treatment it receives. Communities have widely varying water utility treatment systems depending on the public resources to maintain current water-safety standards.

The content of drinking water is regulated by the Environmental Protection Agency (EPA). The EPA monitors more than eighty substances in water, including toxic chemicals and biological contaminants, including viruses, bacteria, and parasites. The National Primary Drinking Water Regulations, drafted and enforced by the EPA, determines which substances are required by law to be tested for and controlled. In its first annual national assessment of drinking water compliance in

1996, the EPA said that 86 percent of this country's tap water met their tough federal standards.

However, scientists from the Washington, D.C.–based Environmental Working Group (EWG), a nonprofit environmental research organization, are a group that contends federal regulations are not as strict as they should be. This group has worked to prove the need for tougher water-quality standards. One of the EWG's primary concerns is that there are some toxic chemicals such as perchlorate (a substance used in rocket and missile fuel that has been found in groundwater and/or soil in forty-three states) that public water systems aren't required to test for. Therefore, the public may not even be aware that these substances are in their drinking water. Also, the levels of certain contaminants that the utility companies are required to monitor may be purposely low, which creates a false sense of security among an unsuspecting public. Another problem with drinking water is that some of the chemicals such as fluoride and chlorine added to our water for supposedly beneficial reasons may themselves pose health risks. (To increase your awareness of potentially harmful substances in water that are not presently monitored by the EPA, log on to the EWG's website at www.ewg.org.)

There are many substances of concern to be aware of when examining the quality of your tap water. Water-treatment plants intentionally add chemicals to kill bacteria, balance pH, and eliminate cloudiness. Other toxic substances enter our water supplies from industrial dumping of chemicals. Runoff from agricultural areas may leach into water, adding herbicides, pesticides, and fertilizers (nitrates/nitrites, phosphates). Water can also contain harmful microorganisms such as viruses, bacteria, and parasites that can also cause illness. And you don't have to *drink* the water to be affected by the contaminants in it—many of these contaminants can be absorbed through the skin while bathing or showering.

To help you understand what may be in your water and what impact that water may have on your health, an adaptation of the National Primary Drinking Water Regulations is shown in Table 14.1. For the specific threshold levels for each of these contaminants, see www.epa.gov/ebtpages/water.html. The number of states violating these regulations is shown in Figure 14.1 on page 356.

COMMON IMPURITIES IN TAP WATER

Let's take a more in-depth look at some of the substances commonly found in drinking water and their effects on your health.

Chlorine: An Intentional Additive

The strong smell and offensive taste of most tap water can be attributed to chlorine. The experimental use of chlorine began in the 1890s in order to combat waterborne diseases such as cholera and typhoid. This was the beginning of the sanitization of public water supplies.

Table 14.1. Current Drinking Water Standards

National Primary Drinking Water Regulations (NPDWRs or primary standards) are legally enforceable standards that apply to public water systems. Primary standards protect public health by limiting the levels of contaminants in drinking water. This table divides these contaminants into microorganisms, antibacterial agents and byproducts, inorganic chemicals, organic chemicals, and radionuclides.

MICRO-ORGANISMS	POTENTIAL HEALTH EFFECTS FROM INGESTION OF CONTAMINATED WATER	SOURCES OF CONTAMINANT IN DRINKING WATER
Cryptosporidium	Gastrointestinal illness (for example, diarrhea, vomiting, cramps)	Human and animal fecal waste
Giardia lamblia	Gastrointestinal illness (for example, diarrhea, vomiting, cramps)	Human and animal fecal waste
Heterotrophic plate count (HPC)	HPC has no health effects, but can indicate how effective treatment is at controlling microorganisms	HPC measures a range of bacteria that are naturally present in the environment
Legionella	Legionnaire's disease (pneumonia)	Found naturally in water; multiplies in heating systems
Total coliforms (including fecal coliform and *E. coli*)	Used as an indicator that other potentially harmful bacteria may be present; disease-causing microbes (pathogens) in these wastes can cause gastrointestinal illness (for example, diarrhea, nausea, cramps) headaches, or other symptoms, and pose a special health risk for infants, young children, and people with severely compromised immune systems.	Coliforms are naturally present in the environment; fecal coliforms and *E. coli* come from human and animal fecal waste
Turbidity	Turbidity is a measure of the cloudiness of water. It is used to indicate water quality and filtration effectiveness. Higher turbidity levels are often associated with higher levels of disease-causing microorganisms such as viruses, parasites and some bacteria. These organisms can cause symptoms of gastrointestinal illness.	Soil runoff
Viruses (enteric)	Gastrointestinal illness (for example, diarrhea, vomiting, cramps)	Human and animal fecal waste
ANTIBACTERIAL AGENTS & BYPRODUCTS	**POTENTIAL HEALTH EFFECTS FROM INGESTION OF CONTAMINATED WATER**	**SOURCES OF CONTAMINANT IN DRINKING WATER**
Bromate	Increased risk of cancer	Byproduct of drinking water disinfection
Chloramines (as Cl_2)	Eye/nose irritation; stomach discomfort, anemia	Water additive used to control microbes
Chlorine (as Cl_2)	Eye/nose irritation; stomach discomfort	Water additive used to control microbes
Chlorine dioxide (as ClO_2)	Anemia; infants & young children: nervous system effects	Water additive used to control microbes
Chlorite	Anemia; infants & young children: nervous system effects	Byproduct of drinking water disinfection

ANTIBACTERIAL AGENTS & BYPRODUCTS	POTENTIAL HEALTH EFFECTS FROM INGESTION OF CONTAMINATED WATER	SOURCES OF CONTAMINANT IN DRINKING WATER
Haloacetic acids (HAA5)	Increased risk of cancer	Byproduct of drinking water disinfection
Total trihalomethanes (TTHMs)	Liver, kidney or central nervous system problems; increased risk of cancer	Byproduct of drinking water disinfection
Inorganic chemicals	Potential Health Effects from Ingestion of Water	Sources of Contaminant in Drinking Water
Antimony	Increase in blood cholesterol; decrease in blood glucose	Discharge from petroleum refineries; fire retardants; ceramics; electronics; solder
Arsenic	Skin damage; circulatory system problems; increased risk of cancer	Erosion of natural deposits; runoff from glass & electronics production wastes
Asbestos (fiber >10 micrometers)	Increased risk of developing benign intestinal polyps	Decay of asbestos cement in water mains; erosion of natural deposits
Barium	Increase in blood pressure	Discharge of drilling wastes; discharge from metal refineries; erosion of natural deposits
Beryllium	Intestinal lesions	Discharge from metal refineries and coal-burning factories; discharge from electrical, aerospace, and defense industries
Cadmium	Kidney damage	Corrosion of galvanized pipes; erosion of natural deposits; discharge from metal refineries; runoff from waste batteries and paints
Chromium (total)	Some people who use water containing chromium well in excess of the maximum contaminant level (MCL), the highest level of a contaminant that is allowed in drinking water), over many years could experience allergic dermatitis	Discharge from steel and pulp mills; erosion of natural deposits
Copper	Short term exposure: Gastrointestinal distress. Long-term exposure: Liver or kidney damage. People with Wilson's disease should consult their personal doctor if their water systems exceed the copper action level.	Corrosion of household plumbing systems; erosion of natural deposits
Cyanide (as free cyanide)	Nerve damage or thyroid problems	Discharge from steel/metal factories; discharge from plastic and fertilizer factories
Fluoride	Bone disease (pain and tenderness of the bones); Children may get mottled teeth.	Water additive which promotes strong teeth; erosion of natural deposits; discharge from fertilizer and aluminum factories

ANTIBACTERIAL AGENTS & BYPRODUCTS	POTENTIAL HEALTH EFFECTS FROM INGESTION OF CONTAMINATED WATER	SOURCES OF CONTAMINANT IN DRINKING WATER
Lead	Infants and children: Delays in physical or mental development. Adults: Kidney problems; hypertension	Corrosion of household plumbing systems; erosion of natural deposits
Mercury (inorganic)	Kidney damage	Erosion of natural deposits; discharge from refineries and factories; runoff from landfills and cropland
Nitrate/Nitrite (measured as Nitrogen)	"Blue baby syndrome" in infants under six months—life threatening without immediate medical attention. Symptoms: Infant looks blue and has shortness of breath.	Runoff from fertilizer use; leaching from septic tanks, sewage; erosion of natural deposits
Selenium	Hair or fingernail loss; numbness in fingers or toes; circulatory problems	Discharge from petroleum refineries; erosion of natural deposits; discharge from mines
Thallium	Hair loss; changes in blood; kidney, intestine, or liver problems	Leaching from ore-processing sites; discharge from electronics, glass, and pharmaceutical companies

Figure 14.1. Community Water Systems Violating Maximum Contaminant Levels

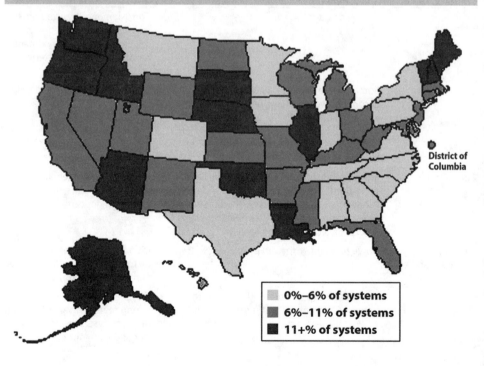

District of Columbia

- 0%–6% of systems
- 6%–11% of systems
- 11+% of systems

Due to its low cost and effectiveness, chlorine has been the most widely used disinfectant in the United States. It is used in 98 percent of public water utilities and is the primary disinfectant for drinking water in the world. Chlorine effectively kills a large variety of microbial waterborne pathogens (disease-causing organisms), including those that can cause typhoid fever, dysentery, cholera, and Legionnaires' disease. Chlorine is widely credited with virtually eliminating outbreaks of waterborne disease in the United States and other developed countries.

Chlorine, however, can combine with naturally occurring substances in water such as leaves, bark, and other sediment to create some undesirable byproducts called *trihalomethanes* (THMs). These are now known to be potential carcinogenic (cancer-causing) byproducts. THMs have also been reported to cause pregnancy- and birth-related complications such as small for gestational age (SGA), low birth weight, preterm birth, birth defects, spontaneous abortions, and fetal deaths.

In 1994, the National Primary Drinking Water Regulations on Disinfection and Disinfection Byproducts limited the allowable level of THMs in drinking-water supplies. However, THMs continue to be one of the contaminants that public utilities must monitor.

Chloramine, a chlorine and ammonia compound that is currently in use in some municipalities, may be used solely or in addition to chlorine. It is thought to produce fewer THMs. However, when THM's amine group combines with nitrates found in water (from fertilizers), it forms nitrosamines, which are known potent human carcinogens.

Another form of chlorine used by some municipalities to disinfect drinking water is called *chlorine dioxide.* Like all forms of chlorine, chlorine dioxide creates THMs. It is also well documented to cause hypothyroidism in animals and is suspected to have a similar effect in humans.

While it's important that public water supplies are treated to prevent microbial growth, chlorine is one of the substances in water that might be interfering with your metabolism. It is wise to decrease intake of chlorine by drinking water filtered by one of the water treatment methods listed in Table 14.2 on page 366.

Fluoride: A Water Additive of Questionable Benefit

Fluoride is a mineral that is abundant in the earth. Like all minerals, it can enter groundwater as the water flows through the soil and rock. Fluoride is present in varying amounts in some foods such as fish, fruits, vegetables, and in the leaves of tea. Fluoride is considered an essential nutrient for the formation of bone and tooth. The fluoride that leeches into groundwater and food is different from the form of fluoride that is added to water supplies. This is known as *sodium fluoride.*

When fluoride's benefits in preventing tooth decay became known in the 1940s, the United States embarked upon a public fluoridation program, and sodium fluoride began to be added to the public drinking water and to toothpaste products to prevent tooth decay. According to the World Health Organization (WHO), fluoride is an effective agent for preventing dental caries if taken in "optimal" amounts. But a single level for daily intake can be difficult to determine. And, although the body needs fluoride, an excess of this mineral is known to cause health problems such as *dental fluorosis* and *skeletal fluorosis.*

People have different levels of tolerance. One factor that accounts for these differences is a person's nutritional status. Nutritional status greatly affects fluoride's absorption by the body. For example, a low vitamin C intake increases the body's absorption of fluoride and a low calcium intake increases the body's retention of fluoride.

In addition, climate and weather affect how much water a person drinks. Countries with hot climates—in which the body's requirements for fluid are increased—may not add as much fluoride to their water as another country. This assumes, however, that a person in a hotter climate drinks more water than someone from a cooler climate, which may not always be the case. Each country that accepts the WHO's position on fluoridation (as most do) determines their own appropriate level of added fluoride. In the United States, where we have varied climates, each community must determine what is an appropriate level of added fluoride. The largest problem with fluoridating water supplies is that it makes it very easy for people to consume too much.

The EPA's Headquarters Professionals' Union (a group of doctors, engineers, lawyers, scientists, and other professionals) has advised the EPA, state and community officials, and consumers against fluoridating water supplies based upon their review of the scientific study and data on fluoride's effectiveness. They feel the negative consequences—some of which are discussed below—far outweigh any possible benefit. Based on the studies of dental caries rates in fluoridated and non-fluoridated countries, they claim that there is no apparent benefit. Furthermore, there are other more effective ways to prevent dental caries such as by eating a nutritious diet (thereby guarding against deficiencies) and by practicing good oral hygiene. After reviewing all of the data on fluoride, many are choosing not to add fluoride to their water supplies.

Fluoride's negative effects are caused by its ability to inhibit enzymes in the body. One type of enzyme that fluoride inhibits breeds acid-producing bacteria, which eats away tooth enamel. So, in theory, by inhibiting this enzyme, fluoride can prevent dental caries. However, not only does fluoride inhibit this enzyme, it also inhibits an estimated sixty-four other, useful enzymes in the body.

Moreover, it is believed that fluoride binds with calcium ions to form a matrix that strengthens tooth enamel as it forms in children. However, according to a report issued by UNICEF, conflicting studies from several other countries are questioning this supposed benefit. According to a UNICEF report on fluoridation, it is well known that "excessive fluoride intake leads to loss of calcium from the tooth matrix (the inner part of the teeth), aggravating cavity formation throughout life rather than remedying it, and can also cause *dental fluorosis.* Severe, chronic and cumulative overexposure can cause the incurable crippling of *skeletal fluorosis.*" Dental fluorosis is characterized by discolored, blackened, mottled, or chalky-white teeth, and it occurs in children who have taken in excessive fluoride. Excessive fluoride intake does not affect the teeth of adults because they are already fully formed. It can, however, have the unseen effects of enzyme inhibition or, with long-term intake, can lead to the hardening or overcalcification of joints and bones known as *skeletal fluorosis.* Since early symptoms including sporadic pain and stiffness of joints, headaches, stomachaches, and muscle weakness, are also associated with other diseases, diagnosis of skeletal fluorosis may be missed. Many scientists believe that the levels currently added to water are sufficient to cause skeletal fluorosis over a period of years, the symptoms of which may be indistinguishable from certain forms of arthritis.

Fluorosis is an irreversible condition that cannot be cured. The only way to control its incidence is to prevent it. Many organizations and public officials have come to the conclusion that drinking fluoridated water is not necessary or beneficial. In order to prevent the long-term problems that can develop from excessive fluoride intake, I recommend drinking non-fluoridated water. Adequate calcium intake is clearly associated with a reduced risk of dental fluorosis and vitamin C may also safeguard against the risk. So pay attention to your nutritional intake to guard against this disease.

Although the American Dental Association (ADA) still firmly supports the use of fluoride, I think it is wise to listen to the many scientists who are now seriously questioning whether risks outweigh the benefits of these fluoridation methods.

Microorganisms

There are many microorganisms that can be found in water supplies, some of which are pathogenic (disease-causing). Most of these organisms are contaminates from animal and human waste. Waterborne microorganisms are a threat to everyone, but are particularly dangerous for people with compromised immune systems, such as those with AIDS or cancer patients. *E. coli, Shigella, Giardia, Salmonella,* and *Cryptosporidium* are examples of microorganisms that can make a home in our water. Although chlorine kills many of these microorganisms, some microorganisms are unaffected. In addition, some microorganisms are becoming resistant to chlorine.

Cryptosporidium and *Giardia lamblia* are examples of two organisms that are not killed by disinfection. In 1993, more than 400,000 people in Milwaukee, Wisconsin, were affected by an outbreak of illness from *Cryptosporidium* in the city's water supply. Up to 100 deaths were attributed to this outbreak. Other outbreaks from *Cryptosporidium* and other microorganisms in the early 1990s led the EPA to require more thorough municipal filtration systems. Estimates are that current systems can remove more than 97 percent of *Cryptosporidium* oocysts (sporelike form of the organism).

Even though municipal water systems are trying to protect against ever more virulent microorganisms by improving water filtration methods, you can further reduce your risk of becoming ill from pathogenic bacteria by using a home water filter designed to remove these microorganisms.

Heavy Metals

Heavy metals present some of the worst health risks of any water contaminants. As you learned in Chapter 10, heavy metals, including mercury, lead, cadmium, aluminum, and arsenic, inactivate enzymes in the body and increase free-radical damage, which can lead to increased risk of cardiovascular disease and cancer. You also learned that some of these metals interfere with hormones in the body. For example, cadmium is a direct competitor of thyroid hormone in the body; therefore, cadmium toxicity can lead to hypothyroidism.

Water is one of the most likely routes of exposure to heavy metals. Heavy metals can get into water supplies from erosion of natural deposits in the ground, but the bigger problem is the heavy metals that get into water from industrial and other pollution. For example, mercury gets into water from oil refineries, factories, and runoff from landfills.

Almost 17 percent of Americans—more than 44 million people—drink water that is contaminated with lead. Lead damages the attention span in children and negatively affects intelligence quotient (IQ) and the immune system. Lead usually gets into water from old plumbing. Over time, the water running through the pipes dissolves the lead, which then gets carried along into the drinking water. Cadmium can also get into drinking water through old galvanized plumbing or it can enter water supplies from the industrial wastes of metal refineries.

It is extremely important for your metabolism and overall health to remove any heavy metals from your drinking water.

IMPURITIES IN WELL WATER

Thus far, this discussion has been in reference to tap water from public water-utility companies. While well water may have been considered to be preferable to tap water at one time, that is no longer the case. Due to extensive pollution in most groundwater supplies, drinking unfiltered well water is also risky.

According to a 1995 U.S. Geological Survey, approximately 42 million people in the United States obtain water from wells, streams, or cisterns. The EPA does not oversee private wells, although some state and local governments do set rules for contractors digging wells as one measure to protect people who drink well water. The EPA encourages households supplied by well water to take special precautions to ensure the protection of those using and drinking the water. The EPA also offers information for what to do with your well after a flood. You can read this information on their website (www.epa.gov/safewater/privatewells/booklet).

Hard Water versus Soft Water

Hard water is water that has a high content of minerals, such as carbonates, sulfates, calcium chloride, magnesium, and iron, with a calcium level of more than 250 parts per million (ppm). Hard water can cause wear and tear on appliances such as washing machines and dishwashers and decreased energy efficiency in appliance operation. It also forms scale on pipes, and causes clothing washed in it to wear out more quickly.

There are regional differences across the country in water hardness. Water along the East Coast and in the Northwest tends to be soft, whereas water in central areas of the country tends to be hard. In some areas, water utilities soften hard water at the treatment plant. If not softened at their water-treatment plant, many people will opt to soften it themselves with household or industrial water softeners.

Soft water is water with a low-mineral content. If hard water is softened by a softener system, the minerals are replaced primarily with sodium. Soft water can be of benefit when it comes to appliances or water pipes, but drinking softened water is not a good idea. Soft water contributes to an increased incidence of hypertension and heart disease, while hard water seems to have just the opposite effect.

Soft water can cause problems if you have old lead pipes because the lead and cadmium contained in them is more easily dissolved by the soft water, which then becomes a source of these toxic minerals to anyone who drinks it. People who live or work in old buildings should run the tap water for a full minute before drinking it. This allows any water that may have been in the pipes awhile (collecting the lead and cadmium) to be flushed out. If you live in an area that has soft water, it is advisable to have your tap water tested for lead and cadmium.

Private water supplies should be tested annually for contaminants, such as *nitrate* (found in intensively farmed areas due to runoff from fertilizers or livestock wastewater) and coliform bacteria (present in large numbers in the intestines and feces of warm-blooded animals, and also as naturally occurring organisms in soil). If you suspect a problem exists, test your well more frequently and for more potential contaminants, including *radon* (a naturally occurring radioactive element), nitrate, or pesticides. Local health departments can provide you with information on testing.

If you have a well, know that anything that is sprayed, dumped, or put into the ground will eventually find its way into the groundwater. You can protect your water supply by carefully managing activities near the water source. Do not dump oil or gasoline onto the ground. Avoid mixing or using pesticides, fertilizers, herbicides, degreasers, fuels, and other pollutants near the well. Great care should be used with the use and disposal of any hazardous chemicals; they also should be kept out of septic systems. Periodically inspect exposed parts of the well for problems, including cracked, corroded, or damaged well casing; broken or missing well cap; and settling and cracking of surface seals.

WATER-TREATMENT METHODS

By now you understand that the water you drink may contain some disease-producing and even life-threatening toxins. Is there any way to prevent those toxins from getting into our bodies? The best we can do is try to purify our water with some of the filtration systems that are available today. Consider some of the following modes of treating water to make it safe for consumption.

Reverse Osmosis

Reverse osmosis (RO) systems use high pressure to force water through a series of semipermeable membranes to reduce inorganic minerals. RO systems vary widely in their ability to filter nitrates, chlorides, and other contaminants. Water pressure, water temperature, pH, bacteria, dissolved solids, and the chemical contaminant level of the water being filtered can all affect their performance. An RO system creates its pressure with additional quantities of water. For this reason, it requires a lot of water to get the job done—one criticism of the RO system. Another is that in order to keep an RO system working optimally, the filters need frequent changing. As the substances filtered out of the water collect in the membranes, the effectiveness of the system declines. This can also create a breeding ground for bacteria. So, it is important to follow the manufacturer's suggestions and to be diligent in the maintenance of an RO system. Despite these drawbacks, a five-stage reverse osmosis system probably provides the most consistent and best water-filtration results at a price that is affordable to the average person.

Deionization (Ion Exchange)

Ions are electrically charged atoms or molecules. Ion exchange is a chemical reaction wherein an ion from one solution is exchanged for a similarly charged ion from another solution. In the deionization process, the water is first treated with reverse osmosis. Then, the disagreeable ions in the water (nickel, sodium, sulfates, chromates, and chlorides, among others) are exchanged with positively or negatively charged hydrogen ions, and are then attached to an immobile solid particle. A variety of synthetic organic resins are used as the source of solid particles because different types can be tailored to specific applications. The result of the ion exchange treatment is relatively pure, neutral water.

Steam Distillation

Steam distillation is not a filtering system, per se. It takes water from the source, heats it into water vapor (steam), and then recondenses it into pure water. The heat kills harmful bacteria, viruses, and all foreign particles, such as inorganic minerals, heavy metals, chlorine, and most volatile organic chemicals (VOCs) that are collected in other chambers or left behind in the boiling chamber. Although distilled water is very pure, most experts feel that its lack of ionization and minerals causes it to draw minerals from the body and, therefore, do not recommend it. People who recommend drinking distilled water for the purity usually also advise supplementing with minerals to safeguard the minerals in the body tissues.

Water Filtration

Filtering occurs when water passes through a layer of materials (usually carbon-containing materials) that trap or chemically alter a limited range of contaminants in water. While carbon filters are inexpensive and can reduce disagreeable tastes and odors like chlorine, they are not effective in removing such contaminants as arsenic, copper, lead, nitrates, parasites, sodium, and sulfate. These contaminants are not removed due to the flow rate of the water through the filter. In most carbon-filter systems, the water passes through the layer in less than one minute. Studies have shown that water must be held in a filter for seven to eighteen minutes to remove some contaminants.

Once again, it is important to know how often to change the filter and to make sure you do it. Otherwise, the filters not only stop filtering substances (some substances trapped in the filter can actually dislodge and get back into your water), but also they can become a breeding ground for bacteria as the organic material that remains in the filter begins to decay.

Table 14.2 on page 366 summarizes the contaminants most commonly found in water and the varying success of water treatment methods to eliminate them.

BOTTLED WATER OPTIONS

The use of bottled water has exploded in the last ten years. More than half of all Americans drink bottled water, and about one-third consume it regularly. Sales of this magnitude are no doubt occurring because of concerns over the safety and health effects of tap water. Bottled water also tastes better. There are two main criticisms of bottled water, however. One, the cost is astronomical compared with the cost per gallon of tap water; and two, it is difficult to identify whether the water is really any better than water from the tap.

There are several different varieties of bottled water. These products may be labeled as *bottled water, drinking water,* or any of the following terms. Is bottled water really safer? The best way to determine this is to familiarize yourself with the Food and Drug Administration's (FDA) product definitions for bottled water below:

Artesian Water/Artesian Well Water

Artesian water, or artesian well water, is water from a well that taps a confined aquifer (a water-bearing underground layer of rock or sand) in which the water level stands at some height above the top of the aquifer.

Table 14.2. Comparison of Water Treatment Technologies

POLLUTANT	SEDIMENT FILTER	CARBON FILTER	DEIONIZATION	REVERSE OSMOSIS	STEAM DISTILLATION
Arsenic	Ineffective	Ineffective	Complete	Significant	Complete
Bacteria	Ineffective	Ineffective	Ineffective	Significant	Complete
Cadmium	Ineffective	Ineffective	Complete	Complete	Complete
Calcium	Ineffective	Ineffective	Complete	Complete	Complete
Chloride	Ineffective	Ineffective	Complete	Complete	Complete
Chlorine	Ineffective	Complete	Ineffective	Complete*	Complete*
Copper	Ineffective	Ineffective	Ineffective	Significant	Complete
Cryptosporidium	Ineffective	Ineffective	Ineffective	Complete	Complete
Detergents	Ineffective	Significant	Complete	Complete	Complete
Fluoride	Ineffective	Ineffective	Complete	Complete	Complete
Lead	Ineffective	Ineffective	Complete	Complete	Complete
Magnesium	Ineffective	Ineffective	Complete	Complete	Complete
Mercury	Ineffective	Ineffective	Ineffective	Significant	Complete
Nitrate	Ineffective	Ineffective	Significant	Significant	Complete
Organics	Ineffective	Complete	Ineffective	Complete*	Complete*
Pesticides	Ineffective	Complete	Ineffective	Complete*	Complete*
Phosphates	Ineffective	Ineffective	Complete	Complete	Complete
Radon	Ineffective	Ineffective	Complete	Complete	Complete
Sediment	Complete	Significant	Complete	Complete	Complete
Sodium	Ineffective	Ineffective	Complete	Complete	Complete
Sulfates	Ineffective	Significant	Complete	Complete	Complete
Viruses	Ineffective	Ineffective	Ineffective	Ineffective	Complete

* Plus Carbon Filtration

Drinking Water

Drinking water is water that is sold for human consumption in sanitary containers and contains no added sweeteners or chemical additives (other than flavors, extracts, or essences). The water source may or may not be listed on the label. It must be calorie-free and sugar-free. Flavors, extracts, or essences may be added to drinking water, but they must comprise less than 1 percent by weight of the final product or the product will be considered a soft drink. Drinking water may be sodium-free or contain very low amounts of sodium. Although the water in bottled water must conform to FDA and state regulations for restrictions on contaminants, if the label states simply "bottled water" without specifying that its source is spring water, or mineral water, or one of the other categories of water defined here, then it could be just filtered tap water.

Mineral Water

Mineral water containing not less than 250 ppm total dissolved solids (minerals) may be labeled as mineral water. Mineral water is distinguished from other types of bottled water by the constant level and relative proportions of mineral and trace elements that are in the water at the point of emergence from the source. No minerals can be added to this product.

Ozonated and Ultraviolet (UV) Light Purified Water

Ozonated and ultraviolet (UV) light purified water is water that has undergone one of these two purification methods. *Ozonation* kills pathogenic organisms by, in a sense, hyperoxygenating *the water.* UV-light *exposure also kills many pathogens.*

Purified Water

Purified water is water that has been produced by distillation, deionization, reverse osmosis, or other suitable processes and that meets the definition of purified water in the *United States Pharmacopoeia.*

Sparkling Water

Sparkling water is water that, after treatment and possible replacement with carbon dioxide, contains the same amount of carbon dioxide that it had at emergence from the source. (*Note:* soda water, seltzer water, and tonic water are not considered bottled waters. They are regulated separately, may contain sugar and calories, and are considered soft drinks.)

Spring Water

Spring water derived from an underground formation that flows naturally to the surface of the earth. Spring water must be collected only at the spring or through a borehole that taps into the spring. Spring water collected with the use of an external force must be from the same underground stratum as the spring and must have all the physical properties, before treatment, and be of the same composition and quality as the water that flows naturally to the surface of the earth.

Well Water

Well water is water from a hole bored, drilled, or otherwise constructed in the ground, which taps the water of an aquifer.

The problem with bottled waters is that it is legal to bottle tap water. According to government and industry estimates, about one-fourth of all bottled water is bottled tap water. Sometimes bottled tap water has received additional treatment, but sometimes not. Waters that are most likely to be bottled tap water are those labeled "drinking water." Your best bet is to buy water that is labeled "purified" and that identifies its methods of purification. Some people may also prefer to drink mineral water if they know the source of the water and trust it to be pure.

There is one catch, however. The FDA's rules completely exempt 60 to 70 percent of the bottled water sold in the United States from the agency's bottled water standards, because the FDA says its rules do not apply to water packaged and sold within the same state. Nearly forty states say they *do* regulate such waters, although, generally, few resources are dedicated to this regulation.

Another problem with bottled waters may be the container the water is in. Have you ever noticed that some bottle water tastes like the plastic container? This occurs because the water is packaged in low-grade plastic, which may leach toxins, such as methyl chloride (a carcinogen), from the container. To avoid this, buy water that is in the clear polyethylene containers.

Although bottled water is expensive, I appreciate the convenience of having a better tasting (if not more pure) source of water available almost anywhere. Because bottled water is now available in convenience stores, fast food restaurants, amusement parks, and sporting events, we now have a much healthier drinking alternative than bottled juice, sports drinks, or soft drinks, which are too high in concentrated and refined sugars. For most people, it is a huge relief to finally be able to buy water as an alternative.

For home use, if you can afford the up front cost, it is more economical in the long run to buy a water-filtration system. If you cannot afford the lump sum, you can sometimes find reverse osmosis machines that will fill gallon containers for a much more reasonable cost than buying the water already in the gallon jug. Purified-bottled water in my mind is preferable to taking your chances on the water from the tap.

STRUCTURED WATER: THE FUTURE OF MEDICINE?

One of the significant areas of research concerning water is in the area of *structured* or *biologically active* water. The famous water of Hunza, in the Himalayas, associated with longevity, has been found to be highly structured water. Henri Coanda, Ph.D., the Romanian father of fluid dynamics and a Nobel Prize winner at seventy-eight years old, spent six decades studying the Hunza water to determine what it was in this water that caused such beneficial effects for the body. His research revealed that this water had a different freezing and boiling point than ordinary water, a different viscosity, and a different surface tension.

The "structured" nature of this water refers to its ability to form liquid crystal structures known as *clathrates*. Supposedly, structured water holds more oxygen, may be more alkaline, and has a decreased surface tension—all properties that would allow it to function better in the body.

Most water that comes out of our taps has approximately 5 to 10 ppm of oxygen. Fresh mountain stream water has 15 ppm oxygen. On the other hand, structured water can contain up to 40 to 60 ppm dissolved oxygen—that's up to 600 percent more oxygen in drinking water. Research has already reported good response from patients (suffering from diseases of the heart, intestines, and lungs, as well as some cases of hypertension) who were treated with superoxygenated water. Structured water has also been reported to improve the oxygen supply to the brain, to stop migraines, to stimulate the immune system, and to help in the prevention and treatment of cancer. Thus far, however, the evidence to prove any claims for structured waters is preliminary.

There are several different types of structured water on the market. Not all companies "structure" water in the same way. Structured water is presently very expensive. If you can afford structured water and feel you could derive benefit from it, there is nothing wrong with drinking it.

HOW MUCH WATER SHOULD YOU DRINK?

The current medical guidelines for estimating water needs are based on calorie intake and body weight. Using caloric intake to estimate your optimum water intake, you need to drink one milliliter (ml) of water for every calorie you consume. For example, if you consume 1,500 calories a day, you need approximately 1,500 ml of water (250 ml per cup of water), or about 48 ounces of water a day.

Using body weight to estimate water needs, divide your body weight by 2.2 to get your weight in kilograms (kg). Then multiply your weight in kg by 30. This will

---

Testing Your Water Quality

If you want to know what's in the water in your particular area, here are some suggestions:

• Call your local water utility and ask for a copy of the "Municipal Drinking Water Contaminant Analysis Report."

• If you have a private well, contact your local health department and ask for a list of the typical well-water contaminants in your area.

• Contact an independent laboratory to have your drinking water tested. Your local health department can provide you with the names of laboratories certified by your state that can perform the tests for you.

• Contact your local water authority to find out if they test water at no charge; if not, contact a certified testing lab to test only those contaminants you're concerned about. This can cost $50 and up for analysis.

• Visit the EPA's "Surf Your Watershed" site (www.epa.gov/surf/) for information on your community watershed.

give you the amount of water in milliliters that you should consume daily. For example, 150 pounds divided by 2.2 equals 68 kg; 68 multiplied by 30 is about 2,000 ml, or 64 ounces of water.

So, now you can see where the general recommendation of drinking six to eight glasses of water a day comes from! I generally encourage people to start from where they are. Meaning, if a patient tells me that he or she drinks no water at all, then even consuming two glasses of water a day is better than before. At first, having to drink additional water makes many people feel water logged. You do not have to down an entire 8 ounces at one time. In fact, it is better to drink water 2 or 3 ounces at a time, because anything over that goes straight to the bladder anyway.

Inevitably people want to know whether tea, coffee, or any other liquid counts toward daily water intake. The answer is no. Both coffee and alcohol have dehydrating effects on the body, so you end up having a net loss of water after drinking them. Tea also has a mild diuretic effect from the caffeine in it; however, if the tea is watered down with about equal amounts of water, you will get a net water gain.

You may also read or hear advice on the proper temperature at which to drink water. There are some reports that cold water increases calorie burning in the body. Or, Oriental medicine, for instance, advises drinking different temperatures of water according to your health problem. People have very different preferences on water temperature; some like their water ice cold, some room temperature. My advice is to drink what suits you, but just drink it!

The final question that comes up is "Can you drink too much water?" The answer is yes. It's possible to drink so much water that you dilute the sodium levels in the body and the cells become too full of water. Athletes are at particular risk of over-hydration because they sweat out a lot of salt. This can be avoided by increasing your sodium intake, by adding a pinch of salt to the fluids that you take in. Sports drinks have sodium in them, but the electrolytes are too concentrated. If you use sports drinks, dilute half the drink with equal parts water. Batmanghelidj recommends that everyone increase their salt intake a little as water intake increases. His guideline is a pinch of salt (preferable high-quality sea salt) for every ten glasses of water you drink.

So, start from where you are and gradually increase your intake. First get used to drinking one or two more glasses a day than you currently drink, then slowly increase your daily intake to around five or six glasses for women and eight glasses for men. Drink water even if at first you don't feel thirsty. I find that once people get used to drinking more water, most reestablish a normal thirst for water and actually miss it if they don't drink it.

WATER IS KEY

Water is the most important nutrient you can put into your body. The bottom line is that you should drink plenty of it for optimal metabolism, striving for six to eight 8-ounce glasses of water daily. Alcohol, coffee, tea, and caffeine-containing beverages and sodas don't count as water. Consider installing one of the home-water treatment methods discussed in this chapter to ensure the water you drink is clean and free of contaminants.

Try to drink the majority of your water between meals. Drinking too much water with a meal can dilute digestive juices, making digestion less complete. Drink only small amounts with meals and the rest in between. Try to pay attention to your body's thirst signals. Do not ignore a dry mouth; it is trying to tell you something. The more water you drink, the more efficient your thirst mechanism becomes.

Be aware of conditions that will increase your need for water. People who exercise strenuously or live in hot climates lose 50 to 100 percent more water through the lungs and skin, and will need to drink more water. People experiencing illnesses such as diarrhea and vomiting will have an increased need for water (consult your doctor as severe vomiting and diarrhea can lead to critical dehydration). Fevers increase your need for water. Also, people on high-protein diets will benefit from larger intakes of water.

When you're tired, drink water. When you're feeling mentally foggy, drink water. When you want to reach for that soft drink, drink water. And when you're feeling hungry, but know you should not eat, drink water. To take in pure water is to take in life itself. So drink freely.

Now, onward for Key Nine . . .

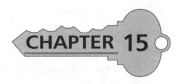

CHAPTER 15

KEY NINE:
Understanding the Two Sides of Oxygen—Breath of Life or Harbinger of Inflammation, Aging, and Disease?

I f you had lived at the turn of the twentieth century, your hope for an average life span would have been just fifty years. People would have laughed at you if you told them that in just over a century, the average life span would be almost eighty years. However, these days, seventy-eight is the average life span. Now, what if I told you that you could possibly live to be one hundred and twenty years old? Would you laugh? It's no joke. Scientists specializing in genetics now believe that we can, and soon will, increase the average life span to one hundred and twenty years.

But the fact is, without oxygen, we can't live to be one day old, much less one hundred twenty years old. Without adequate oxygen intake and utilization, our bodies cannot function. The body uses oxygen to break down protein, carbohydrate, and fat from food—thus, oxygen has a tremendous impact on our metabolism. In fact, the intake of oxygen is so important that there are programs available to retrain people to breath properly to improve oxygen levels in their bodies. Since the body also uses oxygen to build and repair cells, and for immune function, nervous system function, in reproduction, and numerous other activities, improved breathing capacity can have many benefits.

Oxygen is a double-edged sword, however. If your body is not properly utilizing oxygen, it will produce free radicals and can contribute to the development of diseases and affect how well you age. In addition, polluted air can contribute to free-radical production in the body, so while we need to improve oxygenation of tissues, we need to do everything possible to improve the purity of the air we breath and to improve our bodies' ability to deal with increased free radicals.

OXYGEN AS ALLY AND ENEMY

Oxygen is essential to survival of all life. Yet, if it is not properly controlled, it can wreak metabolic havoc, disease, and death. Molecular biology is the study of how molecules in the body interact to produce life. Molecules, once considered the smallest structures of life, are made up of atoms. Atoms, in turn, consist of *protons, neutrons,* and *electrons*—electrically charged particles that give atoms their defining characteristics. Electrical charge determines how atoms will come together to form molecules.

Electrons revolve around the inner structure of the atom (the nucleus) in layers, called *orbitals.* Electrons must exist in pairs in order to be stable. A molecule that has a single or unpaired electron is highly reactive and will attempt to snatch a complementary electron from any nearby molecule. A molecule with an unpaired electron in its outer orbital is called a *free radical.* Free radicals are highly destructive to the molecules and the tissues surrounding them, because, when they rob electrons, they damage the "donor" molecule, sometimes destroying it entirely.

Free-radical damage is a chain of events. Once a free radical has robbed a molecule of an electron, another free radical is created. This cascade of free-radical formation can lead to widespread damage to cells in the body. One unchecked free radical may ultimately generate hundreds of thousands of additional free radicals before it is stopped. Because free-radical damage is the result of the removal of electrons through oxidation reactions, it is also known as *oxidative stress.*

Oxygen cannot be prevented from generating free radicals. There are many types of free radicals that occur in the body. The most common are made from oxygen molecules, or reactive oxygen species (ROS), such as *superoxide radicals, hydroxyl radicals, hydrogen peroxide, singlet oxygen, nitric oxide,* and *peroxynitrite,* among others.

Because these oxygenated free radicals are highly reactive and react instantaneously with surrounding molecules, they have short life spans. Their effect, however, is far-reaching. Each free radical has the potential to trigger a chain reaction of new free radicals anywhere in the body, which can disrupt your endocrine system, alter immune function, and impair the nervous and digestive systems, and more. Thus, the damaging effects of one free radical can be multiplied by more than a millionfold.

Internal Sources of Free-Radical Production

Free radicals are produced naturally in the body as consequences of normal metabolism. Since oxygen is so intricately involved in cellular respiration, your body will produce a certain amount of free-radical activity simply by performing its daily functions. As we just mentioned, a significant source of free-radical formation in the cells comes from *the electron transport chain* during the process of energy production.

The electron transport chain takes place in the mitochondria, the energy center of the cells. It consists of a chain of enzymes that pass electrons from one to another. At the end of the chain is an oxygen molecule that essentially "pulls" electrons down the line. This flow of electrons generates energy in the form of ATP (adenosine triphosphate). Free radicals are formed when electrons are inadvertently pulled off the chain by free-roaming oxygen molecules.

When this happens, oxygen is transformed into the harmful *superoxide radical.* Approximately 2 percent of the oxygen that enters the mitochondria becomes superoxide radicals, which can damage cellular DNA. In the DNA, oxidative damage to the mitochondria is a known causative factor in aging. This damage is not easily repaired since there are few repair defense mechanisms built in to the mitochondrial DNA.

Inflammation, a natural protective function of the immune system, is another considerable source of internal free-radical production. When cells are damaged, several biochemical reactions are initiated. One of these reactions is the release of inflammatory mediators known as *chemotactic factors.* Chemotactic factors dilate capillaries and mobilize white blood cells (neutrophils and macrophages) to the areas of damage, stimulating them to engulf and digest damaged tissue and foreign agents. The process, known as *phagocytosis,* can generate substantial free-radical damage to the surrounding tissue. Neutrophils utilize oxygen to destroy foreign substances, such as bacteria, that cause inflammation. In the process, there is a frenzy of free-radical activity. Neutrophils are relatively short lived. Macrophages are an elegant host defense and survive longer and generate further oxidative damage in their continued fight against foreign invasion.

C-reactive proteins are messengers that get sent out in the body and that cause another form of body-wide inflammation. These and other messengers, which are discussed later in this chapter, are called inflammatory cytokines.

We now know that inflammation and the intense free-radical activity it generates play an important role in the development of cardiovascular disease, as well as in a host of other disorders, including Alzheimer's disease, cancer, diabetes, neurologic disorders, autoimmune disorders, and even obesity. Aside from the obvious stress on the heart that excessive weight provokes, the true nature of this greater risk is rooted in the inflammation process. Belly fat generates hormones, cytokines, glycation (another source of cellular damage), and other inflammatory compounds that increase free-radical load and negatively impact metabolism.

Scientists are finding that, in most cases, the metabolic rate of a species is inversely related to its life expectancy. In other words, the faster free radicals are generated through cellular metabolism, the quicker the aging and death of the species.

External Sources of Free-Radical Production

Unfortunately, the free-radical load in the body is not limited to what it produces internally. Increasingly, *exogenous* (external) free radicals are taking a greater toll on the body. The major sources of external free-radicals include pollution, food and water, oxidized fats, stress, excessive exercise, sunlight, cigarette smoke, and drugs. All of these can contribute to free-radical load, aging, and degenerative disease.

Pollution has become a major threat to health in the last fifty years. Never before in history has the use of toxic chemicals been as prolific as in the last half of the twentieth century. Both the number of chemicals used and the amounts used are at all-time highs. Automobile exhaust, factory waste, fertilizers, pesticides, and fossil fuels have had significant impact on the quality of our air, water, and soil. In some cases, damage to the environment has been irreversible. Many of these pollutants generate free radicals that when breathed, absorbed through the skin, or ingested are highly reactive and damaging to our body chemistry.

Environmental toxins are detoxified by *endogenous* (internal) enzymes known as the cytochrome P-450 system. These enzymes can produce free radicals in the process of detoxification. Sometimes, toxins are only partially inactivated. They are temporarily transformed into even more metabolically active substances before final elimination. During this intermediary step, these transformed molecules can steal electrons off the electron transport chain and wreak free-radical havoc within the cells. If the detoxification process is not completed, then an increased level of phase-one intermediates, known as reactive intermediates, can build up and increase their dangerous free-radical load to body tissues.

Oxidized and rancid fats in the foods we eat are another powerful source of free radicals. Exposure to heat and oxygen cause unsaturated fats to oxidize. This causes the fat to spoil, generating free radicals that quickly pass from molecule to molecule in a chain reaction. Since dietary fat is an essential source of lipids within the body, consumption of oxidized fats introduces free-radical damage directly. Therefore, cooking high-fat foods in intense heat should be avoided, or at least limited, to special occasions. The worst offenders are deep-fried foods (cooked in oil at high temperatures) and cooked meats (especially meats that are high in fat).

Smoking generates free radicals through inhalation of heat from the tip of the burning cigarette. This high heat produces lone electrons that are inhaled in the smoke, generating millions of free radicals with every puff. In addition, tobacco contains free-radical-generating chemicals, such as nitrogen dioxide. Smoking has been shown to significantly increase serum lipid peroxides, and lower the available concentration of antioxidant nutrients like beta-carotene and vitamin C. Cigarettes are particularly harmful because exposure is frequent and repeated. In addition, smokers tend to accumulate cadmium in their tissues, especially the kidneys, which can eventually lead to other health problems such as hypertension and kidney disorders.

Stress increases the release of cortisol from the adrenal glands, which alters cellular metabolism. Chronic stress increases the basal metabolic rate, which in turn speeds up the electron transport chain in the mitochondria and heightens the rate of oxidative damage. Furthermore, the stress hormones epinephrine and norepinephrine break down into free radicals and generate oxidative damage on their own.

Exercise can increase oxygen consumption by ten to twenty times that of the resting state. Individual muscle fibers may require 200 times the resting oxygen levels. When exercising, the activity of the mitochondria accelerates to keep up with the energy demands of the muscles. This increases the generation of free radicals and depletes the antioxidant defense system. Regular, moderate exercise improves your overall health by helping you to oxygenate tissues, burn off excessive stress hormones, and improve insulin regulation. High-intensity training requires an increase in antioxidant intake to reduce the accumulation of free-radical damage. So, the trick is to make exercise a regular part of your life, but not to become too aggressive in your exercise regimen such that your body takes on a dramatically heightened free-radical load. Triathletes—that is, runners and other athletes who are seriously training to participate in events—should take note. The greater the free-radical damage, the greater the chance for injury.

Another mechanism of exercise-induced oxidative damage comes from what is known as reperfusion injury. When blood and oxygen are temporarily diverted from tissue, the return of normal blood flow generates extensive free-radical injury. During exercise, blood flow to the heart and muscles is increased, while other major organs (kidneys, spleen, liver, and others) are temporarily short-changed. After exercise, the blood and oxygen rush back to these organs and free radicals are generated in larger amounts. If you exercise, it is critically important to take antioxidant nutrients.

Ultraviolet light is known to generate free-radical damage directly to the skin. Free radicals from the sun damage protein in the collagen of skin, leading to wrinkles and decreased elasticity. This is why those exposed to excessive amount of sunlight over the years have skin that appears older. Sunlight and other forms of radiation, including X rays and radiation therapy for cancer, react with water molecules in the body, forming hydroxyl radicals. These free radicals can damage proteins, lipoproteins, and DNA.

HOW FREE RADICALS AFFECT METABOLISM

Recent scientific research has begun to show us the effects of oxygen on how we age, as well as what causes cellular deterioration. One theory presently gaining popularity is that damage to the mitochondria triggers cellular disruption and death. I hope you remember from previous chapters that, inside each of our cells, are structures called *mitochondria*. They are the cell's energy source. They generate the energy needed for each cell in your body to function. How well the mitochondria function and their efficiency in delivering energy throughout the body, determine the level of overall energy in every cell, tissue, and organ.

The process of energy production in the mitochondria constantly generates free radicals. Our mitochondria are also constantly under attack from free radicals generated by environmental, physical, and emotional stressors. If mitochondria do not have adequate protection, or fuel, over time, they get damaged or destroyed.

Accelerated damage or destruction of the mitochondria can lead to accelerated aging, or at the very least, increased susceptibility to a wide variety of diseases. The type of mitochondria that is most sensitive to destructive forces is called *mitochondrial DNA*. Mitochondrial DNA is the powerhouse behind the blueprint (DNA) of the future cells that you build. Cells that are built correctly are integral to an optimally functioning body.

When the mitochondrial DNA get damaged, the body starts to manufacture misguided messengers that miscommunicate what functions the cells need to perform. You can think of poor cellular communication as if you were playing a party game and you whispered a secret in someone's ear. You know the game—by the time the secret gets to the last person at the table, the message has become terribly confused.

The bad news is that mitochondrial DNA do not have extensive DNA-repair enzymes to combat the continued free-radical assault. By contrast, the mitochondria in the nucleus of the cells have built-in repair processes to combat the effects of the environment and internal oxidative stress. So, free-radical damage to mitochondrial DNA is long-term damage to the cell's ability to produce energy to drive the function and future of your cells.

A similar theory on aging has been proposed by Anthony Linnane, Ph.D., of the Center for Molecular Biology and Medicine in Melbourne, Australia. This theory suggests that aging is primarily due to cumulative damage to mitochondrial DNA, which causes cells to lose their ability to generate energy. When energy production declines, eventually cells die or at the very least lose the ability to function properly. This, in turn, leads to tissue destruction, loss of organ function and, eventually, the destruction of the whole being. Unlike the previous theory, which attributes aging to

Types of Free-Radical Damage

Oxidative stress mainly targets DNA, cell membranes, lipoproteins, proteins and enzymes that make up cells, tissues, and organs. Free radicals generate essentially five types of damage:

- The first type of free-radical damage is *lipid peroxidation*. Lipids are fats found throughout the body. The most important structural lipids are found in cell membranes. When fat molecules in the cell membranes are damaged by free radicals, the lipid-peroxide free radical is formed. These free radicals initiate a chain reaction in which cell membranes are destroyed and the activities of the cell are inhibited.

- The second type of free-radical destruction is called *membrane damage*. Membrane damage occurs when free radicals destroy the integrity of the cell membrane, which in turn interferes with the ability of the cell to take in nutrients and to release waste products.

- The third type of free-radical damage is *cross-linking* in which proteins and/or DNA molecules are joined together. Since the body's tissues are made of protein, this has far-reaching effects. The "cross-linking theory" was conceived by Professor Johan Bjorksten, who observed that changes in aging skin and other tissues were

direct cellular insult, Dr. Linnane's theory is based on a decrease in cellular energy production.

Whichever of these two theories proves correct, you need to realize that your health begins at the cellular level. You have to be proactive in protecting your mitochondrial DNA. "Genetic expression" means that your genes can take you down either a path that builds proteins and peptides that promote homeostasis (balance), energy production, and a healthy biochemistry, or a path of dysfunction that leads to the development of inflammation and toxic intermediate metabolites, which will slowly poison body chemistry and can lead to cardiovascular disease, cancer, diabetes, or other disorders.

Research is published daily on the effects of drugs and nutrition on genetic expression. Regulating genetic expression and proteomic expression (expression of protein codes that run body chemistry) will be the new frontier in prevention and wellness. Environmental toxins, excessive free-radical damage, stress, poor nutrition status, drugs, and other factors influence our health on a cellular level.

The cumulative effect of these influences create each person's bio-individuality, which can be researched, mapped out, and acted on. Understanding your bio-individuality along with your personal metabolic code means understanding what influences affect you and then taking the steps to create change in your cellular health.

---

similar to the hardening of gels and other flexible substances over time (such as the tanning of leather). These changes were due to permanent tissue alterations caused by the formation of intra- and intermolecular linking, which causes a loss of elasticity in the collagen of different tissues—for example, skin, arterial blood vessel walls, the lens of the eye, ligaments, tendons, and intervertebral discs. In other words, because of oxidative stress and free-radical attack, our collagen eventually gets damaged and "binds" together and starts the aging process of skin and other tissues.

- The fourth type of free-radical destruction originates from the rupture of cellular lysosomal membranes. *Lysosomes* are digestive substances found in each cell. They are designed to digest and eliminate waste from the cell. When the membranes are ruptured prematurely, cell contents are digested and destroyed.

- The fifth type of free-radical damage is known as *lipofuscin*, the accumulation of lipid pigment. Free radicals contribute to the accumulation of *lipofuscin*. Lipofuscin is most commonly found in the muscle, heart, skin, liver, brain, and nerve cells, and is a sign of cellular wear and tear. Lipofuscin is also known as *age pigment* or *age spots* because it increases with age. Lipofuscin is thought to somehow interfere with cellular function, but it is not yet clear how this happens.

DEFENDING AGAINST FREE RADICALS

Since we all have to breathe in order to live, our gradual destruction by free radicals may seem inescapable. This is not so. A healthy body produces energy efficiently without generating excessive quantities of harmful forms of oxygen. When your cells are performing optimally, the body has the internal resources to defend itself by detoxifying these damaging forms of oxygen. To counteract this naturally occurring free-radical damage, the body produces an impressive arsenal of antioxidant enzymes. The most abundant of these biological antioxidants are *glutathione peroxidase, superoxide dismutase,* and *catalase.*

Antioxidant enzymes neutralize the lone electrons in oxygen molecules by monitoring oxidation and reduction reactions. They help to promote optimal oxygen function and utilization, and as such, decrease the damage the free radicals can cause. Recent research even points to their ability to help protect and guide healthy genetic expression. However, the built-in defenses of the body do not completely protect against deterioration from the continual onslaught of free radicals. Fortunately, other antioxidants can be derived from the foods we eat. You can get this protection by eating lots of fresh vegetables and fruits in a wide variety of colors (the natural pigments in foods contain a variety of beneficial antioxidants and phytochemicals). Chief among the dietary antioxidants are the vitamins A, C, E, and selenium. Other nutrients, such as carotenoids (plant pigments found mostly in yellow and orange fruits and vegetables), alpha lipoic acid, and coenzyme Q_{10} (CoQ_{10}), have been proven to provide substantial antioxidant protection when consumed from either foods or supplements. (Specific details about the types and amounts of antioxidants to use are covered in the next chapter.)

Combating free-radical damage is dependent on the availability of antioxidants, both internal and external. In most cases, the body is able to defuse free radicals sufficiently with these antioxidants. However, the more oxidative stress one is exposed to—whether it is disease, stress, or other health problems—the more antioxidants are needed. If you are not eating a plant-rich diet and do not have enough antioxidant enzymes and phytonutrients, then your body will become much more susceptible to the harmful effects of oxygen and other free radicals.

MAJOR CONDITIONS ASSOCIATED WITH OXIDATIVE STRESS

Although the body uses oxygen and generates free radicals as a result of normal metabolic processes, scientific research clearly shows us that free radicals such as *superoxide radicals, hydroxyl radicals, hydrogen peroxide, singlet oxygen, nitric oxide,* and *peroxynitrite,* among others, are a major source of accelerated aging and disease.

Oxidative stress is a factor in the following degenerative conditions:

* Aging of the skin
* Diabetes

- Alzheimer's disease
- Arthritis
- Cancer
- Cardiovascular disease
- Depressed immune function
- Endocrine dysfunction
- Insulin resistance and diabetes
- Macular degeneration
- Neurological dysfunction/Parkinson's disease
- Obesity

According to the free-radical theory of disease, all of these conditions and many more begin at the molecular level. Oxygen radicals interact with cell membranes, proteins, and DNA, generating damage and destruction of the cells. Over time, the molecular damage interferes with the function of tissues, organs, and entire systems, until disease is evident.

According to the free-radical theory of disease, diseases that seem totally unrelated can share the same origin. It is obvious that obese individuals, who have metabolic syndrome that has progressed to full-fledged diabetes and cardiovascular disease, have greatly increased free-radical activity. One hidden source of this increased free-radical activity and the damage it causes may be subclinical hypothyroidism (discussed in detail in Chapter 4). When the thyroid is sluggish, oxygen is not burned in the cells quickly enough. This generates an increased free-radical load on the cells. It is no wonder low thyroid function is associated with so many symptoms and conditions!

Now, let's take a closer look at the major degenerative and inflammatory conditions that can occur when massive amounts of free radicals damage healthy cells.

Alzheimer's Disease and Neurological Degeneration

Alzheimer's disease is a degenerative disorder of the brain, leading to memory loss, cognitive impairment, behavioral disturbances, and premature death. Once a rare condition, Alzheimer's disease is now considered the leading cause of senile dementia, affecting as many as 1 percent of the population in developed countries.

As Alzheimer's disease progresses, the central nervous system develops *plaques,* fibrous deposits within the nerve cells. Along with degeneration of the nerve terminals, there is also a decline in the production of *acetylcholine,* a reduced product of the metabolism of glucose, and abnormally high levels of aluminum. Current research is currently pointing to mercury toxicity as another initiator of destruction of the nerve branches known as *tubulin.* The cause of Alzheimer's disease is not known, although free-radical pathology is strongly being suggested as one of the significant contributing factors. This hypothesis proposes that oxidative stress results in excessive lipid peroxidation and neuronal degeneration in certain parts of the brain. Free radical-induced mitochondrial DNA damage has also been proposed as a mechanism of cell loss in Alzheimer's disease.

Recently, scientists have been able to measure brain levels of oxidative damage through identification of compounds known as *isoprostanes.* Isoprostanes are formed when *arachidonic acid,* a naturally occurring fatty acid, is oxidized by free radicals.

A 1998 study found that isoprostane concentrations were markedly elevated in tissue samples from patients with Alzheimer's disease. Isoprostane elevation is also seen in diabetics. Recently a correlation was found between people with "belly fat," or potential type 2 diabetics, and an increased risk for developing Alzheimer's disease. Getting your weight under control and working on your insulin resistance, before you develop metabolic syndrome, could have a significant long-term impact on the quality of your life and your risk of developing Alzheimer's disease.

According to researchers Cranton and Frackelton as reported in the *Journal of Holistic Medicine,* "Research in senility, dementia, brain ischemia, stroke, and spinal cord injury provides a wealth of evidence incriminating free radicals as a cause of nervous system disease, and also provides a rationale for treatment." Ongoing research, as well as a more complete understanding of free-radical pathology and the role of antioxidant nutrients may eventually offer hope for the prevention of degenerative conditions of the nervous system. For example, in the not-too-distant future, vitamin C may prove to be a protective nutrient in the prevention of Alzheimer's disease. An important function of vitamin C is to protect the central nervous system from oxidative damage to fatty tissues. The central nervous system not only contains the highest concentrations of fat of any organ, but it also contains fifty times more vitamin C than that found in any other tissue in the body. Vitamin E has proven to be of benefit to Alzheimer's patients, as well.

Cancer

Although cancer can manifest in hundreds of forms and in every tissue in the body, the underlying pathology for all cancers is the same. Cancer cells are normal cells that have lost what is known as *differentiation.* Differentiation is the genetic transcription of cellular activity—the code that dictates the task it is supposed to perform. All cells contain the same DNA, but what differentiates muscle cells from brain cells, for example, is the expression of particular genes.

Cancer cells are those cells that have lost the ability to differentiate, becoming incapable of carrying out specific cellular functions. It is thought that free radicals, particularly *singlet oxygen,* may be responsible for the damage to DNA that leads to loss of differentiation.

Recent research indicates that the value of antioxidants may be in their ability to control genetic expression, even more so than their free-radical-quenching activity. Since the early 1990s, the anticancer properties of antioxidant nutrients have been the subject of considerable attention. Although this area of science is still new, some exciting knowledge has been ascertained. The intake of certain foods and nutrients, for example, has been associated with a reduced risk of cancer. Because of the limited understanding of how food is converted into micronutrients, more evidence exists for the protective activities of certain whole foods. A 1995 Italian study demonstrated that intake of fish, raw vegetables, and milk was inversely related to breast cancer. Meaning that higher intakes of those foods were associated with lower cancer incidence.

Vitamin A (retinol) is an essential nutrient found in animal foods. Its ability to regulate cell differentiation may play an important role in the prevention of tumor formation. Vitamin A has demonstrated protective effects against skin, head, neck, breast, liver, and other forms of cancer. Beta-carotene, a plant carotenoid (found in carrots) that is converted to vitamin A in the body, appears to neutralize free radicals, particularly singlet oxygen. Beta-carotene has been found to comprise approximately 15 to 30 percent of carotenoids, making it the most nutritionally abundant of the carotenoids. In epidemiological studies, diets high in carotenoid-rich plant foods (carrots, kale, broccoli, spinach, and tomatoes) have been correlated with protection from certain cancers, particularly lung cancer. Similarly, low beta-carotene levels appear to increase the risk of lung and other cancers.

An even more powerful free-radical quencher than beta-carotene is the carotenoid *lycopene*. Lycopene has demonstrated significant protection in the prevention of prostate and breast cancer. Cooked tomato products are the richest source of lycopene. Another important antioxidant compound for defending against cancer is vitamin E. There are about eight common forms of vitamin E: four of them are known as tocopherols and four are tocotrienols. Tocopherols and tocotrienols can be found naturally in almonds and in fruits and vegetables, including asparagus, red chili peppers, grapes, tomatoes, and spinach and other leafy green vegetables, and can be derived synthetically. Vitamin E has demonstrated a protective role against ultraviolet damage to the skin, as well as the oxidative damage associated with environmental pollution. In addition, natural vitamin E (d-alpha-tocopherol) does seem to absorb better and last longer than its synthetic counterparts (dl-alpha-tocopherol). The tocotrienol form of vitamin E is relatively new on the scene, but some research shows it may offer even more antioxidant protection than vitamin E in tocopherol form.

Cardiovascular Disease

A great deal of scientific attention has been focused on the role of free radicals in cardiovascular disease. More than 57 million Americans suffer from cardiovascular disease. Out of this research, some surprising new facts are emerging about the true origin of cardiovascular disease and the benefits of antioxidant protection. While the knowledge of the underlying mechanisms of cardiovascular disease has not changed, there has been a shift in the understanding of how these mechanisms occur.

It is known that a significant cause of myocardial infarction (heart attack) is *ath-*

erosclerosis. Atherosclerosis is a progressive narrowing of the vessels that transport blood caused from a thickening of the vessel wall. Deposits of fatty molecules, known as *fatty streaks* or *plaque,* cause the thickening. Fatty streaks are formed from lipid-rich cells known as *foam cells.* Atherosclerosis develops most frequently in medium-sized arteries, such as the coronary and carotid vessels that carry oxygenated blood to the heart and brain. Hence, this disease is also known as *arteriosclerosis.*

Progressive atherosclerosis has long been associated with certain risk factors, including smoking, hypertension, diabetes, and high cholesterol. The exact mechanisms by which these factors contribute to the development of fatty streaks have not been explained until now. Recent research has found that foam cells are formed when particular cells (monocyte-macrophage cells) engulf low-density lipoprotein (LDL) cholesterol circulating in the blood. Further investigation has led researchers to surmise that the macrophage cells specifically engulf LDL that have been *oxidized,* or damaged by free radicals. This is an important step forward in our understanding of the etiology of atherosclerosis, the role of free radicals, and the potential for antioxidants in the prevention of cardiovascular disease.

Some experimental evidence suggests that vitamin E may protect against the oxidation of LDL and, therefore, has a potentially important role in preventing the formation of fatty streaks. Vitamin E is a critical antioxidant that neutralizes free radicals before they can oxidize LDL. Vitamin E may also alter the LDL itself, making it more resistant to free-radical damage. However, there are other studies that have not shown vitamin E alone to be protective in cardiovascular disease; this may be due to study flaws or it may be due to the fact that we have not yet found the most biologically active form of vitamin E (most studies use d-alpha-tocopherol).

Unlike vitamin E, two other powerful antioxidants have strong studies behind them showing an important role in the prevention of the oxidation of LDL cholesterol and in slowing down the development of atherosclerosis: CoQ_{10} and Policosanol. CoQ_{10} is a vitaminlike substance manufactured by the body from vitamin B_5 (and available in supplement form) that is transported throughout the body on LDL and VLDL cholesterol (very low density lipoproteins) molecules where it prevents damage from free radicals and is used by cells for the production of energy. Policosanol is a natural mixture of chemicals taken from sugar-cane wax. In supplement form, it has demonstrated profound cholesterol-lowering effects. This ability to lower cholesterol has been reported in many laboratory studies and in patients with high cholesterol levels. An added benefit of Policosanol is that it seems to lower the "bad" or LDL cholesterol and triglycerides while raising the "good" or HDL cholesterol.

Keep in mind that there are many risk factors that can contribute to cardiovascular disease. Exercise and diet alone will not necessarily prevent you from this fate. Micro-infections, heavy metal toxicity, low thyroid performance, and stress can also deal a significant blow to your cardiovascular health.

Diabetes

It is known that diabetics with poor glycemic (blood sugar) control have decreased antioxidant defenses and increased oxidative stress. Increased glucose levels in the mitochondria, and the subsequent increase in cellular metabolism, increases the body's free-radical activity and depletes antioxidant enzymes.

The oxidative stress associated with diabetes is linked to the long-term complications of diabetes, including vascular insufficiency, renal disease, cardiovascular disease, high cholesterol levels, and retinopathy. Yet, not only is this increased free-radical activity a result of diabetes, it may also be a factor leading to the development of diabetes. The imbalance between oxidative stress and antioxidant defenses associated with high levels of glucose in the blood, which we find in insulin resistance, appears to worsen free-radical-induced damage of the pancreatic beta cells. Beta cells are responsible for synthesizing and regulating insulin. Free-radical damage, therefore, may be a contributing factor in the progression from hyperinsulinemia (too much insulin in the bloodstream) to overt type 2 diabetes.

Also, continued exposure to high glycemic loads, such as that encountered after eating high-carbohydrate foods, can lead to an increase in inflammatory mediators such as the *isoprostanes*. Isoprostanes, as discussed earlier, cause oxidative stress, thereby damaging fragile arteries and leading to a host of problems. These and other inflammatory mediators are being implicated in almost all of the diseases we encounter as we age (cardiovascular disease, Alzheimer's disease, diabetes, high cholesterol levels, arthritis, weight gain), and many other diseases related to accelerated and unhealthy aging.

Research indicates that antioxidants may protect against free-radical damage associated with type 1 and type 2 diabetes. In one recent study, administration of N-acetyl-L-cysteine (NAC) and vitamins C and E to diabetic mice provided protection against free-radical damage to the pancreatic beta cells. Treatment with NAC also preserved glucose-stimulated insulin secretion and moderately lowered blood glucose levels. In another study with human subjects, diabetic patients receiving 600 milligrams (mg) of alpha lipoic acid (ALA) for more than three months had lower plasma lipid hydroperoxides (markers of free-radical damage) than those without treatment.

Many scientists believe that ALA may be our most important antioxidant. One of its key characteristics is that it is both fat soluble and water soluble, enabling it to provide antioxidant protection in a much wider range of body systems. Some scientists refer to ALA as the "universal" antioxidant. ALA provides antioxidant protection throughout the body. It may also facilitate the production of energy for cells and helps to regenerate and revitalize other antioxidants in the body. ALA may not only benefit individuals with diabetes, but also those with eye problems such as cataracts and glaucoma. For diabetics, ALA supplementation may help maintain blood sugar levels while treating some of the neurological side effects of the disease such as diabetic neuropathy.

In contrast to many food sources of antioxidants, red meat is the best dietary source of ALA. Smaller amounts occur in the leaves of some plants and in potatoes, carrots, yams, and sweet potatoes. But don't go building up your red meat stores yet. An excess intake of meat is also associated with higher insulin-growth factor-1 (IGF-1) levels in your blood, which means you may be increasing your risk of cancer, especially breast cancer in women. If you want the benefits of ALA without the risks, the best way to ensure an adequate intake for now is supplement form.

Chronic Inflammation

Evidence is emerging that many of our most debilitating chronic diseases have a common underlying factor: inflammation. Inflammation is a vascular and cellular response to illness or injury that causes pain, redness, swelling, and tissue damage. The various compounds in the body that cause inflammation, such as histamine, cytokines, and prostaglandins, are called the *mediators of inflammation.*

Inflammation in and of itself is not a disorder. Inflammation is part of the body's process of self-healing. Excessive prolonged production of inflammatory mediators (chronic inflammation), however, is problematic. Chronic inflammation is now known to play a role in many, if not most, chronic diseases and conditions, including auto-immune disease, which now affects one in five Americans, and cardiovascular disease, diabetes, Parkinson's disease and Alzheimer's disease, in addition to many other diseases and conditions.

Thus far, I have shown how a diet high in sugar and low in phytochemicals, fiber, and other nutrients contributes to the downward spiral of your metabolism and excessive free-radical production in the body. Free radicals can cause various types of damage to tissues as we just learned and, therefore, are thought to be an initiator of chronic inflammation and the conditions and diseases that are caused, or exacerbated, by this inflammation. While the causes of cardiovascular disease and diabetes have always had obvious lifestyle components, we are only now realizing the connection of lifestyle-induced inflammatory processes to chronic and autoimmune diseases.

Most people know of the autoimmune diseases lupus and Sjögren's syndrome; however, many are not aware that rheumatoid arthritis, multiple sclerosis (MS), some types of pancreatitis, Crohn's disease, chronic fatigue syndrome (CFS), and psoriasis also have autoimmune components. In autoimmune conditions, it was thought that the immune system perceived normal cells as invaders and attacked them. Now it is becoming evident that part of the problem may be that the body is not attacking normal cells, but rather cells that have become glycated, or otherwise damaged by free radicals.

Rheumatoid arthritis is a classic example of an autoimmune disorder. In rheumatoid arthritis, the white blood cells of the body attack the collagen tissue in the joints. It is now theorized that this tissue is being damaged by free radicals and/or glycated; thus, the body sees it as foreign and attacks it. Once the white blood cells are mobilized, helper T cells begin producing cytokines, inflammatory proteins that allow white blood cell communication. Excess levels of cytokines such as *tumor necrosis factor alpha* (TNF alpha), *interleukin-6* (IL-6), *interleukin-1B* (IL-1B), and/or *leukotriene B4* (LT-B4) are known to cause the inflammation in this condition.

Free radicals are both a cause and a result of inflammation. While damage to cells from free radicals can cause inflammation, conditions marked by chronic inflammation then go on to generate large numbers of free radicals. It becomes a catch-22, because those free radicals then go on to stimulate more inflammation.

In chronic inflammatory disease, many systems of the body are affected, and a series of other destructive forces are put into motion. Other organs or glands can be damaged, such as the thyroid, the pancreas, or the heart. And once inflammation starts into motion, it is like a forest fire raging out of control in your body.

Cytokines and other inflammatory mediators increase production of *fibrinogen* and *C-reactive protein,* substances that are known to greatly increase risk of cardiovascular disease. Fibrinogen is a protein in blood that assists in the formation of blood clots. Fibrinogen levels are increased from thromboxanes (inflammatory substances produced from arachidonic acid that increase not only blood clotting, but also constriction of blood vessels). The inflammatory mediator C-reactive protein (CRP) is produced in the liver by the inflammatory cytokines IL-6, IL-1B, and TNF alpha. The presence of C-reactive protein indicates an increased risk for destabilized *atherosclerotic* plaque and abnormal arterial clotting. When arterial plaque becomes destabilized, it can burst open and block the flow of blood through a coronary artery, resulting in an acute heart attack. Studies have reported that people with high levels of C-reactive protein were almost three times as likely to die from a heart attack.

Homocysteine is a breakdown product of methionine (an amino acid needed to help produce ATP in cells). It is associated with an increased risk of cardiovascular disease, as well as Alzheimer's disease, depression, cervical cancer, and even increased risk of miscarriage. Homocysteine is known to increase free radicals in the blood vessels, the heart, and other tissues and to increase production of the inflammatory prostaglandins thromboxanes. As long as there is adequate folate and vitamins B_6 and B_{12} in the body, homocysteine gets converted back into methionine. If not, homocysteine levels increase and start causing inflammation.

Prostaglandins (PGEs) also act as mediators of inflammation and are another example of how dietary factors contribute to inflammation. Remember, PGE-2s are the prostaglandins that lead to increased inflammation and blood platelet aggregation (clots). These PGEs are excessively produced in the presence of several dietary factors, including increased insulin levels and inadequate intakes of omega-3 fatty acids.

Leptins are another source of inflammatory compounds in the body. Leptins are hormones made in fat cells. They send satiety signals (a signal that a person is full and no longer needs to eat) to the brain. However, when too much fat is present in the body, it actually starts to act like an organ, secreting inflammatory chemicals such as aromatase, IL-6, TNF alpha, estrogen, cortisol, and angiotensinogen, an enzyme that contributes to hypertension. These inflammatory chemicals, in turn, induce chronic low-grade systemic inflammation in people with excess body fat. So, the thought that fat is just a passive, jellylike substance with no real activity is completely mistaken. Through these byproducts of fat metabolism, obesity is a risk factor for hypertension, cardiovascular disease, glucose intolerance, diabetes, Alzheimer's disease, cancer, and other inflammation-based conditions.

Although medicine is beginning to acknowledge that lifestyle factors are implicated in inflammatory disease, it is still exploring other possible means of treating these conditions. One recent medical approach has been the use of anti-inflammatory drugs. There are two pathways, the *cyclooxygenase* (COX-1 and -2 enzyme pathways) and the *lipoxygenase* pathways, that produce many of these mediators of inflammation.

In the cyclooxygenase pathways, the inflammatory mediators, prostaglandins, *thromboxanes,* and *prostacyclins* are made. Thromboxanes are made in platelets and cause constriction of vascular smooth muscle (contained in the walls of the blood vessels) and platelet aggregation leading to the formation of clots. Prostacyclins are the "good guys" produced by blood vessel walls, which counter thromboxanes by inhibiting platelet aggregation and the ultimate formation of clots. They are made in the COX-1 pathways, and are important because they also play an important role in the protection of stomach and intestinal linings. Lipooxygenase pathways form leukotrienes, which are inflammatory substances produced in white blood cells.

Nonsteroidal anti-inflammatory drugs (NSAIDs) such as aspirin and ibuprofen inhibit production of the COX-2 enzyme and decrease the inflammation response in the body. The problem is that NSAIDs and aspirin also inhibit production of the COX-1 enzyme, which makes the mucosal barrier of the intestine more prone to ulceration and inflammation. When COX-1 enzymes are inhibited along with COX-2 enzymes, the lipoxygenase pathways become more active because arachidonic acid, which is a substrate (a substance acted upon by an enzyme) for both pathways, is then freed up for the production of leukotrienes.

Recently, a new generation of anti-inflammatory drugs called the COX-2 *inhibitors* was introduced. These drugs were expected to be better than the traditional NSAIDs for people with arthritis as they target COX-2 enzymes only and, therefore, should leave stomach linings intact. The best known of these drugs is celecoxib (Celebrex), which quickly became the fastest-selling drug in history.

Because of the ability of COX-2 inhibitors to control pain and inflammation, research suggests that the drugs can also prove useful in preventing cancer and Alzheimer's disease—two other conditions in which the enzyme COX-2 is found to be unregulated, or to have increased activity. Several studies have demonstrated that the use of COX-2 inhibitors is able to reduce the incidence of colon cancer—and deaths from the disease—by nearly half. Initial studies also suggest that the use of

COX-2 inhibitors may be effective in reducing the incidence of Alzheimer's disease. Heightened COX-2 enzyme activity has also been linked to breast cancer as well as to several other cancers. In fact, researchers recently have linked higher levels of COX-2 activity in breast cancer cases with increased mortality.

Although the COX-2-inhibiting prescription drugs were supposed to decrease the incidence of gastrointestinal ulcers and bleeding too, newer studies have found that some people taking COX-2 inhibitor drugs have an increased incidence of heart and kidney problems, upper respiratory infections, and other negative side effects, including diarrhea, headaches, indigestion, and gastrointestinal ulcers. While COX-2 inhibitors are great at controlling the pain associated with inflammatory conditions such as rheumatoid arthritis, they do not address the underlying problems that are causing inflammation.

Because of the side effects of prescription COX-2 inhibitors, many health practitioners are looking for safer alternatives for alleviating pain or for addressing inflammatory conditions. Several herbs, for example, have been discovered to have COX-2 inhibiting qualities, but without the side effects. These include Nexrutine (from *Phellodendron amurense*), turmeric, holy basil, and feverfew, which are discussed in the next chapter.

Enhancement of human growth hormone (HGH) is also proving to be an important component in the struggle to limit the aging and inflammatory processes associated with excessive free-radical activity. HGH is one of key players in maintaining metabolism as we age.

HGH is the most abundant hormone produced by the pituitary gland. HGH triggers IGF-1 (insulin growth factor-1) production in the liver, which then circulates throughout the body. IGF-1 is the factor that is thought to be responsible for many of the activities of HGH, and is the primary anabolic (tissue-building) hormone in the body. IGF-1 plays a huge role in the uptake of carbohydrates, proteins, and fats into the cells.

HGH secretion reaches its peak in the body during adolescence. This makes sense because HGH helps stimulate growth of the body. HGH secretion does not stop after adolescence, however. Many of the physical and personal changes that are associated with the aging process are the result of the age-related decline in HGH and IGF-1, and, therefore, can be greatly impacted by making sure that HGH production is not compromised or inhibited.

Our bodies continue to produce HGH in adulthood usually in short bursts during deep sleep. HGH is known to be critical for tissue repair, muscle growth, healing, brain function, physical and mental health, bone strength, enzyme production, blood sugar regulation, and sexual function, as well as energy and metabolism. Because HGH is responsible for the growth and maintenance of muscle tissue, it is key to maintaining metabolism as we age. Muscle is metabolically more active than other types of tissue. So, the higher the body's percentage of muscle, the higher its resting energy expenditure (resting metabolic rate) will be. Declining rates of HGH production that occur in aging are one of the key reasons we lose muscle as we age.

For this reason, substances that increase HGH have become very popular for the promise of increasing muscle, decreasing fat, and improving energy. From injections of the hormone to scores of dietary supplements that claim to "boost" HGH release, people are looking for the fountain of youth. Although the claims made on some products may be exaggerated, the health benefits that can be attained by optimizing HGH as we age are real, and this is a legitimate and highly pursued area of research.

A cell's ability to function depends on the genetic codes for all the proteins, hormones, and enzymes that make the cell run. Free radicals, in excess, can impair the ability of cells to replicate and/or function normally. Up until now, antioxidant supplements such as vitamin C and E have been a primary focus to help limit the damage to the DNA and bolster our immunities. HGH can help the DNA in cells to repair itself and therefore goes a step further than antioxidants, which simply prevent damage to the cells. So, you may be thinking, "Why not take growth hormone and stay young forever?" (See the inset "Natural Agents that Mimic Growth Hormone.")

The good news for those concerned with oxidative stressors and their health is that it's never too late to start taking steps to reverse free-radical related pathology. One way to slow down the degenerative process caused by chronic inflammation is to increase your intake of antioxidant nutrients and antioxidant-rich foods, as early as possible in your life. By the time the diseases of chronic inflammation typically show up, you're probably seven to ten years into the process.

No matter your age or condition, the disease prevention strategies presented in the next chapter will significantly reduce the inflammatory cascade. Diet, as well as nutritional supplementation, including vitamins, minerals, nutraceuticals, and herbs, can help those suffering from chronic inflammation and potentially slow down the deadly processes associated with aging. And now with the availability of cytokine blood profile tests, it is possible to ascertain the underlying causes of chronic inflammatory disease. The appropriate drugs, nutrients, dietary changes, and/or hormones can then be used to take back control of the secretion of specific cytokines that are promoting the inflammatory cascade.

KEY INFLUENCES ON OXIDATIVE STRESS

The following keys are among the various conditions that determine whether the body uses oxygen for metabolic activity or produces increased levels of destructive forms of oxygen.

Nutrition

An unhealthy diet and insufficient levels of antioxidant protector nutrients will exacerbate the effects of the harmful forms of oxygen and fuel oxidative-stress reactions. No diet should be without a lineup of foods containing important antioxidants and

Natural Agents That Mimic Growth Hormone

Because of the many benefits of HGH for the body, supplement manufacturers and other research and development firms are racing to find ways to facilitate the body's own production of HGH and/or to get HGH into the body. Growth hormone cannot be taken in its intact form because, being a protein, it is broken down during the digestive process. Injections of HGH are available by prescription, and until recently were highly sought after due to their ability to burn fat, improve musculature, increase libido, improve ability to sleep, and other benefits.

Excess growth hormone may make you look great, but it can create some problems. What has scared many healthcare professionals from becoming advocates of HGH is the number of studies showing that increases in IGF-1 are correlated with the potential for stimulating cancer-cell growth; therefore, some healthcare professionals have been hesitant to recommend injections of HGH. In addition, these injections are costly, need careful monitoring, and must be used regularly for continued benefits.

For years, measuring IGF-1 was assumed to be the most accurate method for measuring the effects of various growth hormone therapies. While IGF-1 levels do increase in the blood with HGH injections, research conducted by Rashid Buttar, D.O., and Dean Viktora, Ph.D., has helped elucidate the relationship between HGH and IGF-1 levels. Their research showed that IGF-1 levels were lower in young athletes. IGF-1 should have been higher in the younger population, because HGH hormones are known to be higher in youth and to decrease with age. This indicated that measurement of IGF-1 levels in the blood may not be the best indicator of HGH levels.

The fact is various conditions lead to decreased production of HGH, which leads to the acceleration of the aging process. However, until recently, good options for safe HGH support simply were not available.

There are a variety of natural agents currently on the market that claim to improve growth hormone secretion. The agent with the strongest claim to being able to do this is alpha glycerophosphocholine (alpha GPC). Alpha GPC is a derivative of lecithin that readily crosses the blood-brain barrier, so you don't need to take it in large amounts to get a physiologic effect. Alpha GPC has several important characteristics. It increases the brain's "memory molecules" called *acetylcholine* and helps cognitive problems resulting from short-term memory loss, dementia, and even Alzheimer's disease. Alpha GPC also appears to increase the release of endogenous growth hormone and improve coordination and reflex time. This has become one of my favorite supplements to recommend for people over the age of fifty, children with learning disorders, and athletes.

Another exciting antiaging agent that I have used over the last five years is Trans-D Tropin. Trans-D Tropin consists of a combination of amino acids that when administered transdermally (through the skin) mimic or act as an analog to endogenous growth hormone releasing hormone (GHRH). GHRH from Trans-D Tropin has been shown in studies to improve growth hormone release, but does not increase IGF-1. In fact, it lowers IGF-1. This is significant because in clinical trials it showed a 1,700 percent increase in HGH over baseline. Because IGF-1 was not increased, it is theorized that the IGF-1 receptor sites are increased, so there is less free IGF-1 (in the blood) to excite cells into uncontrolled growth. Trans-D Tropin, therefore, raises HGH enough to get the positive anabolic effects and regenerative effects without the negative feedback or increased risks.

A gentle boost in HGH results in improved lean mass; improved mood; better memory and concentration; reduced fatigue and belly fat; fewer wrinkles; heightened cellular repair; improved sleep; better libido; enhanced blood sugar regulation; improved DHEA to cortisol relationships; healthier skin, hair, and nails; and most relevant to this chapter, reduced inflammatory chemistry. Although alpha GPC and Trans-D Tropin make a significant contribution to wellness and health, do not look to them to be superheroes; they alone will not overcome all aging processes. Both substances work more effectively in a body that is nourished well and has as much toxic waste products removed as possible; they are a wonderful adjunct to diet in fighting the free-radical damage and other processes of aging.

Are there other ways to increase growth hormone production? There are numerous products on the market that claim to increase HGH, homeopathic preparations, oral dietary supplements, and amino acid blends, among others. However, most of these agents, though they may have a logical reason for why they may work in theory, have no studies to back their claims. To date, healthcare physicians are hesitant to provide injections of HGH because of the risks associated with it. So, while there may be other products that will eventually prove their efficacy at increasing HGH, the two with the best study behind them to date are alpha GPC and Trans-D Tropin. However, because the studies on Trans-D Tropin have shown that it down-regulates IGF-1, this product could also have profound effects on the insulin resistant chemistry that leads to metabolic syndrome, cardiovascular disease, obesity, and polycystic ovarian syndrome in women.

phytonutrients. Fresh fruits such as blueberries, strawberries, and red raspberries, red and green grapes, and grapefruit, as well as vegetables, including yellow squash, broccoli, Brussels sprouts, green kale, red and yellow peppers, red and gold beets, carrots, cauliflower, cabbage, leafy green vegetables, onions, and white garlic are all abundant in antioxidants and phytonutrients.

Attempt to minimize the amount of free radicals introduced into the body from the diet. Avoid rancid and hydrogenated oils and dietary sources of trans-fatty acids, whenever possible. One of the largest problems with the modern American diet is the extreme temperature used to cook fatty foods, including meats, eggs, and cheeses. Cooking polyunsaturated fats and cholesterol at a high temperature (above 300°F) oxidizes these fats and introduces free radicals into the body as they are eaten. Frying, grilling, broiling, and charring meats or cheeses should be avoided also. Instead, poaching, stewing, braising, and slow roasting are preferred cooking methods if we are to decrease the formation of potentially damaging free radicals.

Throughout this book, I have been on the soapbox preaching about the dangers of too much sugar consumption, but it has been for a good reason. One of the most damaging byproducts of metabolism that generate free radicals in the body is known as advanced glycation end products (AGEs). Briefly discussed in earlier chapters, AGEs are formed when sugars (glucose, fructose, and galactose) react in a non-enzymatic way to proteins to produce what are known as *glycated proteins*. As these sugars break down, they generate compounds such as *glyoxal, methylglyoxal,* and *3-oxyglucosone*. Glycated proteins and fructosamine (proteins with fructose attached) are broken down by oxidative and non-oxidative pathways to form AGEs. While some glycation is a normal part of metabolism, the standard American diet contributes to excessive amounts of glycation. This sounds like a lot of chemistry but bear with me for a minute.

Glycation of hemoglobin, glutathione, and albumin, as well as collagen, can dramatically accelerate damage to your cells. Hemoglobin A_1C is a measure of how much glycation of hemoglobin is taking place and is considered the principle marker of how well a diabetic is able to control their disease.

The formation of AGEs through glycation generates massive amounts of free radicals, leading to the formation of superoxide, hydrogen peroxide, and hydroxyl radicals, which are associated with accelerated aging and wrinkling of the skin. AGEs have been linked to arthritis, diabetic complications, amyotrophic lateral sclerosis (ALS), and Alzheimer's disease, among other conditions.

Key nutrients known to maintain glycation at a manageable rate of production include alpha lipoic acid, vitamins B_2 and B_6, carnitine, carnosine, chromium, cobalamin, folic acid, glycine, glutamic acid, magnesium, potassium, N-acetyl cysteine, pyruvate, resveratrol, and taurine. The next chapter discusses how to use these nutrients to help manage glycation.

Nutritional Supplements

Even when you are eating a healthy, whole-foods diet, it is difficult to obtain a level of antioxidant intake that provides optimal protection against the levels of oxidative stress that are introduced into our bodies from the environment. Therefore, it makes good sense to take an antioxidant-rich nutritional supplement. Make sure that, at the very least, it includes the carotenoids (beta-carotene, lutein, lycopene, and zeaxanthin), mixed natural tocopherols, vitamin C, alpha lipoic acid, CoQ_{10}, and N-acetyl cysteine, and the minerals selenium, manganese, copper, and zinc. Some of these nutrients serve as cofactors for the synthesis of antioxidant enzymes, which increase detoxification pathways for carcinogens, hormones like estrogen, and other toxins; some protect cell membranes from oxidative damage, and others quench circulating free radicals and help protect and repair DNA.

Do not underestimate the value of nutraceuticals. In one small pilot trial at the Living Longer Institute, we measured several markers of brain biochemistry using brain spectroscopy (scanning) and measured the free-radical levels in the blood of ten men and women, aged fifty-five to seventy. The individuals were then asked to follow a supplement program for one month that included antioxidants and cognitive-specific nutraceuticals such as vinpocetine, bacopa, ginkgo, and phosphatidylserine. At the end of thirty days, we once again scanned their brains and measured their blood. The end result was a decrease in oxidative stress and a reduction in brain glutamate levels, as well as an increase in N-acetylcholine levels, indicators of free-radical activity, potential for brain cell death, and brain cell health. In a short time, we were able to preserve cognitive function and reduce free-radical stress, which are associated with cognitive decline. Even though this was a small trial, it highlights the protection nutraceuticals can offer and the power that they can have on our metabolic code for health and vitality.

Enzymes

Free radicals can also damage enzymes in the body. Enzymes are cofactors in almost every biological function within the body. There are thousands of known enzymes, and many that have yet to be identified. These compounds are subject to destruction by a variety of toxins, known collectively as toxic inhibitors. Many of these inhibitors are free radicals that destroy enzymes by robbing them of electrons.

The fight against cellular oxidative damage is dependent upon a healthy level of antioxidant enzymes. An imbalance of antioxidant enzymes in relationship to free-radical load is known as *oxidative stress.* The most important antioxidant enzymes are *glutathione peroxidase, superoxide dismutase,* and *catalase,* although several other less powerful enzymes play a role. As free-radical activity in the body increases, these enzymes are depleted and must be replenished by the liver. In order for the body to synthesize these enzymes, it must have a steady supply of nutrient cofactors, including vitamins, minerals, and amino acids. For example, the production of glutathione peroxidase is dependent upon ample vitamin B_2 (riboflavin), as well as zinc and selenium, which are also important cofactors in the synthesis of a variety of other enzymes.

In addition, some enzymes such as delta-6-desaturase control inflammatory reactions throughout the body. If these enzymes are inactivated or have reduced function, inflammation increases, along with free-radical activity.

Endocrine Function

A poorly functioning endocrine system intensifies free-radical reactions. The interplay between thyroid hormone, cortisol, and the pancreas will help determine metabolic rate. If metabolism is geared too high, there is excess catabolism, which produces excess free radicals. If metabolism is too low, oxygen is not utilized fully, and itself becomes a free radical. In addition, these endocrine factors affect growth hormone, an important antioxidant, and affect immune cells. A poorly functioning endocrine system also leads to excess production of the mediators of inflammation.

Adrenals

Stress and increased cortisol production by the adrenal glands increase free-radical activity in several ways. First, cortisol increases blood glucose and mitochondrial activity. When you are under stress, the energy demands of your cells increase, forcing the electron transport chain to increase its production of ATP. As already noted, anything that increases mitochondrial activity also increases free-radical production.

Excess cortisol decreases resistance to infection, which may be another source of oxidative stress. Cortisol also increases blood lipid levels, where they may be readily oxidized. Chronic stress eventually leads to adrenal exhaustion, which increases inflammation and therefore free-radical activity throughout the body. Cortisol may also increase the production of pro-inflammatory cytokines such as IL-6, causing inflammation, increased free-radical damage, and, potentially, weight gain.

Pancreas

The pancreatic beta cells, which produce insulin, are subject to free-radical damage that leads to type 1 and type 2 diabetes. There is a strong correlation between hyperglycemia, hyperinsulinemia, and oxidative stress.

Thyroid

People with low thyroid function have a reduced "burn rate" for oxygen due to their lowered metabolism. Over time this will increase free-radical damage due to the increased levels of reactive oxygen species available for free-radical interaction. By contrast, if you have hyperthyroidism your body will burn oxygen too quickly and will create accelerated damage from the fire being turned up too high.

Bowel Terrain

Another mechanism of increased free-radical activity occurs through food allergies. Consumption of foods to which you are allergic can cause inflammation in various tissue sites of the body, and generate a cascade of free-radical activity as part of the natural immune function. Many of the symptoms of food allergy are characterized by inflammation: runny nose, gastrointestinal discomfort, asthma, eczema, and difficulty breathing.

Yeast overgrowth and dysbiosis can also contribute to the body's free-radical load. When yeast, normally present in the bowel, proliferates, it upsets the balance of the normal intestinal flora. Yeast overgrowth can affect immune function and can occur under several conditions, including abnormally high blood sugar and destruction of healthy intestinal flora from the use of antibiotics. As the organisms continue to proliferate, the yeast actually transform into a fungus, which grows rhizomes (roots) that penetrate the bowel wall. These roots damage the mucosal cell membranes, causing inflammation and initiating a cascade of free-radical damage. Symptoms can appear wherever the yeast proliferates, including the mucous membranes of the mouth, vagina, rectum, or intestinal wall.

Detoxification

In addition to its other many functions, one of the primary responsibilities of the liver is to process environmental and endogenous toxins. Detoxification of compounds by the liver is critical to overall health. However, some toxins are metabolized in two phases, generating free radicals as intermediary byproducts. If the two phases of detoxification are not synchronized, these free-radical intermediaries build up and generate tissue damage.

The body relies on the liver to produce endogenous antioxidant enzymes in enough quantity to meet the free-radical load. If the liver cannot perform this vital function, oxidative stress results.

TESTS FOR MEASURING OXIDATIVE STRESS

Each person has a slightly different susceptibility to oxidative stress. Various blood and urine tests are available, which measure your level of oxidative stress, but they must be ordered by a healthcare professional. Smokers and people who work around toxic chemicals, live in cities, and/or are under high stress have a higher level of oxidative stress. You can't avoid having some degree of oxidative stress.

There is a simple over-the-counter urine test that can be used to determine your antioxidant status called OxiData by Optimal Health Systems (800-890-4547; www.optimalhealthsystems.com). Or ask your healthcare practitioner for one of several blood tests available for measuring antioxidants levels. Of these, I recommend the erythrocyte antioxidant test from Metametrix (Metametrix Clinical Laboratory, 4855 Peachtree Blvd., Norcross, GA 30092; 770-441-2237), which measures levels of CoQ_{10}, beta-carotene, vitamins C and E, selenium, and zinc. A new technology that uses a light beam to determine antioxidant status within seconds will soon be on the market.

OXYGEN AS ALLY IS KEY

Oxygen is vital to life, and yet it can be the source of its destruction. All of us can get involved in environmental efforts to improve our outdoor air quality, but many people may not realize that the quality of their indoor air may actually be worse than the air outside your home. This is due to many factors such as outgassing of chemicals from furniture, carpet, and other building materials, from cleaning chemicals, insecticide use, cigarette smoke, molds, and more. It is obvious that the air quality that you have direct control over is indoor air. You can improve your indoor air quality by limiting your use of chemicals in the home by choosing home building and flooring products carefully, and by filtering your air.

There are all kinds of air-filtration systems on the market in all price ranges. If you have a forced air furnace, at the very least, go to a local hardware store and get high-efficiency filter replacements that will trap more dust, mold spores, and harmful substances called volatile organic chemicals (VOCs). If you want to add more to the filtration capabilities, there are air filtration units that can be installed in the ductwork that will ultra-purify the air. Many of these units feature high-efficiency particulate arresting (HEPA) filtration (found in hospitals) and UV-sterilization (ultraviolet light), which remove 99.7 percent of pollen, dust, mold spores, dust mites, bacteria, and animal dander from the air. Some units ozonate the air to further cleanse it and destroy microbes.

Other units are freestanding. These can be plugged into an outlet and left in the corner of a room. These units clean and circulate air for a single room; larger units may clean the air of nearly the entire floor of a home. Many of these products also send ions into the air, which attach to airborne dust and send it to the ground. Sources for various air filters are listed in the "Healthy Home Products" on page 534 of the resources section. Many home building and decorating items are sources of VOCs. These substances are released, or "outgassed," over time from items such as paint, paneling, carpeting, and vinyl flooring. In addition, carpets can hold dust and moisture and be a source of mold growth in the home.

If you are remodeling or building a new home, choose creative flooring that doesn't hold on to dust and is low in VOCs to minimize outgassing. Linoleum-type flooring made from natural materials (Marmoleum), cork flooring, hard wood, and tile are great options. There are even safer carpets that you can purchase. Paints with low emissions after application can also be purchased. Safer options are even available in subflooring and dry wall. There are safer options for virtually every building material. It just takes a little time to search them out. Again, look at our listing on page 534 of the resources section to get you started. More and more books are being published on environmentally friendly products. As people are becoming more educated on the effects of indoor pollution, they are seeking products that contribute to a "total health" lifestyle for their families.

Another way to improve indoor air quality is to have houseplants. Plants remove toxins from the air, such as formaldehyde and benzene, by absorbing them through microscopic openings in their leaves and using them for food. Plants breathe in carbon dioxide and create more oxygen for our home environment. Although all houseplants absorb toxins and increase the oxygen levels in the home, philodendrons, spider plants, and pothos are reported to be the most efficient in the removal of formaldehyde. Place at least one plant in every room and enjoy the beauty and the cleaner air!

Dianna's Story

When I was twenty-three, I underwent my first surgery for female-related problems. Between 1993 and 1998, I had five surgeries: one for a dermoid cyst, two for endometriosis, and two for miscarriages.

With each surgery I endured came a myriad number of prescription drugs to take. Synarel or Lupron were prescribed before I underwent surgery for endometriosis, followed by a contraceptive. Propoxyphene and Naproxen were prescribed for pain before and after my surgery. I was prescribed Prozac when I miscarried the second time and my doctor felt I was slipping into depression. Still feeling unhappy and emotionally drained, my doctor referred me to a fertility specialist.

Starting the fertility process by using a needle, my husband injected me with Repronex every day for one month. This was followed by one injection of Profasi at the doctor's office. After one cycle of fertility treatment, I picked up my prescription for progesterone, and my husband and I prepared to take a vacation to relax and unwind.

Shortly after arriving at the resort, I took a pregnancy test only to find that the result was negative. Visibly upset over the results, my husband reassured me and we made plans for dinner. After eating that night I became nauseated and began to hyperventilate and experience diarrhea. The rest of the vacation was spent in our hotel room or at the hospital. Every other day, I was in the hospital being treated for dehydration. Dreading the trip home, I tried to tell myself that the doctor at the hospital was right and that I just have the flu.

Happy to be home, I went straight to bed. My body ached so severely I would scream when my husband bumped me. Diarrhea, insomnia, panic attacks, dehydration, loss of appetite, and significant weight loss continued well after arriving home. Frustrated after going from doctor to doctor, filling prescription after prescription, and reaping no results, my husband and I went to the Mayo Clinic in Rochester, Minnesota.

During my weeklong stay, I was diagnosed with fibromyalgia and severe irritable bowel syndrome (IBS). I was also prescribed an antidepressant. Part of my required treatment involved attending classes for fibromyalgia and IBS. Going over the ever-popular USDA food pyramid with the dietitian did not help me. Months after arriving home, I was still experiencing the same problems with pain and IBS. My panic attacks became more frequent. So my local doctor increased my medication and added a new antidepressant. Expressing my concern to my husband about the long-term effects of the antidepressants, I convinced him we should take an integrative approach to my illnesses by making an appointment with Dr. LaValle.

Today, I have no symptoms of fibromyalgia, no IBS, and no pain from endometriosis. I was able to become pregnant and have a child. Gone are the hours and days spent in and out of the doctor's office for chronic bronchitis and urinary tract infections. Simple pleasures that I used to take for granted such as taking long walks, playing with my son, enjoying food, laughing with my husband, gardening, and more are all possible now. Looking back, I can say that even the emotional issues concerning my health have been resolved. When I was sick I became self-absorbed and obsessed with my illness, and my family suffered because of it. Having my life back allows healing to take place because the focus is shifted off me now and on the important things in life: family and friends.

Dianna is a great example of just how metabolically dysfunctional someone can become at a very early age. She had problems in virtually all of the nine keys areas. Due to the number of prescriptions she had taken, we concentrated on supporting her liver function. Also, as Dianna started to try and eat a healthy diet, simply following the USDA Food Guide Pyramid was not enough. She needed to individualize her diet and use supplements to balance her intestinal terrain—which was key to solving many of the other problems that she had. Although we had to work on all nine keys, she was able to regain her health gradually. This is where a person's commitment to regaining her health really shows. But for Dianna, the lifestyle changes were worth the rewards.

I do not recommend any one particular breathing program, but I do often recommend Hatha yoga as a means of reducing stress and improving breathing capacity and oxygenation of tissues. However, we must make sure that our bodies can properly deal with oxygen to guard against the ravages of excessive free radicals.

All forms of toxicity—disease, diet, stress, and even oxygen—contribute to oxidative stress. Oxygen, however, becomes harmful only when the body is unable to completely detoxify the free radicals—whether from these toxic conditions or generated by normal metabolic processes.

The most important defense against free-radical damage is a good offense, of which a well-functioning metabolic system is key. Antioxidants are critical in helping to protect against the adverse effects of free radicals. Without the protection that antioxidants supply, there is an increased production of these metabolic toxins that increase the risk of metabolic malfunction, immune problems, inflammation, cancer, cardiovascular disease, and other degenerative conditions.

So, if you are interested in optimizing your health, fighting the good fight against a disease with which you have been challenged or are just trying to age gracefully, you have to consume an antioxidant-rich diet to counteract the effects of free-radical damage. Because it is sometimes difficult to consume enough antioxidants in the foods we eat to keep free radicals in check (especially when we're under any type of physiological or psychological stress), it is wise to include antioxidants or an antioxidant-rich supplement in your diet. The next chapter discusses how to decrease free-radical damage through proper diet and nutritional supplementation.

CHAPTER 16

Key Foods and Supplements to Power Your Health

The foods we eat, the air we breathe, and the water we drink can have profound positive effects on our metabolism and our health. However, unless these substances are pure, all three can have profound negative effects on our metabolism and health. The truth is, we can't always guarantee the quality of these basic staples of health. Poor food choices and a lack of selection, unclean or chemically altered water, and impure air all contribute to the downward spiral from optimal metabolism to a path of accelerated aging and metabolic chaos.

How many times have you been driving behind a diesel truck and wished you could stop that foul-smelling air from entering your vehicle? How many times have you had a drink of water and it tasted so much like chlorine that you could not bear to finish the glassful? How many times have you gone to the local fast food restaurant for convenience sake, even though you know the food lacks the nutrients your body needs or that you may have to deal with the indigestion that comes with continual reliance on fast food?

All of us have experienced the negative side effects of foods, water, and air, but the chance to clean up your act and make healthier choices is here. Your metabolism, your very life, and the health of your family depend on your taking control of what enters your body.

SUPPORTING NUTRITIONAL HEALTH WITH POWER FOODS

Macronutrients are the whole foods—carbohydrate, fat, protein—that are broken down by our bodies for energy and sustenance. Micronutrients are nutrients needed in lesser amounts by the body—although this should not imply that they are less important. Vitamins and minerals are the principal micronutrients.

First, and foremost, you should strive to eat whole foods as much as possible. These foods will naturally supply you with a wide range of macro- and micronutrients and minimize your consumption of processed ingredients. If chosen wisely, these foods (along with water) supply all the calories, vitamins, minerals, essential nutrients, and enzymes your body needs to run efficiently.

This is truly the foundation for optimal health. The Guidelines for Healthy Living presented in Chapter 13 show you how to lay a foundation for health with whole foods. In addition, special attention should be given to the following power foods. They are foods with specific health benefits and should be regularly incorporated into your diet.

Blueberries

Blueberries contain one of the highest known levels of *anthocyanins,* a group of antioxidant phenols (compounds) found in many red and blue fruits. These compounds are believed to fight cancer, strengthen the immune system, and reduce LDL cholesterol.

In a recent U.S. Department of Agriculture (USDA) study, blueberry extract demonstrated an ability to correct free-radical-induced capillary permeability (leaky vessels) and alterations in antioxidant capacity. Anthocyanins appear to be especially attracted to collagen, where they actively protect against destructive inflammatory conditions like macular degeneration and diabetic retinopathy. *Ellagic acid,* also found in blueberries, may have anticancer properties.

Blueberries should be eaten fresh or frozen for maximum benefits. Pure blueberry juice is also an acceptable alternative—just remember to dilute all fruit juices with pure water.

Cultured Dairy Products

Cultured dairy products, such as *yogurt, kefir,* and *buttermilk* are abundant in friendly intestinal bacteria. *Lactobacillus acidophilus, L. bulgaricus,* and *L. bifidus* are among the most beneficial bacteria found in cultured dairy products. They help to maintain optimal digestion, and prevent constipation, and diarrhea. *L. acidophilus* reside primarily in the small intestine, supporting digestion and absorption of nutrients. *L. bifidus* inhabit the large intestine, where it helps to synthesize some vitamins. Certain strains of *L. bifidus* have been used experimentally in cancer treatment and immune fortification.

In phase one of the Healthy Living Guidelines, you are asked to avoid dairy products. But as you achieve your goals and move on to phase two, these foods can be invaluable sources of nutrients and beneficial organisms that promote health. Watch for the hidden sugars in many of the fruited yogurts on the market. Adding all that sugar and sweetened fruit negates the "power" you get out of consuming natural yogurts and kefirs.

Fermented Foods

Fermented foods, including *miso, tempeh,* and *raw sauerkraut,* are naturally rich in enzymes and probiotics (beneficial bacteria normally present in the digestive tract). They are staples of a macrobiotic diet, a diet that emphasizes vegetables, grains, protein from fish and chicken, and is low in dairy, red meat, eggs, and sugar. The nutrients from fermented foods are easily absorbed. They are easily digested and can help to fortify the intestinal tract environment.

Fish Oils

Fish oils are an excellent source of the omega-3 fatty acids: They are a must in your diet. Adequate fish oil intake has been found to reduce the risk of stroke and heart disease, as well as to decrease the risk of developing Alzheimer's disease. From regulating an inflamed chemistry, to supporting immune function, to building neurologic tissues such as the brain, to nourishing cell membranes so that they can perform their intended functions, omega-3 fatty acids have proven to be incredibly important for your health. If you are not a sardine or anchovy lover, this could limit your options. Many of the larger fish rich in omega-3s are polluted with mercury. If this is the case, my advice is to take a fish oil supplement, from 2–5 grams daily. Make sure that the supplement is free of mercury.

Flaxseeds

Flaxseeds are a rich source of omega-3 fatty acids. (However, the omega-3s in flaxseed oil are not a good source of usable omega-3 in the body. You need to rely on fish oils to accomplish this.) Flaxseed is an excellent source of fiber and can help prevent constipation. It is rich in lignans, which help to regulate sex hormone-binding globulin and to reduce circulating free estrogens, and is my favorite food to recommend for the prevention of breast cancer. The seeds can be ground in any coffee grinder or bought as a pre-ground meal. The meal can then be sprinkled on yogurt, cereals, or soups, or even added to a morning protein drink. I recommend one to two tablespoons of flaxseeds per day.

If you prefer, you can take one to two tablespoonfuls of flaxseed oil. The oil can be mixed in drinks or incorporated into a salad dressing. My preference is that you first use the meal and then supplement with the oil if you choose. Do not heat flaxseed oil, because it is high in polyunsaturated fatty acids and the heat will make the fats become rancid. Flaxseeds are a good addition to any weight-loss program, and they also help to improve estrogen metabolism in the body.

Garlic and Onions

Garlic and onions (vegetables in the *allium* family) contain antioxidant compounds in their oils that have a variety of protective roles. Garlic and onion oils are thought to decrease lipid peroxidation (the damaging of fats by oxidation) and increase the activities of antioxidant enzymes in the body.

In a case-controlled study conducted in France, the consumption of garlic and onion was shown to contribute to a reduced risk of breast cancer. Garlic has demonstrated significant inhibition of platelet aggregation in human plasma. Garlic can reduce serum cholesterol levels. Onion consumption is associated with a reduced risk of stomach cancer.

If fresh garlic does not agree with you, try Kyolic aged-garlic capsules. Personally, my Italian heritage leads to copious fresh garlic use!

Green Tea

Green tea (*Camellia sinensis*) is an evergreen shrub that has long been used in much of the world as a popular beverage and a respected medicinal agent. An early Chinese *Materia Medica* lists green tea as an agent to promote digestion, improve mental faculties, decrease flatulence, and regulate body temperature. The earliest known record of consumption is around 2700 B.C. Ceremonies, celebrations, relaxation time, and ordinary meals usually consist of tea in most parts of the world, except the United States, where coffee has become the most popular beverage.

Green tea is one of the most potent antioxidants in the plant kingdom and is commonly used in helping maintain a healthy heart and blood vessel system and in nutritionally supporting healthy cholesterol levels in laboratory animals and humans. The antioxidant effects of green tea also contribute to its role as nutritional support in various cancers. One cup of green tea can provide the same antioxidant capacity as around 150 milligram (mg) of pure vitamin C. There have been positive reports in human clinical studies of green tea's antioxidant potential. Several studies have reported that green tea may decrease the potential damage (including cancer) caused by cigarette smoking. Green tea has also been reported to help decrease the development of some infectious diseases and dental caries, to help maintain a healthy immune system, and to help nutritionally support a healthy body weight and weight loss.

Green tea also is reported to help with metabolism. It has COX-2-inhibiting activity, which results in mild anti-inflammatory effects. It is truly a superfood. Drink green tea daily and take one capsule of green tea standardized to contain 50 percent epigallocatechin gallate extract, the equivalent of four cups of green tea.

Shiitake Mushrooms

Shiitake mushrooms (*Lentinus edodes*) are considered medicinal Japanese mushrooms by traditional healers, and are used extensively in eastern medicine. Their active constituent, *lentinan* stimulates the immune system, defends against viral and chemical carcinogens, attacks cancer, and prevents the metastasis and recurrence of cancer.

Mushrooms can be used fresh or dried and rehydrated. However, they should be avoided in all forms during phase one and reintroduced in phase two of the Healthy Living Guidelines. Shiitake mushroom supplements are available in capsule, pill, and extract form as well.

SUPPORTING NUTRITIONAL HEALTH WITH DIETARY SUPPLEMENTS

Because a number of variables of a whole-foods diet are beyond individual control—such as freshness, growing conditions, soil quality, and methods of preparation, for example, your diet may not be able to supply you with enough of the nutrients you need for optimal health.

Twenty minerals and fifteen vitamins facilitate thousands of chemical reactions in the body. Vitamins and minerals also serve as coenzymes and provide structural components for tissue. Minerals have the additional tasks of regulating acid/alkaline (base) and fluid balances, conducting nerve transmission, running enzymatic reactions, and facilitating muscle contractions.

The study of how nutrients work in the body is absolutely fascinating, but it encompasses a body of research too vast to include here. Instead, I summarize each nutrient's functions and contributions to metabolism and health. For more detailed information, read *The Nutrition Desk Reference* by Robert Garrison M.A., R.Ph., and Elizabeth Somers M.A., R.D. (Keats Publishing, 1995) or *The Nutritional Cost of Prescription Drugs* (Morton Publishing, 2001), which I coauthored with Ross Pelton, R.Ph.

RDA versus ODA

The Food and Nutrition Review Board of the National Academy of Sciences (NAS) first established the Recommended Dietary Allowances (RDA) for nutrients in 1943. A six-page document entitled "The Recommended Dietary Allowances" has since served as a nutritional guideline for health professionals, food suppliers, consumers, and the government.

However, the RDAs were never intended as guidelines for wellness or optimal health. They were originally established as the level of nutrient intake that is required to prevent nutritional deficiencies. In other words, meeting the RDAs will avert diseases associated with nutritional deficiencies, such as scurvy, pellagra, and beriberi. In most cases, the RDAs are substantially lower than the nutrient intake required for optimal health and wellness. Many health professionals are beginning to question the limitations of the RDAs.

Concern about the limitations of the RDAs has given rise to the proposal for a new standard of nutrient intake called the "Optimal Daily Allowances (ODAs)." For example, consider the need for a different standard in regards to vitamin C intake. A 10 mg intake of vitamin C is enough to prevent scurvy. However, studies suggest that much higher levels, 1,000 mg daily, could reduce risk of developing cardiovascular disease and some types of cancer. Most practitioners of complementary medicine are already recommending many nutrients in amounts in excess of the RDAs for this very reason.

Health professionals do not always agree on the importance of taking vitamin and mineral supplements. I believe nutritional supplements are needed for the following reasons:

1. Optimal daily intakes of nutrients are difficult to obtain on low-calorie levels. Most women, for example, consume less than 1,700 calories a day. Even a fairly nutrient-dense diet will not provide the RDA for several nutrients on this calorie level. Calcium, iron, magnesium, and zinc intake are all likely to be less than the RDA on less than a daily intake of 1,700 calories.

2. Many prescription drugs deplete nutrients. Oral contraceptives, for example, deplete folate along with several other nutrients. Supplements are the only feasible way to replenish these nutrients. The calorie levels needed to replenish all the lost nutrients would be too high.

3. Extra nutrients are needed to fuel the enzyme pathways for detoxification, as well as to supply the nutrients needed under conditions that place extra demands on the body such as stress.

While some people fear that higher doses of vitamins and minerals may be dangerous, most experts agree that there is a fairly wide margin of safety for most nutrients. Moreover, most problems caused by excessive intake of nutrients are reversible once the vitamin or mineral is no longer taken.

Despite the safety of nutrients, high doses of any supplement should be supervised by a healthcare professional. Overdosing on vitamins and minerals does propose some risks. Although it has been my experience that occurrences are rare, overdoses of different vitamins and minerals can cause a variety of problems or symptoms in adults. However, much more caution should be used in children, who are more susceptible to problems. The fat-soluble vitamins A, D, and K, in particular, can accumulate in the liver and become toxic to it. Accidental ingestion of iron pills or multivitamin and mineral formulas that contain iron are very dangerous for children. Iron pills are the most common poisoning in young children; as little as five pills containing 60 mg of elemental iron in iron pills, for instance, can be fatal in children twenty-two pounds or under. So be careful if you have young children in the house to keep all supplements capped and out of their reach.

Lastly, it is important to understand that nutritional supplements cannot take the place of a nutrient-rich diet, exercise, and healthy lifestyle choices. Nor can they ameliorate the health-damaging effects of habits like smoking, excessive alcohol consumption, or a sedentary lifestyle.

With that said, let us begin with vitamins. *Vitamins* are organic (carbon-containing) compounds, which are classified as water soluble and fat soluble. Make sure that your multivitamin and -mineral supplement supplies a variety of the following nutrients. If your multivitamin formula falls short of the suggested optimum daily amounts in Table 16.1 below, consider taking additional supplements to fill the gap.

The recommendations below do not include the total daily intake needed for every nutrient. No one pill can contain them all. For example, it is recommended that women take between 1,000 and 2,000 mg of calcium each day for bone health. Table 16.1 suggests 500 mg of calcium. You might need another tablet to supply the remainder of your daily requirements depending on the foods in your diet. The multivitamin and mineral formula assumes that you will be starting to eat more healthfully. Almonds, broccoli, sardines, and sesame seed butter (tahini) are very good nondairy sources of calcium. Once you can tolerate dairy (some people never will), yogurt is a whopping 421 mg of calcium per cup. Also, the formula below does not include iron. Premenopausal women should make sure iron is included in the formula; however, men and postmenopausal women do not need supplemental iron. All men and women should take additional minerals for supporting bone density. The better that you eat, the fewer pills you need to take.

Table 16.1. Suggested Optimal Daily Allowances of Important Nutrients in a Multivitamin and Mineral Formula for Healthy Individuals

NUTRIENT	DOSE	NUTRIENT	DOSE
Beta-carotene (natural mixed carotenoid)	15,000 IU	Pantothenic acid (d-calcium pantothenate)	400 mg
Biotin	300 mcg	Potassium (aspartate-ascorbate complex)	99 mg
Boron (aspartate-citrate)	2 mcg	Selenium (amino-acid complex)	200 mcg
Calcium (citrate, amino-acid chelate, calcium hydroxyapatite)	500 mg	Vanadium (vanadyl sulfate)	200 mcg
Choline (bitartrate)	150 mcg	Vitamin A (D_3 or cholecalciferol-cholecalciferal from fish liver oil)	4,000 IU
Chromium (GTF)	200 mcg	Vitamin B_1 (thiamine monohydrate)	100 mg
Citrus bioflavonoids	100 mg	Vitamin B_{12} (ion exchange resin, methylcobalamin, or cyanoco-balamin)	500 mcg
Copper (optional; amino-acid chelate)	2 mg		
Folic acid (with a portion as 5-MTHF)	800 mcg	Vitamin B_2 (riboflavin with a portion as riboflavin-5-phosphate)	50 mg
Inositol	50 mg	Vitamin B_6 (pyridoxine HCL with a portion as pyridoxal-5-phosphate)	50 mg
Iodine (from kelp)	150 mcg	Vitamin C (L-ascorbic acid, corn-free)	1,200 mg
Magnesium (aspartate-ascorbate complex, citrate, malate)	500 mg	Vitamin D (fish liver oil)	400 IU
Manganese (amino-acid chelate)	20 mg	Vitamin E (d-alpha tocopheryl succinate or mixed tocopherols)	400 IU
Molybdenum (amino-acid chelate)	150 mcg		
Niacin/Inositol hexaniacinate	50 mg	Vitamin K (phytonadione)	60 mcg
Niacinamide	150 mg	Zinc (amino acid chelate)	30 mg
PABA (para-amino benzoic acid)	50 mg		

WATER-SOLUBLE VITAMINS FOR NUTRITIONAL SUPPORT

Water-soluble vitamins are *hydrophilic,* meaning they are attracted to water. These are the B vitamins and vitamin C. Water-soluble vitamins are absorbed directly into the blood and are excreted in the urine. The body does not store water-soluble vitamins; therefore, they must be replenished daily in the diet.

Vitamin B Complex

The B vitamins are known for their role in converting food to metabolic energy. Taking B vitamins does not provide an independent boost of energy—rather, they are cofactors in the processes that turn food into energy. B vitamins are needed for the formation of new cells, especially those cells that proliferate quickly, such as red blood cells. The B vitamins work best in synchrony, which is why most forms of vitamin B supplements are available as a *vitamin B complex.*

Sometimes it is necessary to use a therapeutic level of a specific B vitamin. This need can be caused by a condition or disease that creates a greater demand on B vitamin-related systems or a certain drug therapy that could accelerate the depletion of certain B vitamins from the body.

Vitamin B_1 (Thiamine)

Vitamin B_1 (thiamine) was the first of the B vitamins to be discovered. It was isolated in 1926 as a water-soluble, crystalline yellowish white powder with a salty, slightly nutty taste. Scientists now know that thiamine plays an important role in producing energy for the body's cells.

Because it is water soluble, thiamine is not stored in the body and must be supplied daily.

In adults, chronic dieting, alcoholism, and diets consisting primarily of highly processed, refined foods are causes of thiamine deficiency. All plant and animal foods contain thiamine, but only in low concentrations. The richest sources are brewer's yeast and organ meats, but whole cereal grains are the most common and easily accessible source of thiamine.

In addition to its role in converting blood sugar to energy for cells, thiamine supplementation nutritionally supports nerve tissues and nerve function. It is also necessary for maintaining healthy muscle function, especially in the heart. What is even more important in my estimation is that thiamine is involved in the conversion of fatty acids and amino acids into hormones, proteins, and enzymes.
Recommended dose. 100 mg of thiamine HCl.

Vitamin B_2 (Riboflavin)

Vitamin B_2 (riboflavin) is an essential nutrient for normal growth and development, helping the body to maintain reproduction, physical performance, and provide a general sense of well-being. It also nutritionally helps to keep skin, nails, and hair healthy.

Riboflavin is water soluble and is not stored in the body. It must therefore be supplied daily. Riboflavin belongs to a group of yellow fluorescent pigments called *flavins.* When excreted, it gives the urine a characteristic bright yellow color. Riboflavin is instrumental in the metabolism of fatty acids and amino acids while playing a key role in energy production for the body. It is also essential to the production of glutathione, one of the most important antioxidants.

The best sources of riboflavin are dairy products, liver, and milk. Other sources include avocados, dark-green vegetables, eggs, fish (especially salmon and tuna), meats, mushrooms, and oysters.

Recommended dose. 50 mg of riboflavin with a portion as riboflavin-5-phosphate.

Vitamin B₃ (Niacin)

Vitamin B_3 (niacin) is a water-soluble vitamin that can be produced in the body. It is instrumental in producing two of the body's important coenzymes, nicotine adenine dinucleotide (NAD) and nicotine adenine dinucleotide phosphate (NADH). These two coenzymes are involved in more than 200 chemical reactions in the body. It is also important for metabolism of carbohydrates, fatty acids, and amino acids, as well as energy production on the cellular level.

There are three forms of niacin on the market today, all with potential health benefits. The first, which is known as *nicotinic acid,* has been reported to be beneficial in maintaining healthy blood levels of cholesterol. The second is called *nicotinamide,* which helps in healthy bones and blood sugar levels. The third, *inositol hexaniacinate,* shares similar benefits with nicotinic acid. However, it does not produce the unpleasant tingling and redness commonly associated with nicotinic acid. This supplement is recommended for controlling cholesterol and helping to lower lipoprotein a, a protein in the blood that transports cholesterol, triglycerides, and other lipids to various tissues.

Foods that contain niacin and its precursor, tryptophan, are considered sources of the vitamin. Brewer's yeast, legumes, milk, organ meats, peanuts, and peanut butter are the best sources of niacin. Meanwhile, fish, lean meats, peanuts and poultry, are good sources of both niacin and tryptophan.

Recommended dose. 50 mg as niacin, niacinamide, or inositol hexaniacinate.

Vitamin B₅ (Pantothenic Acid)

Vitamin B_5 (pantothenic acid) was discovered in 1933 by Roger Williams, Ph.D. Because it is present in all cells, Williams, named this vitamin after the Greek word *pantothen,* meaning "everywhere."

Pantothenic acid plays a number of essential metabolic roles, including the production of some hormones and neurotransmitters. It is also involved in the metabolism of all carbohydrates, fats, and proteins, and has been reported beneficial in helping maintain healthy blood cholesterol. Pantothenic acid is useful in wound healing and adrenal gland stress. (A deficiency may lead to fatigue and other health issues if not corrected.)

The best food sources of pantothenic acid include cereals, chicken, eggs, fish, legumes, liver, and whole-grain breads. Other good sources are broccoli, cauliflower, lean beef, white and sweet potatoes, and tomatoes.

Recommended dose. 400 mg as d-calcium pantothenate.

Vitamin B₆ (Pyridoxine)

Vitamin B_6 (pyridoxine) is a water-soluble vitamin that is instrumental in more than 100 enzyme reactions in the body. These activities are mostly related to nutritional support of the metabolism of amino acids and proteins. Pyridoxine also has benefits in maintaining a healthy heart because it is a cofactor in regulating homocysteine production in the body. Pyridoxine is a key nutrient in healthy adrenal function and stress response. It is also an important cofactor in manufacturing serotonin from the amino acid tryptophan. It also plays a role in nerve health. Many people have overcome carpal tunnel syndrome by taking 100–200 mg of pyridoxine. If you take a high dose of pyridoxine, make sure that you are taking other B vitamins with it, and do so under the supervision of a healthcare provider.

The best sources of pyridoxine are bananas, brewer's yeast, legumes, organ meats (especially liver), peanuts, potatoes, and wheat germ. Bacteria in the human intestinal tract also synthesize pyridoxine. Pyridoxine deficiency is one of the most common nutritional deficiencies. Much of this can be blamed on the fact that a lot of vitamin B_6 is lost during cooking and food processing. A USDA study reported that 80 percent of Americans consume less than the RDA for pyridoxine.

Recommended dose. 50 mg of as pyridoxine HCl with a portion as pyridoxal-5-phosphate.

Vitamin B₁₂ (Cobalamin)

Cobalamin is the common name of vitamin B_{12} because it contains the heavy metal cobalt, which gives this water-soluble vitamin its red color. Cobalamin is essential for growth and plays a role in metabolism within cells, especially those of the gastrointestinal tract, bone marrow, and nervous tissue. Cobalamin is produced in the digestive tract of animals. Therefore, animal protein products are the only source of this nutrient. Organ meats are the best source of cobalamin, followed by clams, oysters, beef, eggs, milk, chicken, and cheese.

On the cellular level, cobalamin plays an important role in the replication of DNA while nutritionally supporting growth of the body's cells.

The vitamin is also vital for the function and maintenance of the nervous system and red blood cells, and has been reported recently to be beneficial in maintaining cognitive health. A little known fact is that the first thing a doctor will do when assessing dementia and cognitive function in an elderly patient is to investigate their cobalamin and folic acid status. In my experience, tissue levels of cobalamin do not always directly correlate to people's needs.

Cobalamin is also important nutritionally in the body's metabolism of protein, fat, and carbohydrates. Recently, cobalamin depletion was found to increase the risk of forming elevated homocysteine levels and, therefore, to increase the risk of cardio-vascular disease. Diabetics may be particularly at risk for low cobalamin if they are on biguanide (antidiabetic) drug therapy. Low cobalamin status in the diabetic increases the risk of developing neuropathy, in addition to the other conditions listed here. Low levels of cobalamin can also lead to anemia and tiredness. One of the great-est cobalamin-depleting drugs is oral contraceptives. Today, girls are taking birth control pills at earlier and earlier ages. Combine the poor diet of most teenage girls with the use of a drug that is very efficient at depleting nutrients from the body and you have a recipe for fatigue, depression, and a whole host of other long-term health issues. In some cases, cobalamin injections may be required, in which case a doctor administers a shot.

Recommended dose. 500 micrograms (mcg) as methylcobalamin, ion exchange resin, hydroxycobalamin, or cyanocobalamin.

Biotin

Biotin is one of the more recently discovered water-soluble B vitamins. Since 1942, it has been studied for its role in the production of many enzymes. Biotin is also known as the vitamin that produces healthy hair and helps prevent graying. Biotin also is ben-eficial in supporting the special nutritional needs of people with diabetes. It plays a vital role in the production of energy from the metabolism of carbohydrates and fats.

Biotin is found abundantly in many plant and animal foods. Bacteria in the intes-tines also produce a considerable amount of biotin. The best food sources include bananas, brewer's yeast, grapefruit, liver, milk, peanuts, strawberries, and water-melon.

Recommended dose. 300 mcg of biotin.

Folate (Folic Acid)

Folate (folic acid) is a member of the water-soluble B vitamin group. Isolated in 1946 from spinach leaves, its name comes from *folium,* the Latin word for leaf. In the body, folic acid is converted to a more biologically active form. Our "friendly" intes-tinal bacteria also produce folic acid.

Folic acid occurs in a wide variety of foods. Best sources include brewer's yeast, dark-green leafy vegetables, eggs, and liver. Other good sources are beets, broccoli, Brussels sprouts, cabbage, cantaloupe, cauliflower, kidney, lima beans, orange juice, wheat germ, and whole-grain cereals and breads.

Like cobalamin, folic acid is necessary for the production and repair of both DNA and RNA. It is therefore essential for regulating cellular division and the transmission of the genetic code to all newly formed cells. Folic acid deficiency has been strongly correlated to colon cancer and breast cancer as well as to cervical dysplasia. Folic acid is also essential for the health of red blood cells and the production of proteins and various amino acids. Like pyridoxine, folic acid benefits cardiovascular health by its ability to decrease the formation of homocysteine.

If you are low in folic acid you could become fatigued, anemic, have a greater risk of giving birth to a child with birth defects, increased risk of cervical dysplasia, breast and colon cancer, and increase your risk of cardiovascular disease and depression.

Some people are genetically less able to convert folic acid to an active, usable form. A new folic acid derivative known as 5-methyltetrahydrofolate, or 5-MTHF, is an active metabolite that has been found to ensure folic acid gets converted in the body.

Recommended dose. 800 mcg of folic acid, folinic acid, and 5-MTHF.

Vitamin C (Ascorbic Acid)

Vitamin C has two significant general functions, but in truth, it would take an entire book to cover its complete value. Vitamin C is both a traditional vitamin (an enzyme cofactor) and an antioxidant.

As an antioxidant, vitamin C readily donates electrons to free radicals, stabilizing them and preventing free-radical damage. It also recycles other antioxidants such as vitamin E to keep them charged. In the intestine, vitamin C stabilizes iron (a free radical) and promotes its absorption. Vitamin C helps form the structural protein collagen, which is used to strengthen connective tissue, bone, and teeth. Vitamin C helps metabolize certain amino acids. It is thought to play a role in the formation of certain hormones, particularly *norepinephrine* and *thyroxin.* The adrenal glands, which house more vitamin C than any other organ, release large amounts of the vitamin under stress. The need for vitamin C increases when metabolic demand increases, and, therefore, the need for more thyroxin increases as well. It is also intimately involved in the body's immune response, helping to fuel white blood cell function during times of stress.

The body does not make vitamin C; therefore, it must be supplied through the diet or taken as supplements. Vitamin C is most abundant in berries, citrus fruits, and green vegetables.

Recommended dose. 1,200 mg as buffered ascorbate powder, ester-C, ascorbyl palmitate, or ascorbic acid.

FAT-SOLUBLE VITAMINS FOR NUTRITIONAL SUPPORT

The fat-soluble vitamins are *hydrophobic,* meaning they do not mix with water. Fat-soluble vitamins are absorbed from the intestines by the lymph, where protein carriers carry them to the blood. Because fat-soluble vitamins are stored in fatty tissue throughout the body, they do not need to be replenished as often as water-soluble vitamins. But, because they stay stored in the body, they can reach levels at which they become toxic more quickly, as well.

The fat-soluble vitamins are vitamins A, D, E, and K.

Vitamin A

Vitamin A is active in three forms: *retinol, retinal,* and *retinoic acid.* Each form of vitamin A has it own binding protein and specific function at the cellular level. Carotenoids, plant pigments found mostly in yellow and orange fruits and vegetables, can be converted to vitamin A in the body. The best-known carotenoid is beta-carotene.

Vitamin A is important for the health of the eyes, skin, immune system, and mucous membranes. It helps maintain cell membranes and the protective layer surrounding nerve cells. Vitamin A also assists in manufacturing cortisol, thyroxin, and red blood cells. Recent evidence has pointed to the possibility that excessive vitamin A intake can lead to brittle bones; therefore, it is important to monitor your intake and not exceed recommended levels. Vitamin A intake should also be restricted during pregnancy. If pregnant, do not exceed 4,000 IU daily; an average adult intake is 5,000 IU daily unless there is a specific need as determined by a healthcare provider.
Recommended dose. 4,000–5,000 IU as fish liver oil.

Vitamin D

Vitamin D is distinct from all the other vitamins in that the body can synthesize it from cholesterol and direct sunlight. It is structurally different, as well, resembling the chemical makeup of a hormone. It is able to permeate cellular membranes, interact with intracellular DNA, and help to synthesize proteins. It is toxic at relatively low levels. Ingestion of as little as four times the RDA can cause symptoms of toxicity.

Vitamin D is important for the absorption and utilization of minerals that are required for bone formation. Vitamin D increases absorption and utilization of calcium and phosphorus from the intestine. It also helps release calcium from bones and stimulates retention of calcium by the kidneys. The interaction between calcium and vitamin D is critical for the process of bone mineralization, and is regulated by the *parathormone* from the parathyroid gland and *calcitonin* secreted by the thyroid.

Dairy products, eggs, fish oil (especially cod liver oil), and saltwater fish all include vitamin D. Many multivitamin and -mineral formulas contain at least 400 IU of vitamin D daily, so it is important to monitor any vitamin D in fish oil supplements to make sure that its tolerable upper limit, an amount which once you exceed you run the risk of harmful side effects. The tolerable upper limit of vitamin D has been established at an intake of 25 mcg (1,000 IU) for infants up to twelve months of age and 50 mcg (2,000 IU) for children, adults, pregnant, and lactating women.
Recommended dose. 400 IU of vitamin D_3 or cholecalciferol from fish oil.

Vitamin E

Although it was discovered and isolated in the 1930s, vitamin E's function in the body has come to light only recently. Modern research has shown us that vitamin E could be the most important fat-soluble antioxidant. As such, it insures the stability and integrity of cellular tissues and membranes throughout the body by preventing free-radical damage.

In addition to its antioxidant activity, vitamin E may nutritionally support cardio-vascular and cognitive function. It is beneficial in maintaining a healthy immune system and vision. During heavy exercise, vitamin E reduces the amount of exercise-induced free-radical damage to the blood and tissues while helping the body reduce the incidence of exercise-induced muscle injury.

Good sources of vitamin E include vegetable oils, wheat germ oil, seeds, nuts, and soybeans. Other adequate sources are asparagus, avocados, Brussels sprouts, leafy greens, spinach, whole-wheat products, and whole-grain breads and cereals.

The names of all types of vitamin E begin with either "d" or "dl," which refer to differences in chemical structure. The "d" form is natural and "dl" is synthetic. Natural vitamin E is more active and has a substantially greater ability to be absorbed into the body than synthetic vitamin E. Little is known about how the "un-natural" "l" portion of the synthetic "dl" form affects the body, although no toxicity has been discovered. After the "d" or "dl" designation, often the Greek letter "alpha" appears, which also describes the structure. Synthetic "dl" vitamin E is found only in the alpha form—as in "dl-alpha tocopherol." Natural vitamin E can be found as alpha—as in "d-alpha tocopherol"—or in combination with beta, gamma, and delta—this combination is labeled "mixed" (as in mixed natural tocopherols). Natural mixed tocopherols also may be more potent and offer a wider range of protection than vitamin E alone. Recent studies indicate that higher doses of vitamin E (2,000 IU) may have a protective effect on the progression of Alzheimer's disease. This is most likely due to the reduction of oxidative stress in the neuronal tissue of the brain. For general health purposes, however, 400 IU a day of a mixed tocopherol is sufficient.

Tocotrienols are members of the vitamin E family. Like vitamin E, tocotrienols are potent antioxidants against lipid peroxidation. Human studies indicate that, in addition to their antioxidant function, tocotrienols have other important functions, specifically with regard to the normalization of cholesterol levels.

Recommended dose. 400 IU of d-alpha-tocopherol succinate or mixed tocopherols (d-alpha, d-beta, d-gamma, and d-delta).

Vitamin K (Phytonadione)

Vitamin K is primarily involved in the clotting of blood. Vitamin K also has an important role in bone formation. Without it, the bones are less able to bind with mineral deposits. Food sources include spinach, artichokes, dry roasted peanuts, pistachios, coriander, and Swiss chard.

Recommended dose. 60 mcg of phytonadione.

MINERALS FOR NUTRITIONAL SUPPORT

Minerals are elements found in foods that are themselves taken in from plants. They are essential, meaning that the body cannot manufacture them. The *macrominerals,* required in relatively large quantities, include calcium, chloride, magnesium, phosphorus, potassium, sodium, and sulfur. The *microminerals* (known as *trace elements*) are boron, chromium, cobalt, copper, fluoride, iodine, iron, manganese, selenium, and zinc.

Minerals compete for absorption in the body. For example, calcium competes with iron, and copper competes with zinc, for absorption. Each mineral in the body has an effect on every other mineral, and as such, a proper balance of minerals must be maintained for good health.

Taking high doses of mineral supplements can lead to deficiencies in other minerals. Minerals are in their most biologically available forms in foods. Dark-green leafy vegetables, fruits, nuts, and legumes are usually good sources of minerals. However, because of current agricultural practices, described in previous chapters, our mineral intakes still may not be adequate. I highly recommend that you supplement your diet with a balanced multivitamin and mineral formula, or a separate multimineral supplement. Mineral deficiency symptoms are some of the most common symptomatic complaints in my practice.

Boron

Boron is a trace mineral that has been recognized as an essential nutrient for plants for almost 100 years, but the need for boron in humans was not discovered until the mid-1980s.

The highest concentration of boron in humans is found in bones and dental enamel. Recent research suggests that the mineral plays a role as a necessary nutrient involved in metabolism and bone health. Osteoarthritis, rheumatoid arthritis, and osteoporosis are leading diseases in women and men. Regions of the world in which there is little boron in the agricultural soil have a far higher incidence of arthritis. While boron is sold in supplement form, individually and in multivitamin and mineral formulas, it is also readily available and easily absorbed from fruits and vegetables. Good sources of boron are apples, carrots, grapes, dark-green leafy vegetables, and pears. **Recommended dose.** 2 mcg as boron aspartate (amino-acid chelate) or aspartate-citrate. Boron like many other minerals is often *chelated,* that is, by attaching a mineral to an amino acid or peptide, or to a protein, increases its absorption and availability.

Calcium

The most common question women ask me is what kind of calcium to take? There is so much misinformation and confusion that in the end they resort to taking TUMS, a popular over-the-counter antacid, which neutralizes the very acid needed to break down the calcium.

Calcium is the most abundant mineral in the human body. The body of an average healthy man contains about two and a half to three pounds of calcium while a healthy woman's body has about two pounds. Approximately 99 percent of calcium is present in the bones and teeth, which leaves only about 1 percent in cells and body fluids.

Cow's milk and dairy products are the major source of dietary calcium for most people. But many people are finding out that they do not tolerate dairy products and need to seek alternative sources for calcium. Although many alternative health practitioners do not believe dairy foods should be eaten, I do not believe that we can make a blanket statement that dairy is bad for everyone. Finding quality cow's milk dairy products that are organic is becoming easier. In fact, they can be found in most large supermarket chains. Other non-cow dairy sources of milk and cheese that are also good sources of calcium include goat, buffalo, and sheep. Many of the milks such as almond, rice, soy, and others are also fortified with calcium. Other great sources are broccoli, dark-green leafy vegetables, legumes, nuts, and whole grains.

As most people know, calcium is crucial for the development and long-term health of bones and teeth. What you may not know, however, is that the body's need for calcium is greatest during periods of rapid growth, including childhood, pregnancy, and lactation. Where do you think those minerals are coming from that build a baby's bones? From his or her mother, and possibly from her bones. If you have been pregnant more than once, have your bone density checked (along with your amino acids). Also, if you have children who complain of joint pain during growth spurts, or restless, fidgety legs, give them more calcium (and magnesium). In my experience, many of these complaints resolve themselves quickly when minerals, specifically calcium and magnesium, are added to the diet.

Calcium is also necessary for a wide array of other functions. Calcium initiates muscle contractions, thereby playing a vital role in maintaining a healthy heartbeat. It is also involved in the body's blood-clotting process. On the cellular level, calcium is a major factor in the regulation of the passage of nutrients and wastes through cell membranes. It is also involved in the regulation of various enzymes that control muscle contraction, fat digestion, and metabolism. Low-calcium levels in the body are also correlated with an increased risk of developing certain cancers, in particular colon cancer. Finally, calcium helps in maintaining proper transmission of nerve impulses.

Calcium has received much attention for its role in supporting healthy bones in women and men. Research suggests that supplementing the diet with calcium may aid the body in slowing, but will not completely stop, the progression of bone loss as we age.

In the average adult, only approximately between 10 and 40 percent of dietary calcium intake is absorbed. Calcium from milk and milk products is absorbed more easily than that from most vegetables. However, cow's milk may cause allergies in some individuals, contributing to gas, bloating, and symptoms of sinusitis (nasal stuffiness, runny nose), among other symptoms.

Also, not all forms of calcium are absorbed and utilized by the body effectively. One form of calcium, *microcrystalline hydroxyapatite* (MCHC), has been reported to be more readily available for absorption and use in the body than most other forms. MCHC allows for a more complete absorption of calcium, and has been reported in studies to nutritionally support the body to maintain cortical bone mass in post-menopausal women.

It has always amazed me that so many healthcare professionals recommend antacid calcium that, in general, contains calcium carbonate. There are two reasons that this is not a good choice. First of all, it is well established that calcium carbonate, although high in elemental calcium, is relatively poorly absorbed. Second, calcium absorbs in an acidic environment, so using an antacid or something that lowers acidity in the stomach will decrease the ability of the body to absorb calcium.

If you have some bone loss or if you are on drugs that may increase the risk of osteoporosis, such as corticosteroids, then you have to take a calcium supplement that has better absorption and bone-building properties.

Recommended dose. 500–1,000 mg as MCHC (calcium hydroxyapatite), calcium citrate-malate-glycinate, calcium aspartate (amino-acid chelate), calcium citrate, or d-calcium glucarate. (Take into account any calcium in your multivitamin and mineral formula.)

Chromium

Chromium was first discovered as an essential trace element in 1955. The body of an average healthy individual contains only 7 mg. However, this small amount plays important roles in metabolism. It is a central cofactor in insulin's ability to bind to insulin receptor sites and to regulate blood sugar levels. Chromium also nutritionally supports the activation of various enzymes for energy production and can assist indirectly in weight control. Chromium also plays a role in helping the body regulate blood cholesterol levels.

Researchers have also noted that patients with coronary heart disease have significantly lower chromium levels than do healthy people. Other studies suggest that chromium supplementation may support healthy vision and help fight glaucoma. Chromium plays a role in the conversion of thyroid hormones thyroxine (T4) to the more active triiodothyronine (T3) in the peripheral tissues, thereby helping to regulate metabolism.

A recent survey in England showed that, with age, tissue, urinary, and blood levels of chromium decreased and contributed to increasing the incidence of type 2 diabetes.

Good food sources of chromium include cheeses, lean meats, whole-grain breads and cereals, and some spices, such as black pepper and thyme. Brewer's yeast is also rich in chromium.

Recommended dose. 200 mcg as chromium polynicotinate (GTF chromium).

Copper

Copper is an essential trace mineral that is involved in the support of several key body functions, including tissue health and oxygen transport in the blood. Copper is required for the production and function of hemoglobin, which is responsible for transporting oxygen through the body. Copper is one of the building blocks for collagen and elastin, the proteins that provide structural integrity and elasticity for tissues, organs, and bones. Copper is helpful in maintaining skin integrity and useful in wound healing.

Targeted applications for copper supplementation include helping the body maintain healthy bones, as arthritis and osteoporosis are very prevalent diseases in today's society. Copper is also an antioxidant and has proven beneficial for controlling outbreaks of herpesvirus infections. Copper lysinate is an amino-acid chelate mineral that increases copper's absorption and availability. I do not recommend supplementing with copper separately as it is typically in multivitamin and -mineral formulas.

Copper-containing foods include oysters, organ meats, whole-grain breads and cereals, shellfish, dark-green leafy vegetables, dried legumes, nuts, and chocolate.

Recommended dose. 2 mg (optional) as copper lysinate or other amino-acid chelate.

Iodine

Iodine is a trace element that is vital to the health of the thyroid gland. It also provides the building blocks for the hormones secreted by the thyroid. The availability of iodized salt in the marketplace has made iodine deficiency and its accompanying disorder, *goiter,* very rare in the United States.

Iodine's only known function is the role it plays in the thyroid gland. Without it, the thyroid cannot function properly, which leads to abnormal metabolism, oxygen consumption, and energy production. The iodine-dependent hormones produced by the thyroid control such functions as body temperature, physical growth, reproduction, and the growth of skin and hair.

A simple method for testing for iodine deficiency is to get a bottle of liquid iodine from the natural foods store. Drop one drop on your abdomen. If it takes less than twenty-four hours to completely absorb into the skin and disappear, then most likely you are deficient in iodine.

Iodized salt is our most common source of iodine. Iodine-rich foods include seafood, sea vegetables (seaweed), and vegetables grown in iodine-rich soils.

Recommended dose. 150 mcg from kelp.

Manganese

Manganese is involved in the production of a wide variety of enzymes. These enzymes influence such biological processes as the production of collagen and the metabolism of protein and cholesterol. Manganese is also necessary for normal bone growth and the metabolism of amino acids.

The average human body only contains approximately 20 mg of manganese, most of which is stored in the bones.

Manganese is necessary for the growth and maintenance of tissues, cartilage, and bones. It also plays a role in the regulation of blood clotting. What's more, manganese makes up part of one of the body's most important antioxidants, superoxide dismutase. It also supports the production of certain hormones and neurotransmitters while aiding in the metabolism of fats. Manganese supplementation may be of nutritional support in maintaining the health of blood sugar levels.

The best food sources of manganese include dried beans and peas, nuts, pineapple, raisins, vegetables, and whole-grain breads and cereals.

Recommended dose. 20 mg of manganese glycinate or other amino-acid chelate.

Magnesium

People in our culture are sorely deficient in magnesium. A USDA study found that 75 percent of Americans do not get an adequate supply of magnesium in their diet. This is probably due to the absence of magnesium in many processed foods and the depletion of magnesium from agricultural soils.

I'm a big advocate of magnesium supplements. In fact, it is the supplement that I most often recommend in my practice. I have seen hundreds of people benefit after starting magnesium supplementation. Magnesium helps with many conditions from palpitations, arrhythmias, leg cramps and fatigue, and restless leg syndrome to insomnia, nervousness, anxiety, endurance, and stamina.

Magnesium is involved in the interaction of more than 300 enzymes in the body, making it a necessary nutrient for the transmission of nerve impulses, temperature regulation, detoxification, and energy production (ATP formation). As a key player in calcium metabolism, magnesium is also important for the health and development of bones and teeth. It helps maintain the integrity of bones and helps bind calcium to tooth enamel, thus creating a barrier to tooth decay. Magnesium also plays a vital role in helping the body maintain a healthy cardiovascular system.

The body needs magnesium to metabolize carbohydrates, proteins, and fats. As part of magnesium's role in the activity of enzymes, it is involved in the transmission of nerve impulses and muscle contractions. As already mentioned, magnesium plays a crucial role in maintaining cardiovascular function. There are scores of people with heart conditions who could improve significantly if they supplemented with magnesium. From arrhythmias to blood pressure, magnesium plays a central role in cardiovascular function and insulin regulation. It is involved in the relaxation of blood vessels and keeping blood thickness in balance.

Magnesium also plays a role in the processing of lactic acid. A buildup of lactic acid can interfere with the biochemical reactions needed for muscle contraction. So, if you have sore muscles longer than expected from exercise or have muscle tension for any other reason, such as stress or fibromyalgia, you will benefit from taking magnesium malate.

Good food sources of magnesium include dark-green leafy vegetables, legumes, and nuts, as well as whole grains.

Recommended dose. 500–1,000 mg of magnesium aspartate, magnesium citrate, magnesium glycinate, and magnesium malate. A loose stool is a sign that you are taking too much magnesium. Build up your tolerance to 500–1,000 mg a day gradually. For muscle tension, take one to two 600-mg capsules twice a day.

Molybdenum

Molybdenum is one of the rarest substances on earth, yet small amounts of this mineral are found in nearly all tissues of the human body. Molybdenum is a component of several important interactions that lead to phase one and phase two of the liver's detoxification process. It is also vital for the function of several enzymes, one of which has an important role in regulating urinary excretion.

Some research has focused on the role of molybdenum as nutritional support for those with cancer. Studies have reported that there has been a 30 percent increase in cancer of the esophagus in areas of the United States where there is no molybdenum in the drinking water and in areas where food is grown in molybdenum-poor soils. Molybdenum intake has also been associated with a decrease in dental cavities.

This trace mineral is found in beans, beef liver, cereal grains, dark-green leafy vegetables, legumes, and peas.

Recommended dose. 150 mcg of molybdenum amino-acid chelate.

Potassium

Potassium is one of the body's three major *electrolytes* (the other two being *sodium* and *chloride*). Electrolytes are involved in *intracellular osmosis,* which means that they control the flow of body fluids into and out of tissues and cells.

As part of its role as an electrolyte, potassium controls the distribution and balance of water throughout the body. Potassium also helps maintain pH (acid-alkaline) balance throughout the body. What's more, blood pressure is partially regulated by potassium, and studies suggest that potassium supplementation may be beneficial in maintaining healthy blood pressure. Diets containing foods that are good sources of potassium and low in sodium may reduce the risk of hypertension and stroke. Finally, individuals with a diet high in potassium may have a lower risk of developing kidney stones.

Potassium is plentiful in the diet. Potassium-rich foods include fresh fruits (bananas especially) and vegetables, peanuts, meat, and milk.

Recommended dose. 99 mg of potassium citrate or aspartate-ascorbate complex.

Selenium

Until the late 1950s, selenium was thought to be toxic. Although it can indeed be toxic at high doses, it is now recognized as an important nutritional trace mineral.

Selenium plays important roles in detoxification and antioxidant defense mechanisms in the body. Selenium is itself an antioxidant, but it also plays a role in the formation of glutathione peroxidase, one of the body's key antioxidants. This antioxidant activity is believed to be responsible for selenium's reported ability to help maintain a healthy cardiovascular system. A decreased cardiovascular risk has been associated with adequate selenium intake. Also, studies have linked low dietary selenium intake with higher rates of several types of cancer, including prostate cancer. Selenium may also be beneficial in maintaining immune-system health, warding off viruses and other potential pathogens. It also helps rid the body of heavy metal toxins, such as mercury and cadmium.

Selenium is present in whole grains and is extremely plentiful in Brazil nuts. In fact, just a few Brazil nuts contain the daily requirement of selenium.

Recommended dose. 200 mcg as an amino-acid complex, selenomethionine, or sodium selenide.

Vanadium

In the late 1960s, vanadium was found to be an essential trace mineral for plant nutrition, and in the early 1970s, research suggested it to be an essential nutrient for animals. There is still some debate on whether vanadium is essential in humans, however, and as such, no RDA has been established for this trace mineral. Nonetheless, interest in vanadium as a nutritional substance has been steadily building over the past twenty years, especially since it has been discovered that it may be beneficial in helping maintain healthy blood sugar levels. Vanadium may also be a building material for the development of bones and teeth, and it may assist the body in maintaining healthy cholesterol levels.

Be sure to use caution when supplementing with vanadium. Vanadium's safety in doses higher than trace amounts is questionable at this time. More research is still needed. Currently, many bodybuilders and some people trying to improve insulin function take relatively high levels of vanadyl sulfate—sometimes as much as 15 mg tablets three times a day. I strongly caution against this. Do not take much more than the NAS's established UL (tolerable upper intake) of 1.0 mg a day for this trace mineral.

Fats and vegetable oils are the richest food sources of vanadium. Vanadium also occurs in fish, grains, meats, and nuts. Black pepper, dill seeds, parsley, and mushrooms may also contain vanadium depending on the vanadium content of the soil the plants were grown in.

Recommended dose. 200 mcg as vanadium chelate or vanadyl sulfate.

Zinc

Zinc is necessary for the functioning of more than 300 different enzymes. As such, it plays a vital role in an enormous number of biological processes. Much attention has been placed on this mineral for its role in the immune system and wound repair. In humans, the highest concentrations of zinc are found in the liver, pancreas, kidneys, bone, and muscles. Zinc is also important as a nutritional supplement in men to reduce the risk of prostate cancer.

Zinc is an important component of maturing T cells (immune-mediated cells in the thymus gland that destroy cancer cells, viruses, and microorganisms, such as bacteria and fungi). Zinc is also very important as a key mineral in insulin-receptor activity.

The best dietary sources of zinc are eggs, lean meats, liver, and seafood (especially oysters). Whole-grain breads and cereals are also good sources of zinc.

Recommended dose. 30 mg as zinc citrate.

ANTIOXIDANTS FOR NUTRITIONAL SUPPORT

A dietary antioxidant is a substance in foods or in supplement form that significantly decreases the adverse effects of reactive oxygen species (free radicals), reactive nitrogen species, or both on normal physiological function in humans. Oxidation and the production of free radicals are caused not only by normal body functions, but also by environmental and chemical stresses in our everyday lives. As explained earlier, antioxidants neutralize free radicals by binding to their free electrons.

As you already know, one of the most important dietary changes you can make is to increase the amount of antioxidant-rich fruits and vegetables in your diet. Strive to eat at least five servings of fresh vegetables and two servings of fresh fruit a day. Fresh fruits and vegetables are the richest sources of antioxidants. They also contain other protective phytochemicals (pharmacologically active chemicals naturally present in plant foods) that help to protect DNA from mutation, to metabolize hormones such as estrogen, and to stimulate detoxification pathways for environmental pollutants. In fact, many pharmaceutical drugs are derived from phytochemicals.

Phytochemicals are abundant in fruits and vegetables, but you can also get a rich supply of them from certain herbal compounds. The popularity of herbal products in recent years is a testament to the mild but effective properties of phytochemicals. The *standardization* of herbal products guarantees consumers the exact amount of active ingredients in the formula. This form of quality control has been an important step in the safety and efficacy of over-the-counter phytochemicals. Herbal formulas have a powerful influence over the biological activity in the body. For this reason, it is important to consult a healthcare professional before taking them if you are currently taking prescription medication. Herbs can interact with other herbs and pharmaceuticals and, in rare cases, even cause severe reactions.

Used safely and correctly, phytochemicals can have a large impact on your health and on your ability to regain control of your metabolic function. Among their many benefits, phytochemicals can help to:

- decrease inflammation
- enhance detoxification from environmental toxins
- improve cognitive function
- lower cholesterol
- lower blood pressure
- reduce cortisol levels
- reduce depression

- regulate blood sugar
- relieve menopausal and premenstrual symptoms
- scavenge free radicals
- slow the aging process
- stimulate or modulate immune-system function

The following are the antioxidant dietary supplements (some of which also contain phytochemicals) that I commonly recommend to decrease the formation of free radicals. There are many good multiple antioxidant formulas available that make it easy to take several antioxidants every day, but there is no one "super antioxidant" that will provide all the antioxidants that your body needs. A wide variety of antioxidants are needed to fully operate the body's many protective mechanisms.

At the very least, make sure that you take these antioxidants regularly. Keep in mind that antioxidants work together, so it does no good to take a bunch of green tea leaf extract, for example, if you do not have adequate antioxidants that are essential to run your enzyme and host antioxidant defense systems. The required base antioxidants are carotenoids and flavonoids, alpha lipoic acid, coenzyme Q_{10}, green tea extract, resveratrol, vitamins C and E, and the mineral selenium. They all make each other work more efficiently and extend each other's life in the body.

Alpha Lipoic Acid (ALA)

As mentioned earlier, alpha lipoic acid (ALA) is an essential nutrient for modern industrialized living. Many scientists believe that ALA is one of our most important antioxidant nutrients. Its key characteristic is that it is both fat soluble and water soluble, which enables it to provide antioxidant protection in a much wider range of body systems. Some scientists refer to ALA as the "universal" antioxidant. ALA provides antioxidant protection throughout the body. It may also facilitate the production of energy for cells and enhance the effectiveness of other antioxidants. ALA has been reported beneficial in nutritionally supporting health in individuals with diabetes and eye problems such as cataracts and glaucoma. For diabetics, ALA supplementation may help the body maintain healthier blood sugar levels while treating some of the neurological side effects of the disease such as diabetic neuropathy.

Good food sources of ALA include spinach, broccoli, beef, brewer's yeast, and liver, but food alone will not provide enough ALA for you to reap its antioxidant benefits. **Recommended dose.** 25–600 mg a day (preferably at least 300 mg per day).

Carotenoids and Flavonoids

There are various compounds in plants known as carotenoids and flavonoids that research is finding to be responsible for many of the health benefits associated with plant foods such as fruits, vegetables, spices, and teas. Carotenoids and flavonoids provide most of the flavor and color to fruits, vegetables, and other plants. Many carotenoids and flavonoids have antioxidant properties. Carotenoids are substances that effectively protect the fatty components of our cells, and flavonoids, being water soluble, protect the watery portions. Flavonoids are actually the largest group of antioxidants found in plants.

Carotenoids. The carotenoids are red, yellow, and orange pigments that are widely distributed in nature, including many fruits and vegetables. The major carotenoids are *beta-carotene, alpha-carotene, lutein, zeaxanthin, lycopene,* and *cryptoxanthin.* Approximately 80 to 90 percent of the carotenoids present in leafy green vegetables such as broccoli, kale, spinach, and Brussels sprouts are xanthophylls (a subclass of carotenoids), whereas 10 to 20 percent are carotenes (another subclass of which beta-carotene is the most well known). Conversely, yellow and orange vegetables, including carrots, sweet potatoes, and squash contain predominantly carotenes. Up to 60 percent of the xanthophylls and 15 percent of the carotenes in these foods are destroyed during microwave cooking. Of the xanthophylls, lutein appears to be the most stable. The effects of freezing and other storage conditions on carotenoids are unknown.

Several factors influence the differential absorption of carotenoids from food. First, although cooking reduces the carotene content of food, it also disrupts cellular membranes and liberates nutrients. Therefore, carotenoids are absorbed more efficiently from cooked versus uncooked foods. This is especially true of lycopene, which finds its greatest concentration in cooked tomato products.

Secondly, with regard to the source of carotenoids, serum levels of beta-carotene have been found to be almost 20 percent higher in people who consume purified beta-carotene in a capsule compared with those ingesting an equal amount from cooked carrots. However, foods contain a wide variety of mixed carotenoids, so an individual's primary source of carotenoids should come from the consumption of various orange, red, green, and yellow fruits and vegetables.

The established efficacy of beta-carotene in being an efficient antioxidant makes it part of the diverse antioxidant defense system in humans. Free radicals have been implicated in the development of many diseases such as heart disease (including elevated cholesterol and hypertension), various cancers, cataracts, and macular degeneration. Experiments have demonstrated that lycopene, alpha-carotene, zeaxanthin, lutein, and cryptoxanthin quench singlet oxygen and inhibit lipid peroxidation, thereby decreasing the damaging effects of free radicals. In addition to their antioxidant capability, other biological actions of carotenoids include the ability to enhance immunity and possibly reduce or inhibit cancer.

Recommended dose. Mixture of 15,000 IU a day of natural carotenoids. If you have prostate cancer, make sure this mixture contains 10–300 mg a day of lycopene. If you have an eye disorder, make sure this mixture contains 6–30 mg of lutein.

Flavonoids. Flavonoids are another term for bioflavonoids. The major flavonoids are hesperidin, rutin, and quercetin, which are also known as polyphenols, a particularly potent group of antioxidants. Polyphenols form the deep red and blue pigments in grapes and berries. They have recently been identified as being responsible for the health benefits of red wine. As another example, anthocyanins are some of the flavonoids that are found in green tea. Flavonoids and the other antioxidants protect against heavy metal toxicity, strengthen the immune system and suppress the release of inflammatory compounds such as leukotrienes. Additionally, flavonoids help prevent conditions such as bruising, hemorrhoids, varicose veins, and nose bleeds by improving the integrity of the capillaries.

Recommended dose. Broad-spectrum mixtures of natural flavonoids are available for comprehensive antioxidant protection. Most flavonoid complexes will include lemon, orange, and/or citrus flavonoids in amounts anywhere from 200–500 mg each, with quercetin and rutin in 50 mg amounts. Specialty products such as green tea extracts and resveratrol are discussed below.

Coenzyme Q_{10}

Coenzyme Q_{10} (CoQ_{10}) is an important vitaminlike compound that is present throughout the body. It is found in highest concentrations in the heart, followed by the liver, kidneys, and pancreas. While there are ten other CoQ_{10}-type compounds present in nature, CoQ_{10} is the only one present in humans. It plays a vital role in energy production within the mitochondria, where it helps to break down fats and carbohydrates. It also functions as a powerful fat-soluble antioxidant. One of the most important applications for CoQ_{10}, however, is in the nutritional support of a healthy cardiovascular system.

Current studies suggest that CoQ_{10} may be important in reducing the progression of Parkinson's disease and Alzheimer's disease. In these neurodegenerative diseases, dosages as high as of 1,200 mg per day have been used.

CoQ_{10} may also benefit those with diabetes, as this nutrient may enhance insulin production and regulation. Also, because CoQ_{10} deficiency has been linked to periodontal problems, such as gingivitis and periodontitis, it has been used successfully as a nutritional supplement in many people with unhealthy gums.

People who take prescription medications may have depleted stores of CoQ_{10}. Blood pressure drugs such as beta-blockers, anticonvulsant drugs, and cholesterol-lowering medications have been reported to decrease levels of CoQ_{10} in the body.

CoQ_{10} may provide special nutritional benefits in men. As a nutritional supplement, CoQ_{10} has been reported to aid the body in increasing sperm motility and decreasing the negative effects of oxidation on sperm cells.

The last benefit of CoQ_{10} relates to the aging process. As we age, the mitochondrial DNA continues to get assaulted by free radicals. The repair processes are poor for mitochondrial DNA and there are few supplements that help protect and repair it. CoQ_{10} seems to be one of the rare agents to support mitochondrial repair and protection.

Although CoQ_{10} occurs in the cells of all plants and animals, dietary sources do not provide adequate levels of this nutrient. Food sources of CoQ_{10} are limited. Organ meats, vegetable oils such as expressed soybean and sesame, and spinach and broccoli are the best food sources. However, foods do not contain enough CoQ_{10} for clinical benefit.

Recommended dose. 30–1,200 mg a day. Typically for cardiovascular support in heart failure or hypertension the dose is 150–225 mg per day. (Purchase "a lipid-soluble form" of CoQ_{10}. Some forms claim higher absorption, but to date studies to support this are limited and costly. Soybean oil gel caps of CoQ_{10} are equally effective.) If you are taking these pharmaceutical drugs, CoQ_{10} supplementation is a must! Consider a minimum of 100 mg per day.

Green Tea Leaf Extract

Green tea (*Camellia sinensis*) is one of the most potent antioxidants in the plant kingdom and is commonly used in helping maintain a healthy cardiovascular system and in nutritionally supporting healthy cholesterol levels in laboratory animals and humans. Green tea contains several polyphenols, potent antioxidant compounds, of which the most active is thought to be *epigallocatechin-3-gallate* (EGCG). The antioxidant effects of green tea also contribute to its role as nutritional support in various cancers. One cup of green tea can provide the same antioxidant capacity as around 150 milligram (mg) of pure vitamin C. There have been positive reports in human clinical studies of green tea's antioxidant potential. Several studies have reported that green tea may decrease the potential damage (including cancer) caused by cigarette smoking.

Recommended dose. 250–500 mg of a standardized green tea extract with 90 percent polyphenols minimum. Make sure to ask your healthcare provider before you take green tea supplements if you are taking anticoagulants and/or antiplatelet medications before surgery.

Resveratrol *(Polygonum cuspidatum)*

The root of the polygonum plant has been used for centuries in traditional Chinese medicine and contains the popular antioxidant supplement resveratrol. Resveratrol, also found in other plants including the skins of grapes (and hence, red wine), is a polyphenol or natural antioxidant that protects cells against free radicals. Resveratrol is commonly used as an antioxidant for helping to maintain a healthy cardiovascular system and as nutritional support in various cancers. Polygonum may also be of benefit in helping to maintain proper uric acid levels (increased uric acid levels lead to gout). It also helps reduce the stimulation of the inflammatory cascade and inhibits production of glycation end-products, which accelerate cellular and DNA damage. **Recommended dose.** 200 mg daily, standardized to 8 percent trans-resveratrol.

Selenium

For a discussion of selenium's antioxidant properties and its recommended dosage, see page 421.

Vitamin C

For information on vitamin C's antioxidant properties and its recommended dosage, see page 412.

Vitamin E

For information on Vitamin E's antioxidant properties and its recommended dosage, see page 414.

Other Effective Antioxidant Supplements

In addition to the required base antioxidants, consider strengthening your antioxidant system by including the following antioxidants.

- **Bilberry fruit (*Vaccinium myrtillus*).** This antioxidant is especially beneficial for the eyes. If you have problems with night vision or if you have type 2 diabetes, this is an essential nutrient for you to consider adding to your daily regimen. Also, if you are concerned about macular degeneration, cataracts, or glaucoma, add bilberry fruit to your daily routine. **Recommended dose.** 80 mg, two to three times a day, standardized to 25 percent anthocyanosides.

- **Ginkgo (*Ginkgo biloba*).** This antioxidant is especially beneficial for the brain. Doctors in Europe use ginkgo quite frequently. It has outstanding antioxidant properties and, in addition, helps improve circulation to the brain and helps improve the use of oxygen and glucose in brain tissue. It is invaluable for the preservation of cognitive function and for the treatment of peripheral vascular diseases. Although ginkgo thins the blood, it is not contraindicated with warfarin (Coumadin). In one long-term, randomized, double-blind study, researchers observed no alteration on the anticoagulant warfarin in twenty-four people who were taking both ginkgo and the anticoagulant. However, if you are on a blood thinner, you may want to check with your physician before taking ginkgo. **Recommended dose.** 40–80 mg, three times a day, standardized to 24 to 27 percent gingko flavone glycosides.

- **Grape seed extract (*Vitis vinifera*).** This antioxidant is invaluable for slowing down allergic responses and helping to control inflammation. **Recommended dose.** 25–100 mg, one to three times a day, standardized to 95 percent proanthocyandin content and at least 90 percent phenols.

- **Milk thistle fruit extract (*Silybum marianum*).** This antioxidant is especially beneficial for the liver. Milk thistle provides conditions that allow for more production or more activity of glutathione in the liver. Glutathione is the body's principle antioxidant. Because it also has a powerful effect on improving detoxification pathways, milk thistle helps to protect and optimize liver function. Taking 300 mg a day of milk thistle (five days on, two days off) is one of the best preventive strategies for modern industrial living. **Recommended dose.** 80–160 mg, one to three times a day, standardized to contain 80 percent silymarin.

- **Rosemary leaf (*Rosmarinus officinalis*).** Although this supplement has not yet become popular in this country, rosemary leaf extracts are powerful antioxidants. It is added to a wide variety of herbal formulas and is also used as a preservative. **Recommended dose.** 100 mg, two to three times a day, standardized to contain a minimum of 6.0 percent carnosic acid, 1.0 percent rosmarinic acid, and 1.5 percent ursolic acid.

Herbal Anti-inflammatories

If you know, or suspect, that inflammatory processes are active in you, consider including the following remedies in your daily regimen. Inflammation is linked to increased free-radical formation, and recent science has associated it with most degenerative disease processes and aging. Traditional therapies for inflammation use NSAIDs such as ibuprofen, and the newer COX-2 inhibitors, such as rofecoxib (Vioxx) and celecoxib (Celebrex). Although effective in some situations, they are expensive and have unwanted side effects.

Many ancient medical traditions have long recognized the effectiveness of several herbs that have recently been reported to demonstrate COX-2 inhibiting properties. Some of these herbs include the following:

- **Ginger (*Zingiber officinalis*).** Ginger has a multitude of uses and is primarily known in the West as a spice and flavoring agent in foods. However, in China, it has been used for thousands of years for medicinal purposes to treat such conditions as fever, nausea, stomachache, rheumatism, toothaches, as well as pains and inflammation. Research has discovered that ginger has powerful antioxidant and anti-inflammatory effects, along with being an effective antiemetic (for nausea). The components of ginger root that are believed to be mainly responsible for its medicinal uses are the gingerols. Ginger is reported to be a COX-2 inhibitor. In studies, it has a clear advantage over pharmaceutical and over-the-counter agents in that significant side effects such as those reported with NSAID use have not been reported. **Recommended dose.** 250 mg, two to four times a day or as needed, standardized to contain 5 percent total pungent compounds, most prominently 6-gingerol and 6-shogaol, or 4 percent volatile oils. There is also a 20 percent extract on the market that is more potent. However, this more potent extract may upset the stomach if not taken with food. If it does cause any unpleasant stomach problems, reduce the dosage.

- **Holy Basil (*Ocimum sanctum*).** In India, this plant is called "tulsi" or "tulasi," which in English means "matchless." References to holy basil are common in Hindu literature. In India, it has been traditionally used for fever, the flu, bronchitis, asthma, malaria, and cancer. In Egypt, this herb is traditionally used for arthritis and inflammation. Holy basil contains phytochemicals (particularly rosmarinic acid) that have reported COX-2 inhibitory effects. One study conducted at Dartmouth Medical School found that it possessed anti-inflammatory activity. French researchers have also shown that holy basil has potent COX-2 inhibitory effects. Studies in India and other nations around the world have confirmed these findings. **Recommended dose.** 400–800 mg, two times a day, standardized to contain 1 percent ursolic acid per dose.

- **Nexrutine.** Nexrutine is an herbal supplement that contains a special extract of phellodendron bark (*Phellodendron amurense*), which has been reported not only to have COX-2 inhibiting qualities, but also to protect the gastrointestinal tract against ulceration.

   Phellodendron has been used for centuries in traditional Chinese medicine for individuals with gastroenteritis, abdominal pain, and diarrhea, and it has been used as an antioxidant as well. A Japanese study of laboratory animals with alcohol- and aspirin-induced gastric ulcers reported that phellodendron actually decreased gastric acid content, protecting the stomach lining and suppressing ulceration. Not only is there now a natural product that can be used for treating inflammatory conditions, but it can also aid in protecting the stomach lining against the main problem with using NSAIDs and conventional COX-2 inhibitors. Nexrutine also works well for post-exercise soreness and soft tissue complaints such as fibromyalgia. **Recommended dose.** 500 mg, two to three times a day.

- **Oregano (*Origanum vulgare*).** This plant has gained tremendous popularity over the years as a medicinal agent. The ancient Greeks used this Mediterranean plant extensively. In Greek, its name means "joy of the mountains." The use of oregano spread throughout all of Europe, where it was frequently used to fight respiratory inflammation. It was also used as a sedative and a diuretic. In China, oregano is used for skin inflammation, for digestive problems, and to reduce fever. It is growing in popularity again. In the United States, the medical literature shows that oregano has been used to treat arthritis, toothache, tinnitus (or ringing in the ears), and anxiety. It has also been reported to have antifungal and antiparasitic activity. The constituent rosmarinic acid (also found in other herbs such as holy basil and rosemary) has been reported in laboratory studies to have COX-2 inhibiting properties comparable to popular anti-inflammatory agents. **Recommended dose.** 250–500 mg of leaf extract, three times a day; or 5–10 drops of concentrated oil extract, three times a day. Products are usually standardized to contain 5 percent thymol. Allergies to oregano may develop or exist in sensitive individuals.

- **Turmeric (*Curcuma longa*).** This herb is cousin to the ginger plant. Well known as a spice in East Indian cooking, turmeric root is widely used in the ancient Ayurvedic and traditional Chinese medical systems as an agent for inflammatory conditions, skin lesions, blood and liver disorders, menstrual problems, and even cancer. Turmeric contains an anti-inflammatory chemical called curcumin, which research has reported to be a powerful COX-2 inhibitor. **Recommended dose.** 150–300 mg, three times a day with meals, standardized to contain 95 percent curcuminoids. Do not use if biliary obstruction is present (gall bladder problems). If you are on anticoagulant or antiplatelet medication or have bleeding disorders, do not use turmeric supplements long-term unless under the supervision of a physician; they may upset the stomach.

QUALITY, QUALITY, QUALITY!

The foods, air, and water you consume are of utmost importance in your life—they provide us the life-giving energy that we require. Without quality, these agents can be detrimental to our health. However, something more important is involved, realizing that you are the one making the choices in your life that affect your health. Yes, fast food is on every corner, but these restaurants aren't forcing us to eat it. We walk in and buy it with our own free will. Use your wisdom and your power of choice: Try to buy high-quality foods—organic if possible. Don't use preserved, processed, and treated foods. Try to limit fast foods. Don't smoke—the air we breathe should be clean and fresh. Enhance and improve your indoor air with filters and plants. Try to keep from breathing in the household chemicals that are generally used to clean. Better yet, look for biologically friendly options. Limit your intake of unfiltered water—drink it only if necessary. By choosing to follow these recommendations and others you may run across in your pursuit of optimal wellness, you should be well on your way to the transformation that can come from eating, breathing, and drinking health!

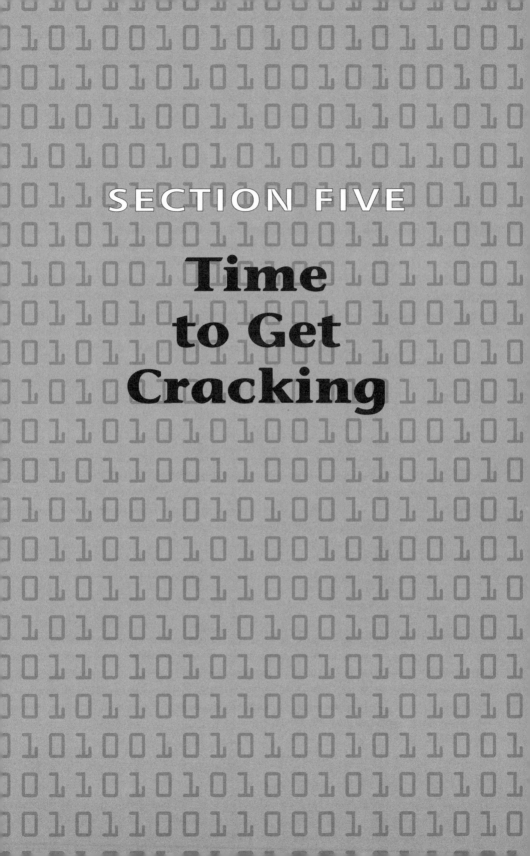

SECTION FIVE

Time to Get Cracking

The System Discovery Questionnaire—A Map to Follow on Your Personal Journey to Optimal Health

Now that you've learned how your body works, it's time to evaluate your general health and that of your individual body systems. Identifying your symptoms and knowing something about their frequency and intensity, and in which system they occur, will help you map your personal path back to optimal health.

Take some time now to complete the questionnaire in this chapter. Be honest with yourself about how you feel. Try not to overstate or understate your symptoms. And remember this is not meant to replace medical treatment or a visit to your healthcare practitioner. You might want to have someone close to you help you complete the questionnaire. Sometimes other people see things in us that we don't see in ourselves. Change takes effort and can be difficult at times, but your desire for improved health and well-being will carry you through. So let's get cracking!

THE SYSTEM DISCOVERY QUESTIONNAIRE

The System Discovery Assessment below is a shortened version of the questionnaire I use in my practice. The assessment is divided into two sections: Section one assesses your overall health habits and lifestyle; section two focuses on the individual key body systems discussed in this book. Each part in this section reveals a tendency or weakness in a given part of your metabolic code. The lifestyle you live, medications you've taken, food selections, effects of chronic stress, exercise, and environmental exposure all can have an impact on how you feel and can influence your chemistry. Your answers to each section of this questionnaire will give you insight into the problem areas that you need to work on in order to restore and optimize your metabolic code for health and longevity.

Each part of the questionnaire proposes a plan of action for you to follow based on your point score, using nutritional supplementation, as well as modifications in diet and lifestyle. Unlike previous supplement recommendations throughout this book that provided you with a minimum to maximum range for a particular nutrient, the supplement protocols here are dose-specific and target varying degrees of metabolic dysfunction within a particular key area.

Once you have filled out the questionnaire, add up the total points from each section to determine your grand total. Your total score at the end of each section will guide you as to which body system(s) need attention. If you have a number of chronic health problems indicated by a grand total of 200 or more, you should see a healthcare practitioner to help you design your own therapeutic program. If your total point score is less than 200 and indicates your symptoms are mild to moderate, although you may benefit from the help of healthcare practitioner, you can also follow the plan of action and revisit the chapters specific to your health complaints, paying special attention to the information in them. It may be that your scores indicate the need to focus on several body systems. It is not only possible, but also advisable, to follow several plans of action at once. However, if you feel overwhelmed, either seek out a healthcare practitioner or prioritize according to the scores.

After three or four weeks of following the plan(s), you can complete the questionnaire again to help you monitor your improvement and to refocus on the most important areas. You may want to complete this questionnaire annually, or any time you feel your body could use a tune-up. Also, keep in mind the other valuable lab tests mentioned throughout the book that can help you assess organ and system function, nutritional needs, environmental exposures, and how your body is utilizing nutrients.

SECTION ONE: GENERAL LIFESTYLE ASSESSMENT

Check the box for each question below to which you answer "yes":

❏ Are you a chronic dieter?

❏ Do you exercise less than three times per week?

❏ Are you under excessive stress?

❏ Are you exposed to chemicals at work or home or do you live in an industrial community?

❏ Do you smoke or are you exposed to cigarette smoke?

❏ Do you eat less than five daily servings of vegetables and fruit?

❏ Do you drink more than ten alcoholic beverages a week?

❏ Does your main source of carbohydrates consist of refined carbohydrates and sugar?

❏ Do you eat packaged food containing partially hydrogenated oils or trans fats?

❏ Are you overweight or do you have excessive belly fat?

❏ Do you feel as if you lack sufficient energy to get through the day?

If you answered yes to any of these questions, it is important that you start to introduce healthier habits into your lifestyle. Most of us don't want to be bothered with changes until a real life crisis hits us or someone we love. If you have children, it is even more important that you begin to take a more proactive approach to your health and your family's health. The earlier children begin to incorporate these changes into their lives and into the environment around them, the healthier their lives will be. Start the process today.

Plan of Action for General Lifestyle

1. Maintain a healthy weight. While this advice is often given, it usually comes without the tools people need to do it. If you have tried various weight-loss methods with little success or you always regain the weight, there is very likely an underlying metabolic interference. Weight management is crucial to health and longevity. The secret to weight control is not found in any one pill. It lies in optimizing all your body systems. Section 2 of the questionnaire will now make it possible for you to do identify the areas that may be keeping you not only from losing weight but also from keeping it off.

2. Follow the Healthy Living Guidelines for eating in Chapter 13. Start with phase two if you want to ease yourself into healthier eating habits. However, if you really want to tailor your diet to the one that is metabolically best for you, then start with phase one. Eat fewer refined carbohydrates and sugars. Americans eat an overabundance of refined carbohydrates and sugars, which sends them spiraling down the path to diabetes, cardiovascular disease, Alzheimer's disease, cancer, and metabolic syndrome.

   If I had a "magic" pill that would decrease cancer risk considerably and had no side effects, most people would take it. That's what a minimum of five to nine servings a day of vegetables and fruit can do for you. Make every attempt to follow the dietary changes recommended in the guidelines, because if you are the typical American, you are a long way from eating a diet that will support health. And while supplements can be very helpful in getting you back to feeling better quickly, some people do not like to take supplements. Many people will feel much better simply by getting the sugar and refined carbohydrates out of their diet, making sure to eat lots of vegetables and a little fruit, drinking more water, and exercising. For many of you, there will be a learning curve in food preparation, but if you persist, you will find that learning to eat healthy actually allows for more fun with food at the same time you are losing weight and feeling better.

3. Learn to manage stress. If you are under stress whether at work or at home you must take steps to make your body more resilient to the negative consequences of chronic stress. Remember, stress weakens your immune system, contributes to weight gain by stimulating cravings for refined carbohydrates and sugar, slows down your metabolic rate, alters your sleep patterns, and more. You can't avoid

stress, but you can learn to manage it better and strengthen your body's defense. Exercise, yoga, or any activity that can take you away from the pressures of daily living is an effective stress-management tool.

4. Exercise. Exercise is critical for reclaiming your health. Exercise increases resting metabolic rate by increasing your lean muscle mass to fat mass ratio. More muscle means more calories per pound of body weight burned even when you're just resting. And remember, fat tissue isn't just hanging off you doing nothing. Fat tissue acts as an endocrine organ, pumping out hormones and cytokines that disrupt your health and contribute to disease. Exercise also helps to stabilize blood sugar and burn off stress hormones that have a negative impact on your metabolism.

5. Limit your exposure to chemical and environmental pollutants. If you are knowingly exposed to chemical and environmental pollutants (for example, in a work environment) and don't do anything to support your body's defense, you are taking big risks. Whether or not you are knowingly exposed to these substances, I strongly encourage you to undergo testing to find out your levels of exposure. Environmental influences on health are associated with increased cancer risk, Alzheimer's disease, Parkinson's disease, and heart disease, among many other health problems. Environmental exposure, especially to heavy metals, is quickly becoming recognized within the medical profession as a contributor to many of our chronic health problems. Remember, that your organs of detoxification are working overtime to keep your chemistry in check in these situations. Sometimes, it could take years before the toxin "trough" fills and begins to alter your metabolism.

6. Assist the body in removing toxins by following a detoxification program of diet and supplementation one to two times a year. This will help to protect the liver from possible damage by toxins and to keep its detoxification pathways running smoothly. Because we are exposed to toxins everywhere—from our air, from our foods, and even from our own metabolism—everyone can benefit from an occasional liver detoxification.

7. Supplement your diet. There are basic nutrient requirements that everyone should meet daily. The nutrients listed below should be part of a daily maintenance supplement regimen just like eating healthy food, drinking clean water, and exercising:

   • An optimal daily intake (ODI) multivitamin and mineral formula. When choosing a multivitamin and mineral formula, try to come as close as you can to matching the nutrient levels indicated in Table 16.1 on page 407.

   • Omega-3 fatty acids derived from fish oil: 1,000–2,000 mg a day.

   • Flaxseed meal, as a fiber supplement: 2 tablespoons a day.

8. The following supernutrients are optional and may be included along with the

daily maintenance supplements to support specific health goals or for overall health insurance:

- Green tea standardized to 50 percent EGCG for antioxidant support: 250–500 mg a day.
- CoQ_{10} for energy and anti-aging: 100–300 mg a day.
- Alpha lipoic acid for detoxification and maintenance of blood sugar: 300–600 mg a day.
- Moducare for immune system and anti-inflammation support: 60 mg a day.
- Alpha GPC for human growth hormone release, memory, and cognition: 1,000 mg a day.
- Chlorella for environmental detox: 3–5 grams a day.
- Cordyceps CS4 extract for stamina and endurance: 2,400 mg a day.

9. Replenish nutrients depleted by medications. In the list below, check off the over-the-counter or prescription drugs you presently take. Refer to Appendix 3, "Prescription and Nonprescription Nutrient Depletions," on page 512 and make a list of all the vitamins and minerals that are depleted by the medication that you are taking. Drug therapy is one factor that can influence the efficiency of your metabolism. It can significantly impact enzyme function, immunity, and the eventual development of symptoms or side effects from the drug or drugs. If you are on multiple drugs, they could alter vitamin and mineral availability and consequently reduce your ability to detoxify environmental and internal toxins. Keep in mind that drugs are not necessarily bad or something that should be avoided. Many times they are necessary. However, there are also times that by implementing lifestyle changes, losing weight, and improving nutritional status, drug therapy can be reduced or even eliminated. One thing that we know is that the more drug therapies you are on, the more chance for complications from potential interactions and side effects. If a drug isn't listed, then it may not have proven nutrient depletions to date.

❏ antacid/H2 blocker/allergy and/or asthma medication

❏ antibiotics

❏ antidepressants

❏ antidiabetic medication/insulin

❏ antifungal medication

❏ anti-anxiety medication

❏ aspirin/acetaminophen/NSAIDs such as ibuprofen/COX-2 inhibitors

❏ blood pressure medication

❑ chemotherapy

❑ corticosteroids

❑ diuretics

❑ estrogen

❑ heart medication

❑ HIV medication

❑ laxatives

❑ oral contraceptives

❑ relaxants/sleeping pills

❑ "statin" drugs/cholesterol-lowering medication

❑ thyroid hormone

❑ ulcer medication

❑ Other:_____

For many people, following the above basic recommendations alone will have a dramatic impact on the way they look and feel. Sometimes, however, more intervention is needed. In these cases, seeking out more specific information about your health and symptoms can give you clues as to what part of your body's chemistry needs extra work.

KNOW YOUR NUMBERS

Don't ignore your health. Regular check ups and laboratory testing can help you get proactive with your health. The chart below shows the guidelines you should be familiar with to help you assess your health risks.

BIOMARKER	BE CONCERNED IF NUMBER IS
Triglyceride	>150
HDL	<40 m <50 w
Glucose	>110
Insulin	>10
Blood Pressure	>130/85
BMI	>27
Waist Circumference	>40" m >30" w
Homocysteine	>10
C-Reactive Protein	1.0–3.0 moderate risk >3.0 high risk
Fibrinogen	> 300

SECTION TWO: BODY SYSTEMS ASSESSMENT

Rank each entry from 0 to 5 based upon the intensity, duration, and frequency of your symptoms within the past year; otherwise, answer yes or no where applicable. When you have finished, total your points for each part.

Point scale:

0 = *Never* have the symptom

1 = *Very infrequently* have the symptom, occurs every few months

2 = *Occasionally* have the symptom, occurs once or twice a month

3 = *Mild,* have the symptom once a week

4 = *Moderate,* have the symptom three or four days a week

5 = *Severe,* have the symptom daily, or when applicable cyclically
    (for example, PMS)

No = 0

Yes = 10

PART 1: PANCREAS FUNCTION (BLOOD SUGAR AND INSULIN BALANCE)						
1. Do you feel shaky or jittery if going too long without eating?	Yes					No
2. Are you irritable if a meal is missed?	Yes					No
3. Do you feel tired or weak if a meal is missed?	Yes					No
4. Do you feel tired one to three hours after eating?	0	1	2	3	4	5
5. Do you crave carbohydrates or sweets excessively?	0	1	2	3	4	5
6. Are you calmer after eating?	0	1	2	3	4	5
7. Do you have headaches that are relieved by eating something sweet?	0	1	2	3	4	5
8. Do you feel stimulated by exercise?	0	1	2	3	4	5
9. Have you been diagnosed with insulin resistance or diabetes?	Yes					No
10. Have you been diagnosed with metabolic syndrome?	Yes					No
11. Are you more than twenty pounds over your ideal weight?	Yes					No
12. Do you eat refined sugar or carbohydrates daily (such as cakes, cookies, candy, and white-flour products)?	0	1	2	3	4	5
13. Do you have sporadic energy "boosts and drops" throughout the day?	0	1	2	3	4	5
14. Is your fasting blood sugar level consistently over 95?	Yes					No
					PART 1 TOTAL:	_____

Plan of Action for Part 1

1. Diet is particularly important for people experiencing any signs of blood sugar dys-regulation. Pay close attention to your carbohydrate intake. While the controversy re-garding the virtues of eating a low-carbohydrate diet versus a high-carbohydrate diet may continue, most health professionals have finally acknowledged the problems that result from an uncontrolled intake of refined sugar and other refined carbohy-drates. Eliminate sugar from the diet almost entirely; reduce your total carbohydrate intake; and make sure that the carbohydrates you do eat are of high nutritional den-sity (whole grains, vegetables, and fruits). This will lead to improved blood sugar bal-ance and will have a significant impact on your ability to optimize your metabolism.

2. Based on your score for part one, add the following nutrients to your daily main-tenance supplements for pancreas support and blood sugar regulation:

   - For scores 15 and higher, add:
     - GTF chromium: 400 micrograms (mcg) a day.

   - For scores 20 and higher, add in addition:
     - Alpha lipoic acid: up to 600 milligrams (mg) a day.

   - For scores 25 and higher, add additional herbal agents:
     - Bitter melon: 200mg, two to three times a day
     - *Gymnema sylvestre:* 250 mg, three times a day.
     - Glucosol: 32–48 mg a day.
     - Milk thistle: 600 mg a day.
     - Relora®: 250 mg, three times a day (if you crave carbohydrates and sugar as a response to stress).
     - Vanadium: 750 mcg a day.

   - If you are diabetic, add:
     - Moducare: three 20–40 mg capsules, twice a day.
     - Cinnamon extract: $1/2$–$3/4$ teaspoon, three times a day, *or*
     - Cyclo-hispro: 300 mg, four times a day.

   Note: These substances may cause alterations in blood sugar levels. Be sure to monitor the changes and report those changes to your healthcare practitioner.

3. If your score is higher than 25, pay particular attention to the following keys and reread the appropriate chapters:

   - Key One: Adrenals (Chapter 5)
   - Key Five: Intestines (Chapter 9)
   - Key Seven: Nutrition (Chapter 13)
   - Key Nine: Oxygen and Oxidative Stress (Chapter 15)

PART 2: THYROID FUNCTION (SUBCLINICAL HYPOTHYROIDISM)						
1. Do you feel exhausted from morning to night?	Yes					No
2. Do you have trouble getting up in the morning?	0	1	2	3	4	5
3. Are you stiff in the morning?	0	1	2	3	4	5
4. Do you have dry skin, brittle hair, or nails?	Yes					No
5. Do you have cold hands and feet?	Yes					No
6. Is your short-term memory failing?	0	1	2	3	4	5
7. Do you go to pieces easily or dislike working under pressure?	0	1	2	3	4	5
8. Do you have difficulty losing weight no matter what diet or exercise plan you follow?	Yes					No
9. Are you depressed?	0	1	2	3	4	5
10. Are you constipated?	0	1	2	3	4	5
11. Do your muscles feel weak as if they can't generate energy?	0	1	2	3	4	5
12. Is your cholesterol over 200?	0	1	2	3	4	5
13. Do you have PMS or menstrual difficulties?	0	1	2	3	4	5
14. Have you had trouble conceiving a child?	Yes					No
15. Is your first morning under arm body temperature less than 97.8°F.?	Yes					No
PART 2 TOTAL: _____						

Plan of Action for Part 2

Over the last few years, it has become more apparent that many people have symptoms of disturbances in thyroid function. However, these symptoms often do not show up in traditional testing methods. If you suspect that your thyroid function is low, or if you can't seem to muster the energy to get through the day, the following plan of action will promote healthier thyroid function. Seek medical attention if you still display many symptoms of low thyroid after taking the following measures to improve thyroid function.

1. Incorporate 1–4 tablespoons of organic, extra-virgin coconut oil into your diet each day. Extra-virgin coconut oil is an excellent cooking oil alternative. Coconut oil promotes healthy thyroid function.

2. Based on your score, add the following nutrients to your daily maintenance supplements for thyroid support:
   - For scores 15 and higher, add:
     - Tyrosine: 250 mg, three times a day.

- For scores 20 and higher, add:
  - *Coleus forskohlii:* 100 mg standardized to contain 10 percent forskolin, three times a day.
  - Guggul: 500 mg, three times a day.
- For scores 30 and higher, add:
  - Thyroid glandular (New Zealand source): 60 mg, one to three times a day.

3. If your score is higher than 25, pay particular attention to the following keys and reread the appropriate chapters:
  - Key One: Adrenals (Chapter 5)
  - Key Five: Intestines and Immunity (Chapter 9)
  - Key Six: Environmental Toxins (Chapter 10)
  - Key Nine: Oxygen and Oxidative Stress (Chapter 15)

PART 3: ADRENAL FUNCTION (ADRENAL EXHAUSTION AND CORTISOL PRODUCTION)

1. Are you under excessive stress at home or at your job?	Yes						No
2. Do you have blue rings under your eyes?	0	1	2	3	4	5	
3. Do you crave sugars and carbohydrates especially at midday and in the evening?	Yes						No
4. Have you gained weight around the belly or waistline?	0	1	2	3	4	5	
5. Do you have increased fat distribution all over your body?	0	1	2	3	4	5	
6. Do you have high blood pressure that may be influenced by stress?	0	1	2	3	4	5	
7. Do you need coffee to get you going in the morning?	0	1	2	3	4	5	
8. Do you have poor concentration and memory?	0	1	2	3	4	5	
9. Are you exhausted physically or does emotional upset bring on exhaustion?	Yes						No
10. Do you feel tired at midday?	Yes						No
11. Do you feel emotionally flat or lacking a zest for living?	0	1	2	3	4	5	
12. Do you consume 50 percent of your calories in the day after 5:00 P.M. and crave carbohydrates in the evening?	0	1	2	3	4	5	
13. Do you feel anxious or nervous?	0	1	2	3	4	5	

14. Do you notice a decrease in your sex drive?	0	1	2	3	4	5
15. Do you have trouble getting to sleep or do you wake in the middle of the night?	Yes					No
16. Do you feel overcommitted in your daily life?	0	1	2	3	4	5

PART 3 TOTAL: _____

Plan of Action for Part 3

Too many people push themselves to exhaustion these days. A person who is adrenally exhausted may cry or tear up more easily, is stressed to the point of memory lapse, feels exhausted, may be emotionally flat, may have gained excess pounds as a result of stress-induced eating, and have slowed down their metabolism such that weight loss is difficult or impossible to achieve. Gaining an understanding of the role that stress plays on your health and doing something about it can truly change your future health and get you feeling better today.

1. Based on your score, add the following nutrients to your daily maintenance supplements for adrenal support. Supplement regimens for adrenal regulation vary according to the stress-related complaint. Here are several different approaches:

   - For scores 15 and higher, and if you are exhausted and have midday fatigue, add:
     - Adrenal glandular (New Zealand): 200 mg, three times a day. (If you notice that you are too awake at night, cut back to twice a day before 4:00 P.M.). If you avoid animal products, try the herbs listed below. The following herbals may also be combined with the adrenal glandular:
     - Holy basil, for anxious feelings: one to two 400-mg capsules, two times a day (may cause drowsiness is some people).
     - Rhodiola rosea, for stress support and when short-term memory is poor: 150–250 mg a day, standardized to 3 to 5 percent rosavins.
     - Moducare, to regulate the negative metabolic effects of stress, including inflammation, alterations in DHEA and cortisol, and cholesterol production: three 20–40 mg capsules, two times a day on an empty stomach.
   - For anxiousness from effects of stress, add:
     - Relora®: 250 mg, three times a day. (If you feel chronically stressed, Relora® may well become a maintenance product for you. In rare cases, Relora® may initially make you drowsy. If so, take it at night only until this effect wears off. Then begin to take it during the day.) *or*
     - Theanine: 100–200 mg, two to three times a day.
   - For lack of sleep from effects of stress, add:
     - Relora®: 250 mg, three times a day.

- 5-HTP, to produce serotonin: 100 mg at bedtime.
- Melatonin: 3–6 mg at bedtime. (As your sleep improves, stop taking the melatonin. Next, stop the 5-HTP, and see whether you can cope with stress well with just the use of Relora®.)

- For increased sugar and carbohydrate cravings and night eating syndrome, add:
  - Chromium GTF , to get blood sugar under control: 600 mcg a day.
  - 5-HTP, to build serotonin and decrease cravings: 50–100 mg, three times a day.
  - Relora®, for normalizing cortisol production: 250 mg, three times a day.
  - Other important nutrients include vitamin C, B-complex, and the mineral magnesium, which should be present in adequate quantities in your multi-vitamin and mineral supplement. Many people may require regular adrenal support, especially people who don't want to slow down.

2. Regardless of your score in Part 3, if any of the questions describe you, reread Chapter 5 on adrenal function. This may be the most important chapter that you read in this book. If your score is higher than 20, pay particular attention to the following keys and reread the appropriate chapters:

- Key One: Pancreas (Chapter 3)
- Key Two: Thyroid (Chapter 4)
- Key Five: Intestines (Chapter 9)
- Key Six: Environmental Toxins (Chapter 10)

PART 4: LIVER FUNCTION (DETOXIFICATION)						
1. Do you have an intolerance to greasy foods?	0	1	2	3	4	5
2. Do you get headaches after eating?	0	1	2	3	4	5
3. Do you have pain under the right side of your ribcage?	Yes					No
4. Is your stool yellow or gold in color?	0	1	2	3	4	5
5. Is there a yellow cast to your tongue?	Yes					No
6. Do you have a sour taste in your mouth or bad breath?	0	1	2	3	4	5
7. Do you have body odor?	0	1	2	3	4	5
8. Are you more than 20 pounds overweight?	0	1	2	3	4	5
9. Do you have diabetes?	0	1	2	3	4	5
10. Do you have skin rashes or other skin disturbances?	0	1	2	3	4	5
11. Is your total cholesterol over 200?	Yes					No

12. Have you had problems with ovarian cysts, fibroids, or breast cancer?	Yes						No
13. Do you sweat profusely?	0	1	2	3	4	5	
14. Do you have allergies?	0	1	2	3	4	5	
15. Are you on prescription medications?	Yes						No
16. Do you use or have you taken recreational drugs?	0	1	2	3	4	5	
17. Do you smoke?	0	1	2	3	4	5	
18. Do you drink alcohol?	0	1	2	3	4	5	

PART 4 TOTAL: _____

Plan of Action for Part 4

1. Based on your score, add the following nutrients to your daily maintenance supplements for liver support and detoxification:

   - For scores 20 and greater, add:
     - Milk thistle: 300 mg, one to two times a day.
     - Artichoke extract: 250 mg, two to three times a day.
   - For scores 30 and greater, add:
     - Alpha lipoic acid: 300 mg, one to two times a day.
     - CoQ_{10}: 100 mg a day.
   - If your cholesterol is high and the suggestions and lifestyle changes above do not lower your cholesterol, add:
     - Policosanol: 30 mg a day until you reach a desirable cholesterol level, then reduce the intake to 10–20 mg a day, *or*
     - Phytosterols*: 500 mg, two times a day.
   - Allergies and skin rashes can also be liver-related. If you have consistent allergies or skin rashes, add the following nutrients:
     - MSM: 1,000–2,000 mg, three times a day.
     - Consider a vitamin C flush (see the inset "Performing a Vitamin C Flush" on page 254 for instructions). Once allergies or rashes clear up, switch to the following nutrients for maintenance:
       - Grape seed extract: 100 mg, three times a day.
       - Moducare: three 20–40 mg capsules, two times a day between meals, for thirty days, then decrease to once a day

2. If your score is higher than 30, pay particular attention to the following keys and reread the appropriate chapters:

---

*Occasionally a supplement may be listed that has not been discussed in previous chapters. These supplements, as well as all the others listed, are readily available in natural food stores.

- Key One: Pancreas (Chapter 3)
- Key Two: Thyroid (Chapter 4)
- Key Three: Adrenals (Chapter 5)
- Key Five: Intestines (Chapter 9)
- Key Six: Environmental Toxins (Chapter 10)
- Key Nine: Oxygen and Oxidative Stress (Chapter 15)

PART 5: INTESTINAL HEALTH (YEAST/DYSBIOSIS/LEAKY GUT)

1. Do you feel mentally foggy, fatigued, bloated, gassy, or gastrointestinal distress after eating a high-sugar or high-carbohydrate meal?	Yes						No
2. Do you have a history of drug use, including chemotherapy, radiation, antibiotics, steroids, NSAIDs or aspirin, H2 blockers, or birth control pills?	Yes						No
3. Do you have allergies, chronic sinusitis, or infections?	Yes						No
4. Do damp, muggy days or moldy places provoke symptoms in you?	0	1	2	3	4	5	
5. Do you crave alcohol, carbohydrates, or sugar?	Yes						No
6. Do you have persistent vaginal yeast, toe nail fungus, skin fungus, or jock itch?	Yes						No
7. Do you have a tendency to feel depressed for no apparent reason?	0	1	2	3	4	5	
8. Do you have trouble losing weight?	0	1	2	3	4	5	
9. Does your belly get distended and uncomfortable on a regular basis?							
10. Do you have trouble with constipation, diarrhea, or pass mucus in your stools?	0	1	2	3	4	5	
11. Do you have rashes or skin allergies?	0	1	2	3	4	5	
12. Do you have an intolerance to certain foods?	0	1	2	3	4	5	
13. Do you have a persistent history of urinary tract infections (UTIs) or cystitis?	0	1	2	3	4	5	
14. Do you suffer from PMS?	0	1	2	3	4	5	

PART 5 TOTAL: _____

Plan of Action for Part 5

If any of this sounds familiar, you need to start making changes to help you over-come the current state of your intestinal health. Heroic efforts are usually not necessary to improve gastrointestinal health. Many times, simply changing the foods that you eat, reestablishing beneficial bacteria in the intestine, and providing nutrients that the body needs to help reduce inflammation or rebuild the integrity of the gut can have a substantial impact on how you feel. Your digestion is truly a principle key to your longevity and well-being.

1. Based on your score, add the following nutrients to your daily maintenance supplements to optimize the flora in your intestines and to restore the integrity of the gut lining.

    * For scores 20 and higher, take:
        ▪ Cat's claw: 500 mg capsules, three times a day, *or*
        ▪ Grapefruit seed extract: one to two 100-mg capsules, three times day, *or*
        ▪ Olive leaf extract: 250–500 mg, three times a day, *or*
        ▪ Oregano extract: 300–500 mg, three times a day.
        ▪ Probiotics: 20 billion CFU (dairy-free) cultures, two times a day.

    * For scores 30 and higher, add:
        ▪ L-glutamine: 500 mg, three times a day, *or*
        ▪ SeaCure: three 500-mg capsules, three times a day.
        ▪ Butyrate: 500 mg, two times a day.

2. If your score is higher than 30, reread Chapter 9 on the gastrointestinal tract, and pay particular attention to the following keys and reread the appropriate chapters:

    * Key One: Pancreas (Chapter 3)
    * Key Two: Thyroid (Chapter 4)
    * Key Three: Adrenals (Chapter 5)
    * Key Four: Liver (Chapter 8)

PART 6: STOMACH ACID (LOW)		
1. Do you constantly need to belch or burp?	Yes	No
2. Do you feel fullness for extended periods of time after meals?	Yes	No
3. Do you feel bloated after eating?	Yes	No
4. Do you pass gas regularly?	Yes	No
5. Do you have known food allergies?	Yes	No
	PART 6 TOTAL:_____	

Plan of Action for Part 6

For scores 10 or higher, follow these suggestions:

1. In addition to your daily maintenance supplements, take a full-range digestive enzyme according to directions on the label. If your symptoms don't resolve, try another brand of enzymes until you find one that works for you.

2. If you still don't get much relief, reread Chapter 9 on the intestines. Keep in mind that as you change your food selection habits and improve the efficiency of your metabolism, these nagging problems may go away and the need for digestive enzymes may no longer exist. Use a digestive enzyme with meals for a period of forty-five to ninety days while improving food selections, and then eat without taking them. If the bloating comes back, continue to take a digestive enzyme for another few weeks, at which time retest yourself at another meal without them. If you start to notice heartburn with the use of digestive enzymes, eliminate them from your program.

PART 7: STOMACH ACID (HIGH)		
1. Do you have chronic stomach pain?	Yes	No
2. Do you have stomach pain just before or after meals?	Yes	No
3. Do you have stomach pain when emotionally upset?	Yes	No
4. Does eating give you relief from stomach pain?	Yes	No
5. Do you need to use antacids regularly?	Yes	No
6. Do you have a history of taking chronic arthritis medication (NSAIDs, such as ibuprofen or aspirin)?	Yes	No
7. Are you currently taking medication to alter your stomach acid production?	Yes	No
PART 7 TOTAL: _____		

Plan of Action for Part 7

For scores 10 or higher, follow these suggestions:

1. Seek advice from a healthcare practitioner. If you have an ulcer, it is treatable.

2. Avoid foods that trigger the pain.

3. Follow the plan of action in Part 5 for rebuilding the integrity of the gut.

4. If necessary, include the additional remedies listed below for healing the lining of the stomach. There are a number of products available that combine several of the following nutrients:

   - L-glutamine: 1,500–5,000 mg a day.

- N-acetyl glucosamine*: 1,000–1,500 mg a day.
- Ginger* (5 percent gingerols extract): 250–500 mg a day.
- Mastic*: 500–1,000 mg twice a day between meals.
- *Saccharomyces boulardii**: 150–300 mg a day.

5. Reread Chapter 9 on the intestines, and also Chapter 11, paying special attention to the bowel terrain protocol recommended for intestinal support.

PART 8: SMALL/LARGE INTESTINAL FUNCTION		
1. Do have abdominal discomfort?	Yes	No
2. Do you have indigestion one to three hours after eating?	Yes	No
3. Do you have chronic gas?	Yes	No
4. Do you have chronic constipation or diarrhea, or both?	Yes	No
5. Do you have skin rashes or allergies?	Yes	No
6. Do you have any known food intolerances or allergies?	Yes	No
7. Do you have mucus in your stools?	Yes	No
8. Do you have dry skin?	Yes	No
9. Do you chronically have hard or difficult bowel movements?	Yes	No
	PART 8 TOTAL: _____	

Plan of Action for Part 8

A score of 10 or higher indicates that you need to work on your colon hygiene.

1. Follow the plan of action in Part 5.

2. Based on your score, add the following nutrients to your daily maintenance supplements to reestablish colon health:

- For scores 20 and higher, add:
  - Omega-3 fatty acids derived from fish oil: 1 teaspoonful or 4–6 1,000mg capsules daily. 2,000–4,000 mg a day.
- For scores 30 and higher, add:
  - Magnesium citrate or aspartate: at least 600 mg a day, if you are constipated and your score is 30 or higher. (Avoid using stimulant laxatives such as *cascara* or *senna* unless it is absolutely necessary.)

*Occasionally a supplement may be listed that has not been discussed in previous chapters. These supplements, as well as all the others listed, are readily available in natural food stores.

- Digestive enzyme, containing a full-range of enzymes. Take according to manufacturers instructions. If you do not notice a difference in your symptoms after eating a meal, the enzymes are ineffective and you should try another brand.
- Peppermint oil: one .2 milliliter (ml) of peppermint oil per capsule, up to three times a day. (Caution: peppermint oil should not be used if you have gastroesophageal reflux.)

PART 9: LOWERED IMMUNE FUNCTION						
1. Do you have chronic infections of the ears, nose, or throat?	0	1	2	3	4	5
2. Do you often get cold sores or fever blisters?	0	1	2	3	4	5
3. Do you catch colds and flu easily?	Yes					No
4. Do you get boils and sties?	0	1	2	3	4	5
5. Do you get chronic swelling of the lymph glands?	0	1	2	3	4	5
6. Do your wounds heal slowly?	0	1	2	3	4	5
7. Have you been diagnosed with chronic fatigue syndrome?	Yes					No
8. Have you been diagnosed with cancer?	Yes					No
9. Have you been diagnosed with HIV or hepatitis C?	Yes					No
10. Do you have rashes or skin allergies?	0	1	2	3	4	5

PART 9 TOTAL: _____

Plan of Action for Part 9

Optimizing your immune response is essential to any longevity program. There is a lot you can do to make your immune system more resilient to the stresses of daily living. Keeping your immune system in good "fighting" condition plays a significant role in helping to combat the effects of the environment, chronic stress, and inflammation on your chemistry.

1. Based on your score, add the following nutrients to your daily maintenance supplements to optimize immune system function:
   - For scores 15 and higher, add:
     - Moducare: three 20–40 mg capsules daily, on an empty stomach.
     - Evaluate your intake of vitamins A and C, and the mineral zinc. Make sure your intake of vitamin A and zinc is at least equal to, or slightly above, the RDA and that your intake of vitamin C is at least 1,000 mg a day.

- For scores 25 and higher, add:
  - Colostrum, to build immunoglobulins: 500–1,000 mg, two times a day.
  - Shiitake, maitake, or a blend of these and other mushrooms to stimulate immune function: 500 mg capsule, two to four times a day.
- For temporary use in overcoming colds or flu, take:
  - Echinacea: 500 mg, twice a day, *or*
  - Andrographis*: 250 mg, three times a day, *or*
  - Elderberry extract: 2 teaspoons, three times a day, *or*
  - Oscillococcinum (*Anas barbariae*), for flu only: as directed on the box.

PART 10: HYPER-IMMUNITY		
1. Do you have allergic symptoms, itching or discharge from eyes, puffiness under the eyes, and/or excessive mucus production?	Yes	No
2. Do you have nasal congestion or sneeze often?	Yes	No
3. Do you get migraine headaches?	Yes	No
4. Have you been diagnosed with an autoimmune disorder?	Yes	No
5. Do you have diabetes?	Yes	No
6. Do you have skin rashes or skin disorders?	Yes	No
7. Do you have multiple chemical sensitivity?	Yes	No
PART 10 TOTAL: _____		

Plan of Action for Part 10

With hyper-immunity, it is important to modulate the overactive immune system and balance inflammatory pathways. A score of 10 or greater can indicate hyper-immunity.

1. Add the following nutrients to your daily maintenance supplements to calm a hyperactive immune system:
   - Alpha lipoic acid: 300 mg, two times a day.
   - DHEA under supervision: up to 100 mg a day only according to healthcare practitioner's advice.
   - Moducare: three 20–40 mg capsules, two times a day between meals.
   - MSM: 2,000 mg, three times a day.
   - Omega-3 fish oils: six to eight 1,000 mg capsules

*Occasionally a supplement may be listed that has not been discussed in previous chapters. These supplements, as well as all the others listed, are readily available in natural food stores.

2. Administer a vitamin C flush (see page 254 for instructions).

3. Incorporate the suggested plan of action for adrenal support in Part 3.

4. Incorporate the suggested plan of action for liver support in Part 4. In addition, follow phase one of the Healthy Living Guidelines, one to two times a year for thirty days, to detoxify the liver.

5. Incorporate the suggested plan of action for intestinal support in Part 5.

6. Incorporate the suggested plan of action for support from environmental toxins in Part 11.

7. If you know that you are in a state of hyper-immunity or have an autoimmune condition, pay particular attention to the following keys and reread the appropriate chapters:
   - Key Three: Adrenals (Chapter 5)
   - Key Four: Liver (Chapter 8)
   - Key Five: Intestines (Chapter 9, focus specifically on dysbiosis)
   - Key Six: Environmental Toxins (Chapter 10, focus specifically on heavy metals)
   - Key Nine: Oxygen and Oxidative Stress (Chapter 15)

PART 11: ENVIRONMENTAL IMPACTS							
1. Do you live in an industrialized area?	Yes						No
2. Do you use pesticides, herbicides, or insecticides in your home or on your lawn?	0	1	2	3	4	5	
3. Do you have six or more amalgam (mercury, silver) fillings in your teeth?	Yes						No
4. Is your water supply chlorinated and fluorinated?	Yes						No
5. Do you drink unfiltered water?	Yes						No
6. Is the water used in your home unfiltered?	Yes						No
7. Do you work in a job that exposes you to various solvents or pollutants?	0	1	2	3	4	5	
8. Have you lived or worked in a new building over the last five years?	Yes						No
9. Do you eat produce without washing it?	0	1	2	3	4	5	
10. Do you eat lake fish or tuna more than once a month?	Yes						No
11. Do you drink from plastic containers regularly?	0	1	2	3	4	5	
12. Do you microwave in plastic containers or with plastic wrap on a regular basis?	Yes						No

13. Do you exercise outdoors in high traffic areas?	0	1	2	3	4	5	
14. Have you been diagnosed with ADHD or have difficulty with memory?	Yes					No	
15. Do you smoke?	Yes					No	
16. Do you use or have you used aluminum cookware?	Yes					No	
17. Do you use aluminum-containing deodorant?	Yes					No	
18. Do you eat canned foods frequently?	Yes					No	
19. Do you get a metallic taste in your mouth?	0	1	2	3	4	5	
20. Do you get your clothes dry-cleaned regularly?	Yes					No	
21. Have you been diagnosed with an autoimmune disorder such as lupus, rheumatoid arthritis, chronic fatigue syndrome, or fibromyalgia?	Yes					No	
22. Have you been diagnosed with cancer?	Yes					No	
23. Have you been diagnosed with Parkinson's disease or Alzheimer's disease?	Yes					No	

PART 11 TOTAL: _____

Plan of Action for Part 11

These are just a few of the most common ways we are exposed to chemicals on a daily basis. It makes sense that our bodies are affected by these potent byproducts of modern living. Don't take the impact that the environment has on your health lightly. Be proactive in protecting yourself. While there is no way to completely avoid environmental toxins, you can take significant steps toward limiting your exposures and strengthening your body's defense to industrial living. Realize that the more chemical burden that your body is challenged with, the more likely it will be that your metabolism will be sent down the path of disruption.

1. Perform phase one of the Healthy Living Guidelines, one to two times a year for thirty days, to detoxify the liver.

2. Toxins build up in the liver over time and periodically should be "cleaned" out. Add the following nutrients to your daily maintenance supplements to optimize your body's ability to detoxify and eliminate environmental pollutants:

   - For scores 30 and higher, take:
     - Chlorella: 3–5 grams a day, *or*
     - Cilantro seed: 400 mg, two to three times a day, *or*
     - Aged garlic: 300 mg, two to three times a day.
     - Alpha lipoic acid: 600 mg a day.

- N-acetyl cysteine: 1,200 mg a day.
- Milk thistle: 600 mg a day.
- For scores 50 and higher, add:
  - DMSA: 100 mg capsule at bedtime for ninety days, then repeat every three months for thirty days, or another alternative is to take 10 mg of DMSA per kilogram of body weight for three days, then stop for eleven days; and repeat.
  - Calcium EDTA: 1,000 mg, three times a day. If using a powder, take one-half to one teaspoon (2.5–5 grams), one or two times a day in water or juice. (Do not take mineral tablets at the same time as DMSA or EDTA; separate by twelve hours.)
  - Have your hair analyzed for heavy metals.
3. If more aggressive detoxification is needed, work under the supervision of a healthcare practitioner.

PART 12: INFLAMMATION AND OXIDATIVE STRESS (CARDIOVASCULAR HEALTH)							
1. Is your C-reactive protein elevated?	Yes						No
2. Do you have more than 20 pounds of excess weight that is distributed mainly around your belly?	Yes						No
3. Is your homocysteine level over 10?	Yes						No
4. Are your cholesterol and triglyceride levels elevated?	Yes						No
5. Are your fibrinogen levels elevated?	Yes						No
6. Are you a diabetic with elevated hemoglobin A_1C?	Yes						No
7. Does your heart pound easily?	0	1	2	3	4	5	
8. Does your heart miss a beat or skip?	0	1	2	3	4	5	
9. Do you get calf cramps when walking?	0	1	2	3	4	5	
10. Do you get swelling in your feet or ankles?	0	1	2	3	4	5	
11. Do you get exhausted with minor exertion?	0	1	2	3	4	5	
12. Do you feel heavy or achy in the legs?	0	1	2	3	4	5	
13. Do you get numbness in your arms or legs?	0	1	2	3	4	5	
14. Do you get vertigo?	0	1	2	3	4	5	
PART 12 TOTAL: _____							

Plan of Action for Part 12

Oxidative stress and inflammation are always present in heart disease. They damage cell membranes, build plaque in your arteries, and disrupt your chemistry. In addition to heart disease, oxidative stress and chronic inflammation have been linked to Alzheimer's disease, diabetes, obesity, and autoimmune disorders. If your goal is to live long and healthy, then you have to be aggressive in the prevention of cardiovascular disease.

If you answered yes to any of the questions in Part 12 and are not currently under a doctor's care, seek medical attention immediately. The nutrition protocols given below are intended to be an adjunct to proper medical care.

1. For scores 10 or greater, increase your daily maintenance intake of omega-3 fish oil to 4,000–8,000 mg a day to reduce oxidative stress and inflammation. In addition:

- For high C-reactive protein, increase:
  - Vitamin E in your daily maintenance intake to 1,200 IU
- For high cholesterol and/or triglycerides, add:
  - Policosanol: 20–30 mg a day, *or*
  - Red yeast rice*: 1,200 mg, two times a day.
  - Chromium GTF : 400–600 mcg a day.
- For high fibrinogen levels, add:
  - Nattokinase*: 800–1,600 fibrinolytic units (FU), two to three times a day.
- For heart arrhythmias (yes to questions 7 and/or 8) or poor circulation (yes to questions 13 and/or 14), add:
  - Hawthorn: 750 mg, a day of a standardized extract.
  - Increase magnesium to 900 mg a day; cut back to 600 mg a day if stools become loose.
- For heart failure (yes to questions 9, 10, 11, and/or 12) or for protection from heart failure, add:
  - CoQ_{10}: 100–300 mg a day.
  - L-carnitine fumarate or malate*: 500 mg, three times a day.
  - Hawthorne: 750 mg a day of a standardized extract.
  - Taurine: 500 mg, two times a day.
- For high blood pressure, add:
  - Arginine: 6–10 grams a day.
  - Hawthorne: 750 mg a day.
  - Magnesium: 600 mg a day.
- For high blood pressure due to stress, add:
  - Relora®: 250 mg, three times a day, *or*
  - Holy basil: one to two 400-mg capsules, two times a day.
- For high homocysteine levels, add:
  - Vitamin B_6: 50–100 mg a day.

---

*Occasionally a supplement may be listed that has not been discussed in previous chapters. These supplements, as well as all the others listed, are readily available in natural food stores.

- Vitamin B$_{12}$: 500 mcg a day.
- Folic acid or 5-MTHF: 800 mcg–1.6 mg a day.

2. Evaluate your heavy metal exposure with hair analysis or a urine heavy metal test.

3. Incorporate the suggested the plan of action for pancreas support in Part 1.

4. Incorporate the suggested the plan of action for adrenal support in Part 3.

5. Lose that belly fat by following the Healthy Living Guidelines in Chapter 13.

6. Exercise, in moderation, but consistently.

7. If you have been diagnosed with heart disease or have a family history of heart disease, reread Chapter 15 on oxygen, free-radical load, and antioxidant use, and pay particular attention to the following keys and reread the appropriate chapters:

- Key One: Pancreas (Chapter 3)
- Key Three: Adrenals (Chapter 5)
- Key Six: Environment Toxins (Chapter 10)

YOUR SCORE

Add up the totals of all parts to get your grand total. If you have a number of chronic health problems indicated by a grand total of 200 or more, you should see a health-care practitioner to help you design your own therapeutic program.

GRAND TOTAL: _____

GETTING THE MOST OUT OF LIFE

Now that you have read the information in all the chapters and have completed the questionnaire, you are now well equipped with an understanding of how your body works as an integrated whole and where the weak spots are in your metabolic chemistry. This information will assist you in mapping your journey back to optimal health. In some cases, combining this information along with the lab tests specified in each chapter will be necessary for a more complete picture of what may be influencing your health.

Look at your scores for each part of the questionnaire. Focus first on those areas where your scores are moderate to high. If more than one area requires attention, try to address them simultaneously. Many times, the areas that had lower scores will resolve themselves after working on the areas with higher scores.

Below is a general list of what works for most of the people who come into my practice who want to feel better, and it should work for you too:

1. Implement the Healthy Living Guidelines.

2. At minimum, take the daily maintenance supplements.

3. Exercise, exercise, exercise.

4. Start by working on the gut, adrenals, and pancreas, and evaluate your need for nutritional thyroid support. Many times, this will quickly improve your digestion, your energy, and your outlook. As your energy and outlook improve, it can empower you to undertake the rest of your needed lifestyle improvements.

5. For sustained health, address the environment and your body's detoxification process. This helps to eliminate toxins from tissues through the liver, kidney, lymph, and the skin. Detoxification is an ongoing process that you should regularly include in your life.

6. Work continuously on gut health and try to identify foods to which you are sensitive.

7. Work continuously to manage the effects of stress.

8. Take additional antioxidants as needed.

Once you understand the changes that need to be made and you have your plan, the next step is just doing it—making those needed changes one by one and dedicating yourself to regaining control of your health. Many times, it takes a feeling of desperation for people to make a change. My hope is that the information in this book will inspire you to act before you reach a health crisis.

Before ending, I would like share with you Kimberly's story of her progression to health. She had the typical set of health complaints that I see over and over again in my practice and which I have addressed throughout this book—adrenal exhaustion, abdominal weight gain, depression, and extreme tiredness—and yet she had no medically diagnosable problem except for high cholesterol. (For those of you with conditions that may have been referred to only briefly in this book, check Appendix 4 "Supplement Protocols for Other Common Conditions" on page 518 for a listing of treatment protocols for other prevalent disorders.)

So, if your healthcare practitioner can't find anything wrong with you from a blood test, nothing must be wrong. Right? Wrong. If you are like Kimberly, you are one of those unfortunate people who can feel that they are falling through the cracks of the medical system. In other words, your metabolism is off balance enough that you know something is wrong, but you can't be diagnosed or helped yet medically. You are the perfect candidate for nutritional help. For Kimberly, regaining control of her health and her metabolic code became a priority in her life. As you now know, there is hope—if you are willing to change some of your lifestyle habits and to support yourself nutritionally.

Kimberly's Story

Forty, fat, and fatigued, with a daily lack of mental clarity and a serious bout of depression is how I felt the day I entered Dr. Jim LaValle's office in September 2001. In fact, that pretty much surmised my physical condition for the four years prior to my visit. Two years later, I can thankfully say my whole life has changed! Today, I am forty-two and a fit size four. My energy level is through the roof and equally matched by my new attitude and fabulous outlook on life. Honestly, I have never looked or felt better! Implementing Dr. LaValle's guidelines for cracking my metabolic code has been absolutely pivotal in changing the direction of my health. As a result of following Dr. LaValle's guidelines, I have been able to achieve positive results and make dynamic changes in my life. My name is Kimberly and this is my story.

Prior to meeting Dr. LaValle, my physical and emotional health was on a slow but steady decline. Because I was a registered nurse, trained to recognize signs of illness, I realized the significance of my suboptimal health and was highly concerned. Undoubtedly, several traumatic events in the past several years had wreaked havoc on my physical and emotional state. Beginning in 1996, I went through a protracted and contentious divorce. As a result of the divorce, I had to transition from being a full-time mother to a working mother in the highly competitive profession of pharmaceutical sales. Additionally, I changed residence and learned to single parent my two wonderful sons, now aged eleven and thirteen. In retrospect, I had experienced three of the top five most stressful life situations in one year. It was no small wonder I was on a pathway of suboptimal health!

In 1996, I was gaining weight, despite my best efforts to exercise and limit calories. Increasingly, I experienced severe fatigue, muscle aches, significant constipation, numbness and tingling in my limbs, headaches, dizziness on standing, difficulty rising in the morning, heart palpitations, hair loss, and poor sleep habits. In addition, my legs felt heavy and achy, I had restless legs at night, and my ears were ringing. I also felt tired after eating and had big time cravings for sugar and carbohydrates.

Most puzzling of all was the concentrated weight gain in my abdominal area. I rapidly moved out of a size eight into size ten. Whether I slept six or twelve hours a night, I was always exhausted when I awoke.

I knew something was terribly wrong and went to multiple internal medicine physicians seeking help. I underwent a battery of medical tests, including several for multiple sclerosis (MS) and lupus, all with normal results. What was most frustrating throughout this process was the fact that my symptoms were disregarded as "hysteria" by the physicians. I was made to believe my physical symptoms weren't real or I was imagining them. Frankly, this added to my miserable state and confusion, because believe me, some days I *did* feel like I was losing my sanity!

By 2000, my weight gain continued and the severe fatigue and depression worsened. Finally, I was prescribed an antidepressant and told by a physician that it was normal for forty-year-old women to be overweight, fatigued, and depressed due to all the stressors I had experienced. Keep in mind, all those events occurred four years earlier. I just wasn't buying the fact that my future health was going to be dictated by past events. I was sick and tired of being sick and tired, as the old saying goes, and increasingly desperate for some concrete answers about my health crisis. Put simply, I wanted my life back.

Finally, a friend from work referred me to Dr. LaValle. I knew that he was a pharmacist as well as a naturopath, but I still had my doubts. Prior to my appointment, I filled out a 300-item lifestyle questionnaire for him to utilize during our initial consultation. During my first appointment, he explained to me that my chemistry was operating out of disharmony and that I may be heading toward multiple metabolic syndrome, also known as Syndrome X. Unknown to me at the time, this biochemical disturbance, in one way or another, affects more than 47 million people in the United States. Dr. LaValle reassured me that my symptoms were both genuine and that many, if not all, of my symptoms could be improved. He was confident I would respond to his therapy and feel the pleasures of life again. Just his reassurance that I was actually experiencing the physical symptoms and pinpointing the root cause for them was a tremendous relief, but it was the promise of getting my health back that was so exhilarating! I left the initial appointment with a recommended change in diet (temporary elimination of wheat, dairy, and simple carbohydrates), several bottles of supplements, and most important of all—hope.

Within two weeks, I was feeling more energetic, and for the first time in many years, I experienced a restful sleep. The dietary changes were a challenge, as I had unknowingly developed an unhealthy addiction to carbohydrates, but the supplements helped to curb my cravings for them. In the past, when the severe fatigue hit (taking naps in my car during lunchtime and being so exhausted I couldn't play outside with my sons), I would search for any carbohydrate to immediately boost my energy level. By resisting the urge to binge on carbohydrates, and by following Dr. LaValle's program religiously, I started seeing and feeling remarkable results.

By the first month, my muscle aches were subsiding, and the constipation and abdominal bloating were minimal. Best of all, the relentless depression I had lived with for so long began to disperse. It seemed so incredible to reexperience the elusive emotion of happiness, however sporadic. I began to exercise two or three days a week, walking thirty minutes a day, even on the days I still had fatigue. I continued to force myself to follow through on the recommendations from Dr. LaValle, reminding myself I would have excellent results.

I incorporated Dr. LaValle's recommendations permanently into my lifestyle. An example of my daily routine included drinking lots of purified water and always having a source of protein with me. Supplements too—lots of vitamins and minerals—are a part of my regimen. I have learned to avoid simple carbohydrates such as cookies, pasta, soda, and candy. The low level of energy and gastrointestinal problems that resulted from any carbohydrate binge was a painful reminder of the punishing effect that these foods had on my body.

By the second and third month of following Dr. LaValle's metabolic program, I continued to drop pounds and inches, especially in the troublesome abdominal area. My self-esteem and positive body image were returning! The depression I had been experiencing had evaporated and I truly had a new and positive outlook on life. My mental clarity at work was improving and I was once again finding my outgoing sales personality. It's amazing how the state of your emotions is so directly connected to your health!

As my physical health improved, Dr. LaValle changed my program with my improving metabolic needs. I never doubted his recommendations or suggestions on continuing to reach for my optimal health. After six months, I was in a size six and felt better than I had in years. Most of my dehabilitating symptoms were gone. I had the energy and mental acuity to increase my activity on all levels. I joined a gym and began working out four to five times a week, in addition to lifting weights and taking an occasional Pilates class. Moreover, I was waking up before the alarm clock rang and was excelling in my job performance—I even got a coveted promotion in my sales position. Best of all, I was able to enjoy quality time with my sons. I found myself initiating games of basketball with the boys, instead of sitting on the porch due to fatigue and lack of energy. My body was again finding the proper and normal way of functioning and it reflected in my attitude and activity. Interestingly, I continued to have the same stressors in my life, but my body was now responding in a healthier way. I was able to meet all of life's challenges successfully, something I couldn't have imagined just a few short months earlier.

I recall reviewing all my initial symptoms with Dr. LaValle—thinning hair and eyebrows, sadness, depression, weight gain, water retention, constipation, fatigue, muscle aches, lack of mental concentration (I actually once tried to put the blender carafe into the coffeemaker and was dazed and confused as to why it wouldn't fit), and lack of sexual desire. As I reflect on these symptoms, it truly is amazing that a subclinically functioning thyroid, burned out adrenal glands, and insulin resistance can create such havoc in one's body. More amazing still was the fact I had to endure the dehabilitating effects of an "out-of-sync" metabolism (in Dr. LaValle's terms) for four long years. How many of you readers have walked this same path? I am so thankful for the opportunity to regain my health that Dr. LaValle offered me. I truly have my life back and look forward to longevity and many years of happiness and success.

Today, because I realize there are many factors that can contribute to a dysfunctional metabolism, I have trained myself to always be aware of my changing metabolic needs. I still occasionally have challenges with slight fatigue and weight gain. A few months ago, I noticed some of the old symptoms trying to creep back and I immediately went to see Dr. LaValle. By slightly increasing my nutritional thyroid supplement, I was able to overcome the fatigue and dropped the last few layers of fat and weight. I am a fit size four and will not hesitate to enjoy sunning in a bathing suit this season. I promise you though, that would never have entered my mind less than two years ago.

Because of my ordeal with multiple metabolic syndrome and the subsequent successful treatment with Dr. LaValle's program for "cracking your metabolic code," I feel an obligation to share my story, in hopes that it might help others who are struggling with the same issues that I was. I have been fortunate to share my success with others through newspaper and magazine interviews. If you are one of the 47 million people in our country who are suffering from multiple metabolic syndrome, please know that there is help and hope for you. Dr. LaValle's guidelines for cracking your metabolic code can change your life! It is easy to follow, gets dramatic results, and most important, will help you reclaim your health and happiness.

In the past two years, I have received many compliments on my positive attitude and physical appearance. Truly, at age forty-two, I have never felt or looked better! I want to share with you one of the best compliments I received recently. It was from one of my physician customers who said, "Kim, I am not sure what you are doing, but you keep looking younger and younger . . . and you always have your 'happy light' on now!" Well put, doctor, I couldn't have said it better myself, but then, what more could I ask for?

What little I have left to say now is by way of benediction. I can only supply you with my experience and give you the facts as I know them. I can, with these written words, hopefully give you hope and a bit of motivation. But only you can take charge of your health. Only you can use these nine keys in order to actually attain optimal health.

While optimal health is something different for each of us, something determined by the quality of your health, your lifestyle, as well as you age, your weight, your gender, and a number of other issues, each of us does have a level of health that can be termed "optimal."

But what does that mean? Well, for me, in large part, health has to do with freedom. When I see my patients getting healthier, I see them living freer lives. No longer are they prisoners in their own bodies. Instead, they are more free to live their lives unencumbered by the common health complaints or more serious health problems that send us into the downward spiral of health.

Try to think of this book as the synthesis of twenty years of knowledge gained that has helped many of my patients achieve a more vibrant health and better quality of life. Now this knowledge is put into your hands with a prayer that it helps you to be healthier, more whole, and free. If this book helps you resolve even one health complaint that has affected the quality of your life, then it has been a success.

Endnotes

Glossary

ablate. to remove especially by cutting, abrading, or evaporating.

acetylcholine. a neurotransmitter that regulates nerve impulse transmission between nerve cells and between nerve and muscle cells.

acupuncture. insertion of needles into living tissues for health and remedy purposes.

acute. severe, but limited in duration.

adaptogen. a substance that helps the body adapt to various physical, chemical, and emotional stressors.

adenosine triphosphate (ATP). chemical compound used by cells to fuel metabolism.

adipose. fat or tissue containing fat cells.

adrenaline. a hormone produced by the brain in response to low blood glucose, exercise, and stress.

adrenocorticotropic hormone. a substance that stimulates the growth of the adrenal cortex and/or secretion of its hormones, including DHEA and cortisol.

aerobic. growing or living in the presence of oxygen.

alpha cells. cells that secrete glucagon, a hormone that increases blood sugar levels.

alveoli. small sacs in the lungs in which oxygen and carbon dioxide are exchanged.

Alzheimer's disease. a progressive, neurodegenerative disease characterized by a loss of function and death of nerve cells in several areas of the brain leading to a loss of cognitive functions such as memory and language.

amalgam, dental. an alloy (a solution) of silver and mercury often used in dental fillings.

ameliorate. to make better; improve.

amino acid. key components in all living things from which proteins are synthesized.

anabolism. a phase of metabolism in which new molecules are synthesized.

anaerobic. growing or living in the absence of oxygen.

analgesic. a pain-relieving substance.

androgen. male hormone.

anemia. a condition in which there are too few red blood cells in the bloodstream, resulting in insufficient oxygen to tissues and organs.

angiotensin. a hormone that causes the blood vessels to constrict, which increases blood pressure.

anion. a negatively charged atomic particle, such as an atom or group of atoms.

antacid. a substance that neutralizes acid in the stomach, esophagus, or the duodenum, the first part of the intestines.

antibody. a protein molecule that reacts with an antigen (foreign substance) in the body; part of the immune system.

antidiuretic hormone. a hormone made by the hypothalamus and released by the pituitary gland; keeps fluid in the body.

antifungal. an agent that destroys fungal infections by inhibiting either their reproduction or their growth.

antigen. a substance capable of inducing a specific immune response in the body and reacting with an antibody. Antigens may be toxins, foreign proteins, or particulates such as bacteria and tissue cells.

antioxidant. a substance found in the body and in plant food that stops the formation of free radicals or oxidation in the body.

antiprotease. a substance that inhibits protein-dissolving enzymes.

apoptosis. a process that takes place in normal cells in which they are programmed to die when they have fulfilled their task.

arachidonic acid. an essential dietary component in mammals and a free acid in the body with a host of biochemical properties; usually a precursor to inflammation.

arteriosclerosis. hardening or thickening of the arteries.

astrocyte. a star-shaped brain cell that supports nerve cells.

asymptomatic. presenting no symptoms of disease.

atherosclerosis. an arteriosclerosis characterized by the buildup of blood fats on the damaged lining of artery walls, leading to plaques that block blood flow.

atopic. of, relating to, or caused by a hereditary predisposition toward developing certain hypersensitivity reactions, such as hay fever, asthma, or chronic urticaria, upon exposure to specific antigens.

autoantibody. an antibody that reacts with an antigen that is a normal component of the body. This reaction can lead to autoimmune disorders (as below) such as lupus and rheumatoid arthritis.

autoimmune disorder. a condition in which the immune system attacks the body's own tissues and interferes with normal functioning—for example, rheumatoid arthritis or lupus.

autonomic nervous system. the part of the nervous system that governs involuntary actions such as digestion and peristalsis.

basal metabolic rate. energy required for internal or cellular work (metabolism) when the body is at rest; heat is the measure of metabolic rate.

beta cells. cells in the pancreas responsible for synthesizing and regulating insulin.

bile. a yellow-green fluid consisting of bile salts, cholesterol, water, bilirubin, and acidic compounds that is released by the liver into the intestines for the digestion of fats.

bilirubin. a yellow-brown waste product that results from the breakdown of old red blood cells.

bioequivalent. having the same strength and similar availability for the body as a similar substance being used for the same purpose; usually refers to pharmaceutical drugs.

blood sugar. a form of sugar known as glucose that is present in the blood and serves as the body's primary source of fuel.

blood-brain barrier. a series of semipermeable partitions monitoring and separating the body and its supply of substances and nutrients from the brain.

B lymphocytes. also known as B cells, white blood cells that are manufactured by, and mature in, the bone marrow, which produce antibodies to protect the body from future viruses, bacteria, yeast, and other organisms.

body mass index. ratio of muscle to fat body mass.

bronchial. pertaining to the large air passages in the lungs.

Burkitt's lymphoma. a form of non-Hodgkin's lymphoma.

calcitonin. a hormone produced by cells in the thyroid that causes a reduction in blood calcium levels.

candidiasis. a fungal infection, or bowel terrain disturbance, caused by the yeast *Candida albicans* or related organisms.

carbon monoxide. a colorless, odorless gas that when inhaled in sufficient quantities enters the bloodstream and combines with the hemoglobin in red blood cells, crowding out needed oxygen.

carcinogenic. cancer-producing.

catabolism. a destructive phase of metabolism in which substances are broken down into their component parts.

catalyst. a substance that accelerates a chemical reaction but is not consumed or changed in the process.

catalyze. speeding up a reaction.

cation. a positively charged atomic particle.

cecum. a pouchlike area of the colon in the right lower quadrant of the abdomen at the end of the small intestine; the appendix extends off the end of the cecum.

cell. a tiny but complex organic unit consisting of a nucleus, cytoplasm, and a cell membrane. All living tissues are composed of cells.

cellular metabolism. the mechanism by which food energy is converted to ATP, the chemical compound used by the cells to fuel metabolism.

chelate. to combine with a metal to form a complex that can either be used by the body or be excreted.

chelating agent. a substance that is capable of displacing a metal bond.

chelation therapy. intravenous infusion of a proteinlike agent that binds with metals in the body, making them soluble in blood and able to be excreted.

chemotactic factors. inflammatory mediators that dilate capillaries and mobilize white blood cells (neutrophils and macrophages) to the areas of damage, stimulating them to engulf and digest damaged tissue and foreign agents.

chemotherapeutic. relating to chemotherapy, chemical agents used to treat cancer.

cholecystokinin (CCK). a hormone released by the gallbladder that signals the brain that a person has eaten enough.

cholesterol. a pearly, fatlike chemical synthesized in the liver, which can also be absorbed from the diet.

cholinesterase. an enzyme needed for the proper functioning of the neurotransmitter acetylcholine.

chronic fatigue syndrome. a complex syndrome that often includes muscle and/or joint pain, headaches, poor sleep, poor memory, and a sore throat.

chronic. persisting over an extended period; when referring to a disease, it may be benign or serious.

chylomicrons. specialized fat globules found in blood or lymph used to transport fat from the intestine to the liver or fat tissue.

chyme. partially digested food that has been acted upon by stomach juices but has not yet been passed on into the intestines.

cofactor. an inorganic player in an enzyme reaction, usually a metal ion, that helps another substance to perform its functions.

cognitive. pertaining to the mental process of knowing, thinking, learning, and judging.

conjugation. joining together of two compounds to produce another compound, such as the combination of a toxic product with some substance in the body to form a detoxified product, which is then eliminated.

corticosteroids. natural hormones produced by the adrenal gland, as well as a group of pharmaceutical drugs that act similarly to the natural hormones to suppress inflammation.

cortisol. a hormone produced by the adrenal glands in response to stress.

Crohn's disease. an inflammatory disease of the digestive tract that seems to have both genetic and environmental causes and is not well understood. Common symptoms include recurrent abdominal pains, fever, nausea, vomiting, weight loss, and diarrhea.

cyclic adenosine monophosphate (cAMP). a messenger chemical that activates other chemicals inside the cells to produce the target cell action.

cyclooxygenase. an enzyme that is necessary for the formation of prostaglandins.

cyst. a closed cavity or sac, normal or abnormal, that is lined by epithelial tissue and may contain liquid or semisolid material.

cytochrome P-450. an enzyme that is the key component responsible for the transformation of foreign compounds in the body to either usable substances or substances to be excreted.

cytokine. small proteins or biological factors, which are destructive cell-signaling chemicals, that are released by cells and have specific effects on cell-to-cell interaction, communication, and behavior. Cytokines contribute to many degenerative diseases.

cytotoxins. chemicals that are directly toxic to cells, preventing their reproduction or growth.

deaminate. the process of metabolism whereby the nitrogen portion of amino acids is removed.

dehydroepiandrosterone (DHEA). a hormone that is produced chiefly by the adrenal glands, and is an important base from which other substances such as testosterone and progesterone are derived.

delta cells. cells that secrete somatostatin, a hormone that inhibits gastric acid release.

dental caries. erosion and decay of the tooth caused by the effects of bacteria in the mouth.

dermatitis herpetiformis. a chronic skin disease characterized by severe itching and extensive eruption of blisters that occur in groups; it may be associated with a malignancy in the elderly patient.

detoxification. the process of removing and metabolizing unwanted chemical compounds that can disrupt normal bodily functions so that normal function is restored to the organs or systems being affected.

diverticulitis. inflammation of diverticula.

diverticulum. a small saclike structure that sometimes forms in the walls of the intestines; it can trap particles of food and become very inflamed and painful.

down regulation. decreased production.

duodenum. the first portion of the small intestine.

dysbiosis. imbalance in the natural flora of the gastrointestinal tract, leading to an overgrowth of yeast (*Candida*) or other disruptive microbes.

dyspepsia. impairment of digestion usually applied to the upper central region of the abdomen (epigastric area).

ecology. the scientific study of the relationship of organisms to each other and to their environment.

ecosystem. the physical and climactic features and all the living and dead organisms in an area that are interrelated in the transfer of energy and material.

eicosanoid. generic term for compounds derived from arachidonic acid, including leukotrienes, prostacyclin, prostaglandins, and thromboxanes.

electrodermal. pertaining to electric properties (acupuncture meridians) of the skin, usually referring to altered resistance; electrodermal screening is a prediagnostic method for health problems used by clinicians.

electrolyte. substances that separate into charged ions when dissolved in water.

endocrine. pertaining to internal hormonal secretions.

endogenous. developing or originating within the organism or arising from causes within the organism.

endometriosis. a condition in which tissue more or less perfectly resembling the uterine mucosal membrane (the endometrium) and containing typical cells of the endometrium occurs aberrantly in various locations in the pelvic cavity.

endotoxins. metabolic byproducts that are disruptive to the body's metabolism; internal toxins that are actually produced by the body as a result of normal biochemical processes.

enzyme. a protein molecule produced by living organisms that speeds up a chemical reaction of other substances without itself being destroyed or altered upon completion of the reaction(s).

epithelial. pertaining to the covering of internal and external surfaces of the body, including the lining of the blood vessels and other small cavities.

erythematosus. reddening of the skin produced by congestion of the capillaries.

erythropoietin. a hormone released by the kidneys in response to a deficiency of oxygen in the blood such as in anemia. Erythropoietin increases the production of red blood cells in an attempt to increase the oxygen-carrying capacity of the blood.

etiology. cause or origin of disease, in medical science.

ex vivo. a biological process that takes place outside a living cell.

exotoxins. toxins that enter the body from without; products of the external environment.

extracellular. occurring outside the cell.

exudates. material such as fluid, cells, or cellular debris that has escaped from blood vessels and has been deposited in tissues or on tissue surfaces, usually as a result of inflammation.

fasting blood glucose levels. glucose levels obtained after no calories are consumed for at least eight hours prior to the drawing of blood.

fat-soluble. susceptible to being dissolved in fat.

fibromyalgia. a disorder characterized by muscle pain, stiffness, and easy fatigability that has no obvious physical cause.

follicle-stimulating hormone. a hormone secreted by the anterior pituitary gland; in women, it stimulates the development of ovarian eggs and the release of estrogen; in men, it stimulates the production of sperm.

free radicals. chemically active atom or molecular fragment, containing a negative charge from a deficient or excess electron, resulting in a negative charge; free radicals attack healthy cells in the body in the hopes of finding another electron to stabilize themselves. This process can cause damage to healthy cells.

fungicide. a chemical agent that destroys fungus.

gene. a unit of DNA, the biochemical information that carries the complete instructions for making all the proteins in a cell. Each gene contains specific instructions for making a cell.

genetic. inherited.

glomeruli. a network of tiny blood vessels in the kidneys where the blood is filtered and waste products are removed.

glomerulonephritis. a condition caused by inflammation of the glomeruli.

glucagon. a hormone secreted by cells in the pancreas in response to low blood sugar levels. It serves to increase blood glucose concentrations; it has the opposite effect of insulin, and also regulates the conversion of amino acids to glucose.

gluconeogenesis. the synthesis of glucose from non-carbohydrate sources, such as amino acids, which takes place largely in the liver and serves to maintain blood glucose levels under conditions of starvation or intense exercise.

gluten. a protein found in many grains, including wheat, rye, barley, and oats.

glycation. the uncontrolled non-enzymatic reaction of sugars with proteins; chemical glycation is important in the cellular damage related to diabetics when their sugar levels rise above normal and in damage done to critical proteins of long-lived nerve cells in aging.

glycemic. pertaining to sugar value.

glycemix index. glycemic index of a food measures the rate at which a carbohydrate breaks down into glucose in the bloodstream.

glycogen. the main form in which glucose is stored in the body, primarily in the liver and muscles. Glycogen synthesis causes a decrease in blood glucose.

glycogenolysis. the breaking down process of glycogen into sugar molecules of glucose and of glucose-1-phosphate within the body by enzymes; the enzymes are controlled by nerve impulses and hormones.

goblet cell. cell of the epithelial lining of the small intestine that secretes mucus.

hemodialysis. removal of certain elements (usually toxins) from the blood by a machine or filter; used in individuals with kidney disease.

hemoglobin. the oxygen-carrying components of red blood cells. There are about 200 hemoglobin molecules in each red blood cell. The hemoglobin molecule consists of *heme,* an iron portion, and *globin,* a protein.

hepatic. pertaining to the liver.

hepatocytes. important epithelial cells in the liver, active in the detoxification of drugs, heavy metals, chemicals, alcohol, and hormones.

herbicide. chemical used to kill or control the growth of plants.

high-density lipoprotein (HDL). form of cholesterol, the type that is called the "good" cholesterol, because it carries cholesterol from the bloodstream to the liver for elimination. Raised HDL levels have been correlated with a lower risk for cardiovascular disease.

hippurate. a metabolic byproduct of benzoic acid conjugation. Benzoic acid (benzoate) is a common food additive.

hirsutism. abnormal hairiness.

histamine. a chemical formed when the immune system is activated; causes symptoms of allergies such as the reddening of the skin along with red, itching and watery eyes.

homeostasis. state of balance in an organism.

hormone binding. a situation in which a hormone disrupter binds with a hormone, rendering it unable to carry out its hormonal message.

hormone masking. a situation in which chemicals bind with receptor sites and blocks the hormone's activity at the cellular level.

hormone mimicry. a situation in which a chemical mimics a hormone by binding with receptors and stimulating cellular activity. This mimicry tricks the body into thinking it has sufficient levels of certain hormones, which signals the hypothalamus to stop its hormone production.

hydration. the addition of water.

hydrochloric acid (HCL). a strong stomach acid necessary for the breakdown and digestion of many foods.

hydrogenation. a process used to make oil more solid, as is commonly done in the production of margarine.

hydrolysis. the process of breaking a compound into smaller fragments by the addition of water.

hyperglycemia. abnormally high levels of glucose in the blood, usually associated with diabetes.

hyperinsulinemia. too much insulin in the bloodstream.

hyperproliferation. an abnormally high rate of cell division, occurring in tumors and cancers, for example.

hypersensitivity. a state of altered reactivity in which the body reacts with an exaggerated immune response to a foreign substance.

hyperthyroidism. excessive function of the thyroid gland marked by an increased metabolic rate, enlargement of the thyroid gland, rapid heart rate, and high blood pressure, among other symptoms.

hypoglycemia. low blood sugar levels.

hypothyroidism. deficiency of the thyroid gland most commonly found in women and characterized by a decreased basal metabolic rate, tiredness and lethargy, sensitivity to cold, and menstrual disturbances.

hypovolemic. a condition in which there is abnormally low levels of blood plasma in the body, such that the body is unable to properly maintain blood pressure, cardiac output of blood, and normal amounts of fluid in the tissues.

idiopathic. arising from an unknown cause.

ileum. the last portion of the small intestine that communicates with the large intestine.

immunosuppressant. anything that suppresses the immune system, such as a drug or chemical pesticide.

immunotoxic. toxic to the immune system.

inflammation. an immune reaction to illness or injury characterized by swelling, warmth, and redness.

inorganic. not of organic origin.

insulin. a hormone produced by the pancreas that regulates the metabolism of glucose (sugar) in the body.

interleukin. a variety of naturally occurring polypeptide proteins that are members of the family of cytokines, which affect functions of specific cell types and are found in small quantities. They are produced by lymphocytes, monocytes, and various other cell types of the immune system and are released by cells in response to antigenic and non-antigenic stimuli. Interleukins help in the modulation of inflammation.

intracellular. occurring inside the cell.

intradermal. in the skin.

intrauterine. in the uterus.

ion. an atom or molecule that has lost or gained an electron, and thus acquired an electrical charge, such as hydrogen in the water molecule.

irritable bowel syndrome (IBS). a condition characterized by recurrent crampy abdominal pain and diarrhea, or alternating constipation and diarrhea.

irritant. any substance that causes inflammation following immediate, prolonged, or repeated contact with skin or mucous membrane.

isoflavone. a type of plant estrogen that occurs abundantly in soy.

isoprostanes. inflammatory mediators formed when arachidonic acid, a naturally occurring fatty acid, is oxidized by free radicals.

jejunum. a portion of the small intestine that extends from the duodenum to the ileum.

ketoacidosis. acidosis accompanied by the accumulation of ketone bodies in the tissues and fluids, as in diabetic ketoacidosis.

ketogenic. giving rise to ketone bodies in metabolism.

ketogenic diets. diets that recommend starving the body of carbohydrates, which forces the body to convert fat stores to glucose, thereby stepping up the metabolism of body fat.

ketone. waste products of partially burned (or metabolized) fat.

Kupffer cells. large star-shaped or pyramidal cells found in the liver.

lactose intolerance. an inability to digest milk proteins.

leaky gut syndrome. a condition in which minute particles of undigested or partially digested protein pass through the intestinal wall into the bloodstream, causing allergic reactions and other systemic symptoms due to inflammation.

lectin. a protein obtained particularly from the seeds of leguminous plants but also from many other plant and animal sources that has binding sites for specific cells and which agglutinates, or glues together, human red blood cells or particular blood groups.

lethargy. abnormal drowsiness or stupor; a condition of indifference.

lipid peroxidation. damaging oxidation by free radicals on fatty substances in the body.

lipids. term for the family of fats that includes triglycerides, cholesterol, and phospholipids.

lipogenesis. the formation of lipids.

lipophilic. having an affinity for lipids (fats).

low-density lipoprotein (LDL). form of cholesterol, the type that is called the "bad" cholesterol, because it acts as a carrier for cholesterol in the blood but is easily oxidized, or damaged, by free radicals. High levels of LDL are considered a positive risk factor for the development of coronary artery disease.

lupus. a systemic disease that results from an autoimmune mechanism. Individuals with lupus produce antibodies to their own body tissues, resulting in inflammation that can cause kidney damage and arthritis among other problems.

lymph. the almost colorless fluid that bathes body tissues and is found in the lymphatic vessels that drain the tissues of the fluid across the blood vessel walls from blood.

lysosome. digestive substances found in each cell.

macronutrition. intake of carbohydrates, protein, and fat.

macrophages. immune system scavengers that engulf particles, bacteria, and viruses, and are also capable of detoxifying some chemicals.

malabsorption. impaired intestinal absorption of nutrients.

mast cell. a resident cell of connective tissue that contains primarily histamine and heparin (an anticoagulant). The release of histamine from mast cells is responsible for the immediate reddening of the skin.

metabolism. the physical and chemical processes necessary to sustain life, including the production of cellular energy, the synthesis of important biological substances, and degradation of various compounds.

metabolites. any substance produced by metabolism or by a metabolic process.

methylation. a process in which methyl groups conjugate circulating estrogens.

microflora. natural bacteria or fungi that inhabit an area; pertaining to the bacterial colonies that normally inhabit the gut, which help in nutrient absorption and proper digestion and usage of foods.

microgram (mcg). unit of mass (weight) of the metric system being one millionth of a gram or one thousandth of a milligram.

micronutrition. intake of vitamins and minerals.

microorganism. a microscopic organism.

microvascular. pertaining to a very small blood vessel.

milligram (mg). unit of measure equal to one thousandth of a gram.

mitochondria. a small cellular component that is responsible for energy production and cellular respiration.

mitochondrial. pertaining to mitochondria.

mitochondrial DNA. DNA within the mitochondria.

monocytes. one of three types of white blood cells, or cells, that are part of the immune system.

motility. exhibiting movement.

mucous membrane. lubricated inner lining of the mouth, nasal passages, vagina, and urethra that contains mucus-secreting glands.

mucus. slimy, ropy, or stringy and lubricous substance.

multiple chemical sensitivity syndrome (MCS). an acquired disorder characterized by recurrent symptoms occurring in response to exposure to many chemically unrelated compounds (such as milk, drugs, foods, pesticides, perfumes, and other chemicals) at doses far less than established in the general population to cause harmful effects.

mutagen. any substance that causes a genetic mutation.

myasthenia gravis. a disorder in which eye muscles weaken.

mycoplasma. a microorganism that is a causative agent in pneumonia and is resistant to many conventional antibiotics.

mycotoxin. metabolic byproduct (waste) produced by a fungus.

nasopharyngeal carcinoma. cancer of the nose and throat.

natural killer cells (NK). immune cells that destroy cancer and virus-infested cells.

negative feedback mechanism. the process by which the body turns off hormones after they've done their job.

nephrons. functional units of the kidney that contain tiny filters that are used in detoxification.

neurologic. pertaining to the nervous system.

neuropeptide Y. a chemical messenger that turns off the body's natural killer cell activity (part of a healthy immune system).

neuroprotective agent. a substance that is protective of the nervous system.

neurotoxic. toxic to the nervous system.

neurotransmitters. a group of substances known as "chemical messengers" that are released on excitation from a nerve that travel to excite or inhibit target cells throughout the body.

neutralize. to render neutral; not engaged on either side.

neutrophil. white blood cell of the immune system.

nucleic acid. complex molecular substances, such as DNA and RNA, that are found in every cell and that contain the cell's genetic code or are responsible for protein synthesis.

nutraceutical. a vitamin, mineral, herbal, or other natural substance with medicinal value.

opportunistic. being or caused by a microorganism that does not normally cause disease but under certain circumstances (for example, impaired immunity) becomes disease causing.

organochlorine pesticides. fat-soluble compounds that are well absorbed orally and topically that are known to cause endocrine disruption in birds, fish, and mammals, and also interfere with hormone regulation in humans.

oxidation. a biochemical reaction that inactivates or destroys chemicals by the transfer of oxygen and loss of electrons.

ozonation. act of treating with a specific form of oxygen.

parasite. an organism that lives on or in another organism from which it obtains food and shelter.

Parkinson's disease. a progressive neurological disorder characterized by a shuffled gait, stooped posture, tremors at rest, speech impediments, moving difficulties, and an eventual slowing of mental processes.

particulate. having the form of a tiny mass of material.

peristalsis. wormlike movement by which the digestive canal or other tubular organs propel their contents.

peritoneum. smooth membrane that lines the abdominal cavity.

peritonitis. inflammation of the peritoneum leading to abdominal pain, tenderness, constipation, vomiting, and moderate fever.

permeability. capable of being passed through or penetrated.

pH. symbol relating the hydrogen ion concentration or activity of a solution to that of a standard solution.

phagocytosis. uptake of material, such as microorganisms or cell fragments, into a cell.

pharmacology. medical science dealing with the discovery, chemistry, effects, uses, and manufacture of drugs.

phenolic compounds. phytochemical compounds found in fruits, vegetables, and other foods.

phosphatase. an enzyme needed for bone formation.

phospholipid. fat molecule.

photosensitivity. an abnormal skin reaction involving the interaction between substances that increase sensitivity to sunlight or artificial light. Some drugs and herbs, such as St. John's wort and griseofulvin, can cause this sensitivity.

phytochemicals. biologically active substances in plants such as flavonoids and carotenoids that protect the body against illness. They are the naturally occurring substances from which many pharmaceutical drugs are derived.

pigment. any one of the colored substances found in animal and vegetable tissues and fluids.

polycystic. having or involving many cysts.

polyphenols. potent antioxidants found abundantly in green tea, which prevent free radicals from damaging healthy cells.

polysaccharide. many simple sugars joined together to form a new molecule.

polysymptomatic. having many symptoms.

portal vein. the large vein that carries blood from the stomach and intestines to the liver.

predisposition. susceptibility to disease that may be activated by certain conditions such as stress.

probiotic. a substance that promotes the growth of friendly microorganisms normally present in the digestive tract.

prolactin. a pituitary hormone that causes lactation.

proliferation. reproduction or multiplication of cells or cysts.

prophylactic. guarding from or preventing a disease, such as with the use of a drug.

prostatitis. a condition characterized by inflammation of the prostate.

proteases. inflammatory enzymes that are released when particles are inhaled.

proteolytic. the act of cleaving proteins by enzymes.

psychosis. mental disorder characterized by a gross impairment in reality testing as evidenced by delusions, hallucinations, markedly incoherent speech, or disorganized and agitated behavior.

reactive intermediate metabolite. a compound that has not been processed completely during phase-one detoxification in the liver. These metabolites are more dangerous than the original compound.

rehydration. to hydrate; the addition of water.

renin. an enzyme secreted by the kidneys that helps regulate blood pressure. Renin calls on plasma proteins to release a substance called angiotensin that causes the blood vessels to constrict, which increases blood pressure.

retroviruses. a large group of viruses that contain RNA and the enzyme *reverse transcriptase*. Reverse transcriptase transforms viral RNA to DNA in the process of replication, which is the reverse of the normal transcription from DNA to RNA.

rheumatoid arthritis. chronic inflammatory disease in which there is destruction of the joints; considered to be an autoimmune disorder.

rodenticide. a chemical that kills rodents such as rats and mice.

salicylate. a group of chemical substances with anti-inflammatory properties, including aspirin and magnesium salicylate.

scleroderma. an autoimmune disorder characterized by hardening of the skin.

secretagogue. a substance that stimulates a gland to secrete a particular hormone.

secretory. to secrete or release specialized fluids from body parts such as glands.

septicemia. a systemic problem associated with the presence and persistence of disease-causing bacteria and their toxins in the blood.

serotonin. a neurotransmitter found primarily in the brain that is considered essential for relaxation, sleep, concentration, and satiety.

singlet oxygen radical. an energized but uncharged form of oxygen that is produced in the metabolic bursts of leucocytes (white blood cells of the immune system) that can be toxic to cells.

slow detoxifier. a person who has a compromised detoxification system that slows phase-one of the liver's detoxification process.

spasm. a sudden, violent involuntary contraction of a muscle or group of muscles; usually accompanied by pain and interference with function.

spasmodic. relating to or characterized by a spasm.

standardization. sufficient amount of an herb's primary active ingredients needed to be present in order for the herb to have a beneficial effect.

substrate. a substance on which an enzyme acts.

sulfation. the process by which sulfur molecules from cysteine conjugate substances like bacterial toxins from the gut and hormones.

syndrome X. also known as "multiple metabolic syndrome." Name given to a set of factors that includes elevated triglycerides, elevated cholesterol, elevated blood pressure, above ideal body weight, and elevated blood glucose or diabetes.

synovial. pertaining to or secreting a transparent, thick, lubricating fluid.

synovial fluid. lubricating material of the joint, which is almost all water, along with some protein-carbohydrate molecules.

synthesis. the building up of a chemical compound by the union of its elements or from other suitable materials.

T cells. immune-mediated cells, also called T lymphocytes, in the thymus gland that destroy cancer cells, viruses, and microorganisms like bacteria and fungi.

thermogenesis. the ability of the body to convert caloric energy to heat.

thromboembolism. obstruction of a blood vessel with material that actually clogs the vessel.

thyroid stimulating hormone. a polypeptide hormone secreted by the anterior pituitary gland that activates cyclic adenosine monophosphate (cAMP), a messenger chemical, production in thyroid cells, leading to the production and release of thyroid hormones.

thyroxine. hormone produced by the thyroid gland that increases metabolic rate and is used to treat thyroid disorders.

tinnitus. a condition characterized by ringing in the ears.

toxin. a substance that causes irritation, harm, or destruction in the body.

transdermal. entering through the skin, as in the administration of a drug applied to the skin in ointment or patch.

triglycerides. primary form of fat. They comprise the bulk of fat in foods, the storage of fat in the body, and the primary form of fat in the blood. Only triglycerides provide calories or energy to the body. Elevated triglyceride levels are associated with the development of hardening of the arteries eventually leading to stroke or heart attack.

tropic hormones. hormones that control the levels of other hormones.

tubulins. nerve branches.

ulcerative colitis. inflammation of the colon and rectum.

urticaria. reddening and itching of the skin usually caused by an allergic reaction.

very low-density lipoprotein (VLDL). a combination of fat and protein that acts as a carrier for cholesterol and fats (particularly triglycerides) in the bloodstream. Elevated VLDL levels are associated with an increased risk of hardening of the arteries.

villi. small fingerlike folds on certain vascular membranes usually thought of as in the intestines that increase the absorption of nutrients; the overgrowth of yeast degrades the villi.

virulence. the degree or ability of a disease-causing organism to cause disease.

viscous. having a thick, syrupy consistency.

water soluble. being able to be dissolved in water.

xenobiotic. a completely synthetic chemical compound that is foreign to the body and does not naturally occur on earth.

xenoestrogen. a chemical toxin that acts like estrogen and disrupts hormonal activity in the body.

Nutrient
Reference Guide

5-HYDROXYTRYPTOPHAN (5-HTP)

RDA: None established.

Dosage Range: 50–100 mg, 1–3 times a day.

Uses

- Anxiety[1]
- Depression[2]
- Fibromyalgia[3]
- Headaches[4]
- Migraines[5]
- Obesity[6]
- Sleep disorders[7]
- Sugar cravings

Metabolic Functions

- Precursor to serotonin
- Influences the synthesis of melatonin
- Reported to increase levels of brain dopamine and norepinephrine
- Influences activities controlled by serotonin, which include mood regulation (anxiety and depression), impulse control (aggression and obsessive behavior), appetite, pain control and sleep

Symptoms of Nutrient Deficiency

- Deficiency studies in humans have not been conducted.
- Symptoms may include anxiety, depression, sleep disturbances, and cravings for carbohydrates and sugars.

Contraindications/Side Effects

- 5-HTP should be used cautiously and under the supervision of a healthcare professional when taken with antidepressants, such as tricyclics; select serotonin reuptake inhibitors (SSRIs); and monoamine oxidase inhibitors (MAOIs) under the supervision of a healthcare professional.
- 5-HTP has been reported to occasionally cause gastrointestinal upset.
- Use cautiously if you have an autoimmune disorder.

ACETYL-L-CARNITINE (ALC)

RDA: None established.

Dosage Range: 500–2,000 mg daily, in divided doses.

Uses

- Alzheimer's disease[8]
- Depression[9]
- Improves peripheral nerve function in diabetes[10]

Metabolic Functions

- Enhances energy production in the mitochondria
- Enhances cellular oxygenation and helps prevent damage from hypoxia or a lack of oxygen
- Promotes the synthesis and release of acetylcholine in the brain
- Protects and enhances the activity of neurotransmitters in the brain
- Increases the number of nerve growth hormone (NGH) receptors and the amount of nerve growth hormone that is produced

Symptoms of Nutrient Deficiency

- Deficiency studies in humans have not been conducted.

- Deficiency may cause age-related memory loss.

Contraindications/Side Effects

- No known toxicity or serious side effects.
- Occasional reports of mild abdominal discomfort, restlessness, vertigo (dizziness), and headache.

ADRENAL GLANDULAR EXTRACT (New Zealand)

RDA: None established.
Dosage Range: 100–300 mg, 1–3 times a day.

Uses

- Fatigue and stress[11]

Metabolic Functions (anecdotal)

- Supports adrenal function
- Promotes energy production
- Enhances immune function
- Improves stamina, midday fatigue

Symptoms of Nutrient Deficiency

- Deficiency studies in humans have not been conducted.

Contraindications/Side Effects

- May cause excitability in large doses.

ALPHA GPC

RDA: None established.
Dosage Range: 500–3,000 mg daily.

Uses

- Alzheimer's and dementia
- ADHD
- Growth hormone secretagogue
- Enhances acetylcholine production
- Improves reaction time and tactile coordination

Metabolic Functions

- Improves cognition and mental function/short term memory
- Improves growth hormone release resulting in improved metabolic function and rejuvenation of tissue

Symptoms of Nutrient Deficiency

- None known.

Contraindications/Side Effects

- None known.

BETAINE HYDROCHLORIDE

RDA: None established.
Dosage Range: 325–650 mg, 3 times a day with meals that contain protein.

Uses

- Aids in digestion (hypochlorhydria and achlorhydria)[13]

Metabolic Functions

- Digestive aid

Symptoms of Nutrient Deficiency

- Imbalances in stomach acid content are common digestive problems, including allergies and asthma.

Contraindications/Side Effects

- Too high of a dosage can cause gastric irritation.
- Not to be taken by individuals with ulcers.

BIFIDOBACTERIA (*BIFIDUS*)

RDA: None established.
Dosage Range: 5–20 billion CFUs daily.

Uses

- Maintains healthy microflora in the colon[14]
- Important for use during chemotherapy, radiation, and prescription drug use such as NSAIDs, antibiotics, birth control pills, or corticosteroids

Metabolic Functions

- Produce short-chain fatty acids (SCFAs) in the colon, which creates a slightly acidic environment that is unfavorable for the growth of pathological bacteria, yeasts, and molds
- Short-chain fatty acids formed by bifidobacteria are the main source of energy for the cells that form the inner surface of the colon

Symptoms of Nutrient Deficiency

- Gas, bloating, diarrhea or constipation, bad breath, chronic vaginal yeast infections.

Contraindications/Side Effects

- No known toxicity or serious side effects.

BIOTIN

RDA: 0.3 mg daily.
Dosage Range: 0.3–3 mg daily.

Uses

- Brittle nails[15]
- Helps metabolize glucose[16]
- Diabetic peripheral neuropathy[17]
- Seborrheic dermatitis[18]
- Uncombable hair syndrome[19]

Metabolic Functions

- Coenzyme during the metabolism of protein, fats, and carbohydrates
- Activity in protein metabolism reportedly promotes healthy skin, nails, and hair

Symptoms of Nutrient Deficiency

- Deficiency in humans is rare.

Contraindications/Side Effects

- No known toxicity or serious side effects.
- Excess is eliminated via urination.

BISMUTH

RDA: None established.
Dosage Range: 120 mg, 4 times a day, 20 minutes before meals for ulcer therapy.

Uses

- Treatment of ulcers[20]

Metabolic Functions

- Protective coating for inflamed surfaces such as ulcers
- May suppress growth of bacteria such as *Campylobacter pylori* and *Helicobacter pylori*

Symptoms of Nutrient Deficiency

- Bismuth is not considered to be a nutrient and there is no deficiency condition associated with it.

Contraindications/Side Effects

- Possible neurological toxicity with long-term use.
- Treatment should not last longer than 6–8 weeks.

BRANCHED-CHAIN AMINO ACIDS (BCAAS) LEUCINE/ISOLEUCINE/VALINE

RDA: None established.
Dosage Range: Isoleucine: 900 mg daily.
Leucine: 1,200 mg daily.
Valine: 1,050 mg daily.

Uses

- Assist in building muscle and lean body mass[21]

Metabolic Functions

- Serve as a direct source of energy for skeletal muscles
- Promote protein synthesis in muscle and they regulate protein metabolism throughout the body
- Reportedly play a role in helping to regulate insulin secretion
- Decrease the rate of protein catabolism under stressful conditions

Symptoms of Nutrient Deficiency

- Human deficiencies are rare.
- Severe valine deficiency is reported to cause neurological defects in the brain.
- Isoleucine deficiency may cause muscle tremors.
- There are no reports of leucine deficiencies.

Contraindications/Side Effects

- No known toxicity or serious side effects.

BORON

RDA: None established.
Dosage Range: 3–6 mg daily.

Uses

- Osteoarthritis[22]
- Reduces urinary calcium excretion[23]
- Rheumatoid arthritis[24]

Metabolic Functions

- Influences the mobilization of calcium
- May influence the synthesis of vitamin D, which plays a role in the prevention of bone loss
- Plays an important role in the metabolism of magnesium
- Has a regulatory effect on the production of estrogens and testosterone

Symptoms of Nutrient Deficiency

- Deficiency may cause urinary loss of calcium and magnesium.
- Deficiency is also associated with an increased rate of bone demineralization, which may influence the development of osteoporosis in postmenopausal women.

Contraindications/Side Effects

- Excessive intake can cause nausea, vomiting, diarrhea, skin rashes, and fatigue.
- No health or medical problems have been reported in areas of the world where the daily diet supplies up to 41 mg daily of boron.

CARNITINE
(Fumerate or Tartrate)

RDA: None established.

Dosage Range: 200–4,000 mg daily, in divided doses.

Uses

- Congestive heart failure[25]
- Lowers elevated cholesterol and triglycerides[26]
- Enhances athletic performance[27]
- Renal failure
- Weight Loss
- Male infertility[28]

Metabolic Functions

- Supports heart function (affects the production of energy in muscle tissue)
- Regulates fat metabolism by facilitating the transport of fats across cell membranes into the mitochondria (part of the cell that produces energy)
- Helps the body oxidize amino acids to produce energy when necessary

- Helps metabolize ketones
- Increases energy and endurance
- Increases the oxidation of fats

Symptoms of Nutrient Deficiency

- Deficiencies are rare because the body produces carnitine relatively easily.
- Symptoms include elevated blood lipids, abnormal liver function, muscle weakness, reduced energy, and impaired glucose control.

Contraindications/Side Effects

- No known toxicity or serious side effects.
- May experience loose stools in doses exceeding 2,000 mg per day.

CHITOSAN

RDA: None established.

Dosage Range: 750–1,500 mg (of a 90% deacetylation product), 2 to 3 times a day, 1 hour before meals.

Uses

- Weight reduction[29]

Metabolic Functions

- Potentially inhibits intestinal absorption of dietary fat
- May chelate and eliminate heavy metals; used in detoxification

Symptoms of Nutrient Deficiency

- Deficiency studies in humans have not been conducted.

Contraindications/Side Effects

- May inhibit absorption of fat-soluble dietary supplements (vitamins, fatty acids, and lipid-containing herbs), so do not take at the same time lipid-soluble or lipid-dispersible dietary supplements are taken—ask your pharmacist.

CHONDROITIN SULFATE

RDA: None established.

Dosage Range: 300–1,500 mg daily.

Uses

- Osteoarthritis[30]

Metabolic Functions

- Aids in improving cartilage function
- Used as nutritional support in sports injury, acute traumatic injury, and other connective tissue injuries
- Supports joint and connective tissue health in combination with glucosamine

Symptoms of Nutrient Deficiency

- Deficiency studies in humans have not been conducted.

Contraindications/Side Effects

- No known toxicity or serious side effects.

CHROMIUM GTF (Glucose Tolerance Factor)

RDA: None established.
Dosage Range: 200–800 mcg daily.

Uses

- Diabetes/insulin resistance[31] (supports blood sugar regulation and sugar cravings)
- Elevated cholesterol[32]
- Elevated triglycerides[33]
- Low blood sugar levels[34]
- Weight loss[35]

Metabolic Functions

- Pancreas regulation
- A component of glucose tolerance factor, which reportedly enhances the blood-sugar lowering effects of insulin by facilitating the uptake of glucose into cells
- May help insulin bind to its receptors, thereby increasing the activity of insulin and reducing the amount of insulin required to control blood sugar
- Influences the metabolism of carbohydrates and fats
- Component to conversion of T4 to T3

Symptoms of Nutrient Deficiency

- Deficiency symptoms parallel those of diabetes, including elevated blood sugar, numbness and tingling in the extremities, nerve disorders in the limbs, and glucose intolerance.
- Disturbances in protein and lipid metabolism have also been reported in conjunction with deficiency.

Contraindications/Side Effects

- Toxicity risk is low in humans.

COENZYME Q$_{10}$

RDA: None established.
Dosage Range: 30–1,200 mg daily.

Uses

- Angina[36]
- Antioxidant
- Cancer
- Congestive heart[37]
- Diabetes[38]
- Component to energy production
- High blood pressure[39]
- Mitral valve prolapse[40]
- Muscular[41]
- Obesity[42]
- Parkinson's disease
- Periodontal disease[43]

Metabolic Functions

- Involved in the manufacture of ATP, the primary source of energy for humans
- Functions as an antioxidant
- Has the ability to enter mitochondria (the area of a cell where energy is produced) and provides protection against free-radical damage

Symptoms of Nutrient Deficiency

- Cardiovascular problems are the most frequent sign of deficiency, including elevated blood pressure, congestive heart failure, mitral valve prolapse, and angina pectoris.
- Deficiency increases the incidence of periodontal disease.

Contraindications/Side Effects

- No known toxicity or serious side effects.

COLLAGEN (TYPE II)

RDA: None established.
Dosage Range: 200–400 mg, 3 times a day.

Uses

- Topical application for wound healing
- Pressure ulcers
- Venous stasis ulcers
- Diabetic ulcers
- Ulcers resulting from arterial insufficiencies
- Surgical wounds
- Traumatic wounds
- First and second degree burns[44]

Metabolic Functions

- Supports collagen production
- Functions as an anti-inflammatory
- Improves joint flexibility
- Reduces destruction of collagen

Symptoms of Nutrient Deficiency

- Deficiency studies in humans have not been conducted.

Contraindications/Side Effects

- No known toxicity or serious side effects.

COLOSTRUM

RDA: None established.
Dosage Range: 500–1,000 mg, 1–3 times a day.

Uses

- Antidiarrheal[45]
- Immune system support[46,47]
- Enhances endurance and stamina
- Growth hormone secretagogue
- Antiviral properties[48]

Metabolic Functions

- Supports immune function
- Aids energy production

Symptoms of Nutrient Deficiency

- Deficiency studies in humans have not been conducted.

Contraindications/Side Effects

- No known toxicity or serious side effects.

CONJUGATED LINOLEIC ACID (CLA)

RDA: None established.

Dosage Range: 1,000–2,000 mg, 3 times a day, in divided doses.

Uses

- Increases metabolism and decreases body fat[49]

Metabolic Functions

- Helps transport glucose and reduce body fat
- Antioxidant
- Enhances the immune system

Symptoms of Nutrient Deficiency

- Deficiency studies in humans have not been conducted, but weight gain would be a result of deficiency.

Contraindications/Side Effects

- No known toxicity or serious side effects.

CREATINE

RDA: None established.

Dosage Range: 10 grams (g) daily, in divided doses, for 1 week during the loading phase, then 5 g daily during the maintenance phase; should be cycled 2 weeks on and 1 week off.

Uses

- Improves ATP production
- Useful in the elderly for improving lean mass and strength
- Athletic performance: enhances energy production and protein synthesis for muscle building[50]

Metabolic Functions

- Enhances the production of energy and muscle building
- Building muscle equates to increased metabolic rate
- An immediately available source of energy for muscle contraction
- Promotes protein synthesis

Symptoms of Nutrient Deficiency

- Deficiency studies in humans have not been conducted.

Contraindications/Side Effects

- No known toxicity or serious side effects.

CYCLO-HISPRO

RDA: None established.

Dosage Range: 200–300 mg of powdered prostate extract containing cyclo-hispro, 2–4 times a day.

Uses
• Type 2 diabetes, blood sugar regulation, and hypoglycemia[51]

Metabolic Functions
• Pancreas regulation
• Helps control glucose metabolism in individuals with non-insulin dependent diabetes
• Stimulates intestinal absorption of zinc

Symptoms of Nutrient Deficiency
• Deficiency studies in humans have not been conducted.

Contraindications/Side Effects
• No known toxicity or serious side effects.

DEHYDROEPIANDROSTERONE (DHEA)

RDA: None established.

Dosage Range: 25–50 mg daily.

Doses of 100 mg daily are sometimes prescribed for elderly individuals.

Uses
• Anti-aging[59]
• Depression[60]
• Diabetes[61]
• Lupus[62]
• Weight loss/metabolism

Metabolic Functions
• Precursor for the synthesis of more than fifty other hormones in the human body
• Estrogen and testosterone are two of the main hormones that are made from DHEA
• Stimulates the production of insulin growth factor-1 (IGF-1), which stimulates anabolic metabolism, accelerates muscle growth and maintenance, improves insulin sensitivity, and enhances energy production
• Has been reported to decrease the need for insulin doses

Symptoms of Nutrient Deficiency
• Low blood levels may be associated with an increased risk for many of the common diseases of aging.
• Low levels are associated with high blood pressure, elevated cholesterol levels, and increased platelet aggregation (blood clot formation).

Contraindications/Side Effects
• No known toxicity or serious side effects (long-term human studies have not yet been conducted).
• Should not be used by individuals with a history of prostate or breast cancer.

DHA (DOCOSAHEXAENOIC ACID)

RDA: None established.

Dosage Range: 125–500 mg, 1–3 times a day.

Uses
• Crohn's disease[52]
• Diabetes[53]
• Eczema[54]
• Elevated blood pressure[55]
• Elevated triglycerides[56]
• Psoriasis[57]
• Rheumatoid arthritis[58]

Metabolic Functions
• Important for eye and brain development in infants
• Lowers serum triglycerides
• Most abundant fat in brain cells
• May play a role in cellular electrical communication

Symptoms of Nutrient Deficiency
• Vision problems.
• Lower IQ.
• Slower rate of learning.

Contraindications/Side Effects
• No known toxicity or serious side effects.

DIINDOLEMETHANE (DIM)

RDA: None established.

Dosage Range: 75–600 mg a day daily in divided doses; 75–150 mg for PMS;

150–450 mg for fibroids and PCOS; 300–600 mg for weight loss and prostate cancer.

Uses

- Improves estrogen metabolism to friendly metabolites
- Helps with estrogen-related disturbances, fibroids, cancers, polycystic ovarian syndrome, and improves other hormonal relationships in the body
- May reduce the incidence of breast cancer[160,161]

Metabolic Functions

- Detoxification
- Improves estrogen metabolism
- Weight loss

Symptoms of Nutrient Deficiency

None.

Contraindications/Side Effects

- Do not use if taking hormonal replacement therapy unless under the supervision of a healthcare professional.

FISH OILS OR MARINE LIPIDS (EPA)

RDA: None established.

Dosage Range: 1,000–2,000 mg, 2 times a day.

Uses

- Crohn's disease[63]
- Diabetes[64]
- Eczema[65]
- Elevated blood pressure[66]
- Elevated triglycerides[67]
- Psoriasis[68]
- Rheumatoid arthritis[69]
- Stroke risk reduction

Metabolic Functions

- Mediates inflammatory response
- Source of essential fatty acids necessary for nerve tissue, hormone, and cell membranes
- Protection against high blood pressure, elevated cholesterol and triglycerides,

plaque formation, arthritis, eczema, psoriasis

Symptoms of Nutrient Deficiency

- Increased risk of cardiovascular disease.
- Inflammatory problems.

Contraindications/Side Effects

- No known toxicity or serious side effects.

FLAXSEED OIL

RDA: None established.

Dosage Range: 1–2 Tbsp daily, which contains approximately 58–60% omega-3; may also use flaxseed meal for fiber at 1–2 tablespoons daily added to food or protein drink.

Uses

- Source of omega-3 essential fatty acid, also known as alpha-linolenic acid or ALA.
- An integral part of the structure of cell walls and cellular membranes;
- Necessary for the transport and oxidation of cholesterol; and
- Precursors for an important group of chemicals called the prostaglandins[70]
- Increases sex hormone binding globulin to help bind estrogen
- Inhibits beta glucuronidase

Metabolic Functions

- Omega-3 is a primary structural component of cellular membranes throughout the body
- Omega-3 is converted into longer-chain fatty acids, which are precursors for prostaglandins (regulatory chemicals) that control a variety of body functions including pain, inflammation, swelling, blood pressure, cholesterol levels, digestive processes, synthesis of sex hormones, smooth muscle activity, fluid retention, blood clotting, nerve transmission, and the immune system

Symptoms of Nutrient Deficiency

- Symptoms may include cardiovascular problems, elevated blood pressure, increased platelet stickiness, increased inflammation, asthma, allergies, problems with skin and hair.

- Other problems can develop from a deficiency because it upsets the synthesis of prostaglandins.

Contraindications/Side Effects

- No known toxicity or serious side effects.

GLUCOSAMINE
(Sulfate or Hydrochloride)

RDA: None established.
Dosage Range: 500 mg, 3–4 times a day.

Uses

- Osteoarthritis[71]

Metabolic Functions

- Protective against joint damage and improves joint mobility
- Building block to connective tissues like cartilage and collagen
- Component to the natural lubricant found in joints

Symptoms of Nutrient Deficiency

- Deficiency studies in humans have not been conducted.

Contraindications/Side Effects

- No known toxicity or serious side effects.
- Occasional reports of mild stomach discomfort.

GLUTAMINE

RDA: None established.
Dosage Range: 500–4,000 mg, 3 times a day.

Uses

- Alcoholism[72]
- Enhances growth hormone release/recovery from exercise
- Peptic ulcers[73]
- Post-surgical healing[74]
- Inhibits mucositis induced from chemotherapy
- Ulcerative colitis and other forms of inflammatory bowel disease[75]

Metabolic Functions

- Source of energy for cells of the gastrointestinal tract
- Promotes protein synthesis and muscle growth
- Alternative brain fuel
- Blocks cortisol-induced protein catabolism
- Conditionally essential in gastrointestinal disorders and tissue-wasting phenomena

Symptoms of Nutrient Deficiency

- Deficiency studies in humans have not been conducted.

Contraindications/Side Effects

- No known toxicity or serious side effects.

GLUTATHIONE

RDA: None established.
Dosage Range: 500–3,000 mg daily, in divided doses.

Uses

- May protect against alcohol-induced liver damage[76]
- Strengthen immune system[77]
- Ulcers[78]

Metabolic Functions

- Detoxifies many compounds in the body, especially in the liver
- Helps protect the body against toxins from cigarette smoke, excess alcohol, overdoses of aspirin, and exposure to radiation
- Helps support the immune system
- Helps transport certain amino acids across cellular membranes
- Involved in the synthesis of fatty acids

Symptoms of Nutrient Deficiency

- Decreased macrophage activity and a weakened immune system.
- Increase in free-radical damage throughout the body, especially in the membranes of red blood cells and mitochondria.
- Decreases the body's ability to detoxify many compounds in the liver.
- Could result in hair loss and baldness.

Contraindications/Side Effects

- No known toxicity or serious side effects.
- Oral absorption of this supplement is questionable.

HYDROXYMETHYL BUTYRATE (HMB)

RDA: None established.

Dosage Range: 1,500–3,000 mg daily, in divided doses.

Uses

- Used to increase muscle mass during intense exercise[79]

Metabolic Functions

- An anticatabolic agent that may reduce protein/muscle breakdown by shifting protein turnover in favor of new muscle growth resulting in greater gains in muscle size and strength
- Increases the body's ability to build muscle and burn fat with intense exercise
- Increases endurance
- Helps to promote basal metabolism improvement

Symptoms of Nutrient Deficiency

- Deficiency studies in humans have not been conducted.

Contraindications/Side Effects

- No known toxicity or serious side effects.

ISOFLAVONES
(Genistein and Diadzein)

RDA: None established.

Dosage Range: 500–1,000 mg of soy extract daily (13–17% genistein).

Uses

- Cancer prevention[80]
- Lower elevated cholesterol[81]

Metabolic Functions

- Phytoestrogenic
- Lowers LDL and raises HDL
- Stimulates bone remodeling

Symptoms of Nutrient Deficiency

- Deficiency studies in humans have not been conducted

Contraindications/Side Effects

- Women who are on estrogen medications should consult their physician.
- Individuals with estrogen positive breast cancershould use with caution.

LACTOBACILLUS ACIDOPHILUS
(Dairy Free)

RDA: None established.

Dosage Range: 5–20 billion CFUs daily.

Uses

- Recolonize the gastrointestinal (GI) tract with beneficial bacteria following antibiotics[82]
- Adjunct support for chemotherapy, radiation, and drug therapy such as NSAIDs, antibiotics, birth control pills, or corticosteroids
- Enhance immunity[83]
- Infant use for immune support, allergies, colic [84]
- Lower elevated cholesterol[85]
- Lactose intolerance[86]
- Vaginal yeast infection [87]
- Candida-related complex
- Children's allergies

Metabolic Functions

- Act as a barrier against infection by producing natural antibiotics in the gastrointestinal tract
- Produce a wide range of B vitamins and vitamin K in the intestinal tract
- Essential nutrient in combating dysbiosis, candida imbalances, leaky gut
- Improves chronic constipation and diarrhea

Symptoms of Nutrient Deficiency

- Gas, bloating, diarrhea or constipation, bad breath and chronic vaginal yeast infections.

Contraindications/Side Effects

- No known toxicity or serious side effects.

LIVER GLANDULAR EXTRACT
(New Zealand)

RDA: None established.
Dosage Range: 500 mg, 1–3 times a day.

Uses

- Functions as a liver tonic[88]

Metabolic Functions

- Supports liver function
- Rich source of the antioxidant superoxide dismutase (SOD)
- Builds red blood cells

Symptoms of Nutrient Deficiency

- Deficiency studies in humans have not been conducted.

Contraindications/Side Effects

- No known toxicity or serious side effects.

LIPOIC ACID (ALPHA LIPOIC ACID)

RDA: None established.
Dosage Range: 25–600 mg daily.

Uses

- Powerful antioxidant effects
- Improves nerve blood flow, reduces oxidative stress and improves nerve conduction in diabetic neuropathy[89]
- Prevention of cataracts[90]
- Promotes healthy skin, reduces rate of aging of skin
- Protection against stroke and other brain disorders[91]

Metabolic Functions

- Antioxidant against water-soluble and fat-soluble free radicals
- Provides antioxidant protection both inside and outside of cells
- As a cofactor, plays a role in the production of cellular energy (ATP)
- Prevents the symptoms that accompany vitamin E deficiency
- Increases insulin receptor sensitivity; helps in pancreas function
- Chelates heavy metals
- Supports detoxification

Symptoms of Nutrient Deficiency

- Alpha lipoic acid deficiency in humans has not been reported.
- Deficiency would likely result in higher levels of lactic acid, which could cause muscle fatigue.

Contraindications/Side Effects

- No known toxicity or serious side effects.
- Diabetics should monitor blood sugar if using lipoic acid to improve glucose regulation.

LUTEIN

RDA: None established.
Dosage Range: 2–60 mg daily.

Uses

- Cataracts[92]
- Macular degeneration[93]

Metabolic Functions

- Antioxidant and a member of the carotenoids
- Strengthens capillaries
- Concentrates in the eye, filters out blue light and prevents macular degeneration

Symptoms of Nutrient Deficiency

- Development of cataracts and macular degeneration.
- Weak capillaries and easy bruising.

Contraindications/Side Effects

- No known toxicity or serious side effects.

LYCOPENE

RDA: None established.
Dosage Range: 5–300 mg daily.

Uses

- Atherosclerosis (hardening of the arteries)[94]
- Cancer prevention[95]
- Macular degeneration[96]

Metabolic Functions

- Antioxidant and a member of the carotenoids

- Reported to protect against macular degeneration, atherosclerosis and several types of cancer, especially prostate cancer

Symptoms of Nutrient Deficiency

- Deficiency studies in humans have not been conducted.

Contraindications/Side Effects

- No known toxicity or serious side effects.

LYSINE

RDA: None established.
Dosage Range: 500–1,000 mg daily.

Uses

- Angina pectoris[97]
- Herpes simplex[98]
- Osteoporosis[99]

Metabolic Functions

- Essential amino acid involved in synthesis of connective tissue, neurotransmitters, and carbohydrate metabolism

Symptoms of Nutrient Deficiency

- Seldom deficient in humans.

Contraindications/Side Effects

- No known toxicity or serious side effects.

MALIC ACID

RDA: None established.
Dosage Range: 500 mg, 3–4 times a day with food.

Uses

- Fibromyalgia[100]
- Aluminum toxicity[101]

Metabolic Functions

- Promotes cellular production of energy
- Detoxification of aluminum

Symptoms of Nutrient Deficiency

- Deficiency studies in humans have not been conducted.

Contraindications/Side Effects

- No known toxicity or serious side effects.
- Occasionally produces gastrointestinal (GI) disturbance.

MELATONIN

RDA: None established.
Dosage Range: 0.5–6 mg at bedtime.

Uses

- Insomnia[102]
- Jet lag[103]

Metabolic Functions

- Functions as a hormone that regulates on 24–hour circadian rhythm
- Regulates the sleep/wake cycle
- Possesses antioxidant activity
- Controls the output of growth hormone and sex hormones
- Supports adrenal function

Symptoms of Nutrient Deficiency

- Insomnia and other sleep disturbances.

Contraindications/Side Effects

- No known toxicity or serious side effect (long-term human studies have not been conducted).
- Taking too much can cause morning grogginess and undesired drowsiness.

METHIONINE

RDA: None established.
Dosage Range: 500–3,000 mg daily.

Uses

- The active form of methionine (S-adenosyl-methionine; SAM-e) has been reported to exert anti-depressant activity[104]

Metabolic Functions

- Precursor for the synthesis of cystine, cysteine, and taurine
- Enzymatically converted into S-adenosyl-methionine (SAM-e) or "active methionine," which participates in many biochemical reactions
- Involved in the detoxification of organochlorines and many other toxic substances in the liver
- Precursor for the synthesis of glutathione, which plays a role in maintaining proper levels of the antioxidant enzyme glutathione peroxidase

- Helps metabolize homocysteine
- One of three amino acids needed by the body to manufacture creatine monohydrate, which is essential for energy production and muscle building

Symptoms of Nutrient Deficiency

- Symptoms of deficiency include hair loss, poor skin tone, toxic elevation of metabolic waste products, and liver malfunction.

Contraindications/Side Effects

- Elevated methionine can create toxic conditions, but this is unlikely from excess dietary intake.
- Supplementation without adequate intake of folic acid, vitamin B_6, and vitamin B_{12}, can increase the conversion of methionine to homocysteine and increase risk for cardiovascular disease.

METHYL SULFONYL METHANE (MSM)

RDA: None established.
Dosage Range: 2,000–15,000 mg daily.

Uses

- Allergy relief
- Pain relief[105]
- Interstitial cystitis[106]
- Lupus[107]
- Osteoarthritis[108]

Metabolic Functions

- Anti-inflammatory agent
- Influences inflammatory mediators
- Improves detoxification especially phase two processes

Symptoms of Nutrient Deficiency

- Deficiency studies in humans have not been conducted.

Contraindications/Side Effects

- No known toxicity or serious side effects.

N-ACETYL CYSTEINE (NAC)

RDA: None established.
Dosage Range: 200–1,500 mg daily.

Uses

- Improves glutathione production in the liver
- Acetaminophen (Tylenol) toxicity[109]
- AIDS[110]
- Asthma: functions as a mucolytic agent and an antioxidant[111]
- Bronchitis[112]

Metabolic Functions

- A sulfhydryl compound that is a powerful detoxifying agent capable of detoxifying heavy metals such as mercury, cadmium, and lead
- Increases the body's stores of glutathione
- Functions as an antioxidant in two ways:
  1. Neutralizes hydrogen peroxide, hypochlorous acid, and the hydroxyl radical; and
  2. Enhances glutathione formation
- Functions as an antiviral agent

Symptoms of Nutrient Deficiency

- Deficiency would compromise the immune system by decreasing liver detoxification capabilities, reducing antioxidant activity, and lowering the body's ability to eliminate heavy metal toxins.

Contraindications/Side Effects

- No known toxicity or serious side effects.
- Large doses (5–6 g daily) have been reported to cause diarrhea.
- Some antibiotics may become inactivated if taken in conjunction with N-acetylcysteine.

NICOTINAMIDE ADENINE DINUCLEOTIDE (NADH)/COENZYME 1

RDA: None established.
Dosage Range: 2.5–5 mg, 1–4 times a day

Uses

- Parkinson's disease[113]
- Stamina and energy[114]

Metabolic Functions

- Essential coenzyme in the production of cellular energy
- Facilitates DNA-repair mechanisms

- Antioxidant
- Stimulates the production of dopamine and adrenaline

Symptoms of Nutrient Deficiency

- Deficiency studies in humans have not been conducted.

Contraindications/Side Effects

- No known toxicity or serious side effects.

PARA-AMINOBENZOIC ACID (PABA)

RDA: None established.
Dosage Range: 100–400 mg daily.

Uses

- Peyronie's disease[115]
- Scleroderma[116]
- Vitiligo[117]

Metabolic Functions

- Facilitates the breakdown and utilization of proteins
- Aids in the production of red blood cells
- Promotes skin health, hair pigmentation, and health of the intestines

Symptoms of Nutrient Deficiency

- PABA deficiency has not been reported in humans.

Contraindications/Side Effects

- No known toxicity or serious side effects at doses below 400 mg daily.
- Can cause low blood sugar, rash, fever, and liver damage in large doses.

PHENYLALANINE (DL-FORM)

RDA: None established.
Dosage Range: 250–500 mg, 3 times daily.

Uses

- Depression[118]
- Pain relief[119]
- Reward deficiency craving patterns
- Vitiligo[120]

Metabolic Functions

- Precursor for tyrosine, epinephrine, norepinephrine, dopamine, thyroxine, and melanin

- Influences the synthesis of many important brain neuropeptides including vasopressin, ACTH, somatostatin, enkephalin, angiotensin II, and cholecystokinin (CCK), a hormone that seems to induce a feeling of fullness that may reduce the desire for food
- Converted to phenylethylamine, a chemical that occurs naturally in the brain and appears to elevate mood
- Inhibits the breakdown and extends the activity of enkephalins and endorphins, which are the body's natural analgesics
- Stimulates the release in the stomach of cholecystokinin

Symptoms of Nutrient Deficiency

- Deficiency rarely occurs in humans.
- Symptoms include behavioral changes, eye disorders, poor vascular health, increase in appetite, and weight gain.

Contraindications/Side Effects

- Hyperactive children and individuals that suffer from migraine headaches have been found to have elevated plasma phenylalanine.
- Phenylketonuria (PKU) a genetic abnormality causing toxicity from elevated phenylalanine results in severe mental retardation.
- Ingestion of the artificial sweetener aspartame causes a rapid increase in brain levels of phenylalanine.

PHOSPHATIDYLSERINE

RDA: None established.
Dosage Range: 100 mg, 1–3 times a day.

Uses

- Alzheimer's disease[124]
- Cortisol regulation
- Depression[125]
- Memory enhancement[126]

Metabolic Functions

- Helps provide cell membranes with their fluidity, flexibility, and permeability
- Stimulates the release of various neuro-

transmitters, such as acetylcholine and dopamine
- Enhances ion transport and increases the number of certain neurotransmitter receptor sites in the brain
- May reduce cortisol levels and have an antistress effect; used in adrenal support

Symptoms of Nutrient Deficiency

- Depression, loss of memory, and cognitive decline.

Contraindications/Side Effects

- No known toxicity or serious side effects.

PREGNENOLONE

RDA: None established.
Dosage Range: 5–30 mg daily depending on age and gender.

Uses

- Natural precursor for the production of DHEA, cortisol, progesterone, estrogens, and testosterone in the body
- Arthritis[127]
- Improved mental performance[128]

Metabolic Functions

- Precursor for DHEA and steroid and sex hormones

Symptoms of Nutrient Deficiency

- Deficiency studies in humans have not been conducted.

Contraindications/Side Effects

- No known toxicity or serious side effects, but caution is advised because pregnenolone can stimulate the synthesis of many hormones.

PROGESTERONE (Natural Topical)

RDA: None established.
Dosage Range: Dosage for topical progesterone depends on the strength of the extract; follow manufacturer's directions.

Uses

- Menopause symptoms[129]
- PMS symptoms[130]

- Prevention of breast cancer[131]

Metabolic Functions

- Hormone replacement
- Aids bone remodeling
- Energy production

Symptoms of Nutrient Deficiency

- Increased symptoms of PMS or menopause with edema weight gain, emotional problems.
- Possible increased risk of breast cancer.

Contraindications/Side Effects

- No known toxicity or serious side effects.
- Women taking hormone medication should check with their physician.
- May cause excitability.

PYRUVATE (CALCIUM)

RDA: None established.
Dosage Range: 500–750 mg, 3 times a day, preferably with meals; dosages from 2,500–5,000 mg daily have been used for weight loss.

Uses

- Improves athletic performance[132]
- Obesity and weight loss[133]

Metabolic Functions

- Facilitates the transport of glucose into muscle cells, increasing energy available for the muscles, supports metabolic balance

Symptoms of Nutrient Deficiency

- Pyruvate is not an essential nutrient. There are no studies reporting a deficiency state associated with pyruvate or pyruvic acid.

Contraindications/Side Effects

- Large doses of pyruvate can cause gastrointestinal disturbances, such as gas, bloating, and diarrhea.

QUERCETIN

RDA: None established.
Dosage Range: 300–400 mg, 1–3 times a day.

Uses

- Allergies[134]
- Atherosclerosis[135]
- Cataracts[136]
- Peptic ulcers[137]

Metabolic Functions

- Antioxidant
- Antihistamine
- Anti-inflammatory agent
- Strengthens capillaries

Symptoms of Nutrient Deficiency

- Easy bruising, frequent nosebleeds, or other signs of weak capillaries.

Contraindications/Side Effects

- No known toxicity or serious side effects at normal dosage ranges.

S-ADENOSYLMETHIONINE (SAM-e)

RDA: None established.
Dosage Range: 400–1,600 mg daily.

Uses

- Cardiovascular disease[138]
- Depression[139]
- Fibromyalgia[140]
- Insomnia[141]
- Liver disease[142]
- Rheumatoid arthritis[143]
- Osteoarthritis[144]

Metabolic Functions

- Antidepressant
- Antioxidant
- Necessary for synthesis of glutathione
- Liver detoxification
- Synthesis of, and receptor enhancement for, serotonin, dopamine, and melatonin

Symptoms of Nutrient Deficiency

- Deficiency studies have not been conducted. However, a deficiency would probably result in decreased antioxidant activity and weaken liver detoxification capability.

Contraindications/Side Effects

- No known toxicity or serious side effects.

- Occasional dry mouth, nausea, and restlessness.

TAURINE

RDA: None established.
Dosage Range: 1,000–3,000 mg daily.

Uses

- Congestive heart failure[148]
- Diabetes[149]
- Epilepsy[150]
- Hypertension[151]

Metabolic Functions

- As an amino acid (protein building block)
- Inhibitory neurotransmitter that helps to stabilize nerve cell membranes
- As a component of bile acids helps to regulate the absorption of fats and fat-soluble vitamins
- Regulates the volume of fluid in cells, especially in the kidneys and central nervous system
- Helps regulate the contraction and pumping action of the heart muscle and may provide a cardioprotective effect
- Protects the photoreceptors in the retina of the eye from damage

Symptoms of Nutrient Deficiency

- In pre-term and term infants, taurine insufficiency results in impaired fat absorption, bile acid secretion, vision disturbances, and liver malfunction, all of which can be reversed by taurine supplementation.

Contraindications/Side Effects

- No known toxicity or serious side effects.

THYMUS GLANDULAR EXTRACT (New Zealand)

RDA: None established.
Dosage Range: 250–500 mg, 3 times a day.

Uses

- Immune support[152]

Metabolic Functions

- Immunomodulator
- Provides thymic proteins

Symptoms of Nutrient Deficiency

- Deficiency studies in humans have not been conducted.

Contraindications/Side Effects

- No known toxicity or serious side effects.

THYROID GLANDULAR EXTRACT (New Zealand)

RDA: None established.
Dosage Range: 60 mg, 1–3 times a day.

Uses

- Metabolism, fatigue, immune support[153]

Metabolic Functions

- Regulates metabolism
- Nutritional support for thyroid metabolism
- Fatigue, energy production

Symptoms of Nutrient Deficiency

- Deficiency studies in humans have not been conducted.

Contraindications/Side Effects

- Caution if on thyroid medication.

TYROSINE (L Form)

RDA: None established.
Dosage Range: 250–500 mg 2 times a day.

Uses

- Alzheimer's disease[154]
- Depression[155]
- Phenylketonuria (PKU)[156]
- Substance abuse[157]

Metabolic Functions

- Precursor for the neurotransmitters dopamine, norepinephrine, epinephrine, and cholecystokinin (CCK)
- Necessary for synthesis of melanin and thyroid hormones

Symptoms of Nutrient Deficiency

- Depression and emotional disturbances.
- Underactive thyroid and disturbed metabolism.

Contraindications/Side Effects

- No known toxicity or serious side effects.
- Not to be taken by individuals on MAO-inhibiting antidepressants.

VANADIUM (as Vanadium Pentoxide or Vanadyl Sulfate)

RDA: None established.
Dosage Range: 250–500 mcg, 1–3 times a day.

Uses

- Blood sugar regulation
- Support muscle growth
- Type 1 diabetes[158]
- Type 2 diabetes[159]

Metabolic Functions

- Supports function of the pancreas
- Functions as a cofactor, which enhances or inhibits various enzymes
- Stimulates glucose metabolism and improves glucose control
- At higher dosage levels, reported to assist in lowering elevated serum cholesterol and triglyceride levels

Symptoms of Nutrient Deficiency

- Deficiency studies in humans have not been conducted.

Contraindications/Side Effects

- No dietary toxicity or serious side effects have been reported.
- Industrial exposure has resulted in toxicity.
- Caution for diabetics (may increase the need to regulate blood sugar).

Herbal Reference Guide

ARABINOXYLANE

Dosage

General immune support: 500-mg capsule once daily.

Aggressive therapy: 500 mg, 2 capsules, 3 times a day, for two to four weeks. Then 500 mg, 1 capsule, 2–3 times a day thereafter.

Uses

Enhances immunity[1]; used in HIV infection (only use under the supervision of a health-care provider).[2]

Used as immune support in cancer therapy.[3]

Used as support in chemotherapy and radiation therapy.

Reduces chance of leukopenia.

Enhances NK cells and T cell/B cell activity.

Contraindications/Side Effects

People who are allergic to mushrooms should consult a doctor before use.

Do not use in kidney disorders since the fermentation media is high in phosphorus.

Metabolic Functions

- Immune enhancement
- General health tonic

ARTICHOKE (*Cynara scolymus*) LEAF

Dosage

500 mg extract daily, standardized to contain 15% chlorogenic acid, or 2–5 % cynarin per dose.

Uses

Used to stimulate the flow of bile[4]; useful in eczema and skin disorders and as a liver pro-tective agent,[5,6] and adjunctive agent in high blood cholesterol levels.[7]

Contraindications/Side Effects

Do not use if allergic to plants in the daisy (chrysanthemum) family.

Do not use if bile obstruction is present.[8]

Metabolic Functions

- Detoxification
- Liver and gallbladder health

ASHWAGANDHA (*Withania somniferum*) ROOT

Dosage

450–900 mg daily of standardized extract, standardized to 1.5% with anolides.

Uses

Used as an adaptogen, to enhance mental and physical performance, improve learning ability, and decrease stress and fatigue[9]; general tonic in stressful situations, especially insomnia, overwork, nervousness, and restlessness[10]; chemotherapy and radiation protection and enhancement of these agents.[11,12]

Contraindications/Side Effects

May cause spontaneous abortion. Use with caution in pregnancy and lactation.

Do not use with sedatives and hypnotics such as barbiturates (reported to increase the effects of these drugs).[13]

Metabolic Functions

- Immune enhancement
- Increases stamina under stress and fatigue (adrenal function)

ASTRAGALUS
(*Astragalus membranaceus*) ROOT

Dosage

250–500 mg, 4 times a day, standardized to a minimum of 0.4% 4'-hydroxy-3'-methoxy-isoflavone 7-sug.

Uses

Used as an adaptogen; increases stamina and energy;[14] support for chemotherapy and radiation;[15] improves resistance to disease and immune function;[16] used in oxygen deprivation of tissues.[17]

Contraindications/Side Effects

None known.

Metabolic Functions

- Immune enhancement
- May increase cellular oxygenation

BACOPA (*Bacopa monniera*) LEAF

Dosage

100–150 mg, 2 times a day, standardized to contain 20% bacosides A and B.

Uses

Used for memory enhancement and improving cognitive function.[18]

Contraindications/Side Effects

None known.

Metabolic Functions

- Mental clarity, cognitive function

BILBERRY
(*Vaccinium myrtillus*) BERRY

Dosage

80–160 mg, 2–3 times a day, standardized to 25% anthocyanosides, calculated as anthocyanidins.

Uses

Used in eye disorders including: myopia, diminished visual acuity, dark adaptation, day and night blindness, diabetic retinopathy, cataracts.[19] Excellent antioxidant used in cardiovascular health-helps maintain healthy blood vessels.[20]

Contraindications/Side Effects

Use with caution in pregnancy and lactation.[21] Use with caution if taking anti-coagulants (blood thinning agents).

Metabolic Functions

- Antioxidant
- Eye health
- Cardiovascular health
- Diabetic complications

BITTER MELON
(*Momordica charantia*) FRUIT

Dosage

200 mg, 1–3 times a day, standardized to 5.1% triterpenes.

Uses

Used to regulate blood sugar levels;[22,23] used as an antidiabetic agent and for impaired glucose tolerance (IGT); antiviral.[24]

Contraindications/Side Effects

Do not use in pregnancy. May alter insulin and/or oral medication needs in diabetic individuals.[25] Close monitoring of blood sugar levels is recommended.

Metabolic Functions

- Diabetic complications
- Improves insulin resistance
- Support of pancreas function

BLACK COHOSH (*Cimicifuga racemosa*) ROOT/RHIZOME

Dosage

20–40 mg, 2 times a day, standardized to 1 mg triterpenes (27-deoxyacteine).

Uses

Phytoestrogen action; used in menopausal complaints and PMS; rheumatic complaints.[26,27,28]

Contraindications/Side Effects

Contraindicated in pregnancy and lactation (uterine stimulation reported).[29,30]

Caution if taking hormonal drugs such as estrogen or birth control pills; may alter hormonal therapy. May cause nausea, vomiting, and headache in high doses.

Metabolic Functions

- Female-related hormonal imbalances
- Balances menopausal hormonal shifts

BROMELAIN ENZYME
(*Annas comosus*)

Dosage

One tablet, 3 times a day, with meals containing at least 2,000 mcu/gram per dose.

Uses

Proteolytic agent; used as an anti-inflammatory agent in arthritis[31]; also used as a digestive enzyme.

Contraindications/Side Effects

Do not use if taking anticoagulants.[32]

Use with caution in gastrointestinal ulceration.

Metabolic Functions

- Enzyme function
- Digestion, gas, bloating

CASCARA (*Rhamnus purshiana*) BARK

Dosage

100 mg as needed, not to exceed 3 capsules daily or for more than 2 days, standardized to contain 25–30% hydroxyanthracene derivatives per dose.

Uses

Anthraquinone laxative.[33]

Contraindications/Side Effects

Avoid in children under 12 years of age.

May decrease absorption of oral medications. Excessive use may lead to potassium loss and other electrolyte disturbances and may potentiate the effects of various pharmaceutical drugs—ask your pharmacist before taking laxatives such as cascara.[34]

Metabolic Functions

- Laxative
- Detoxification

CAT'S CLAW
(*Uncaria tomentosa*) ROOT BARK

Dosage

250–1,000 mg, 3 times a day, standardized to contain 3% alkaloids and 15% total phenols; OR TOA (tetracyclic alkaloid) free dose, 20 mg, 3 times a day, for 3 weeks, then 1 time daily.

Uses

Used to improve immunity[35]; antibacterial, antifungal, and antiviral[36,37]; anti-inflammatory[38]; antioxidant.[39]

Contraindications/Side Effects

Should not be used by organ transplant patients.

Do not use during pregnancy.

Do not use in individuals on the following:

- IV Hyper-immunoglobulin therapy
- Insulin
- Immunosuppressant therapy

Use with caution in individuals on the following medications:

- Anticoagulants (may increase the chance of bleeding due to PAF inhibition);
- NSAIDs (may increase the chance of GI bleeding)

Metabolic Functions

- Immune enhancement
- Antioxidant
- Gastrointestinal health
- Bowel terrain protocol
- Anti-inflammatory effect on colon
- Anti-fungal, bacterial

CAYENNE (*Capsicum annuum*) FRUIT

Dosage

400 mg, 3 times a day, standardized to 0.25% or greater capsaicin content; may also be standardized to heat units, with 150,000 being average.

Uses

May stimulate digestion;[42] circulatory support for cardiovascular system,[43] used topically in inflammation and pain.[44,45]

Contraindications/Side Effects

Do not use with peptic or duodenal ulcer.

Use with caution in individuals taking anticoagulant medications due to platelet aggregating inhibition.

May interfere with MAOI and antihypertensive therapies due to increased catechol-amine secretion.

Metabolic Functions

- Anti-inflammatory agent
- Detoxification
- Thermogenic (increases metabolism)

CHAMOMILE
(*Matricaria chamomilla*) FLOWERS

Dosage

400–1,600 mg daily in divided doses, standardized to 1% apigenin and 5% essential oil; may use tea (1 heaping teaspoonful in hot water—steep 10 minutes, drink up to 3 times a day).

Gargle with mouth rinse 2–3 times a day or as needed.

Uses

Used as a carminative (stomach settling), antispasmodic, mild sedative, antianxiety mild inflammation.[47]

Used topically for mild inflammation and other skin disorders.

Used as a mouth rinse and gargle in oral health.

Contraindications/Side Effects

Use with caution in individuals with severe ragweed allergy or allergy to members of the daisy (chrysanthemum) family.

Metabolic Functions

- Digestive tonic
- Stress, especially in children

CHASTE BERRY
(*Vitex agnus-castus*) BERRY

Dosage

200–400 mg every morning, preferably on an empty stomach, either 1 hour before or 2 hours after breakfast, standardized to contain at least 0.5% agnuside and 0.6% aucubin.

Uses

Progesteronelike action with uses in PMS, menopause, corpus luteum insufficiency and other menstrual irregularities;[48,49] insufficient lactation and hyperprolactinemia.[50,51]

Contraindications/Side Effects

May alter hormonal therapy such as birth control and hormone replacement therapy (HRT).[52]

Metabolic Functions

- Female-related hormonal imbalances
- PMS
- Endometriosis
- Menopause
- Hyperprolactenemia
- Sensitizes pituitary to improve hormone relationships

COLEUS (*Coleus forskohlii*) ROOT

Dosage

250 mg, 1–3 times daily, standardized to 1% forskolin, OR 100 mg 1–3 times daily standardized to 10% forskolin.

Uses

Increases intracellular c-AMP; used in asthma, hypertension, congestive heart failure, glaucoma, allergies, eczema, weight loss.[53,54,55]

Contraindications/Side Effects

Use with caution in low blood pressure.

Avoid in peptic ulcer disease.[56] Use with caution in individuals taking the following (may increase the effects of these drugs):

- Antihypertensives
- Decongestants
- Antihistamines

Use with caution in individuals taking blood-thinning agents.[57]

Metabolic Functions

- May help increase tissue oxygenation
- May help with sluggish metabolism
- Support of enzyme function

CORDYCEPS
(*Cordyceps sinensis*) FUNGUS

Dosage

1,000–1,200 mg, 2–3 times a day, standardized to contain 0.14% adenosine and 5% mannitol; higher standardizations are available. Must be CS4 extract.

Uses

Excellent antioxidant[58],supports healthy lung and kidney function;[59] adaptogenic/tonic to support wellness, longevity, and general health;[60] beneficial for athletes in increasing stamina and endurance improving VO2 max 10–13%;[61] increases cellular oxygenation; useful during times of stress; reduces tiredness and fatigue; has immunomodulatory effects;[62] adjunct support for chemotherapy and radiation reduces platelet and stem cell destruction[63]; improves sexual vitality[64]; liver protective.[65]

Contraindications/Side Effects

Use with caution in pregnancy and lactation. Do not take if allergic to fungus.

Use with caution in individuals taking anticoagulants (due to platelet aggregating inhibition).[66]

Do not use if taking MAO inhibitors.[67]

Metabolic Functions

- May increase tissue oxygenation
- Stress; adrenal function
- Immune enhancement
- Liver protection
- Improves energy, endurance and stamina without stimulant effect

DANDELION
(*Taraxacum officinale*) ROOT/PLANT

Dosage

250–500 mg, 3 times a day of whole root, standardized extract, OR 5–10ml, 3 times a day, of liquid extract (1:1 weight/volume fresh plant or 1:4 weight/volume dried plant) in water or juice.

Uses

Used for disorders of bile secretion (choleretic); appetite stimulation; dyspeptic complaints;[68] diuretic.[69]

Contraindications/Side Effects

Do not use if biliary obstruction or gallstones are present.[70]

Metabolic Functions

- Liver detoxification

ECHINACEA (*Echinacea purpurea; Echinacea angustifolia*) FLOWER, HERB, ROOT

Dosage

Acute: 500 mg, 3 times a day for day 1, then 250 mg, 4 times a day.

Prevention: 250 mg daily, 3 weeks on and 1 week off. Products should be standardized to contain 4% echinacosides (angustifolia), or 4% sesquiterpene esters (purpurea); purpurea succus use 60 drops, 3 times a day, with food for 1 day, then 40 drops 3 times a day with food for up to 10 days, standardized to contain not less than 2.4% soluble beta-1,2 D-5 fructofuranosides.

Uses

Increase nonspecific immunity; used in prevention and treatment of colds, flu, minor infections, tonsillitis, sore throat; used in chronic skin complaints.[71,72]

Used topically as an antibacterial, wound healing agent; used as an antiviral agent.

Contraindications/Side Effects

Recommended for no longer than 10 days of therapy in treatment of infections.

Not for use in individuals with chronic immunosuppression.[73]

Use with caution in individuals with kidney disorders.[74]

Metabolic Functions

- Immune enhancement
- Support in colds/influenza

EVENING PRIMROSE
(*Oenothera biennis*) OIL FROM SEED

Dosage

500 mg, 1–2 times a day, depending on severity of condition, standardized to 8% gamma-linoleic acid.

Uses

Rich in omega-6 essential fatty acids; used in atopic eczema, dry skin, popping joints, PMS, menopause, rheumatoid arthritis, diabetic neuropathy, psoriasis.[75,76]

Contraindications/Side Effects

Do not use if currently on phenothiazine

antipsychotics or diagnosed with schizophrenia; contraindicated in epilepsy.[77]
Use with caution in the following:
- Individuals on blood thinning agents.[78]
- Individuals with seizures and/or on seizure medication (may lower seizure threshold).[79]

Metabolic Functions
- Essential fatty acid supplement (omega-6)
- Detoxification
- Enzyme function
- Thyroid, adrenal and pancreas health

FEVERFEW (*Tanacetum parthenium*) LEAF

Dosage
100–250 mg daily, standardized to 250–600 mcg of parthenolide.

Uses
Used in the preventive treatment of migraine headaches.[80]

Contraindications/Side Effects
Do not use in pregnancy.[81]
Do not use if the individual is allergic to the daisy (chrysanthemum) family.
Use with caution in individuals on blood-thinning agents.[82]

Metabolic Functions
- Migraine headache prevention
- Anti-inflammatory

GARLIC (*Allium sativum*) BULB

Dosage
400 mg, 3 times a day, standardized to contain 10–12 mg/gm alliin and/or 4,000 mcg of total allicin potential (TAP) per dose; may also use aged garlic.

Uses
May lower cholesterol and blood fats;[83,84] mild PAF inhibitor;[85] has antibiotic effect, especially against bacteria and fungi;[86,87] beneficial to the immune system.

Contraindications/Side Effects
May cause GI distress in sensitive individuals.
Use with caution with the following medications:

- Blood-thinning agents
- Blood sugar-lowering agents
- Blood pressure-lowering agents
- Anti-retroviral agents

Metabolic Functions
- Liver detoxification
- Enzyme function
- Cholesterol regulation

GINKGO (*Ginkgo biloba*) LEAF

Dosage
40–80 mg, 3 times a day, standardized to 24–27% ginkgo flavone glycosides (heterosides), and 6–7% triterpene lactones.

Uses
Reported to increase peripheral blood flow; used in cerebral vascular insufficiency, peripheral vascular insufficiency, Alzheimer's disease, impotence, tinnitus, resistant depression, memory.[88,89]

Contraindications/Side Effects
Use with caution in individuals on blood-thinning agents.[90,91,92]

Metabolic Functions
- Circulation
- Cognitive function
- Oxygenation of tissues
- Antioxidant
- Helps regulate homocysteine

GINGER (*Zingiber officinalis*) ROOT

Dosage
250 mg, 3 times a day with food, standardized to contain 4 percent volatile oils or 5 percent total pungent compounds, most prominently 6-gingerol and 6-shogaol (20% extract used in arthritis).

Uses
Used as an anti-nausea agent.[93,94]

Contraindications/Side Effects
Use only under the supervision of a health-care provider in pregnancy.

Metabolic Functions
- Gastrointestinal health

• Irritable bowel syndrome

GINSENG, ASIAN
(*Panax ginseng*) ROOT

Dosage
200–600 mg daily, standardized to a minimum of 5% ginsenosides.

Uses
Enhances mental and physical performance; increases energy, decreases stress; improves immune function; adjunct support for chemotherapy and radiation.[95,96]

Contraindications/Side Effects
Do not use in kidney failure.

Do not use in pregnancy.

Use with caution when taking prescription or OTC stimulant products such as caffeine and decongestants.

May interfere with hormonal replacement therapy; use with caution.

Use with caution in the following:

• Digoxin therapy
• Hypertension and hypertensive medications[97]
• Blood-thinning therapy[98,99]

Use with caution in individuals currently on MAO inhibitors, primarily phenelzine.[100]

May cause mastalgia (breast tenderness) in prolonged and high doses.[101]

May cause vaginal breakthrough bleeding.[102]

Metabolic Functions
• Immune enhancement
• Adrenal function

"GINSENG," SIBERIAN (Eleuthero)
(*Eleutherococcus senticosus*) ROOT

Dosage
200 mg, 2 times a day, standardized to contain 0.8% eleutherosides.

Uses
Adaptogen;[103,104] beneficial in athletic performance, decreasing stress and fatigue; reported to increase immune system function.[105]

Contraindications/Side Effects
Use with caution when taking stimulant products such as caffeine and decongestants.

May interfere with antihypertensive, anticoagulant, and hypoglycemic medications.

Should not be taken in high doses during acute phases of infection, especially when accompanied by a high fever.

Do not use in the following:

• Concurrent with digoxin therapy.[106]
• May increase effects of hexobarbital.[107]

Metabolic Functions
• Immune enhancement
• Adrenal function

GOLDEN SEAL (*Hydrastis canadensis*)
ROOT/RHIZOME

Dosage
250 mg, 2–4 times a day, standardized to 10% alkaloids, or 2.5% berberine and 1.5–5% hydrastine.

Uses
Mucous membrane tonifying; antibacterial, antifungal; used in inflammation of the mucosal membranes; treatment of gastritis, bronchitis, cystitis, infectious diarrhea.[108]

Contraindications/Side Effects
Contraindicated in pregnancy.

High doses (2–3 g) may cause low blood pressure.[109]

May have blood sugar-lowering effects.

Metabolic Functions
• Supports upper respiratory tract in colds/influenza
• Antiparasitic effect on GI tract

GRAPE SEED
(*Vitis vinifera*) SEED/SKIN

Dosage
25–100 mg, 1–3 times a day, standardized to procyanidolic value of not less than 80–90% total phenols.

Uses
Antioxidant; treatment of allergies, asthma; improves peripheral circulation; decreases platelet adhesion (thins blood), capillary

fragility; improves general circulation; inflammation[110,111,112]

Contraindications/Side Effects

Use with caution in individuals on blood-thinning therapy due to platelet inhibition.

Metabolic Functions

- Antioxidant
- Cardiovascular health
- Reduces allergic reactions by limiting the release of histamine.

GRAPEFRUIT SEED EXTRACT (*Citrus paradisi*) PULP, JUICE

Dosage

100–200 mg, 2–3 times a day with meals.

Uses

Used as an antifungal, antibacterial, antiparasitic agent; excellent in restoration of bowel health.

Contraindications/Side Effects

Use with caution in individuals with gastrointestinal ulcers.

Metabolic Functions

- Gastrointestinal health
- Bowel terrain, antifungal, antibacterial, antiparasitic

GREEN TEA (*Camellia sinensis*) LEAF

Dosage

250–500 mg daily, standardized to contain 50% catechins (polyphenols, specifically [-] epigallocatechin-3- gallate [EGCG]).

Uses

Used as an antioxidant to aid in cancer prevention, cardiovascular disease[113,114]; support for chemotherapy and radiation treatment;[115] may lower cholesterol;[116] platelet inhibiting action;[117] anticariogenic (reduces dental plaque).[118]

Contraindications/Side Effects

Caffeine-free products are available.

Use with caution in individuals taking anti-coagulant medications due to platelet aggregating inhibition.

Use with caution when taking other stimulants such as caffeine and decongestants.

Metabolic Functions

- Antioxidant
- Cardiovascular health
- Breast health
- Prostate health
- Protective effects against cancer
- Weight loss

GUGGUL (*Commiphora mukul*) RESIN

Dosage

250–500 mg 3 times a day, standardized to 5% guggulsterones.

Uses

Used in lowering blood cholesterol levels and in supporting thyroid function.[119,120,121]

Contraindications/Side Effects

Use with caution in individuals on the following:

- Thyroid-lowering medications
- Blood-thinning agents[122]
- Cholesterol-lowering medications

Reported to interfere with diltiazem and propranolol metabolism, so caution should be used in calcium channel blocker and beta-blocker medications.[123]

Metabolic Functions

- Thyroid metabolic support
- Cholesterol lowering

GYMNEMA (*Gymnema sylvestre*) LEAF

Dosage

250–500 mg, 1–3 times a day, standardized to contain 25% gymnemic acids.

Uses

Regulation of blood sugar levels.[124]

Contraindications/Side Effects

Use only under the supervision of a healthcare professional if taking diabetic medications.

Metabolic Functions

- Pancreas support
- Reduces insulin resistance
- Improves insulin production

HAWTHORN (*Crataegus oxyacantha*) FLOWER/LEAF/BERRY

Dosage
250 mg, 1–3 times a day, standardized to at least 2% vitexin-2-0-rhamnoside.

Uses
Treatment of angina, low or high blood pressure, peripheral vascular diseases, tachycardia; used as a cardio-tonic.[125,126]

Contraindications/Side Effects
Use with caution in individualss on the following:
- Antihypertensives
- Digoxin
- Angiotensin converting enzyme inhibitors (ACE inhibitors)[127]

Metabolic Functions
- Cardiovascular tonic
- Antioxidant

HOLY BASIL (*Occimum sanctum*) PLANT

Dosage
400-800 mg, 1–2 times a day, standardized to contain 1% ursolic acid.

Uses
Anti-inflammatory agent[128]; antioxidant[129]
May decrease cortisol production (stress related)[130]

Contraindications/Side Effects
Use with caution in gastrointestinal ulcers.

Metabolic Functions
- Enzyme function
- Anti-inflammatory
- Adrenal support; cortisol lowering effect
- Blood sugar regulation
- Stress-induced hypertension support

HOPS (*Humulus lupulus*) STROBILES

Dosage
100 mg, 2 times a day as needed, standardized to 5.2% bitter acids and 4% flavonoids.

Uses
Mild sedative and hypnotic.[131,132]

Contraindications/Side Effects
Use with caution in individuals on the following (action may be potentiated):
- Sedatives
- Antianxiety medications
- Hypnotics
- Antipsychotics
- Antidepressants
- Alcohol

Use caution when driving an automobile or operating heavy machinery.

Use with caution while taking sedative medications (reported to increase sleeping time induced by pentobarbital).[133]

Metabolic Functions
- Stress; insomnia

HORSE CHESTNUT (*Aesculus hippocastanum*) SEED

Dosage
300 mg, 1–2 times a day, standardized to 3–13% escin; also may be applied topically: apply 2% escin gel, 1–2 times a day, to swollen areas.

Uses
Treatment of varicose veins, hemorrhoids, other venous insufficiencies, deep venous thrombosis[134,135]; Used topically in the same conditions.

Contraindications/Side Effects
Use with caution in patients on anticoagulants (may increase chances of bleeding due to PAF inhibition).[136,137,138]

Do not use topically if skin is broken.

Metabolic Functions
- Vascular tonic
- Circulation, varicosities
- Hemmorhoids

HORSETAIL
(*Equisetum arvense*) SHOOTS

Dosage

300 mg, 3 times a day as needed, standardized to contain 10% silica.

Uses

Diuretic.[139]

Contraindications/Side Effects

Diuretic effect may cause electrolyte disturbances and may potentiate certain pharmaceutical drugs with narrow therapeutic windows.

May deplete thiamine (vitamin B_1) from the body due to thiaminase activity.[140]

Metabolic Functions

• Detoxification

KAVA KAVA (*Piper methysticum*) ROOT

Dosage

100–250 mg, 3 times a day as needed, standardized to contain 30% kavalactones.

Uses

Used in anxiety, nervousness, sedation, skeletal muscle relaxation[143,144]; reported useful as a skeletal muscle relaxant.[145]

Contraindications/Side Effects

May cause drowsiness or sedation in higher doses; use with caution while driving a car or operating heavy machinery[146]; long-term use has resulted in rash.

Do not use if prone to liver disease or if one has liver dysfunction.

Use with caution in patients on the following (action may be potentiated):

• Sedatives
• Antianxiety medications
• Hypnotics
• Antipsychotics
• Antidepressants

Do not use with the following:

• Alprazolam (Xanax) (may increase sedative effects)[147]
• Ethanol (may increase ethanol toxicity)[148] (conflicting study)[149]

Do not use in Parkinson's disease (has been reported to cause dopamine antagonism).[150]

Metabolic Functions

• Stress, anxiety

LICORICE (*Glycyrrhiza glabra*) ROOT

Dosage

250 mg, 3 times a day, either 1 hour before or 2 hours after meals and at bedtime, standardized to contain no more than 2% glycyrrhizin per dose (DGL); as expectorant, 15–30 drops of liquid extract, 3 times a day as needed, in juice or other beverage.

Uses

Used in adrenal insufficiency[151]; licorice extract beneficial as an expectorant and antitussive[152]; chewable DGL products used in gastric and duodenal ulcer.[153,154]

Contraindications/Side Effects

Do not use in high blood pressure (unless using the DGL licorice).[155]

Use with caution in individuals with hepatic or renal problems.

Licorice may deplete potassium. Use with caution if on the following:

• Thiazide diuretics
• Potassium-sparing diuretics

Do not use in hypertension, liver problems, kidney problems, or obesity due to possible mineralocorticoid effects of licorice (glycyrrhizin content).[156,157]

Metabolic Functions

• Adrenal support
• Gastrointestinal health (DGL form)

MILK THISTLE
(*Silybum marianum*) SEED

Dosage

80–240 mg, 1–3 times a day, standardized to contain 80% silymarin.

Uses

Antioxidant activity specifically for hepatic cells; used in liver diseases; acute/chronic liver inflammation[158,159,160]; liver protective against pharmaceutical drug toxicities including: psychotropics, ethanol and acetaminophen[161]; antidote for death cap mushroom poisoning[162,163]

Contraindications/Side Effects
None known.

Metabolic Functions
• Liver detoxification
• Antioxidant

NEXRUTINE
(from *Phellodendron amurense*)

Dosage
250 mg, 2–3 times a day.

Uses
Anti-inflammatory with COX-2 inhibition; used in arthritis and other forms of inflammation.

Contraindications/Side Effects
None known.

Metabolic Functions
• Inflammation
• Enzyme function

OLIVE (*Olea europaea*) LEAF

Dosage
250–500 mg, 1–3 times a day, standardized to contain 15–23% oleuropein per dose.

Uses
Antibiotic, antifungal, antiviral; has blood sugar regulating and blood pressure lowering activity.[164,165]

Contraindications/Side Effects
None known.

Metabolic Functions
• Gastrointestinal health
• Bowel terrain protocol

PASSION FLOWER
(*Passiflora spp.*) WHOLE PLANT

Dosage
100 mg, 2 times a day for anxiety; 200 mg at bedtime for insomnia; standardized to 3.5% isovitexin.

Uses
Sedative agent.[166,167]

Contraindications/Side Effects
Use caution when driving an automobile or operating heavy machinery.
Use with caution in individuals on the following:
• Sedatives
• Antidepressants
• Hypnotics
• Antianxiety agents
Reported to increase sleeping time induced by hexobarbital.[168]

Metabolic Functions
• Stress and sleeplessness

REISHI MUSHROOM
(*Ganoderma lucidum*)

Dosage
150–300 mg, 3–4 times a day, standardized 4% triterpenes and 10% polysaccharides (-1,3-glucans).

Uses
Used for proper immune function; fatigue, chemotherapy and radiation protection; blood pressure regulating; anticonvulsive.[169]

Contraindications/Side Effects
Use with caution if taking blood-thinning medications.[170]

Metabolic Functions
• Immune system regulation
• Cardiovascular health
• Stamina

RELORA® (from *Magnolia officinalis* and *Phellodendron amurense*)

Dosage
250 mg, 3 times a day.

Uses
Reduce anxiety, irritability, and nervousness.[171]

Contraindications/Side Effects
Use with caution if taking other sedative drugs.

Metabolic Functions
• Adrenal support for stress

- Helps with stress induced appetite increases
- Helps with sleep
- Helps regulate cortisol
- Improves serotonin and GABA relationships in the brain

RHODIOLA, ARCTIC ROOT (*Rhodiola rosea*) ROOT

Dosage
50–250 mg, 3 times a day standardized to contain 1% salidrosid, and/or 40–50% phenylpropenoids and/or 3–5% rosavins

Uses
Adaptogen/tonic, helps the body adapt to various stresses[172]; helps with cognition under stress; helps with immune regulation.

Contraindications/Side Effects
Use with caution if taking anti-arrhythmic medications.[173]

Metabolic Functions
- Adrenal function
- Cognitive function

ROSEMARY (*Rosmarinum officinalis*) LEAF

Dosage
100 mg, 2–3 times a day standardized to contain a minimum of 6.0% carnosic acid, 1.0% rosmarinic acid, and 1.5% ursolic acid.

Uses
Antioxidant[174]; anti-inflammatory.[175]

Contraindications/Side Effects
Use with caution in gastrointestinal ulcers.

Metabolic Functions
- Antioxidant
- Anti-inflammatory
- Enzyme function

SAW PALMETTO (*Serenoa repens*) BERRY

Dosage
160 mg, 2 times a day, standardized to at least 80–90% fatty acids and sterols.

Uses
Used in the treatment of benign prostatic hypertrophy (BPH).[176,177,178]

Contraindications/Side Effects
None known.

Metabolic Functions
- Male hormonal balance

SCHISANDRA (*Schizandra chinensis*) BERRY

Dosage
100 mg, 2 times a day with food, standardized to contain at least 9% schisandrin.

Uses
Adaptogen/health tonic; liver protection and detoxification[179,180]; support for chemotherapy and radiation therapy[181]; increases endurance, stamina, and work performance.

Contraindications/Side Effects
Use with caution in individuals with liver damage.
Do not use in pregnancy.[182]

Metabolic Functions
- Immune enhancement
- Detoxification
- Energy

SENNA (*Cassia senna*) SEED

Dosage
605 mg, 2 capsules 2 times a day, standardized to contain 8–10% total sennosides; take with water approximately 30 minutes prior to mealtimes; do not use more than 10 days consecutively.

Uses
Anthraquinone laxative.[183]

Contraindications/Side Effects
Avoid in children under 12 years of age.
May decrease absorption of oral medications.
Excessive use may lead to potassium loss and other electrolyte disturbances and may potentiate the effects of various pharmaceutical drugs—ask your pharmacist before taking laxatives such as cascara.[184]

Metabolic Functions
• Detoxification

SHIITAKE MUSHROOM (*Lentinus edodes*)

Dosage
100–400 mg, 3 times a day standardized to contain 3.2% KS-2 polysaccharides.

Uses
Immune enhancement[185]; antiviral (used in HIV therapy)[186]; may be used as adjunct in cancer therapy.[187]

Contraindications/Side Effects
Do not use if allergic to mushrooms.

Metabolic Functions
• Immune enhancement

SOY ISOFLAVONES

Dosage
10–300 mg daily.

Uses
Estrogenic effect; used in menopause.[188]

Contraindications/Side Effects
None known.

Metabolic Functions
• Female hormonal replacement

ST. JOHN'S WORT (*Hypericum perforatum*) FLOWERING BUDS

Dosage
300 mg, 3 times a day, standardized to 0.3–0.5% hypericin.

Uses
Used in mild to moderate depression, melancholia, anxiety[189,190,191]; antiviral activity in increased doses.[192]

Used topically in bruises, minor burns, wounds, and muscle soreness and sprains.

Contraindications/Side Effects
Due to possible drug interactions, only use St. John's wort under medical supervision if you are taking prescription and/or OTC medications. Some drugs known to have interactions with St. John's wort include:

• SSRI antidepressants (Prozac, Zoloft, Paxil)[193,194]
• Theophylline[195]
• Digoxin[196]
• HIV drugs (protease inhibitors)[197]
• Blood-thinning agents[198]
• Oral contraceptives[199]
• Immunosuppressive agents (cyclosporin)[200]

Not for use in severe depression.

Avoid tyramine-containing foods.

May elevate reversible liver enzyme function in high doses.[201]

May cause photosensitivity in susceptible individuals.[202]

Metabolic Functions
• Stress and depression

TEA TREE OIL (*Melaleuca alternifolia*) VOLATILE OILS

Dosage
Apply (preferably diluted) as needed.

Uses
FOR EXTERNAL USE ONLY; antifungal; antibacterial; used in mouthwash for dental and oral health; topically for burns, cuts, scrapes, insect bites.[203,204]

Contraindications/Side Effects
May cause allergic dermatitis in sensitive individuals.[205]

Metabolic Functions
• Topical use

TURMERIC (*Curcuma longa*) ROOT

Dosage
100–300 mg, 3 times a day with meals, standardized to contain 95% curcuminoids.

Uses
Antioxidant; anti-inflammatory[206]; used in arthritic problems; may also lower blood lipid levels.[207]

Contraindications/Side Effects
Some individuals may experience GI distress or irritation when beginning use.

Use with caution if peptic ulceration is present.

Use with caution if currently taking anti-coagulant medications.[208]

Do not use if biliary obstruction is present.[209]

Metabolic Functions

- Inflammation
- Enzyme function

VALERIAN
(*Valeriana officinalis*) ROOT

Dosage

200 mg, 1–4 times a day, standardized to 0.8–1% valerenic acids.

Uses

Used as a sedative/hypnotic; used in nervous tension during PMS, menopause; used in restless motor syndromes.[210,211]

Contraindications/Side Effects

May cause drowsiness or sedation.

Use with caution when driving a car or operating heavy machinery.[212]

Use with caution in individuals taking the following:

- Sedatives
- Antidepressants
- Hypnotics
- Antianxiety agents

Reported to increase sleeping time induced by pentobarbital.[213]

Metabolic Functions

- Stress; insomnia

Prescription and Nonprescription Nutrient Depletions

Prescription and nonprescription drugs can deplete the body of specific nutrients. The following is a guide to the most commonly used medications, prescription or otherwise, and the nutrient depletions that can result. Taking the nutrient in supplement form will help replace these nutrients. When taking medications, always check with your pharmacist or healthcare professional for possible side effects or interactions with other substances.

Prescription and Nonprescription Nutrient Depletions

MEDICATION	NUTRIENTS DEPLETED
ANTACIDS/LAXATIVES	
• Aluminum hydroxide (Amphojel, Riopan) • Magnesium hydroxide (Milk of Magnesia) • Magnesium oxide (Mag-Ox) • Magnesium sulfate (Epsom Salts) • Aluminum hydroxide and magnesium hydroxide (Mylanta, Maalox) • Aluminum hydroxide and magnesium carbonate (Algicon, Gaviscon) • Aluminum hydroxide and magnesium trisilicate (Gaviscon) • Aluminum hydroxide, magnesium hydroxide, and simethicone (Mylanta Plus, Gelusil)	• Calcium • Phosphorus
• Sodium Bicarbonate	• Potassium
ANTIBIOTICS	
• Penicillins (Veetids, Amoxil) • Cephalosporins (Keflex, Ceclor, Ceftin) • Fluoroquinolones (Cipro, Floxin, Levaquin) • Macrolides (Macrodantin, Zithromax) • Aminoglycosides (Garamycin,Cleocin)	• Biotin • Inositol • *Lactobacillus acidophilus, Bifidobacteria bifidum (bifidus)* • Vitamin B_1 • Vitamin B_2 • Vitamin B_3 • Vitamin B_6 • Vitamin B_{12} • Vitamin K

MEDICATION	NUTRIENTS DEPLETED
• Tetracyclines, Sulfonamides (Vibramycin, Minocin)	• Biotin • Calcium • Inositol • Iron • *Lactobacillus acidophilus,* *Bifidobacteria bifidum (bifidus)* • Magnesium • Vitamin B_1 • Vitamin B_2 • Vitamin B_3 • Vitamin B_6 • Vitamin B_{12} • Vitamin K
• Neomycin (Mycifradin)	• Beta-carotene • Iron • Vitamin A • Vitamin B_{12}
• Co-Trimoxazole (Bactrim, Septra)	• *Bifidobacteria bifidum (bifidus)* and *Lactobacillus acidophilus* • Folic acid
• Isoniazid (Nydrazid)	• Vitamin B_3 • Vitamin B_6 • Vitamin D
• Rifampin (Rifadin)	• Vitamin D
• Ethambutol (Myambutol)	• Copper • Zinc
ANTICONVULSANTS	
• Barbiturates (Tuinal, Seconal)	• Biotin • Calcium • Folic acid • Vitamin D • Vitamin K
• Phenytoin (Dilantin)	• Calcium • Folic acid • Vitamin B_1 • Vitamin B_{12} • Vitamin D • Vitamin K
• Carbamazepine (Tegretol)	• Biotin • Folic Acid • Vitamin D
• Primidone (Mysoline)	• Biotin • Folic acid
• Valproic Acid (Depakote, Depakene)	• Carnitine • Folic acid
ANTIDIABETICS	

• **Sulfonylureas:**
  Acetohexamide (Dymelor)
  Glyburide (Micronase, Diabeta)
  Tolazamide (Tolinase)
	• Coenzyme Q_{10}

MEDICATION	NUTRIENTS DEPLETED
• **Biguanides:** Metformin (Glucophage)	• Vitamin B_{12}

ANTI-GOUT DRUGS	
• Colchicine	• Beta-carotene • Potassium • Sodium • Vitamin B_{12}

ANTI-INFLAMMATORIES	
• **Salicylates:** Aspirin (Empirin, Ecotrin, Aspergum) Choline magnesium trisalicylate (Trilisate) Choline salicylate (Arthropan) Salsalate (Disalcid)	• Folic acid • Iron • Potassium • Sodium • Vitamin C
• **Nonsteroidal anti-inflammatory agents:** Celecoxib (Celebrex) Diclofenac (Cataflam) Diflunisal (Dolobid) Etodolac (Ultradol) Fenoprofen (Nalfon) Ibuprofen (Motrin, Advil) Ketoprofen (Orudis) Ketorolac (Toradol) Meclofenamate (Meclomen) Mefenamic acid (Ponstan) Nabumetone (Relafen) Naproxen (Nalfon) Piroxicam (Feldene) Sulindac (Clinoril) Tolmetin (Tolectin)	• Folic acid
• Indomethacin (Indocin)	• Folic acid • Iron
• **Corticosteroids:** Betamethasone (Celestone) Budesonide (Entocort) Cortisone (Cortone) Dexamethasone (Decadron) Flunisolide (Aerobid) Fluticasone (Salmeterol) Hydrocortisone (Cortef) Methylprednisolone (Medrol) Mometasone (Nasonex) Prednisolone (Prelone, Delta-Cortef) Prednisone (Deltasone, Orasone) Triamcinolone (Aristocort, Kenacort)	• Calcium • Folic acid • Magnesium • Potassium • Selenium • Vitamin C • Vitamin D • Zinc
• **Anti-inflammatory, Miscellaneous:** Sulfasalazine (Azulfidine)	• Folic acid

ANTIVIRALS	
• **Reverse Transcriptase Inhibitors:** Didanosine (Videx) Lamivudine (Epivir) Stavudine (Zerit)	• Carnitine • Copper • Vitamin B_{12} • Zinc

MEDICATION	NUTRIENTS DEPLETED
Reverse Transcriptase Inhibitors (cont.): Zalcitabine (ddC, HIVID) Zidovudine (Retrovir)	
• **Non-Nucleosides:** Delavirdine (Rescriptor) Nevirapine (Viramune)	• Carnitine • Copper • Vitamin B_{12} • Zinc

BENZODIAZEPINES

• Alprazolam (Xanax) • Diazepam (Valium)	• Melatonin

BRONCHODILATORS

• Theophylline (Slo-Bid, Theolair, Slo-Phylline, Theodur)	• Vitamin B_6

CARDIOVASCULAR DRUGS

• **Vasodilators:** Hydralazine (Apresoline)	• Coenzyme Q_{10} • Vitamin B_6
• **Loop diuretics:** Bumetanide (Bumex) Ethacrynic Acid (Edecrin) Furosemide (Lasix)	• Calcium • Magnesium • Potassium • Vitamin B_1 • Vitamin B_6 • Vitamin C • Zinc
• **Thiazide diuretics:** Hydrochlorothiazide (Esidrex, Hydrodiuril) Indapamide (Lozol) Methyclothiazide (Enduron) Metolazone (Zaroxolyn)	• Coenzyme Q_{10} • Magnesium • Potassium • Zinc
• **Potassium-sparing diuretics:** Triamterene (Dyazide)	• Calcium • Folic acid • Zinc
Hydrochlorothiazide (Esidrex, Hydrodiuril) Triamterene (Dyazide)]	• Calcium • Folic acid • Vitamin B_6 • Zinc
• **ACE inhibitors:** Captopril (Capoten) Enalopril (Vasotec)	• Zinc
• **Centrally-acting antihypertensives:** Clonidine (Catapres) Methyldopa (Aldomet)	• Coenzyme Q_{10}
Chlorthalidone (Hygroton)	• Zinc
• **Cardiac glycosides:** Digoxin (Lanoxin)	• Calcium • Magnesium • Phosphorus • Vitamin B_1
• **Beta-blockers:** Acebutolol (Sectral) Atenolol (Tenormin)	• Coenzyme Q_{10} • Melatonin

MEDICATION	NUTRIENTS DEPLETED
Beta-Blockers (cont.): Betaxolol (Kerlone) Bisoprolol (Cardicor) Carteolol (Cartrol) Carvedilol (Coreg) Esmolol (Brevibloc) Labetalol (Normodyne) Metoprolol (Lopressor, Toprox XL) Nadolol (Corgard) Pindolol (Visken) Propranolol (Inderal) Sotalol (Betapace) Timolol (Blocadren)	

CHOLESTEROL-LOWERING DRUGS

• **HMG-CoA Reductase Inhibitors:** Atorvastatin (Lipitor) Cerivastatin (Baycol) Fluvastatin (Lescol) Lovastatin (Mevacor) Pravastatin (Pravachol) Simvastatin (Zocor)	• Coenzyme Q_{10}
• **Bile Acid Sequestrants:** Cholestyramine (Questran)	• Beta-carotene • Calcium • Folic acid • Iron • Magnesium • Phosphorus • Vitamin A • Vitamin B_{12} • Vitamin D • Vitamin E • Vitamin K • Zinc
Colestipol (Colestid)	• Beta-carotene • Folic acid • Iron • Vitamin A • Vitamin B_{12} • Vitamin D • Vitamin E

ELECTROLYTE REPLACEMENT

• Potassium Chloride (Timed Release)	• Vitamin B_{12}

FEMALE HORMONES

• Oral contraceptives	• Folic acid • Tyrosine • Vitamin B_2 • Vitamin B_6 • Vitamin B_{12} • Vitamin C • Magnesium • Zinc

MEDICATION	NUTRIENTS DEPLETED
• **Estrogen replacement (ERT) and hormone replacement (HRT) therapies:** Conjugated Estrogens (Premarin) Esterified Estrogens (Estratab, Menest) Estrogens (Estrace, Estinyl) Medroxyprogesterone (Provera) Raloxifene (Evista)	• Magnesium • Vitamin B_6 • Zinc
LAXATIVES	
• Mineral Oil	• Beta-carotene • Calcium • Vitamin A • Vitamin D • Vitamin E • Vitamin K
• Bisacodyl (Dulcolax)	• Potassium
PSYCHOTHERAPEUTIC AGENTS	
• **Tricyclic antidepressants:** Amitriptyline (Elavil) Desipramine (Norpramin) Doxepin (Sinequan) Nortriptyline (Aventyl)	• Coenzyme Q_{10} • Vitamin B_2
• **Phenothiazines:** Chlorpromazine (Thorazine) Thioridazine (Mellaril) Fluphenazine (Prolixin)	• Coenzyme Q_{10} • Vitamin B_2
• **Butyrophenones:** Haloperidol (Haldol)	• Coenzyme Q_{10}
ULCER MEDICATIONS	
• **H-2 receptor antagonists:** Cimetidine (Tagamet) Famotidine (Pepcid) Nizatadine (Axid) Ranitidine (Zantac)	• Calcium • Folic Acid • Iron • Vitamin B_{12} • Vitamin D • Zinc
• **Proton pump inhibitors:** Lansoprazole (Prevacid) Omeprazole (Losec)	• Vitamin B_{12}
MISCELLANEOUS MEDICATIONS	
• Methotrexate	• Folic Acid
• Penicillamine (Cuprimine)	• Copper • Magnesium • Vitamin B_6 • Zinc
• Acetaminophen (Tylenol)	• Glutathione

Supplement Protocols for Other Common Conditions

The following ten supplement protocols are provided for common conditions that the body of this book could not address in depth. If you have any of these conditions, the protocols are offered as a starting point to improve your health. Later, you may wish to use the System Discovery Assessment questionnaire on pages 433–456 to fine-tune your supplement use. In addition to using supplements, the Healthy Living Guidelines presented in Chapter 13 should be followed for the best results. (*Note:* If a supplement has not been discussed in the body of this book, refer to Appendix 1, "Nutrient Reference Guide" or Appendix 2, "Herbal Reference Guide," or if necessary, do some independent research on your own before adding it to your supplement regimen.)

ATTENTION DEFICIT DISORDER (ADD)/ATTENTION DEFICIT HYPERACTIVITY DISORDER (ADHD)

Conventional therapies include the use of stimulants such as methylphenidate (Ritalin) and amphetamine (Adderall). However, there is much concern over the long-term impact of these medications on neurotransmitter function. Children on these drugs often end up "graduating" to antidepressants because of serotonin-receptor "burn-out" from continual sympathetic receptor stimuli caused by ADD/ADHD drug therapy.

Although the role of diet is often downplayed in conventional medicine, early studies showed it has a significant effect on the etiology of the condition. Three large trials published in different journals from 1985 to 1994 showed artificial colorings, artificial flavorings, sugar, and common allergens such as dairy, wheat, chocolate, corn, soy, citrus fruits, yeast, egg, and peanuts to be implicated in ADHD. All three trials showed significant improvement in children when the diets eliminated some or all of these foods.

However, diet, along with chromium, magnesium, fatty acid, and other nutrient deficiencies are still only part of the ADD/ADHD picture. Many children with these conditions have significant biochemical disturbances resulting from poor diet, excessive antibiotics and other drug therapy, environmental exposure, and poor nutrient status.

Supplement Protocol for ADD and ADHD	
CATEGORY	**NATURAL PRODUCT**
Herb	Grape seed extract: 25–100 mg, standardized to 95 percent proanthocyandin content and at least 90 percent phenols, one to three times daily.
	Ginkgo: 40–60 mg, two times daily.
	Bacopa: 100 mg, two times daily.
Vitamin/Mineral/Trace Element/Nutraceutical	Alpha GPC: 1,000 mg daily
	Lactobacillus acidophilus/Bifidobacterium: 2–5 billion CFU, daily for one month.
	DHA: For ages three to six, 60 mg, two times daily; for ages six to twelve, 120 mg, two times daily; for ages twelve and older, 240 mg, two times daily.
	Chromium GTF: 200 mcg daily.
	Magnesium: 400–600 mg daily.
	Phosphatidylserine: 100 mg daily
	DMAE: 50–100 mg, two times daily.
Additional Supplements to Consider	Acetyl L-carnitine: 50–250 mg, two times daily.

Key metabolic code considerations:

- Evaluate heavy metal exposure.

- Check for history of antibiotic use, and evaluate intestinal health.

- Check organic acids in urine for dysbiosis and, if needed, work on reestablishing healthy flora in the gut.

- Check amino acid status. If deficient, have an amino acid compound made.

- Evaluate stress and family dynamics.

ALLERGIES

There are a number of natural products on the market that help in treating the symptoms of allergies. Antioxidant and antihistaminic supplements are at the core of these recommendations.

Supplement Protocol for Allergies	
CATEGORY	**NATURAL PRODUCT**
Herb	*First Try*
	Stinging nettle (leaf): Use 3–6 capsules of 300 mg at onset of symptoms, then every four hours as needed. (Use a freeze-dried product if possible.)
	Grapeseed extract: 25–100 mg, one to three times daily, standardized to contain a procyanidolic value of not less than 95% and 90% total phenols.
Vitamin/Mineral/Trace Element/Nutraceutical	*First Try*
	Quercetin: 300–400 mg, 3 times daily
	Vitamin C: 500–1,000 mg, two times daily
	Methyl sulfonyl methane (MSM): 2,000–5,000 mg daily
	Vitamin B_6: 50 mg daily
Homeopathic Remedy	Homeopathic combination formulas are available for many conditions. Listed below are some of the most common single homeopathic remedies for symptom relief from allergies:
	Allium cepa
	Ambrosia artemisia folia
	Arsenicum album
	Arundo mauritanica
	Drosera rotundifolia
	Histaminum
	Kali bichromicum
	Sabadilla
Additional Supplements to Consider	Omega-3 fatty acids derived from fish oils: 1–2 capsules, 500–1,000 mg each, two times daily.

Key metabolic code considerations:

- Check intestinal health and follow protocols for healing leaky gut syndrome.
- Check for environmental and heavy metal toxicity.
- Work on liver detoxification.
- Check adrenal function.
- Test for food allergies.
- Administer vitamin C flush with MSM (see the inset "Performing a Vitamin C Flush" on page 254 for instructions), if needed for severe allergy symptoms.

ALZHEIMER'S AND COGNITIVE FUNCTION

Mild cognitive impairment may be an early predictor of Alzheimer's disease. Prevention of memory loss and cognitive disorders is key in natural therapeutics. It is also important to evaluate the stress in your life. Stress is considered a major contributor to short-term memory loss and cognitive impairment since it increases the release of cortisol, which appears to shrink the hippocampus, the learning center of the brain. Other factors that can affect cognitive function include genetic predisposition; infections, including from prions (small infectious protein particles) and fungus; poor nutritional status of vitamin B_{12}, folic acid, omega-3 fatty acids; heavy metal or environmental toxicity; poor detoxification pathways; and arterial plaque formation.

Supplement Protocol to Improve Cognitive Function	
CATEGORY	**NATURAL PRODUCT**
Vitamin/Mineral/Trace Element/Nutraceutical	Alpha GPC: 1,000 mg, one to two times daily.
	Acetyl L-carnitine: 500 mg, one to two times daily.
	DMAE: 100 mg, two to three times daily.
	Omega-3 fatty acids derived from fish oils: 3–5 grams daily.
	Vitamin B_{12}: 500 mcg, twice daily.
	Vitamin E: 800–2,000 IU daily.
	Folic acid: 800 mcg daily.
Herbs	Bacopa: 150 mg, two to three times daily.
	Ginkgo: 60 mg, two to three times daily.
	Huperzine A: 100–150 mcg daily.
	Relora®: 250 mg, three times daily for stress-related memory loss; *or* Vinpocetine: 10–50 mg daily.

Key metabolic code considerations:

- Check for heavy metals and initiate detoxification process.

- Have an organic acids urine test to make sure that fungal or other microbes are not a contributing factor.

- Control belly fat.

- Work on preventing inflammation chemistry, check levels of C-reactive protein, homocysteine, hemoglobin A_1C, and fibrinogen.

- Exercise regularly.

BENIGN PROSTATIC HYPERPLASIA (BPH)

Several supplements work well to help prevent the development of BPH when taken in combination or alone. Taking steps to modulate estrogen metabolism, inhibit the enzyme 5-lipoxygenase, and decreasing inflammatory chemistry initiators are all essential steps to regaining prostate health.

Supplement Protocol for Benign Prostatic Hyperplasia	
CATEGORY	NATURAL PRODUCT
Herb	Saw palmetto berry: 160 mg twice daily, standardized to 80 to 90% free fatty acids.
	Pygeum bark: 50–100 mg twice daily, standardized to 12% phytosterols.
	Stinging nettle (root): 250 mg twice daily, standardized to 1 to 2% plant silica.
	Pumpkin seed oil: 160 mg, three times daily.
	Green tea extract: 500 mg daily, standardized to contain 50 to 97% polyphenols, containing at least 50% (-) epigallocatechin-3-gallate (EGCG) per dose. Caffeine-free products are recommended.
	Moducare: 3 capsules of 20 mg, two to three times daily for one month, then one 20 mg dose, three times daily thereafter.
	DIM (Bioresponse): 150 mg, two times daily for estrogen metabolism.
	Nexrutine: 500 mg, three times daily
Vitamin/Mineral/Trace Element/Nutraceutical	Zinc: 15–35 mg daily.
	Lycopene: 5 mg, two times daily
Additional Supplements to Consider	Omega-3 fatty acids derived from fish oils: 1–2 500–1,000-mg capsules, two times daily.
	Vitamin E: 400 IU daily.

Key metabolic code considerations:

- Reread Chapters 9 and 10 on the intestines and the environment, respectively.

- Get an amino acid panel done to check for deficiencies.

- Eat several servings of cooked tomato products each week. Cooked tomatoes supply a rich source of the carotenoid lycopene, which is especially beneficial in supporting prostate tissue health.

- Increase intake of soy and vegetables.

- Decrease intake of red meat, nonorganic protein sources (for example, chicken), as well as non-organic dairy products, since these may have hormonal residues that could contribute to the development of a more serious prostate condition.

- Exercise in moderation.

- Reduce stress.

- Evaluate adrenal activity.

CHRONIC FATIGUE SYNDROME (CFS)/FIBROMYALGIA (FM)

Natural therapeutics attempt to correct the chronic disruption of energy production present in both CFS and FM and that is caused by environmental toxins, dysbiosis, infections from yeast or other microorganisms, low thyroid and adrenal function, or in many cases, a combination of these initiators of inflammation. Infrared saunas may also be of value in detoxification of metabolites that are stored in muscle and adipose tissue. Although natural therapeutics can be very effective for treating these conditions, in my experience, they require a wide array of supplements and dedication to a very healthy diet.

Supplement Protocol for CFS and FM	
CATEGORY	**NATURAL PRODUCT**
Herb	*Try first* Cordyceps: two 525-mg capsules, two to three times daily, standardized to contain 0.14% adenosine and 5% mannitol.
	Try first Rhodiola: 50 mg, two times daily, standardized to contain 1% salidrosid and/or 40 to 50% phenylpropenoids.
	If anxious, try Relora®: 250 mg, two to three times daily.
	Schisandra: 100 mg, two times daily, standardized to contain a minimum 9% schisandrins.
	Try first Moducare: three 20 mg capsules, two times daily.
	Chlorella: 3–5 grams daily.
Vitamin/Mineral/Trace Element/Nutraceutical	*Try first* Coenzyme Q_{10}: 50–100 mg, two times daily.
	Try first S-adenosylmethionine (SAM-e): 400–1,600 mg daily.
	Try first Magnesium/malic acid: 2 capsules of 150 mg magnesium and 700 mg malic acid daily.
	NADH: 2.5–5 mg daily.
	L-carnitine: 500–1,000 mg twice daily.
	Adrenal glandular (New Zealand): 200 mg, three times daily.
	Thyroid glandular (New Zealand): 60–400 mg, daily.
	Alpha lipoic acid: 300 mg, two times daily.
	Omega-3 fatty acids derived from fish oils: 3–5 grams daily.
Additional Supplements to Consider	Vitamin B complex: 25–50 mg, two times daily.
	Bowel terrain protocol: includes cat's claw, L-glutamine, olive leaf, grapefruit seed extract, oregano, and probiotics (acidophilus products).

Key metabolic code considerations:

- Evaluate heavy metal intoxication and liver detox pathways.

- Evaluate amino acid deficiencies.

- Initiate detoxification of the intestines; work on dysbiosis.

- Test for infections from microorganisms.

- Test for possible food allergies.

- Evaluate adrenal function.

- Evaluate thyroid function.

- Look at stress as a source of adrenal exhaustion.

- Evaluate magnesium and other mineral loss.

- Improve glutathione function in the body.

DIABETES

Educating yourself about the importance of a healthy lifestyle and diet, and making the neccesary changes are crucial for improving blood sugar control. Weight control is one of the most important ways to reduce the risk of diabetes. Exercising regularly, limiting the amount of refined foods (sugars and foods from the bread and cereal group) and soft drinks you consume, and trying to eat more fiber-rich foods are other important lifestyle factors. It is also important to pay attention to the glycemic index of the foods you eat. Diets very high in sugar may worsen glucose tolerance in non-diabetics and lead to insulin resistance and eventually to type 2 diabetes.

Natural therapeutics for diabetes focus on dietary supplements that help the body keep blood sugar levels in balance. It is important to inform your physician of any dietary supplements you are taking and work together to closely monitor blood sugar levels and to reduce medication if necessary. Also, inform your physician of any supplements you want to take as some supplements may interact with certain medications you have been prescribed.

Supplement Protocol for Diabetes

CATEGORY	NATURAL PRODUCT
Herb	*Gymnema sylvestre:* 250 mg, two times daily standardized to contain 25% gymnemic acids; *or*
	Bitter melon: 200 mg, two times daily, standardized to contain 7% bitter principles and 0.5% charatin.
	Evening primrose or borage oil: 500–1,500 mg daily, standardized to contain 8% GLA content per dose; expeller-pressed oil is preferred.
	Glucomannan (from konjac root): 8–13 grams daily.
	Milk thistle: 600 mg daily, standardized to contain 80% silymarin
	Cinnamon extract: 250–500 mg, three times daily.
Vitamin/Mineral/Trace Element/Nutraceutical	Cyclo-hispro: 200–300 mg, four times daily.
	Vanadyl sulfate: 250 mcg, three times daily.
	Alpha lipoic acid: 300–600 mg daily.
	Omega-3 fatty acids derived from fish oils: 2–6 grams daily.
	Magnesium: 600–1,000 mg daily.
	NAC: 500 mg, two times daily to reduce glycation.
	Chromium GTF: 200–800 mcg daily.
Additional Supplements to Consider	Vitamin B complex: 25–50 mg, two times daily.
	Zinc: 15–35 mg daily.

Key metabolic code considerations:

- Diabetics will often test high in the stress/adrenal section of the System Discovery Assessment questionnaire on pages 433–456 and should complete the entire questionnaire to find other involvements.

- Check for dysbiosis.

- Evaluate heavy metals.

- Evaluate stress and cortisol production.

- Evaluate liver and support its function.

- Exercise to improve blood glucose levels.

HIGH CHOLESTEROL

Natural products that help to regulate and manage cholesterol levels include antioxidants, cholesterol-lowering supplements, and vitamins/minerals that help support the natural conversion of cholesterol into a usable substance for the body.

Supplement Protocol for High Cholesterol	
CATEGORY	**NATURAL PRODUCT**
Herb	*Try first* Policosanol: 15 mg, two times daily until cholesterol is under control, then maintain at 10–20 mg daily
	Garlic: 400 mg (standardized extract), two times daily; *or* 600 mg (standardized, aged extract), two times daily, standardized to 10–12 mg/gm alliin and 4 mg of TAP per dose; aged garlic products standardized to contain 1 mg/gm S-allyl cysteine (SAC) content.
	Olive leaf: 250–500 mg of olive leaf, one to three times a day, standardized to contain 15 to 23% oleuropein per dosage.
	Green tea extract: 500 mg daily, standardized to contain 50% to 97% polyphenols, containing at least 50% (-) epigallocatechin-3-gallate (EGCG) per dose. Caffeine-free products are recommended.
Vitamin/Mineral/Trace Element/Nutraceutical	Chromium GTF: 200–600 mcg daily.
	Try first Inositol-hexaniacinate: 25–100 mg daily.
	L-carnitine: 500–4,000 mg daily in divided doses.
	CoQ_{10}: 30–100 mg, two times daily.
	Vitamin E: 400 IU daily.
	Alpha lipoic acid: 300 mg daily for liver support.
Additional Supplements to Consider	Omega-3 fatty acids derived from fish oils: 1.5 g, two times daily.

Key metabolic code considerations:

- Check for heavy metal toxicity.

- Check for intestinal or gut health, including dysbiosis and digestion.

- Check liver function.

- Check thyroid function.

- Check adrenal glands and stress.

HYPERTENSION (HIGH BLOOD PRESSURE)

High blood pressure is a serious condition; make sure to check your blood pressure regularly, even if you think that it is normal. If your blood pressure is borderline high (equal to or higher than 120–139/80–89 mmHg), aggressive steps using nutrition and exercise to lower it should be taken. Otherwise medication will be needed.

Conventional treatments include a wide array of drugs such as diuretics, beta-blocking agents, calcium channel blocking agents, and ACE inhibitors. If you are taking medication, refer to Appendix 3 "Prescription and Nonprescription Nutrient Depletions" on page 512 to replenish potential nutrient losses. This is especially important in this category of drugs because many of them will deplete CoQ_{10}, potassium, calcium, and magnesium, which are essential to a long-term blood pressure control strategy. Changes may occur in your blood pressure if you are on medication, so make sure that you are being supervised by a healthcare professional.

Supplement Protocol for Hypertension	
CATEGORY	**NATURAL PRODUCT**
Herb	*Try first* Hawthorn: 250 mg, three times daily standardized to 2% vitexin and/or 20% procyanidins per dose.
	Coleus forskohlii: 250 mg (1% standardized extract), two times daily *or* 50 mg (18% standardized extract), two times daily standardized to 1% forskolin.
	Garlic: 400 mg (standardized extract), two times daily *or* 600 mg (standardized, aged extract), two times daily standardized to 10–12 mg/gm alliin and 4 mg of total allicin potential (TAP) per dose; aged garlic products standardized to contain 1 mg/gm S-allyl cysteine (SAC) content.
	Try first if stress is suspected trigger Relora®: 250 mg, three times daily for stress.
	Try if fibrinogen is high Nattokinase: 800–2,400 FU, two to three times daily.
Vitamin/Mineral/Trace Element/Nutraceutical	*Try first* Magnesium: 400–1,000 mg daily.
	Try first (use at least six months) Coenzyme Q_{10}: 100 mg, two to three times daily.
	L-carnitine: One to two 500-mg capsules daily.
	L-arginine: 6–10 grams daily to improve nitric oxide (NO) formation in your blood. (NO is a principle chemical that causes relaxation of constricted vessels.)
Additional Supplements to Consider	Calcium: 1,000–1,500 mg daily.
	Try first Omega-3 fatty acids derived from fish oils: 1–2 500–1,000-mg capsules, two times daily.

Key metabolic code considerations:

- Evaluate heavy metal and environmental exposure.

- Lose weight, if overweight, especially if you have belly fat.

- Exercise regularly.

- At minimum, assess your levels of fasting insulin, homocysteine, C-reactive protein, hemoglobin A_1C, cholesterol, and fibrinogen. Also, consider checking your erythrocyte magnesium level.

- Have a salivary cortisol test to determine the role of stress hormones in your chemistry.

- Evaluate the impact of stress on your blood pressure. Learn meditation or another form of relaxation such as yoga.

- Watch your intake of refined sugar and carbohydrates.

- Quit smoking.

- Initiate liver and environmental detoxification, if appropriate.

- If symptoms of gastrointestinal discomfort are present, work on intestinal health.

OSTEOARTHRITIS

Natural therapies for osteoarthritis include antioxidants, anti-inflammatory agents, COX-2 inhibiting herbs, and substances that protect connective tissues and bone. If you have been on arthritis drugs for any period of time, work on rebuilding the mucosa of the intestine. Taking L-glutamine and probiotics will help. The use of hot soaks, heating pads, and joint support devices can also be of benefit along with a wide array of topical creams.

Natural Therapies for Osteoarthritis	
CATEGORY	**NATURAL PRODUCT**
Herb	*Try first* Nexrutine: 500 mg, two to three times daily; *or* another herbal COX-2 inhibitor such as hops extract and ginger and follow manufacturer's instructions for dose.
	Try first Chondroitin sulfate: 300—1,500 mg daily with glucosamine sulfate or hydrochloride: 1,500–2,000 mg daily.
	Turmeric: 100–300 mg, standardized to contain 95% curcuminoids anti-inflammatory, three times daily.
	Boswellia: 200–400 mg, standardized to contain 65% boswellic acids, three times daily; may also be used as a topical cream.
Vitamin/Mineral/Trace Element/Nutraceutical	*Add, if not successful, try* Methyl sulfonyl methane (MSM): 2,000–5,000 mg daily.
	S-adenosylmethionine (SAM-e): 400–1,600 mg daily.
	Collagen: 200 mg two to three times daily.
Additional Supplements to Consider	*Add first* Omega-3 fatty acids derived from fish oils: 1–2 capsules of 1–2 grams, two times daily.
	Boron: 3–6 mg daily.
	Selenium: 200 mcg daily.
	Vitamin A as mixed carotenoids: 10,000–20,000 IU daily.
	Vitamin C: 500–2,000 mg daily.
	Vitamin E: 400 IU daily.

PARKINSON'S DISEASE

Natural therapeutics can be used to help balance the neurotransmitter dopamine and to support healthy brain function, including memory and blood flow. Supplements can also help to reduce the chronic inflammation that is associated with Parkinson's disease.

Supplement Protocol for Parkinson's Disease	
CATEGORY	**NATURAL PRODUCT**
Herb	Ginkgo: 40 mg, three times daily, standardized to contain either 24% ginkgo flavoglycosides and 6% triterpenes per dose, or to 27% flavoglycosides and 6% triterpenes per dose.
	Grape seed extract: 25–100 mg, two to three times daily, standardized to 95 percent proanthocyandin content and at least 90 percent phenols.
	Bacopa: 100 mg, three times daily, standardized to contain 20% bacosides A and B for dementia associated with Parkinson's disease.
	Chlorella: 3–5 grams daily for heavy metal and environmental detoxification.
	Turmeric: 300 mg, three times daily.
Vitamin/Mineral/Trace Element/Nutraceutical	NADH: 5–10 mg, two times daily.
	Multivitamin and mineral formula
	Selenium: 200 mcg daily.
	Vitamin E: 800 IU
	Vitamin C: 2,000–4,000 mg daily.
	Carotenoids: 25,000 IU daily.
	5 MTHF or folic acid: 400–800 mcg daily.
	Acetyl-L-Carnitine: 500–2,000 mg daily in divided doses
	Alpha lipoic acid: 300 mg, two to three times daily.
	Co-Q$_{10}$: 1,200 mg daily.
	DMSA: Use under supervision of a healthcare practitioner for detoxification of heavy metals
	Fish oils: 5,000 mg daily.
	N acetyl L cysteine: 500 mg, two times daily to improve detoxification.
	EDTA: Available in powder and capsule form. Take $1/4$ teaspoon of powder or a 1,000 mg capsule, three times daily; if lead is high in body, take $1/4$ teaspoon of powder or a 1,000 mg capsule, four to five times daily for a total of 4,000–5,000 mg for 120 days, then reevaluate lead levels.

Key metabolic code considerations:

- Get evaluated for heavy metal or environmental toxicity.

- Get an amino acid assay done to determine whether you have specific amino acid deficiencies. A deficiency indicates that you do not have the building blocks needed to build dopamine- and chemistry-regulating enzymes.

- Get an organic acid urine test to determine whether your body is producing toxic intermediate metabolites, an indicator of heightened oxidative stress, dysbiosis, and poor utilization of vitamins, as well as metabolism of neurotransmitters. Yeast mycotoxins are neurotoxic and dysbiosis can cause malabsorption of nutrients.

- Evaluate stress and adrenal exhaustion, especially if you feel washed out. This could be a hidden trigger of chronic inflammation.

- Consider various IV-treatments such as IV-glutathione, vitamin C, and chelation under a doctor's supervision.

- Follow detoxification guidelines for liver, environment, and yeast (intestine) in Chapter 11.

- Get mild exercise if possible, such as daily walking.

Resources

The following is a list of educational resources and manufacturers of products referred to in this book. This information is provided to enable you to enhance your understanding of health, as well as to contact the companies if you are interested in learning more about their products. Be aware that addresses and telephone numbers are subject to change.

Manufacturers of Herbal and Nutritional Products

There are many companies that make excellent herbal and nutritional supplements. Below are several that have targeted formulas for many of the key health issues discussed in this book. Their inclusion does not constitute an endorsement of one company over another, rather they are listed because I have found their products to be effective or of high quality. Some companies sell to both professionals and stores; other companies sell only to health professionals. Professional products are indicated with an asterisk.*

COMPANY	PHONE NO.	WEBSITE	PRODUCTS
Allergy Research Group*	(800) 545–9960	www.allergyresearch group.com	Quality dietary supplements
Balance Dermaceuticals	(888) 321-1922	www.balancederm.com	Supplier of Trans-D Tropin®
Douglas Laboratories*	(412) 494-0122	www.douglaslabs.com	Quality dietary supplements
Eclectic Institute	(800) FDA-HERB	www.eclecticherb.com	Freeze-dried encapsulated herbs; liquid extracts
Enzymatic Therapy	(800) 783–2286	www.enzy.com	Standardized encapsulated and tableted products
Frontier Natural Products	(800) 669-3275	www.frontiercoop.com	Bulk herbs, encapsulated herbal supplements
Heel/BHI	(800) 621-7644	www.heelusa.com	Quality homeopathic formulations and drainage formulas

COMPANY	PHONE NO.	WEBSITE	PRODUCTS
Herb Pharm	(800) 348–4372	www.herb-pharm.com	Quality liquid herbal extract; children's formulas
Intensive Nutrition	(800) 333–7414	www.intensivenutrition.com	Quality dietary supplements
Marco Pharma International	(800) 999–3001	www.internatural.com (website for distributor of Marco Pharma products)	Quality dietary supplements, homeopathic and drainage herbal formulas
Metagenics*	(800) 962–9400	www.metagenics.com	Full service line of products, herbs, nutraceuticals
Moducare	(877) 297–7332	www.moducare.com	Quality dietary supplements
Next Pharmaceuticals	(949) 450-0203	www.nextpharmaceuticals.com	Specialized Herbal Extracts (Nexrutine, Relora®)
New Chapter	(800) 543–7279	www.new-chapter.com	Herbal compounds, supercritical extracts
Pekana	0049–7563–91160	www.pekana.com	Quality drainage formulas
Perque*	(800) 525–7372	www.Perque.com	Quality vitamin, mineral, and nutraceutical line
Pharmanex	(801) 345–9800	www.pharmanex.com	Standardized encapsulated and tableted products
PhytoPharmica	(800) 376–7889	www.phytopharmica.com	Quality dietary supplements; available through select pharmacies and healthcare professionals
Premiere Research Labs	(512) 238-0610	www.prlabs.com	Quality dietary supplements
Purity Life Distributors Canada	(800) 265–2615	www.puritylife.com	Wide distribution of products
Solgar	(800) 645–2246 or (877) 765–4274	www.solgar.com	Encapsulated herbs; standardized products mixed with raw herb
Thorne Research Labs*	(208) 263–1337	www.thorne.com	Quality dietary supplements, herbal and nutraceutical preparations
Vinco Labs*	(800) 245–1939	www.vincoinc.com	Standardized herbal supplements, specialty combination vitamin/ mineral and nutraceutical formulas

Healthy Home Products

Below are several companies that make products referred to in this book.

COMPANY	PHONE NO.	WEBSITE	PRODUCTS
Abundant Earth Products	(888) 513–2784	www.AbundantEarth.com	Home products
AFM	(619) 239-0321	www.afmsafecoat.com	Non-toxic paints, sealers, finishes, carpet, cleaning materials
Aquacheck Water	(800) 504–5580	www.southwest.net/ aquacheck	Reverse osmosis water-purifying units
Earthweave	(706) 278–8200	www.earthweave.com	Non-toxic carpeting
Eco-Friendly Flooring	(866) 250–3273	www.ecofriendlyflooring.com	Natural flooring
EcoHome	(323) 662–5207	www.ecohome.org	Products and services for sustainable and ecological building
Furnature	(800) 326–4895	www.furnature.com	Chemical-free furniture and organic bedding
LifeKind	(800) 284–4983	www.lifekind.com	Organic bedding
Marmoleum	(866) 627–6653	www.themarmoleumstore.com	Natural linoleum flooring
Natural Cork	(800) 404–2675	www.naturalcork.com	Natural cork flooring
Natural Home Products	(707) 824-0914	www.naturalhomeproducts.com	Natural products for the home
NaturaLawn of America	(800) 989–5444	www.nl-amer.com	Organic lawn care
Watts Premier Water	(800) 752–5582	www.premierh2o.com	Reverse osmosis systems
Weatherbos	(800) 664–3978	www.weatherbos.com	Non-toxic paints, sealants, finishes

Recommended Reading

American Herbal Products Association, *Botanical Safety Handbook* (Boca Raton: CRC Press, 1997)

Bradley, PR, ed., *British Herbal Compendium,* Vol. 1 (Bournemouth, England: British Herbal Medicine Association, 1992)

Brinker, F. *Herb Contraindications and Drug Interactions* (Sandy, OR: Eclectic Medical Publications, 1997)

LaValle, J, Hawkins, EB. *Black Cohosh: Nature's Versatile Healer* (New York, NY: Avery Publishing, 2000)

LaValle, J, Krinsky, D, Hawkins, E, Pelton, R, Willis, N. *Natural Therapeutics Pocket Guide* (Hudson, OH: LexiComp, Inc., 2000, 2002)

LaValle. J. *The COX-2 Connection.* (Brookline, MA: Redwing Book Co., 2001)

Leung, A. et al., *Encyclopedia of Common Natural Ingredients Used in Food, Drugs, and Cosmetics* (New York: John Wiley and Sons, Inc., 1996)

Marz, RB. *Medical Nutrition from Marz.* (Portland, OR: Omni-Press, 1997)

Newall, CA. et al., *Herbal Medicines: A Guide for Health-Care Professionals* (London: The Pharmaceutical Press, 1996)

Pelton, R, LaValle, J. *The Nutritional Costs of Prescription Drugs.* (Morton Publishing Co, 2000)

Pelton, R, Lavalle, J, Hawkins, E, Krinsky, D. *Drug-Induced Nutrient Depletion Handbook* (Hudson, OH: LexiComp, Inc., 1999, 2001)

Schulz, V. et al., *Rational Phytotherapy* (Berlin: Springer-Verlag, 1998)

Weiss, RF. *Herbal Medicine* (Stuttgart: Hippokrates Verlag GmbH, 1988)

Zand, J, LaValle J, Spreen A. *Smart Medicine for Healthier Living: A Practical A-to-Z Reference to Natural and Conventional Treatments for Adults.* (Albuquerque, NM: HealthPress, 2000)

Recommended Journals and Newsletters

HerbalGram
P.O. Box 201660
Austin, TX 78720
(512) 331–8868
www.healthworld.com/library/periodicals/
    journals/HerbalGram/index.html

Nutrition Science News
1301 Spruce Street
Boulder, CO 80302
(303) 939–8440
www.nutritionsciencenews.com

Natural Home Magazine
201 East Fourth Street
Loveland, CO 80537
(800) 272–2193
www.naturalhomemag.com

Townsend Letter
911 Tyler Street
Port Townsend, WA 98368
(360) 385–6021
www.tldp.com

Recommended Internet Sites

Alternative Medicine Homepage
American Board of Chelation Therapy
American Botanical Council
American Herbal Products Association
American Herbalists Guild
Childsake
Dr. Mercola's Natural Health Homepage
Dr. James LaValle

Dietary Supplement Information Bureau
Environlink
Health World Online
Healthwell Health and Healing Articles
Herb Research Foundation
Herbal Bookworm
Herbal Hall
Herbal Resources
HerbMed
International Board of Clinical
  Metal Toxicology
Medline abstract search
Robyn's Recommended Readings

www.pitt.edu/~cbw/altm.html
www.abct.com
www.herbalgram.org
www.ahpa.org
www.healthy.net/herbalists/
www.childsake.com
www.mercola.com
www.doctorlavalle.com
www.metaboliccode.com
www.livinglonger.com
www.supplementinfo.org
www.envirolink.com
www.healthy.net
www.healthwell.com
www.herbs.org
www.teleport.com/~jono/
www.crl.com/~robbee/herbal.html
www.herbsinfo.com/default.htm
www.herbmed.org

www.ibcmt.com
www.ncbi.nlm.nih.gov/PubMed
www.wtp.net/~rrr/journals.html

References

Chapter 1

Dannhardt G, Kiefer W. "Cyclooxygenase inhibitors—current status and future prospects," *Eur J Med Chem,* 36(2) (February 2001): 109–26.

Frankish, H., "Why do COX-2 inhibitors increase risk of cardiovascular events?" *Lancet* 359(9315) (Apr 2002): 1410.

Gerber, G.S., Kuznetsov, D., Johnson, B.C., et al., "Randomized, double-blind, placebo-controlled trial of saw palmetto in men with lower urinary tract symptoms," *Urology,* 58(6): (Dec 2001): 960–4; discussion 964–5.

Howell, E., *Enzyme Nutrition* (New Jersey: Avery Publishing, 1985).

Kawamori T., Rao C.V., Seibert K., Reddy B.S., "Chemopreventive activity of celecoxib, a specific cyclooxygenase-2 inhibitor, against colon carcinogenesis," *Cancer Res,* 58:3 (February 1998): 409–12.

Kelm, M.A., Nair, M.G., Strasburg, G.M., et al., "Antioxidant and cyclooxygenase inhibitory phenolic compounds from Ocimum sanctum Linn," *Phytomedicine,* 7(1) (March 2000):7–13.

Metzker, H. Kieser, M., Hölscher, U., "Efficacy of a combined Sabal-Urtica preparation in the treatment of benign prostatic hyperplasia (BPH),"*Urologe [B],* 36 (1996): 292–300.

O'Toole, M. (Ed), *Miller-Keane Encyclopedia and Dictionary of Medicine, Nursing, and Allied Health* (5th Ed.) (Philadelphia: WB Saunders, 1992).

Peterson, W.L., Cryer, B., "COX-1 sparing NSAIDs: is the enthusiasm justified?" (Editorial), *JAMA* 282(1999): 1961–63.

Professional Health Products, "Actions of metals in the body," *Oligoelements* (Portland, OR: Professional health Products, Ltd., 1992).

Sears, B., *The Zone* (New York: Harper Collins, 1995).

Seibert K., Lefkowith J., et al., "COX-2 inhibitors—is there cause for concern?" *Nat Med,* 5(6) (June 1999): 621–2.

Senozan, N.M., Thielman, C.A.,"Glucose-6-phosphate dehydrogenase deficiency—an inherited disorder that affects 100 million people," *Journal of Clinical Education,* 68(1) (1991): 7–10.

Simon, L.S., Lanza, F.L., Lipsky, P.E., et al., "Preliminary study of safety and efficacy of SC-58635, a novel cyclooxygenase inhibitor," *Arthritis Rheumatism* 41(1998): 1591–1602.

Sugaya, S. et al., "New anti-inflammatory treatment strategy in Alzheimer's disease," *Jpn J Pharmacol* 82(2) (Feb 2000): 85–94.

Thomas, J.A., "Diet, micronutrients, and the prostate gland," *Nutr Rev,* 57(4) (April 1999): 95–103.

Uchiyama T., Kamikawa H., et al., "Anti-ulcer effect of extract from phellodendri cortex," *Yakugaku Zasshi,* 109(9) (September 1989): 672–6.

Urban, M.K.,"COX-2 specific inhibitors offer improved advantages over traditional NSAIDS," *Orthopedics* 23(7s)(Jul 23 2000): 761–4s.

Chapter 3

Adler, J., Kalb, C., "Diabetes: an American epidemic," *Newsweek,* (4 September 2000).

Anderson, R.A., Kozlovsky, A.S., "Chromium intake, absorption, and excretion of subjects consuming self-selected diets," *Am J Clin Nutr,* 41 (1985): 1177–1183.

Arciero, P.J., et al., "Comparison of short-term diet and exercise on insulin action in individuals with abnormal glucose tolerance," *J Appl Physiol,* 86(6) (June 1999): 1930–5.

Ashcroft, F.M., et al., "ATP-sensitive K+ channels in human isolated pancreatic B-cells," *FEBS Lett,* 215(1) (May 1987): 9–12.

Assman, G., Cullen, P., Schulte, H., "Simple scoring scheme for calculating the risk of acute coronary events based on the 10-year follow-up of the prospective cardiovascular Munster (PROCAM) study," *Circulation,* 105(3) (January 2002): 310–5.

Barham, J.B., et al., "Addition of eicosapentaenoic acid to gamma-linolenic acid-supplemented diets prevents serum arachidonic acid accumulation in humans," *J Nutr,* 130(8) (August 2000): 1925–31.

Booyens, J., "The role of unnatural dietary trans and cis unsaturated fatty acids in the epidemiology of coronary artery disease," *Med Hypotheses,* 25(3) (March 1988): 175–82.

Brindley, D.N., "Introduction: perspective on molecular mechanisms of insulin action," *Canadian Journal of Diabetes Care,* 22(3s) (1998): 31s.

Buggy, J.J., Livingston, J.N., Rabin, D.U., et al., "Glucagon.glucagon-like peptide I receptor chimeras reveal domains that determine specificity of glucagon binding," *J Biol Chem,* 270 (1995): 7474–7478.

Cox, J.H., et al., "Effect of aging on response to exercise training in humans: skeletal muscle GLUT-4 and insulin sensitivity," *J Appl Physiol,* 86(6) (June 1999): 2019–25.

Dannhardt, G., Kiefer, W., "Cyclooxygenase inhibitors – current status and future prospects," *Eur J Med Chem,* 36(2) (February 2001): 109–26.

de Valk, H.W., "Magnesium in diabetes mellitus," *Neth J Med,* 54(4) (April 1999): 139–46.

Eades, M.R., Eades, M.D., *Protein Power* (New York: Bantam, 1996): 12–21.

Efendic, S., Luft, R., "Somatostatin: a classical hormone, a locally active polypeptide and a neurotransmitter," *Ann Clin Res,* 12(2) (1980): 87–94.

Eisenbarth, G.S., "Type I diabetes mellitus: a chronic autoimmune disease," *N Engl J Med,* 310 (1986): 1360.

Eriksson, J., Taimela, S., Koivisto, V.A., "Exercise and the metabolic syndrome," *Diabetologia,* 40 (1997): 125–35 [review].

Flegal, K.M., Carrol, M.D., Kuczmarski, R.J., Johnson, C.L., "Overweight and obesity in the United States: prevalence and trends, 1960–1994," *Int J Obes Relat Metab Disord,* 22(1) (January 1998): 39–47.

Forshee, R.A., Storey, M.L., "The role of added sugars in the diet quality of children and adolescents," *J Am Coll Nutr,* 20(1) (February 2001): 32–43.

Fowkes, S.W., "Insulin resistance," *Smart Life News,* 6(7) (29 June 1998): 1–5.

Gerber, G.S., Kuznetsov, D., Johnson, B.C., et al., "Randomized, double-blind, placebo-controlled trials of saw palmetto in men with lower urinary tract symptoms," *Urology,* 58(6) (December 2001): 960–4; discussion 964–5.

Golan, R., *Optimal Wellness,* (New York: Ballantine Books, 1995) 134, 151.

Haffner, S.M., "Obesity and the metabolic syndrome: the San Antonio Heart Study," *Br J Nutr*, 83 (2000): S67–70.

Harris, M.I., Flegal, K.M., Cowie, C.C., "Prevalence of diabetes, impaired fasting glucose, and impaired glucose tolerance in U.S. adults. The Third National Health and Nutrition Examination Survey, 1998–1994," *Diabetes Care*, 21(4) (April 1998): 518–24.

Honeyman, M.C., Coulson, B.S., Stone, N.L., et al., "Association between rotavirus infection and pancreatic islet autoimmunity in children at risk of developing type 1 diabetes," *Diabetes* 49(8) (August 2000): 1319–24.

Howard, B.V., "Insulin resistance and lipid metabolism," *Am J Cardiol*, 84(1A) (8 July 1999): 28J–32J

Howell, E., *Enzyme Nutrition* (Wayne, New Jersey: Avery Publishing, 1985).

Kao, W.H., et al., "Serum and dietary magnesium and the risk for type 2 diabetes mellitus: The Atherosclerosis Risk in Communities Study," *Arch Intern Med*, 159 (18) (11 October 1999): 2151–9.

Karter, A.J., Mayer-Davis, E-J., Selby, J.V., et al., "Insulin sensitivity and abdominal obesity in African-American, Hispanic, and non-Hispanic white men and women: The Insulin Resistance and Atherosclerosis Study," *Diabetes*, 45(11) (November 1996): 1547–55.

Kawamori, T., Rao, C.V., Seibert, K., Reddy, B.S., "Chemopreventive activity of celecoxib, a specific cyclooxygenase-2 inhibitor, against colon carcinogenesis," *Cancer Res*, 58(3) (February 1998): 409–12.

Kendall, P., "Syndrome x and insulin resistance," *Colorado State University Cooperative Extension*, (27 October 1997) (Online: www.colostate.edu/coopext/).

King H., Kriska, A.M., "Prevention of type II diabetes by physical training: epidemiological considerations and study methods," *Diabetes Care*, 15(11) (1992): 1794–9.

Legato, M.J., "Gender specific aspects of body fat," *J Fertil*, 42 (1997): 184–97.

Mackowiak, P., et al., "The influence of hypo- and hyperthyreosis on insulin receptors and metabolism," *Arch Physiol Biochem*, 107(4) (October 1999): 273–9.

Marks, J.B., "The insulin resistance syndrome," *The Monitor*, 1(3) (Spring1996).

Metzker, H., Kieser, M., Hölscher, U., "Efficacy of a combined Sabal-Urtica preparation in the treatment of benign prostatic hyperplasia (BPH)," *Urologe [B]*, 36 (1996): 292–300.

National Diabetes Education Initiative, "Young adults who gain weight are at risk for developing Insulin Resistance Syndrome," *News Watch*, (November 1998): 1–2.

O'Toole, M., (ed.), *Miller-Keane Encyclopedia and Dictionary of Medicine, Nursing, and Allied Health* (Fifth Edition) (Philadelphia: WB Saunders, 1992)

Perry Kelley, C.D., "Understanding syndrome x: what it is and how to prevent it," *Clinician Reviews* 7(10) (1997): 1–14.

Peterson, W.L., Cryer, B., "COX-1 sparing NSAIDs—is the enthusiasm justified? (Editorial)," *JAMA*, 282(1999): 1961–63.

Pleau, J.M., et al., "Prevention of autoimmune diabetes in nonobese diabetic female mice by treatment with recombinant glutamic acid decarboxylase," *Clin Immunol Immunopathol*, 76(1 pt 1) (July 1995): 90–5.

Professional Health Products, "Actions of metals in the body," *Oligoelements*, (Portland, OR: Professional Health Products, Ltd., 1992).

Ruderman, N.B., Schneider, S.J., "Diabetes, exercise, and atherosclerosis," *Diabetes Care*, 15(11) (1992): 1787–93.

Sears, B., *Enter the Zone*, (New York: Harper Collins, 1995): 20.

Sears, B., *The Zone* (New York: Harper Collins, 1995).

Seibert, K., Lefkowith, J., et al., "COX-2 inhibitors—is there cause for concern?" *Nat Med*, 5(6) (June 1999): 621–2.

Senozan, N.M., Thielman, C.A., "Glucose-6-phosphate dehydrogenase deficiency-an inherited disorder that affects 100 million people," *Journal of Clinical Education,* 68(1) (1991): 7–10.

Simon, L.S., Lanza, F.L., Lipsky, P.E., et al., "Preliminary study of safety and efficacy of SC-58635, a novel cyclooxygenase inhibitor," *Arthritis Rheumatism,* 41(1998): 1591–1602.

Singh, B., Prange, S., Jevnikar, A.M., "Protective and destructive effects of microbial infection in insulin-dependent diabetes mellitus," *Semin Immunol,* 10(1) (February 1998): 79–86.

Stearns, D.M., et al., "Chromium (III) picolinate produces chromosomal damage in Chinese hamster ovary cells," *FASEB J,* 9(15) (1995): 1643–48.

Stein, J., "The low-carb diet craze," *Time,* 154 (18) (1 November 1999): 72–80.

Sugaya, S., et al., "New anti-inflammatory treatment strategy in Alzheimer's disease," *Jpn J Pharmacol,* 82(2) (February 2000): 85–94.

Thomas, J.A., "Diet, micronutrients, and the prostate gland," *Nutr Rev,* 57(4) (April 1999): 95–103.

Threlkeld, D.S., ed., "Hormones, antidiabetic agents, insulin," In *Facts and Comparisons Drug Information,* St. Louis, MO: Facts and Comparisons, October 1997, 129F–9J.

Urban, M.K., "COX-2 specific inhibitors offer improved advantages over traditional NSAIDS," *Orthopedics,* 23(7s) (23 July 2000): 761–4s.

Vanhala, M.J., Pitkajarvi, T.K., Kumpusalo, E.A.,Takala, J.K., "Obesity type and clustering of insulin resistance-associated cardiovascular risk factors in middle-aged men and women," *Int J Obes Relat Metab,* 22(4) (April 1998): 369–74.

Varela-Calvino, R., et al., "T-Cell reactivity to the P2C nonstructural protein of a diabetogenic strain of coxsackievirus B4," *Virology,* 274(1) (August 2000): 56–64.

Verity, L.S., Ismail, A.H., "Effects of cardiovascular disease risk in women with NIDDM," *Diabetes Res Clin Prac,* 6(1) (1989): 27–35.

Vincent, J.B., "Mechanisms of chromium action: low-molecule-weight chromium-binding substance," *J Am Coll Nutr,* 18(1) (February 1999): 6–12.

Whitney, E.N., et al., *Understanding Normal and Clinical Nutrition,* (St. Paul: West Publishing Co., 1991): 833–6.

Wolever, T.M., "Dietary carbohydrates and insulin action in humans," *Br J Nutr,* 83 (2000): S97–S102 [review].

Chapter 4

Adeniyi, K.O., Olowookorun, M.O., "Gastric acid secretion and parietal cell mass: effect of thyroidectomy and thyroxine," *Am J Physiol,* 256(6 pt 1) (June 1989): 975G–8.

Barakat-Walter, I., Duc, C., Sarlieve, L.L., et al., "The expression of nuclear 3,5,3' triiodothyronine receptors is induced in Schwann cells by nerve transection," *Exp Neurol,* 116 (2) (1992): 189–97.

Barnes, B.O., Galton, L., *Hypothyroidism: The Unsuspected Illness,* (New York: Harper & Row, 1976).

Barregard, L., et al., "Endocrine function in mercury exposed chloalkali workers," *Occup Environ Med,* 51(8) (August 1994): 536–40.

Benediktsson, R., Taft, A.D., "Management of the unexpected result: compensated hypothyroidism," *Postgrad Med J,* 74(878) (December 1998): 729–32.

Browenstein, D., *Overcoming Thyroid Disorders,* (Medical Alternative Press, Copyright 2002).

Colao, A., Pivonello, R., Faggiano, A., et al., "Increased prevalence of thyroid autoimmunity in patients successfully treated for Cushing's disease," *Clin Endocrinol,* 53(1) (July 2000): 13–9.

Crook, W., *The Yeast Connection and the Woman,* (Jackson, TN: Professional Books, Inc., 1995): 550.

Hak, A.E., Pols, H.A., Visser, T.J., et al., "Subclinical hypothyroidism is an independent risk factor for atherosclerosis and myocardial infarction in elderly women: the Rotterdam Study," *Ann Intern Med,* 132(4) (15 February 2000): 270–8.

Hallengren, B., "Hypothyroidism—clinical findings, diagnosis, therapy: thyroid tests should be performed on broad indications," *Lakartidningen,* 95(38) (September 1998): 4091–6.

Hansen, D., Bennedbaek, F.N., Hansen, L.K., et al., "Thyroid function, morphology and autoimmunity in young patients with insulin-dependent diabetes mellitus," *Eur J Endocrinol,* 140(6) (June 1999): 512–8.

Hole, J.W., Jr., *Human Anatomy and Physiology,* (Dubuque, IA: WC Brown Publishers, 1990): 488.

Hulbert, A.J., "Thyroid hormones and their effects: a new perspective," *Biol Rev Camb Philos Soc, 75* (4) (2000): 519–631.

Kanazawa, K., Konishi, F., Mitsuoka, T., et al., "Factors influencing the development of sigmoid colon cancer: bacteriologic and biochemical studies," *Cancer,* 77(S8) (15 April 1996): 1701–6.

Kasperlik-Zaluska, A., Czarnocka, B., Czech, W., "High prevalence of thyroid autoimmunity in idiopathic Addison's disease," *Autoimmunity,* 18(3) (1994): 213–6.

Konstadoulakis, M.M., Kroubouzos, G., Tosca, A., et al., "Thyroid autoantibodies in the subsets of lupus erythematosus: correlation with other autoantibodies and thyroid function," *Thyroidology,* 5(1) (April 1993): 1–7.

Lonn, L., Stenlof, K., Ottosson, M., et al., "Body weight and body composition after treatment of hyperthyroidism," *J Clin Endocrinol Metabol,* 83(12) (December 1998): 4269–73.

Mackowiak, P., et al., "The influence of hypo- and hyperthyreosis on insulin receptors and metabolism," *Arch Physiol Biochem,* 107(4) (October 1999): 273–9.

Mariani, E., et al., "Vitamin D, thyroid hormones and muscle mass influence natural killer (NK) innate immunity in healthy nonagenarians and centenarians," *Clin Exp Immunol,* 116(1) (April 1999): 19–27.

Porth, C.M., *Pathophysiology: Concepts of Altered Health States,* (Philadelphia: JB Lippincott, 1990) 784.

Queen, H.L., *Chronic Mercury Toxicity: New Hope for an Endemic Disease,* (Colorado Springs: Queen and Company, 1988): 32–40, 47.

Regelson, W., *The Superhormone Promise,* (New York: Simon and Schuster, 1996): 195.

Rosenthal, M.S., *The Thyroid Sourcebook,* (Los Angeles: Lowell House, 1994): 226.

Sundaram, V., et al., "Both hypothyroidism and hyperthyroidism enhance low density lipoprotein oxidation," *J Clin Endocrinol Metal,* 82(10) (October 1997): 3421–4.

Watanabe, C., et al., "*In utero* methylmercury exposure differentially affects the activities of selenoenzymes in the fetal mouse brain," *Environ Res,* 80(3) (April 1999): 208–14.

Zaichick, V., et al., "Trace elements and thyroid cancer," *Analyst,* 120(3) (March 1995) 817–21.

Ziff, S., Ziff, M.F., *Infertility and Birth Defects,* (Orlando, FL: Bioprobe, Inc., 1987) 176–179.

Chapter 5

Bjorntorp, P., Rosmond, R., "Neuroendocrine abnormalities in visceral obesity," *Int J Obes Relat Metab Disord,* 24(S2) (June 2000): 80–5S.

Bjorntorp, P., Rosmond, R., "Neuroendocrine abnormalities in visceral obesity," *Int J Obes Relat Metab Disord,* 24(S2) (June 2000): 80–5S.

Buffington, C.K., Pourmotabbed, G., Kitabchi, A.E., "Case report: amelioration of insulin resistance in diabetes with dehydroepiandrosterone," *Am J Med Sci,* 306(5) (November 1993): 320–4.

Casson, P.R., et al., "Replacement of dehydroepiandrosterone enhances T-lymphocyte insulin binding in postmenopausal women," *Fertil Steril,* 63(5) (May1995): 1027–31.

De Pergola, G., "The adipose tissue metabolism: role of testosterone and dehydroepiandrosterone," *Int J Obes Relat Metab Disord,* 24(S2) (June 2000): 59–63S.

DeFord, H.A., "Medicine and Spirituality," *Tex Med.* 97(4) (April 2001): 10.

Ewers, V., Erbe, R., "Effects of lead, cadmium and mercury on brain adenylate cyclase," *Toxicology,* 16 (1980): 227–237.

Facchini, F.S., et al., "Hyperinsulinemia: the missing link among oxidative stress and age-related diseases?" *Free Radic Biol Med,* 29(12) (December 2000): 1302–6.

Filaire, E., Duche, P., Lac, G., "Effects of amount of training on the saliva concentrations of cortisol, dehydroepiandrosterone, and on the dehydroepiandrosterone: cortisol concentration ratio in women over 16 weeks of training," *Eur J Appl Physiol Occup Physiol,* 78(5) (October 1998): 466–71.

Holmes, T.H., Rahe, R.H., "Booklet for schedule of recent experiences (SRE): Social Readjustment Rating Scale," *J Psychosom Res,* 11 (1967): 213–18.

Keltikangas-Jarvinen, L., Ravaja, N., Raikkonen, K., et al., "Relationships between the pituitary-adrenal hormones, insulin, and glucose in middle-aged men: moderating influence of psychosocial stress," *Metabolism,* 47(12) (December 1998): 1440–9.

Khalil, A., et al., "Age-related decrease of dehydroepiandrosterone concentrations in low density lipoproteins and its role in the susceptibility of low density lipoproteins to lipid peroxidation," *J Lipid Res,* 41(10) (October 2000): 1552–61.

Khayat, A., Denker, L., "Organ and cellular distribution of inhaled metallic mercury in the rat and Marmoset monkey: influence of ethyl alcohol pretreatment," *Acta Pharmacol,* 55(2) (1984): 145–52.

Lesser, M., *Nutrition and Vitamin Therapy,* (New York: Grove Press, Inc, 1980): 69–70.

Levin, J.S., Vanderpool, H.Y., "Is frequent religious attendance really conducive to better health? Toward an epidemiology of religion," *Soc Sci Med,* 24 (1987): 589–600.

Maarin, P., Darin, N., Amemiya, T., Andersson, B., Jern, S., BjAorntorp, P., "Cortisol secretion in relation to body fat distribution in obese premenopausal women," *Metabolism,* 41(8) (1992): 882–6.

Medalie, J.H., Goldbourt, U., "Angina pectoris among 10,000 men, II: Psychosocial and other risk factors," *Am J Med,* 60 (1976): 910–21

Mel'nikova, V.L., Proshliakova, E.V., Calas, A., et al., "Tyrosine hydroxylase expression in differentiating neurons of the rat arcuate nucleus: inhibitory effect of serotoninergic afferents," *Ross Fiziol Zh Im I M Sechenova,* 87(10) (October 2001): 1333–40.

Miller, J.E., et al., "Characterization of 24-h cortisol release in obese and non-obese hyperandrogenic women," *Gynecol Endocrin,* 8 (1994): 247–254.

Mukasa, K., et al., "Dehydroepiandrosterone (DHEA) ameliorates the insulin sensitivity in older rats," *J Steroid Biochem Mol Biol,* 67(4) (November 1998): 355–8.

Niwa, Y., et al., *Protection for Life: How to Boost Your Body's Defenses Against Free Radicals and the Aging Effects of Pollution and Modern Lifestyle,* (Wellingborough: Thorson's Publishers, 1989): 9.

O'Hara, D.P., "Is There a Role for Prayer and Spirituality in Health Care? *Med Clin North Am,* 86(1) (January 2002): 33–46.

Pasquali, R., Anconetani, B., Chattat. R., Biscotti, M., Spinucci, G., Casimirri, F., et al., "Hypothalamic-pituitary-adrenal axis activity and its relationship to the autonomic nervous system in women with visceral and subcutaneous obesity: effects of the corticotropin-releasing factor/arginine vasopressin test and of stress," *Metabolism,* 45(3) (1996): 351–6.

Regelson, W., Colman, C., *The Superhormone Promise,* (New York: Simon & Schuster, 1996) 77.

Schauer, J.E., Schelin, A., Hanson, P., Srtaman, F.W., "Dehydroepiandrosterone and a beta-agonist, energy transducers, alter antioxidant enzyme systems: influence of chronic training and acute exercise in rats," *Arch Biochem Biophys,* 283(2) (December1990): 503–11.

Serafeim, A., Grafton, G., Chamba, A., et al., "5-hydroxytryptamine drives apoptosis in biopsylike burkitt lymphoma cells: reversal by selective serotonin reuptake inhibitors," *Blood,* 99(7) (April 2002): 2545–53.

Veltman, J.C., Maines, M.D., "Alterations in heme, cytochrome P-450, and steroid metabolism by mercury in rat adrenal," *Arch Biochem Biophys,* 248(2) (1987): 467–78.

Wilson, S.K., Kneisl, C.R., *Psychiatric Nursing,* (Redwood City: Addison Wesley, 1992): 80.

Chapter 6

Agarwal, K.C., et al., "Significance of plasma adenosine in the antiplatelet activity of forskolin: potentiation by dipyridamole and dilazep," *Thromb Haemost,* 61(1) (1989): 106–10.

Antonio, J., Colker, C.M., Torina, G.C., et al., "Effects of a standardized guggulsterone phosphate supplement on body composition in overweight adults: a pilot study," *Curr Ther Res,* 60 (1999): 220–7.

Baumann, G., et al., "Cardiovascular effects of forskolin (HL 362) in patients with idiopathic congestive cardiomyopathy—a comparative study with dobutamine and sodium nitroprusside," *Cardiovasc Pharmacol,* 16(1) (1990): 93–100.

Berry, M.J., Larsen, P.R., "The role of selenium in thyroid hormone action," *Endocrine Rev,* 13(1992): 207–20.

Bhat, S.V., et al., "The antihypertensive and positive inotropic diterpene forskolin: effects of structural modifications on its activity," *J Med Chem,* 26 (1983): 486–92.

Bol'shakova, I.V., et al., "Antioxidant properties of a series of extracts from medicinal plants," *Biofizika,* 32(2) (March–April 1997): 480–83.

Bottecchia, D., et al., "Vaccinium myrtillus," *Fitoterapia,* 48 (1977): 3–8.

Brichard, S.M., et al., "The role of vanadium in the management of diabetes," *Trends Pharmacol Sci,* 16(8) (August 1995): 265–70.

Broadhurst C.L., Polansky M.M., Anderson R.A. Insulin-like biological activity of culinary and medicinal plant aqueous extracts in vitro. *J Agric Food Chem,* 48(3) (March 2000): 849–52.

Burkholder, P.R., "Drugs from the Sea," *Armed Forces Chem J,* 17(6) (1963): 12–16.

Cangiano, C., et al., "Eating behavior and adherence to dietary prescriptions in obese adult subjects treated with 5-hydroxytryptophan," *Am J Clin Nutr,* 56(5) (November 1992): 863–67.

Chan, P., Tomlinson, B., Chen, Y.J., et al., "A double-blind placebo-controlled study of the effectiveness and tolerability of oral stevioside in human hypertension," *Br J Clin Pharmacol,* 50(3) (September 2000): 215–20.

Christenson, J.T., et al., "The effect of forskolin on blood flow, platelet metabolism, aggregation and ATP release," *Vasa,* 24(1) (1995): 56–61.

Curro, F., et al., "*Fucus vesiculosis* L. nel trattamento medico dell'obesita e delle alterazioni metaboliche connesse," *Arch Med Interna,* 28 (1976): 19–32.

Dalvi, S.S., et al., "Effects of gugulipid on bioavailability of diltiazem and propranolol," *J Assoc Physicians India,* 42(6) (1994): 454–55.

Darbinyan, V., Kteyan, A., Panossian, A., et al., "Rhodiola rosea in stress induced fatigue—a double blind cross-over study of a standardized extract SHR-5 with a repeated low-dose regimen on the mental performance of healthy physicians during night duty," *Phytomedicine,* 7(5) (October 2000): 365–71.

Delange, F., "The role of goitrogenic factors distinct from iodine deficiency in the etiology of goiter," *Ann Endocrinol (Paris),* 49(4–5) (1988): 302–5.

Divi, R.L., et al., "Anti-thyroid isoflavones from soybean: isolation, characterization, and mechanisms of action," *Biochem Pharmacol,* 54(10) (15 November 1997): 1087–96.

Doi, K., et al., "The effect of adenylate cyclase stimulation on endocochlear potential in the guinea pig," *Eur Arch Otorhinolaryngol,* 247(1) (1990): 16–19.

Duke, J.A., *Handbook of Phytochemical Constituents of GRAS Herbs and Other Economic Plants,* (Boca Raton, FL: CRC Press, 1992).

Duncan, A.M., et al., "Soy isoflavones exert modest hormonal effects in premenopausal women," *J Clin Endocrinol Metab,* 84(1) (January 1999): 192–7.

Ganapathy, S., Volpe, S.L., "Zinc, exercise and thyroid hormone function," *Crit Rev Food Sci Nutr,* 39(4) (July 1999): 369–90.

Gupta, R.P., et al., "Effect of experimental zinc deficiency on thyroid gland in guinea pigs," *Ann Nutr Metab,* 41(6) (1997): 376–81.

Halberstram, M., et al., "Oral vanadyl sulfate improves insulin sensitivity in NIDDM but not in obese nondiabetic subjects," *Diabetes,* 45(5) (May 1996): 659–66.

Holben, D.H., Smith, A.M., "The diverse role of selenium within selenoproteins: a review," *J Am Diet Assoc,* 99(7) (July 1999): 836–43.

Iso, H., Sato, S., Umemura, U., et al., "Linoleic acid, other fatty acids, and the risk of stroke," *Stroke,* 33(8) (August 2002): 2086–93.

Jeppesen, P.B., Gregersen, S., Poulsen, C.R., et al., "Stevioside acts directly on pancreatic beta cells to secrete insulin: actions independent of cyclic adenosine monophosphate and adenosine triphosphate-sensitive K+-channel activity," *Metabolism,* 49(2) (February 2000): 208–14.

Kahn, R.S., et al., "L-5-hydroxytryptophan in the treatment of anxiety disorders," *J Affect Disord,* 8(2) (March 1985): 197–200.

Kakuda, T., Sakane, I., Takihara, T., et al., "Hypoglycemic effect of extracts from Lagerstroemia speciosa L. leaves in genetically diabetic KK-AY mice," *Biosci Biotechnol Biochem,* 60(2) (February 1996): 204–8.

Kreutner, R.W., "Bronchodilator and antiallergy activity of forskolin," *European Journal of Pharmacology,* 111 (1985): 1–8.

Kudoh, K., Shimizu, J., Ishiyama, A., et al., "Secretion and excretion of immunoglobulin A to cecum and feces differ with type of indigestible saccharides," *J Nutr Sci Vitaminol,* (Tokyo). 45(2) (April 1999): 173–81.

Leatherdale, B.A., et al., "Improvement in glucose tolerance due to Momordica Charantia (Karela)," *Br Med J (Clin Res Ed)*, 282(6279) (June 1981): 1823–24.

Molokovskii, D.S., et al., "The action of adaptogenic plant preparations in experimental alloxan diabetes," *Probl Endokrinol,* (Mosk), 35(6) (November–December 1989): 82–87.

Morazonni, P., et al., "Vaccinium myrtillus," *Fitoterapia,* vol. LXVII, no. 1 (1996): 3–29.

Murkakami, C., Myoga, K., Kasai, R., et al., "Screening of plant constituents for effect on glucose transport activity in Erlich ascites tumour cells," *Chem Pharm Bull,* 41(12) (December 1993): 2129–31.

Nagamatsu, M., et al., "Lipoic acid improves nerve blood flow, reduces oxidative stress, and improves distal nerve conduction in experimental diabetic neuropathy," *Diabetes Care,* 18(8) (August 1995): 1160–67.

Newall, C.A., et al., *Herbal Medicines: A Guide for Health Care Professionals* (London: The Pharmaceutical Press, 1996): 124–126.

Ng, T.B., et al., "Insulin-like molecules in Momordica Charantia seeds," *J Ethnopharmacol,* 15(1) (January 1986): 107–17.

Nishiyama, S., et al., "Zinc supplementation alters thyroid hormone metabolism in disabled patients with zinc deficiency," *J Am Coll Nutr,* 13(1994): 62–7.

Saratikov, A.S., et al., "Rhodiola rosea is a valuable medicinal plant," *Tomsk State Medicinal University,* Russia: Russian Academy of Medicinal Sciences. (1987).

Sarkar, S., et al., "Demonstration of the hypoglycemic action of Momordica Charantia in a validated animal model of diabetes," *Pharmacol Res,* 33(1) (January 1996): 1–4.

Satyavati, G.V., "Gum guggul (commiphora mukul)—The success story of an ancient insight leading to a modern discovery," *Indian J Med Res,* 87 (1988): 327–35.

Satyavati, G.V., et al., "Experimental Studies on Hypocholesterolemic Effect of Commiphora Mukul," *Indian J Med Res,* 57(10) (1969): 1950–62.

Scalfi, L., Coltori, A., D'Arrigo, E., et al., "Effect of dietary fibre on postprandial thermogenesis," *Int J Obes,* 11 (Suppl. 1) (1987): 95–9.

Seamon, K.B., et al., "Forskolin: its biological and chemical properties," *Advances in Cyclic Nucleotide and Protein Phosphorylation Research,* vol. 20 (New York: Raven Press, 1986): 1–150.

Sears, B., *Enter the Zone* (New York: Harper Collins, 1995) 32–37.

Shapiro, A.C., et al., "Eicosanoids derived from arachidonic and eicosapentaenoic acids inhibit T cell proliferative response," *Prostaglandins,* 45(3) (March 1993): 229–40.

Sitasawad, S.L., Shewade, Y., Bhonde, R., "Role of bittergourd fruit juice in stz-induced diabetic State *in vivo* and *in vitro*," *J Ethnopharmacol,* 73(1–2) (November 2000): 71–9.

Song, M.K., et al., "Animal prostate extract ameliorates diabetic symptoms by stimulating intestinal zinc absorption in rats," *Diabetes Research,* 31 (1996): 157–70.

Srivastava, Y., et al., "Hypoglycemic and life-prolonging properties of gymnema sylvestre leaf extract in diabetic rats," *Isr J Med Sci,* 21(6) (June 1985): 540–42.

Sufka, K.J., Roach, J.T., Chambliss, W.G., Jr., et al., "Anxiolytic properties of botanical extracts in the chick social separation-stress procedure," *Psychopharmacology,* (Berl), 153(2) (1 January 2001): 219–24.

Sun, Y.H., "Cordyceps sinensis and cultured mycelia," *Chung Yao Tung Pao,* 10(12) (December 1985): 3–5.

Tripathi, Y.B., et al., "Thyroid stimulating action of Z-guggulsterone obtained from Commiphora mukul," *Planta Med,* (1) (1984): 78–80.

U.S. Department of Health and Human Services, Physical Activity and Health: A Report of the Surgeon General, Centers for Disease Control and Prevention, (1996).

Vita, P.M., Restelli, A., Caspani, P., et al., "Chronic use of glucomannan in the dietary treatment of severe obesity," *Minerva Med,* 83(3) (March 1992): 135–9.

Vuksan, V., Jenkins, D.J., Spadafora, P., et al., "Konjac-mannan (glucomannan) improves glycemia and other associated risk factors for coronary heart disease in type 2 diabetes: a randomized controlled metabolic trial," *Diabetes Care,* 22(6) (June 1999): 913–9.

Vulksan, V., Sievenpiper, J.L., Owen, R., et al., "Beneficial effects of viscous dietary fiber from Konjac-mannan in subjects with the insulin resistance syndrome: results of a controlled metabolic trial," *Diabetes Care,* 23(1) (January 2000): 9–14.

Welihinda, J., et al., "Effect of Momordica Charantia on the glucose tolerance in maturity onset diabetes," *J Ethnopharmacol,* 17(3) (September 1986): 277–82.

Zhu, J., et al., "CordyMax Cs-4: a scientific product review," *Pharmanex Phytoscience Review Series,* 1997.

Chapter 7

U.S. Environmental Protection Agency. *Broad scale analysis of the FY 82 national human adipose tissue survey specimens. Volume II: Volatile organic compounds.* EPA 560/5–86-036. Office of Toxic Substances. Washington, D.C., 1986)

Chapter 8

Bettelheim, F.A., March, J., *Introduction to Organic and Biochemistry,* (Philadelphia: Saunders College Publishing, 1990): 296.

Bottiglieri, T., et al., "Cerebrospinal fluid S-adenosylmethionine in depression and dementia: effects of treatment with parenteral and oral S-adenosylmethionine," *J Neurol Neurosurg Psychiatry,* (Eng.) 53(12) (December 1990): 1096–98.

Bressa, G. M., et al., "S-adenosyl-l-methionine (SAMe) as antidepressant: meta-analysis of clinical studies," *Acta Neurol Scand,* Suppl. 154 (1994): 7–14.

Burchell, B., Hume, R., "Molecular genetic basis of Gilbert's syndrome," *J Gastroenterol Hepatol,* 14(10) (October 1999): 960–6.

Chawla, R.K., et al., "Biochemistry of pharmacology of S-adenosyl-L-methionine and rationale for its use in liver disease," *Drugs,* 40(Suppl. 3) (1990): 98–110.

di Benedetto, P., Iona, L.G., Zidarich, V., "Clinical evaluation of S-adenosyl-L-methionine versus transcutaneous electrical nerve stimulation in primary fibromyalgia," *Curr Ther Res,* 53(2) (February 1993): 222.

di Padova, C., "S-adenosylmethionine in the treatment of osteoarthritis: review of the clinical studies," *Am J Med,* 83(5A) (20 November 1987): 60–65.

Edelson, S.B., Candor, D.S., "Autism: xenobiotic influences," *Toxicol Ind Health,* 14(4) (July–August 1998): 553–63.

Fontanari, D., et al., "Effects of S-adenosyl-L-methionine on cognitive and vigilance functions in the elderly," *Curr Ther Res Clin Exp,* (USA) 55(6) (1994): 682–89.

Friedel, H.A., et al., "S-Adenosyl-L-methionine: a review of its pharmacological properties and therapeutic potential in liver dysfunction and affective disorders in relation to its physiological role in cell metabolism," *Drugs,* 38(3) (1989): 389–416.

Glorioso, S., et al., "SAMe impact on hips and knees," *Int J Clin Pharmacol Res,* (Switzerland) 5(1) (1985): 39–49.

Goldwin, B.R., *Dietary Fat and Cancer* (New York: Alan R. Liss, 1986): 655–85.

Grasetto, M., et al., "Primary fibromyalgia is responsive to S-adenosyl-L-methionine," *Curr Ther Res Clin Exp,* (USA) 55(7) (1994): 797–806.

Gutierrez, S., et al., "SAMe and osteoarthritis," *Br J Rheumatol,* (England) 36(1) (January 1997): 27–31.

Han D., et al., "Lipoic acid increases de novo synthesis of cellular glutathione by improving cystine utilization," *Biofactors,* (1997) 6(3):321–38.

Ianniello, A., et al., "S-adenosyl-L-methionine in sjogren's syndrome and fibromyalgia," *Curr Ther Res Clin Exp,* (USA) 55(6) (1994): 699–706.

Kaminski, M., Jr., et al., "AIDS wasting syndrome as an enterometabolic disorder: the gut hypothesis," *Altern Med Rev* 3(1) (February 1998): 40–53.

Konig, B., "A long-term (two years) clinical trial with S-adenosylmethionine for the treatment of osteoarthritis," *Am J Med,* 83(5A) (20 November 1987): 89–94.

Krohn, J., Taylor, F.A., Prosser, J., *Natural Detoxification* (Point Roberts, A: Hartley & Marks Publishers, Inc., 1996).

Lang, C.A., et al., "Blood glutathione decreases in chronic disease," *J Lab Clin Med,* 135(5) (May 2000): 402–5.

LaValle, J., et al., *Natural Therapeutics Pocket Guide 2000–2001* (Hudson, OH: Lexi-Comp, Inc., 2000): 498–500.

Le Sellin, L., "Clinical signs of food allergy," *Allergy Immunol,* (Paris) 29 (July 1997): 11–4.

Lenton, K.J., et al., "Direct correlation of glutathione and ascorbate and their dependence on age and season in human lymphocytes," *Am J Clin Nutr,* 71(5) (May 2000): 1194–200.

Loehrer, F. M., et al., "Low whole-blood S-adenosylmethionine and correlation between 5-methyltetrahydrofolate and homocysteine in coronary artery disease," *Arterioscler Thromb Vasc Biol,* 16(6) (June 1996): 727–33.

Mato, J. M., et al., "S-adenosylmethionine in alcoholic liver cirrhosis: a randomized, placebo-controlled, double-blind, multicenter clinical trial," *J Hepatol,* 30(6) (June 1999): 1081–89.

Miglio, F., et al., "Double-blind studies of the therapeutic action of S-Adenosylmethionine (SAMe) in oral administration, in liver cirrhosis and other chronic hepatitides," *Minerva Med,* 66(33) (1975): 1595–9.

Monaghan, G., et al., "Gilbert's syndrome is a contributory factor in prolonged unconjugated hyper-bilirubinemia of the newborn," *J Pediatr,* 134(4) (April 1999): 441–6.

Reist, M., Jenner, P., Halliwell, B., "Sulphite enhances peroxynitrite-dependent alpha-1 antiproteinase inactivation: a mechanism of lung injury by sulfur dioxide?" *FEBS Lett,* 423(2) (20 February 1998): 231–4.

Sen, C.K., Packer, L., "Thiol homeostasis and supplements in physical exercise," *Am J Clin Nutr,* 72(Suppl. 2) (August 2000): 653S–69S.

Sitaram, B. R., et al., "Nyctohemeral rhythm in the levels of S-adenosylmethionine in the rat pineal gland and its relationship to melatonin biosynthesis," *J Neurochem,* 65(4) (October 1995): 1887–94.

Tavoni, A., et al., "Evaluation of S-adenosylmethionine in primary fibromyalgia: a double-blind crossover study," *Am J Med,* 83(5A) (20 November 1987): 107–10.

Valenzuela, A., et al., "Selectivity of silymarin on the increase of the glutathione content in different tissues of the rat," *Planta Medica,* 55 (1989): 1550–52.

Yanick, P., Jaffe, R., (Eds), *Clinical Chemistry and Nutrition Guidebook: A Physician's Desk Reference,* (Volume I) (R & H Publishing, 1988).

Chapter 9

Abernathy-Carver, K.J., et al., "Milk-induced eczema is associated with the expansion of T cells expressing cutaneous lymphocyte expansion," *J Clin Invest,* 95(2) (February 1995): 913–8.

Ahmed, T., Fuch, G.J., "Gastrointestinal allergy to food," *J Diarrhoeal Dis Res,* 15(4) (December 1997): 211–23.

Antonsson, B.E., Klig, L.S., "Candida albicans phosphatidylinositol synthase has common features with both Saccharomyces cerevisiae and mammalian phosphatidylinositol synthases," *Yeast,* 12(5) (April 1996): 449–56.

Apperloo-Renkema, H.Z., et al., "Host microflora interaction in systemic lupus erythematosus (SLE): circulating antibodies to the indigenous bacteria of the intestinal tract," *Epidemiol Infect,* 114(1) (February 1995): 133–41.

Barnes, R.M., "Serum antibodies reactive with Saccharomyces cerevisiae in inflammatory bowel disease: is IgA antibody a marker for Crohn's disease?" *Arch Allergy Appl Immunol,* 92(1) (1990): 9–15.

Bercault, N., Boulain, T., "Mortality rate attributable to ventilator-associated nosocomial pneumonia in an adult intensive care unit: a prospective case-control study," *Crit Care Med,* 29(12) (December 2001): 2303–9.

Bergstrom, K., Havermark, G., "Enzymes in intestinal mucosa from patients with rheumatoid diseases," *Scan J Rheumatol,* 5(1) (1976): 29–32.

Bjorksten, B., et al., "The intestinal microflora in allergic Estonian and Swedish 2-year-old children," *Clin Exp Allergy,* 29(3) (March 1999): 342–6.

Bolte, E.R., "Autism and clostridium tetani," *Med Hypotheses,* 51(2) (1 August 1998): 133–44.

Boris, S., et al., "Adherence of human vaginal lactobacilli to vaginal epithelial cells and interaction with uropathogens," *Infect Immun,* 66(5) (May 1998): 1985–9.

Borkhsenius, S.N., Chernova, O.A., Chernov, V.M., "Interaction of mycoplasma with immune system of animals and humans," *Tsitologiia,* 43(3) (2001): 219–43.

Brandes, J.W. et al., "Sugar-free diet as long-term or interval treatment in the remission phase of Crohn's disease – a prospective study," *Leber Magen Darm,* 12(6) (November 1982): 225–8.

Brandes, J.W., Lorenz-Meyer, H., "Sugar-free diet: A new perspective in the treatment of Crohn's disease?" *J Gastroenterol,* 19(1)(1981): 1–12.

Brockel, B.J., Cory-Slechta, D.A., et al., "Lead, attention, and impulsive behavior: changes in a fixed-ratio waiting-for-reward paradigm," *Pharmacol Biochem Behav,* 60(2) (June 1998): 545–52.

Buskila, D., "Fibromyalgia, chronic fatigue syndrome, and myofascial pain syndrome," *Curr Opin Rheumatol,* 12(2) (March 2000): 113–23.

Catasi, C., et al., "Is the sugar intestinal permeability test a reliable investigation for celiac disease screening?" *Gut,* 40(2) (February 1997): 215–7.

Chandra, R.K., "Five-year follow up of high risk infants with family history of allergy who were exclusively breast-fed or fed partial whey hydrosylate, soy and conventional cow's milk formulas," *J Pediatr Gastroenterol Nutr,* 24(4) (April 1997): 380–8.

Clark, J.B., et al., *Pharmacologic Basis of Nursing Practice,* (St. Louis: Mosby, 1993): 361–5.

Cummings, J.H., "Fermentation in the human large intestine: evidence an implications for health," *Lancet,* (1208) (1983).

D'Adamo, P.J., Whitney, C., *Eat Right for Your Type* (New York: GP Putnam's Sons, 1996): 23–28.

Dalberg, J. et al., "Colorectal cancer in the Faroe Islands—a setting for the study of the role of diet," *J Epidemiol Biostat,* 4(1) (1999): 31–6.

Darroch, C.J., et al., "*In vitro* lymphocyte proliferation response to a glycoprotein of the yeast Saccharomyces cerevisiae," *Immunology,* 81(2) (February 1994): 247–52.

de Boissieu, D., et al., "Multiple food allergy: a possible diagnosis in breastfed infants," *Acta Pediatr,* 86(10) (October 1997): 1042–6.

De Schepper, L., M.D., *Peak Immunity* (Published by Author: Santa Monica, 1990): 113–114.

DeStefano, F., "Vaccines and autism," *Pediatr Infect Dis J,* 20(9) (September 2001): 887–8.

Egger, J., et al., "Controlled trial of oligoantigenic treatment in the hyperkinetic syndrome," *Lancet,* 1(8428) (9 March 1985): 540–5.

Ekstrand, J., Bjorkman, L., Edlund, C., et al., "Toxicological aspects on the release and systemic uptake of mercury from dental amalga," *Eur J Oral Sci,* 106(2 Pt 2) (April 1998): 678–86.

Ferguson, A., "Immunological functions of the gut in relation to nutritional state and mode of delivery of nutrients," *Gut,* 35(1s) (January 1994): 10–2s.

Forshee, R.A., Storey, M.L., "The role of added sugars in the diet quality of children and adolescents," *J Am Coll Nutr,* 20(1) (February 2001): 32–43.

Galland, L., *Leaky Gut Syndromes: Breaking the Vicious Cycle* (Online: www.healthy.net): 1–15.

Garrison, M.W., Campbell, R.K., "Identifying and treating common and uncommon infections in the patient with diabetes," *Diabetes Educ,* 19(6) (November–December 1993): 522–9.

Geerlings, S.E., Hoepelman, A.I., "Immune dysfunction in patients with diabetes mellitus (DM)," *FEMS Immunol Med Microbiol,* 26(3–4) (December 1999): 259–65.

Geerlings, S.E. and Hoepelman, A.I., et al., "Intraoral candida in Thai diabetes patients," *J Med Assoc Thai,* 81(6) (June 1998): 449–53.

Ghannoum, M.A., Elteen, K.A., Effect of growth of Candida spp.: in the presence of various glucocorticoids on the adherence to human buccal epithelial cells," *Mycopathologia,* 98(3) (June 1987): 171–8.

Goenka, M.K., et al., "Candida overgrowth after treatment of duodenal ulcer: a comparison of cimetidine, famotidine, and omeprazole," *J Clin Gastroenterol,* 23(1) (July 1996): 7–10.

Goldman, L.S., et al., "Diagnosis and treatment of attention-deficit/hyperactivity disorder in children and adolescents," Council on Scientific Affairs, American Medical Association, *JAMA,* 279(14) (April 1998): 1100–07.

Granfors, K., et al., "Yersinia antigens in synovial-fluid cells from patients with reactive arthritis," *New Engl J Med.,* 320(4) (26 January 1989): 216–221.

Grant, B.F., "Alcohol consumption, alcohol abuse, and alcohol dependence: the United States as an example," *Addiction,* 89(11) (November 1994): 1357–65.

Grant, B.F., "Prevalence and correlates of alcohol use and DSM-IV alcohol dependence in the United States: results of the National Longitudinal Alcohol Epidemiologic Survey," *J Stud Alcohol,* 58(5) (September 1997): 464–73.

Greenamyre, J.T., Sherer, T.B., Betarbet, R., et al., "Complex I and parkinson's disease," *IUBMB Life,* 52(3–5) (September–November 2001): 135–41.

Greenamyre, J.T., Sherer, T.B., Betarbet, R., et al., "Mitochondrial dysfunction in Parkinson's disease," *Biochem Soc Symp,* 66 (1999): 85–97.

Gronlund, M.M., et al., "Fecal microflora in healthy infants born by different methods of delivery: permanent changes in intestinal flora after cesarean delivery," *J Pediatr Gastroenterol Nutr,* 28(1) (January 1999): 19–25.

Guggenheimer, J., Moore, P.A., Rossie, K., et al., "Insulin-dependent diabetes mellitus and oral soft tissue pathologies: II. Prevalence and characteristics of Candida and Candidal lesions," *Oral Surg Oral Med Oral Pathol Oral Radiol Endod,* 89(5) (May 2000): 570–76.

Haas, E.M., *Staying Healthy with Nutrition,* (Berkeley: Celestial Arts Publishing, 1992): 869–79.

Hamburger, R., *Proceedings of the First Annual Symposium on Food Allergy,* Vancouver, BC (1982).

Hara, H., et al., "Short chain fatty acids suppress cholesterol synthesis in rat liver and intestine," *J Nutr* 129(5) (May 1999): 942–8.

Hoffman, T., "Analysis of food allergy incidence in children up to 5 years of age in the Wielikopolska region," *Pol Merkuriusz,* 5(30) (5 December 1998): 341–5.

Holt, P.R., "Dairy foods and prevention of colon cancer: human studies," *J Am Coll Nutr,* 18(5s): (October 1999): 379s–91s.

Hornstein, O.P., "Remarks and recommendations on the definition and classification of eczematous diseases," *Z Hautkr,* 61(18) (15 September 1986): 1281–96.

Jantos, M., White, G., "The vestibulitis syndrome: medical and psychosexual assessment of a cohort of patients," *J Reprod Med,* 42(3) (March 1997): 145–52.

Jenkins, A.P., et al., "Do non-steroidal anti-inflammatory drugs increase colonic permeability?" *Gut,* 32(1) (January 1991): 66–9.

Jenkins, R.T., "Increased intestinal permeability in patients with rheumatoid arthritis: a side effect of oral nonsteroidal anti-inflammatory drug therapy?" *Br J Rheumatol,* 26(2) (1987): 102–7.

Johnson, R.K., Frary, C., "Choose beverages and foods to moderate your intake of sugars: the 2000 dietary guidelines for Americans–what's all the fuss about?" *J Nutr,* 131(10) (October 2001): 2766S–2771S.

Juji, F., Suko, M., "Effectiveness of disodium chromoglycate in food-dependent, exercise-induced anaphylaxis: a case report," *Ann Allergy,* 72(5) (May1994): 452–4.

Juntii, H., et al., "Cow's milk allergy is associated with recurrent otitis media during childhood," *Acta Otolaryngol,* 119(8) (1999): 867–73.

Kane, E., "Food allergies," *American Association of Naturopathic Physicians* (online: www.healthy.net): 1–3.

Kaplan, B.J., et al., "Dietary replacement in preschool-aged hyperactive boys," *Pediatrics,* 83(1) (January 1989): 7–17.

Karolus, H.E., "Alcoholism and food allergy," *Illinois Med J,* 119(3) (March 1962): 151–2.

Kidd, P.M., "Attention defecit/hyperactivity disorder (ADHD) in children: rationale for its integrative management," *Altern Med Rev*, 5(5) (August 1998): 133–44.

Kirjavainen, P.V., Gibson, G.R., "Healthy gut microflora and allergy: factors influencing the development of the microbiota," *Ann Med*, 31(4) (August 1999): 288–92.

Kirsner, J.B., "Recent developments in 'non-specific' inflammatory bowel disease," *N Engl J Med*, (306) (1982): 775.

Knibb, R.C., Armstrong, A., Booth, D.A., et al., "Psychological characteristics of people with perceived food intolerances in a community sample," *J Psychosom Res*, 47(6) (December 1999): 545–54.

Kochhar, R., et al., "Invasive candidiasis following cimetidine therapy," *Am J Gastroenterol*, 83(1) (January 1988): 102–3.

Kruzel, T., "Serotyping and diet: D'Adamo serotype panel," *American Association of Naturopathic Physicians* (online: www.healthy.net): 1–3.

Lak, R.L., Saint, S., Chenoweth, C., et al., "Four-year prospective evaluation of community-acquired bacteremia: epidemiology, microbiology, and patient outcome," *Diagn Microbiol Infect Dis*, 41(1–2) (September–October 2001): 15–22.

Lamb, K., Nichols, T.R., "Endometriosis: a comparison of associated disease histories," *Am J Prev Med*, 2(6) (November–December 1986): 324–9.

Lewis, S.J., Heaton, K.W., "The metabolic consequences of slow colonic transit," *Am J Gastroenterol*, 94(8) (August 1999): 2010–6.

Lindberg, E., et al., "Antibody (IgG, IgA, and IgM) to baker's yeast (Saccharomyces cerevisiae), yeast mannan, gliadin, ovalbumin and betalactoglobulin in monozygotic twins with inflammatory bowel disease," *Gut* 33(7) (July 1992): 909–13.

Lindgren, L., et al., "Occurrence and clinical features of sensitization to Pityrosporum orbiculae and other allergens in children with atopic dermatitis," *Acta Derm Venereol* 75(4) (July 1995): 300–4.

Linday, L.A., Dolitsky, J.N., Shindledecker, R.D., Pippenger, C.E., "Lemon-flavored cod liver oil and a multi-vitamin/mineral supplement for the secondary prevention of otitis media in young children: Pilot research," *Annals of Otology, Rhinology & Laryngology,* 111 (2002): 642–652.

Logan, B.K., Jones, A.W., "Endogenous ethanol 'auto-brewery syndrome' as a drunk-driving defense challenge," *Med Sci Law*, 40(3) (July 2000): 206–15.

Louie, J.P., Bell, L.M., "Appropriate use of antibiotics for common infections in an era of increasing resistance," *Emerg Med Clin North Am*, 20(1) (February 2002): 69–91.

Majamaa, H., Isolauri, E., "Probiotics: a novel approach in the management of food allergy," *J Allergy Clin Immunol*, 99(2) (February 1997): 179–85.

McCourtie, J., Douglas, L.J., "Relationship between cell surface composition, adherence, and virulence of Candida albicans," *Infec Immunol*, 45(1) (1984): 6–12.

Melief, M.J., et al., "Presence of bacterial flora-derived antigen in synovial tissue macrophages and dendritic cells," *Br J Rheumatol*, 34(12) (December 1995): 1112–6.

Menzel, I., Holzmann, H., "Reflections on seborrheic scalp eczema and psoriasis capillitii in relation to intestinal mycoses," *Z Hautkr*, 61(7) (1 April 1986): 451–4.

Mielants, H., et al., "Gut inflammation in the spondyloarthropathies: clinical, biologic, and genetic features in relation to the type of histology," *J Rheumatol*, 18(10) (October 1991): 1542–51.

Miura, S., et al., "Modulation of intestinal immune system by dietary fat intake: relevance to Crohn's disease," *J Gastroenterol Hepatol*, 13(12) (December 1998): 1183–90.

Nagler-Anderson, C., "Man the barrier!' Strategic defences in the intestinal mucosa," *Nature Rev Immunol*, 1(1) (October 2000): 59–67.

Nagy, B., Sutka, P., Ziwe-el-Abidine, M., et al., "Candida guilliermondii var. guilliermondii infection in infertile women," *Mycoses*, 32(9) (September 1989): 463–8.

Nissen, D., et al., "IgE-sensitization to cellular and culture filtrates of fungal extracts in patients with atopic dermatitis," *Ann Allergy Asthma Immunol,* 81(3) (September 1998): 247–55.

Pactor, M.L., et al., "Controlled study of oxatomide vs disodium chromoglycate for treating the adverse reactions to food," *Drugs Clin Exp Res,* 18(3) (1992): 119–23.

Pena, A.S., Crusius, J.B., "Food allergy, celiac disease and chronic inflammatory bowel disease in man," *Vet Q,* 20 (3s) (1998): 49s–52.

Person, J.R., Bernhard, J.D., "Autointoxication revisited," *J Am Acad Dermatol,* 15(3) (September 1986): 559–63.

Persson, P.G., et al., "Diet and inflammatory bowel disease: a case control study," *Epidemiology,* 3(1) (January 1992): 47–52.

Peterson, N., "Otitis media (middle ear infections)," *American Association of Naturopathic Physicians* (online: www.healthy.net): 1–2.

Philpott, W.H., Kalita, D.K., *Brain Allergies: The Psychonutrient Connection* (New Canaan, CT: Keats Publishing, 1980): 7, 15–27, 28–49.

Porth, C.M., *Pathophysiology: Concepts of Altered Health States* (Philadelphia: JB Lippincott Co., 1990): 698.

Rapp, D., *Is This Your Child?* (New York: William Morrow & Co., Inc., 1991): 62–63, 167–171.

Reif, S. et al., "Pre-illness dietary factors in inflammatory bowel disease," *Gut,* 40(6) (June 1997): 754–60.

Remington, D.W., Higa, B.W., *Back to Health: A Comprehensive Medical and Nutritional Yeast Control Program* (Salt Lake City: Publishers Press, 1986): 209–210.

Riordan, A.M., et al., "Treatment of active Crohn's disease by exclusion diet: East Anglican multicentre controlled trial," *Lancet,* 340(8880) (6 November 1993): 1131–4.

Rivera, R., Deutsch, R.D., *Your Hidden Food Allergies are Making You Fat,* (Rocklin, CA: Prima Publishing, 1998): 39–40, 285–9.

Roboz, J., "Diagnosis and monitoring of disseminated candidiasis based on serum/urine D/L-arabinitol ratios," *Chirality* 6(2) (1994): 51–7.

Rose, D.P., Connoly, J.M., "Omega-3 fatty acids as cancer chemopreventive agents," *Pharmacol Ther,* 83(3) (September 1999): 217–44.

Rubaltelli, F.F., et al., "Intestinal flora in breast- and bottle-fed infants," *J Perinat Med,* 26(3) (1998): 186–91.

Sartor, R.B., et al., "Animal models of intestinal and joint inflammation," *Baillieres Clin Rheumatol,* 10(1) (February 1996): 55–76.

Savolainen, J., et al., "Candida albicans and atopic dermatitis," *Clin Exp Allergy* 23(4) (April 1993): 332–9.

Schmidt, M.H., et al., "Does oligoantigenic diet influence hyperactive/conduct-disordered children—a controlled trial," *Eur Child Adolesc, Psychiatry,* 6(2) (June 1997): 88–95.

Sesink, A.L., et al., "Red meat and colon cancer: the cytotoxic and hyperproliferative effects of dietary heme," *Cancer Res,* 59(22) (15 November 1999): 5704–9.

Severijnen, A.J., et al., "Cell wall fragments from major residents of the human intestinal flora induce chronic arthritis in rats," *J Rheumatol,* 16(8) (August 1989): 1061–8.

Shapiro, E., "Injudicious antibiotic use: an unforeseen consequence of the emphasis on patient satisfaction?" *Clin Ther,* 24(1) (January 2002): 197–204.

Shaw, W., Kassen, E., Chaves, E., "Increased urinary excretion of analogs of Kreb's cycle metabolites and arabinose in two brothers with autistic features," *Clin Chem,* 41(8) (1995): 1094–1104.

Shoenfeld, Y., Aron-Maor, A., "Vaccination and autoimmunity–'vaccinosis': a dangerous liaison?" *J Autoimmun,* 14(1) (February 2000): 1–10.

Sigthorson, G., Tibble, J., Hayllar, J., et al., "Intestinal permeability and inflammation in patients on NSAIDs," *Gut,* 43(4) (October 1998): 506–11.

Smith, R.S., "The immune system is a key factor in the etiology of psychosocial diseases," *Med Hypotheses,* 34(1) (January 1991): 49–57.

Staines, et al., *Introducing Immunology,* (St. Louis: Mosby, 1993): 93.

Stephanini, G.F., Saggioro, A., Alvisi, V., et al., "Oral cromolyn sodium in comparison with elimination diet in the irritable bowel syndrome, diarrheic type: multicenter study of 428 patients," *Scan J Gastroeneterol,* 30(6) (June 1995): 535–41.

Swank, G.M., Deitch, E.A., "Role of the gut in multiple organ failure: bacterial translocation and permeability changes," *World J Surg,* 20(4) (May 1996): 411–7.

Theron, R. Moss, R., *An Alternative Approach to Allergies,* (New York: Harper & Row, 1989).

Tiwana, H., et al., "Antibody response to gut bacteria in ankylosing spondylitis, rheumatoid arthritis, Crohn's disease, and ulcerative colitis," *Rheumatol Int,* 17(1) (1997): 11–6.

Traub, M., "Food allergy prevention: introduction of solid foods for infants," *American Association of Naturopathic Physicians* (online: www.healthy.net): 1–2.

Tuthill, R.W., "Hair lead levels related to children's classroom attention-deficit behavior," *Arch Environ Health,* 51(3) (May–June 1996): 214–20.

Van Ree, J.M., "Endorphins and experimental addiction," *Alcohol,* 13(1) (January–February 1996): 25–30.

Vanderhaeghe, L., Bouic, P., *The Immune System Cure,* (New York: Kensington Books, 1999): 156–174, 159–60, 166.

Vatn, M.H., Grimstad, I.A., Thorsen, L., et al., "Adverse reaction to food: assessment by double-blind placebo-controlled food challenge and clinical, psychosomatic and immunological analysis," *Digestion,* 56 (1995): 421–28.

Volatier, J.L., Verger, P., "Recent national french food and nutrient intake data," *Br J Nutr,* 81 Suppl. 2 (April 1999): S57–9.

Walker, W.A., Bloch, K.J., "Gastrointestinal transport of macromolecules in the pathogenesis of food allergy," *Ann Allergy,* 51(2 pt. 2) (August 1983): 240–5.

Wilson, C., et al., "Correlation between anti-Proteus antibodies and isolation rates of P. mirabilis in rheumatoid arthritis," *Rheumatol Int,* 16(5) (1997): 187–9.

Winderlin, C., *Candida Related Complex: What Your Doctor Might be Missing,* (Dallas: Taylor Publishing, 1996): 72.

Zeiger, R.S., "Dietary aspects of food allergy prevention in infants and children," *J Pediatr Gastroenterol Nutr,* 30s (2000): 77–86s.

Chapter 10

Abraham, J.E., et al., "The effect of dental amalgam restorations on blood mercury levels," *J Dent Res,* 63(1) (1984): 71–3.

Adonaylo, V.N., Oteiza, P.I., "Lead intoxication: antioxidant defenses and oxidative damage in rat brain," *Toxicology,* 135(2–3) (15 July 1999): 77–85.

Adonaylo, V.N., Oteiza, P.I., "Pb2+ promotes lipid oxidation and alterations in membrane physical properties," *Toxicology,* 132(1) (1 January 1999): 19–32.

Agency for Toxic Substances and Disease Registry, *The Nature and Extent of Lead Poisoning in Children in the United States,* (ATSDR Report to Congress, July 1988).

Agency for Toxic Substances and Disease Registry (ATSDR), *Benzene: Public health statement,* U.S. Department of Health and Human Services/Centers for Disease Control and Prevention, Atlanta, GA, (May 1989).

Agency for Toxic Substances and Disease Registry (ATSDR), *Toxicological Profile for Lead,* (Draft) U.S. Public Health Service, U.S. Department of Health and Human Services, Atlanta, GA, (1993).

Agency for Toxic Substances and Disease Registry (ATSDR), *Toxicological Profile for Cadmium,* U.S. Public Health Service, U.S. Department of Health and Human Services: Atlanta, GA, (1992).

Al Mufti, A.W., et al., "Epidemiology of organomercury poisoning in Iraq. I. Incidence in a defined area and relationship to the eating of contaminated bread," *Bull World Health Organ,* 53(s) (1976): 23–36.

Allen, B., et al., "Declining sex ratios in Canada," *Can Med J,* 156(1) (1 January 1997): 37–41.

Amin-Zaki, L., et al., "Prenatal methylmercury poisoning," *Am J Dis Child,* 133 (1979): 172–77.

Andrews, J.E., Gray, L.E., "The effects of lindane and linuron on calcium metabolism, bone morphometry, and the kidney in rats," *Toxicology,* 60(1–2) (January–February 1990): 99–107.

Baker, M.J., et al., "Renal toxicity in uranium mil workers," *Scand J Work Environ Health,* 11(2) (11 April 1985): 83–90.

Baldi, I., et al., "Prevalence of asthma and mean levels of air pollution: results from the French PAARC survey. Pollution Atmospherique et Affections Respiratoires Chroniques," *Eur Respir,* 14(1) (July 1999): 132–8.

Ballew, C., et al., "Blood lead concentration and children's anthropometric dimensions in the Third National Health and Nutrition Examination Survey," *J Pediatr* 134(5) (May 1999): 623–30.

Bellinger, D.C., et al., "Low-level lead exposure, intelligence and academic achievement: a long-term follow-up study," *Pediatrics,* 90(1992): 855–61.

Berglund, M., et al., "Intestinal absorption of dietary cadmium in women depends on iron stores and fiber intake," *Environ Health Perspect,* 102(12) (December 1994): 1058–66.

Bishop, N.J., Morley R., Day J.P., et al., "Aluminum neurotoxicity in preterm infants receiving intravenous-feeding solutions," *N Engl J Med,* 336(22) (May 29 1997): 1557–61.

Bland, J.S., et al., "A medical food-supplemented detoxification program in the management of chronic health problem," *Altern Ther Health Med,* 1(5) (1 November 1995): 62–71.

Bludovska, M., et al., "The influence of alpha-lipoic acid on the toxicity of cadmium," *Gen Physiol Biophys,* 18(October 1999): 28–32.

Borja, V.H., et al., "Blood lead levels measured prospectively and risk of spontaneous abortion," *Am J Epidemiol,* 150(6) (15 September 1999): 590–7.

Bourgoin, B.P., et al., "Lead content in 70 brands of dietary calcium supplements," *Am J Pub Health,* 83(8) (August 1993): 1155.

Brockel, B.J., Cory-Sclechta, D.A., "Lead, attention, and impulsive behavior: changes in a fixed-ratio waiting-for-reward paradigm," *Pharmacol Biochem Behav* 60(2) (June 1998): 545–52.

Brody, D.J., et al., "Blood lead levels in the US population. Phase I of the Third National Health and Nutrition Examination Survey," *JAMA,* 272(4) (July 1994): 277–83.

Brys, M., et al., "Zinc and cadmium analysis in human prostate neoplasms," *Biol Trace Elem Res,* 59(1–3) (Winter 1997): 145–52.

Brzoska, M.N., Moniuszko-Jakoniuk, J., "The influence of calcium content in the diet in cumulation and toxicity of cadmium in the organism," *Arch Toxicol,* 72(2) (1998): 63–73.

Buchet, J.P., et al., "Renal effects of cadmium body burden of the general public," *Lancet,* 336(8717) (22 June 1991): 1554.

Buckley, J.D., et al., "Occupational exposures of parents of children with acute nonlymphocytic leukemia: a report from the Children's Cancer Study Group," *Cancer Res,* 49(14) (15 July 1989): 4030–7.

Campbell, C.G., et al., "Chlorpyrifos interferes with cell development in rat brain regions," *Brain Res Bull,* 43(2) (1997): 179–89.

Campbell, A., "The potential role of aluminum in Alzheimer's Disease," *Nephrol Dial Transplant* 17 Suppl 2 (2002): 17–20.

Carmignani, M., et al., "Kininergic system and arterial hypertension following chronic exposure to inorganic lead," *Immunopharmacology,* 44(1–2) (15 October 1999): 105–10.

Centers for Disease Control and Prevention, *Chronic Fatigue Syndrome,* (online: www.cdc.gov/).

Centers for Disease Control and Prevention, *Cytomegalovirus (CMV)* (Online: www.cdc.gov/ncidod/diseases/cmv.htm) (Revised 8 September 1999).

Centers for Disease Control and Prevention, *Epstein-Barr virus (EBV)* (Online: www.cdc.gov/ncidod/diseases/ebv.htm) (Revised 8 September 1999).

Chan, T.Y., "The prevalence use and harmful potential of some Chinese herbal medicines in babies and children," *Vet Hum Toxicol,* 36(3) (June 1994): 238–40.

Clark, M., et al., "Interaction of iron deficiency and lead and the hematologic findings in children with severe lead poisoning," *Pediatrics,* 81(2) (February 1988): 247–54.

Clarkson, T.W., "The three modern faces of mercury," *Environ Health Perspect,* 110 (Suppl. 1) (February 2002): 11–23.

Colborn, T., et al., "Developmental effects of endocrine-disrupting chemicals in wildlife and humans," *Environ Health Perspectives,* 101(1993): 378–84.

Davis, D.L., et al., "Reduced ration of male to female births in several industrial countries: a sentinel health indicator?" *JAMA,* 279(13) (1 April 1998): 1018–23.

Dawson, E.B., et al., "Amniotic fluid B12, calcium, and lead levels associated with neural tube defects," *Am J Perinatol* 16(7) (1999): 373–8.

deCastro, F.J., Medley, J., "Lead in bone and hypertension," *Matern Child Health,* 1(3) (September 1997): 199–200.

Deitrich, K.N., et al., "The developmental consequences of low to moderate prenatal and postnatal lead exposure: intellectual attainment at the Cincinnati Lead Study Cohort following school entry." *Neurotoxicol Teratol,* 15(1993): 37–44.

Desi, I., et al., "Experimental model studies of pesticide exposure," *Neurotoxicology,* 19(4–5) (August–October 1998): 611–6.

Dich, J., et al., "Pesticides and cancer," *Cancer Causes Control,* 8(3) (May 1997): 420–43.

Droge, W., et al., "Glutathione augments activation of cytotoxic T lymphocytes *in vivo,*" *Immunobiol,* 172 (1–2) (1986): 151–6.

Eggelston, D.W., "Effect of dental amalgam and nickel alloys on T-lymphocytes: preliminary report," *J Prosthet Dent,* 51(5) (May 1984): 617–23.

Ellis, K.J., et al., "Cadmium: *in vivo* measurements in smokers and non-smokers," *Science,* 205(4403) (20 July 1979): 323–5.

El-Missiry, M.A., "Prophylactic effect of melatonin on lead-induced inhibition of heme biosynthesis and deterioration of antioxidant systems in male rats," *J Biochem Mol Toxicol,* 14(1) (2000): 57–62.

El-Sokkary, G.H., Karnel, E.S., Reiter R.J., "Prophylactic effect of melatonin in reducing lead-induced neurotoxicity in the rat," *Cell Mol Biol Letter,* 8(2) (2003): 461–70.

Environmental Protection Agency, (Online: www.epa.gov).

Environmental Working Group, "A shopper's guide to pesticides in produce," (Online: www.ewg.org/pub/home/reports/Shoppers/shop_short.html).

Environmental Working Group, "Government finds excessive risks in widely used insecticide," (27 October 1999) (Online: http://www.ewg.org/pub/home/reports/bandursban/bandursban.html): 1–3.

Eskenazi, B., Bradman, A., Castorina, R., "Exposures of children to organophosphate pesticides and their potential adverse health effects," *Environ Health Perspectives,* 107(3S) (June 1999): 409–41.

Esteban, E., et al., "Hair and blood as substrates for screening children for lead poisoning," *Arch Environ Health*, 54(6) (November–December 1999): 436–40.

Factor-Litvak, P., et al., "Hyperproduction of erythropoietin in non-anemic lead-exposed children," *Environ Health Perspect* 106(6) (June 1998): 361–4.

Fagin, D., Lavelleby, M., "Why let Col. Klink manage the EPA?" *Newsday*, (12 June 1997): A49.

Fenske, R.A., et al., "Potential exposure and health risks of infants following indoor residential pesticide applications," *Am J Pub Health*, 80(6) (June 1990): 689–93.

Fernandez, M., Bell, I.R., Schwartz, G.E., "EEG sensitization during chemical exposure in women with and without chemical sensitivity of unknown etiology," *Toxicol Ind Health*, 15(3–4) (April–June 1999): 305–12.

Fisher, B.E., "Most unwanted," *Environ Health Perspect*, 107(1) (January 1999): A18–23.

Fisher, M., "Environmental poisons in our food," *NOHA News*, 18(3) (Summer 1993): 1–3.

Fujita, E., "Experimental studies of organic mercury poisoning on the behaviors of Minamata disease: causal agent in the maternal bodies and its transference to their infants via either placenta or breast milk," *J Kumamoto Igakkai Zasshi*, 43(1) (25 January 1969): 47–62.

Fulton B., Jeffery E.G. "Absorption and retention of aluminum from drinking water: One Effect of citric and ascorbic acids on aluminum tissue levels in rabbits," *Fundam Appl Toxicol*, 14(4) (May 1990): 788–96.

Galland, L., "Biochemical abnormalities in patients with multiple chemical sensitivities," *Occup Med*, 2(4) (October–December 1987): 713–20.

Gilliland, F.D., et al., "Uranium mining and lung cancer among Navajo men in New Mexico and Arizona, 1969 to 1993," *J Occup Environ Med*, 42(3) (March 2000): 278–83.

Golan, R., *Optimal Wellness*, (New York: Ballantine Books, 1995).

Gomez, G., Rawson, N.E., Hahn, C.G., et al., "Characteristics of odorant elicited calcium changes in cultured human olfactory neurons," *J Neurosci*, 62(5) (December 2000): 737–49.

Goodbred, S.L., Gilliom, R.J., Gross, T.S., Denslow, N.P., Bryant, W.L., Schoeb, T.R., "Reconnaissance of 17b-estradiol, 11-ketotestosterone, vitellogenin, and gonad histopathology in common carp of United States Streams—Potential for contaminant-induced endocrine disruption," *US Geological Survey Open-File Report*, 96–627, (1997): 47.

Grant, W.B., Campbell A., Itzhaki R.F., et al., "The significance of environmental factors in the etiology of Alzheimer's disease," *J Alzheimers Dis*, 4(3) (June 2002): 179–89.

Graziano, J.H., et al., "Depressed serum erythropoietin in pregnant women with elevated blood lead," *Arch Environ Health*, 46(6) (November–December 1991): 347–50.

Gruber, S.J., Munn, M.D., "Organochlorine pesticides and PCBs in aquatic ecosystems of the Central Columbia Plateau," *USGS Fact Sheet*, FS-170–96 (September 1996) (Online: http://water.usgs.gov/nawqa/nawqa_home.html): 1–6.

Gurer, H., et al., "Antioxidant effects of N-acetylcysteine and succimer in red blood cells from lead exposed rats," *Toxicology*, 128(3) (17 July 1998): 181–9.

Gurer, H., et al., "Antioxidant role of alpha-lipoic acid in lead toxicity," *Free Radic Biol Med*, 27(1–2) (July 1999): 75–81.

Haas, E.M., *Staying Healthy With Nutrition* (Berkeley, CA: Celestial Arts, 1992).

Halder, C.A., et al., "Hydrocarbon nephropathy in male rats: identification of the nephrotoxic components of unleaded gasoline," *Toxicol Ind Health*, 1(3) (November 1985): 67–87.

Hayes, R.B., et al., "Benzene and the dose-related incidence of hematologic neoplasms in China," Chinese Academy of Preventive Medicine—National Cancer Institute Benzene Study," *J Natl Cancer Inst*, 89(14) (16 July 1997): 1065–71.

Hirokawa, K., Hayashi, Y., et al., "Acute methyl mercury intoxication in mice—effect on the immune system," *Acta Pathol Japan,* 30(1) (January 1980): 23–32.

Houston, D.K., Johnson, M.A., "Lead as a risk factor for hypertension in women," *Nutr Rev,* 57(9 Pt 1): 277–9.

Hu, H., "Bone lead as a new biomarker of lead dose: recent findings and implications for public health," *Environ Health Perspect,* 106(4s) (August 1998): 961–7.

Hu, H., et al., "The relationship between bone lead and hemoglobin," *JAMA,* 272(19) (16 November 1994): 1512–7.

Hu, H., et al., "The relationship of bone and blood lead to hypertension: The Normative Aging Study," *JAMA,* 275(15) (17 April 1996): 1171–6.

Irgens, A., et al., "Reproductive outcome in offspring of parents occupationally exposed to lead in Norway," *Am J Ind Med,* 34(5) (November 1998): 431–7.

James, J.A., et al., "An increased prevalence of Epstein-Barr virus infection in young patients suggests a possible etiology for systemic lupus erythematosus," *J Clin Invest,* 100(12) (15 December 1997): 3019–26.

Jansson E.T., "Aluminum exposure and Alzheimer's disease," *J Alzheimers Dis,* 3(6) (Dec 2001): 541–549.

Jarup, L., et al., "Health effects of cadmium exposure—a review of the literature and a risk estimate," *Scand J Work Environ, Health,* 24(1s) (1998): 1–51.

Jo, W.K., Song, K.B., "Exposure to volatile organic compounds for individuals with occupations associated with potential exposure to motor vehicle exhaust and/or gasoline vapor emissions," *Sci Total Environ,* 269(1–3) (2001): 25–37.

Johnson, D.E., et al., "Early biochemical detection of delayed neurotoxicity resulting from developmental exposure to chlorpyrifos," *Brain Res Bull,* 45(2) (1998): 143–7.

Johnson, F.M., "The genetic effects of environmental lead," *Mutat Res,* 410(2) (April 1998): 123–40.

Kim, R., et al., "A longitudinal study of low-level lead exposure and impairment of renal function. The Normative Aging Study," *JAMA,* 275(15) (17 April 1996): 1177–81.

Kipen, H.M., et al., "Prevalence of chronic fatigue and chemical sensitivies in Gulf Registry Veterans," *Arch Environ Health,* 54(5) (September–October 1999): 313–8.

Kneip, T.J., et al., "The effects of anemia on heme synthesis parameters during lead exposure," *Am Ind Hyg Assoc,* 37(10) (October 1976): 578–85.

Knobil, E., et al., *Hormonally Active Agents in the Environment,* Washington, D.C., National Academy Press, (July 1999).

Koller, L.D., et al., "Neoplasia induced in male rats fed lead acetate, ethyl urea, and sodium nitrite," *Toxicol Pathol,* 13(1) (1985): 50–7.

Kreutzer, R., et al., "Prevalence of people reporting sensitivities to chemicals in a population-based survey," *Am J Epidemiol,* 150(1) (1 July 1999): 1–12.

Krohn, J., Taylor, F.A., Prosser, J., *Natural Detoxification,* (Point Roberts, WA: Hartley & Marks Publishers, Inc., 1996).

Lamphere, D.N., et al., "Reduced cadmium body burden in cadmium-exposed calves fed supplemental zinc," *Environ Res,* 33(1) (February 1984): 119–29.

Lange, G., et al., "Psychiatric diagnoses in Gulf War veterans with fatiguing illness," *Psychiatry Res,* 89(1) (13 December 1999): 39–48.

Langford, N., Ferner, R., "Toxicity of mercury," *J Human Hypertens,* 13(10) (October 1999): 651–6.

Lanphear, B.P., et al., "Lead-contaminated house dust and urban children's blood lead levels," *Am J Public Health,* 86(10) (October 1996): 1416–21.

Lauwerys, R., et al., "Does environmental exposure to cadmium represent a health risk? Conclusions from the Cadmibel Study," *Acta Clin Belg,* 46(4) (1991): 219–25.

Leggett, R.W., "The behavior and chemical toxicity of U in the kidney: a reassessment," *Health Pys* 57(3) (September 1989): 365–83.

Loghman-Adham, M., "Renal effects of environmental and occupational lead exposure," *Environ Health Perspect,* 105(9) (September 1997): 928–39.

Lorscheider, F.L., Vimy, M.J., et al., "Mercury exposure from "silver" tooth fillings: emerging evidence questions a traditional dental paradigm," *FASEB J,* 9(7) (April 1995): 504–8.

McLachlan, D.R.C., et al., "Aluminum and the pathogenesis of Alzheimer's disease: a summary of the evidence," Ciba Foundation Symposium 160, *Aluminum in Biology and Medicine* (New York: John Wiley & Sons, 1992).

Miller, C.S., Prihoda, T.J., "A controlled comparison of symptoms and chemical intolerances reported by Gulf War veterans, implant recipients, and persons with multiple chemical sensitivity," *Toxicol Ind Health,* 15(3–4) (April–June 1999): 386–97.

Miller, L.J., Kubes, K.L., "Serotonergic agents in the treatment of fibromyalgia syndrome," *Ann Pharmacothe,* 36(4) (April 2002): 707–12.

"Multiple chemical sensitivity: a 1999 consensus," *Arch Environ Health,* 54(3) (May–June 1999): 147–9.

Munger, R., et al., "Intrauterine growth retardation in Iowa communities with herbicide-contaminated drinking water supplies," *Environ Health Perspect,* 105(3) (March 1997): 308–14.

National Research Council, *Toxicity Testing,* Washington: National Academy Press, (1984).

National Resource Defense Council, "Our children at risk: the five worst environmental threats to their health," (online: www.nrdc.org).

National Resource Defense Council, *Pesticide Fact Sheets: Highest Risk Pesticides,* (online: www.nrdc.org).

National Resource Defense Council, *The Food Quality Protection Act of 1996,* (online: www.nrdc.org).

Niemeyer, S., et al., "Handling wastes: household solvents," *NebFacts,* (Nebraska Cooperative Extension: UNL: NF94–193, August 1994): 1–5.

Nogawa, K., et al., "Critical concentration of cadmium in kidney cortex of humans exposed to environmental cadmium," *Environ Res,* 40(2) (August 1986): 251–60.

Nordt, S.P., Chew, G., "Acute lindane poisoning in three children," *J Emerg Med* 18(1) (January 2000): 51–3.

Nowell, L., "National summary of organochlorine detections in bed sediment and tissues for the 1991 NAWQA study units," *USGS National Water Quality Assessment Program: Pesticide National Synthesis Project,* (14 June 1999) (Online: http://water.wr.usgs.gov/pnsp/rep/bst/): 1–3.

Ornaghi, F., et al., "The protective effects of N-acetyl-L-cysteine against methyl mercury embryotoxicity in mice," *Fundam Appl Toxicol,* 20(4) (May 1993): 437–45.

Oteiza, P.I., et al., "Cadmium-induced testes oxidative damage in rats can be influenced by dietary zinc intake," *Toxicology,* 137(1) (10 September 1999): 13–22.

Ott, W.R., Roberts, J.W., "Everyday exposure to toxic pollutants," *Scientific American,* (February 1998): 1–9.

Paulozzi, L.J., et al., "Hypospadias trends in two US surveillance systems," *Pediatrics,* 100(5) (November 1997): 831–4.

Pellmar, T.C., et al., "Electrophysiological changes in hippocampal slices isolated from rats imbedded with depleted uranium fragments," *Neurotoxicology,* 20(5) (October 1999): 785–92.

Pena, A., Iturri, S.J., "Cadmium as hypertensive agent: effect on ion excretion in rats," *Comp Biochem Physiol,* 106(2) (October 1993): 315–9.

Pertowski, C.A., *Lead Poisoning,* (Division of Environmental Hazards and Health Effects, Centers for Disease Control and Prevention, Atlanta, GA).

Petit, T.L., LeBoutillier, J.C., "Zinc deficiency in the postnatal rat: implications for lead toxicity," *Neurotoxicology,* 7(1) (Spring 1986): 237–46.

Pirkle, J.L., et al., "Exposure of the U.S. population to lead, 1991–1994," *Environ Health Perspect,* 106(11) (November 1998): 745–50.

Piyasirisilp, S., Hemachudha T., "Neurological adverse events associated with vaccination," *Curr Opin Neurol,* 15(3) (June 2002): 333–8.

Pizzichini, M., Fonzi, M., Sugherini, L., et al., "Release of mercury from dental amalgam and its influence on salivary antioxidant activity," *Sci Total Environ,* 284(1–3) (2002): 19–25.

Porter, W.P., Jaeger, J.W., Carlson, I.H., "Endocrine, immune, and behavioral effects of aldicarb (carbamate), atrazine (triazine), and nitrate (fertilizer) mixtures at groundwater concentration," *Toxicol Ind Health,* 15(1–2) (January–March 1999): 133–50.

Presidential Advisory Committee on Gulf War Veterans Illnesses: Final Report (December 1996), *Frontline: The Last Battle of the Gulf War,* (online: http://www.pbs.org/).

Puri, V.N., "Cadmium induced hypertension," *Clin Exp Hypertens,* 21(1–2) (January–February 1999): 79–84.

Queen, H.L., *Chronic Mercury Toxicity: New Hope Against an Endemic Disease,* (Colorado Springs: Queen and Company, 1988): 36–38.

Redwood, L., Bernard, S., Brown, D., "Predicted mercury concentrations in hair from infant immunizations: cause for concern," *Neurotoxicology,* 22(5) (October 2001): 691–7.

Rogan, W.J., et al., "Polychlorinated biphenyls (PCBs) and dichlorodiphenyl dichloroethene (DDE) in human milk: Effects on growth, morbidity, and duration of lactation," *Am J Public Health,* 77(10) (Oct 1987): 1294–7.

Rogers, M.A., Simon, D.G. "A preliminary study of dietary aluminum intake and risk of Alzheimer's disease," *Age Aging,* 28(2) (March 1999): 205–9.

Rossi, J., III, "Sensitization induced by kindling and kindling-related phenomena as a model for multiple chemical sensitivity," *Toxicology,* 111(1–3) (17 July 1996): 87–100.

Sakai, T., "Biomarkers of lead exposure," *Ind Health,* 38(2) (April 2000): 127–42.

Shaikh, Z.A., Vu, T.T., Zaman, K., "Oxidative stress as a mechanism of chronic cadmium induced hepatotoxicity and renal toxicity and protection by antioxidants," *Toxicol Appl Pharmacol,* 154(3) (February 1999): 256–63.

Shenker, B.J., et al., "Low-level methylmercury exposure causes human T-cells to undergo apoptosis: evidence of mitochondrial dysfunction," *Environ Res,* 77(2) (May 1998): 149–59.

Siblerud, R.L., Kienholz, E., "Evidence that mercury from silver dental fillings may be an etiological factor in multiple sclerosis," *Sci Total Environ,* 142(3) (March 1994): 191–205.

Smith, T., et al., "Bacterial oxidation of mercury metal vapor, Hg (0)," *Appl Environ Microbiology,* 64(4) (April 1998): 1328–32.

Staessen, J.A., et al., "Public health implications of environmental exposure to cadmium and lead: an overview of epidemiological studies in Belgium. Working groups," *J Cardiovasc Risk,* 3(1) (February 1996): 26–41.

Steven, I.D., et al., "General practitioners' beliefs, attitudes and reported actions towards chronic fatigue syndrome," *Aust Fam Physician,* 29(1) (January 2000): 80–5.

Suplido, M.L., Ong, C.N., "Lead exposure among small-scale battery recyclers, automobile radiator mechanics, and their children in Manila, the Philippines," *Environ Res,* 82(3) (March 2000): 231–8.

Telisman, S., et al., "Semen quality and reproductive endocrine function in relation to biomarkers of lead, cadmium, zinc and copper in men," *Environ Health Pespect,* 108(1) (January 2000): 45–53.

Thrasher, J.D., et al., "Immunologic abnormalities in humans exposed to chlorpyrifos: preliminary observations," *Arch Environ Health,* 48(2) (March–April 1993): 89–93.

Thun, M.J., et al., "Mortality among a cohort of U.S. cadmium production workers: an update," *J Natl Cancer Inst* 74(2) (1985): 325–33.

Tomera, J.F., et al., "Divalent cations in hypertension with implications to heart disease: calcium, cadmium interactions," *Methods Find Exp Clin Pharmacol,* 16(2) (March 1994): 97–107.

Tuthill, R.W., "Hair lead levels related to children's classroom attention-deficit behavior," *Arch Environ Health,* 51(3) (May–June 1996): 214–20.

U.S. Department of Housing and Urban Development, "Comprehensive and workable plan for the abatement of lead-based paint in privately owned housing," *Report to Congress,* (Washington, DC: 1990).

U.S. Environmental Protection Agency, "Methyl Parathion," *The HED Chapter of the Reregistration Eligibility Decision Document (RED),* (FIFRA Docket OPP-34161/0008, 1998).

U.S. Environmental Protection Agency, *Endocrine Disrupter Screening Program Web Site,* (10 February 1999) (Online: www.epa.goc/scipoly/oscpendo/index.htm): 1–2.

U.S. Environmental Protection Agency, *Intergrated Risk Information System (IRIS) on Cadmium,* (Environmental Criteria and Assessment Office, Office of Health and Environmental Assessment, Office of Research and Development: Cincinnati, OH, 1993)

U.S. Environmental Protection Agency Office of Pesticide Programs, *Organophosphate Pesticides: Documents for Chlorpyrifos,* (18 October 1999) (Online: www.epa.gov/pesticides/op/clorpyrifos.htm): 1–68.

U.S. Environmental Protection Agency Office of Pesticide Programs, "Organophosphate pesticides in food: a primer on reassessment of residue limits," (May 1999) (Online: www.epa.gov/pesticides): 1–5.

U.S. Food and Drug Administration, "Mercury in fish: cause for concern?" *FDA Consumer,* (September 1994) (Online: http://vmcfsan.fda.gov/~dms/mercury.html).

Verschoyle, R.D., et al., "A comparison of the acute toxicity, neuropathology, and electrophysiology of N,N-diethyl-m-toluamide and N,N-dimethyl-2,2-diphenylacetamide in rats," *Fundam Appl Toxicol,* 18(1) (January 1992): 79–88.

Videla, L.A., et al., "Mechanisms of lindane-induced hepatotoxicity: alterations of respiratory activity and sinusoidal glutathione efflux in the isolated perfused rat liver," *Xenobiotica,* 21(8) (August 1991): 1023–32.

Vimy, M.J., Lorscheider, F.L., "Intra-oral air mercury released from dental amalgams." *J Dent Res,* 64(8) (August 1985): 1069–71.

Vimy, M.J., Lorscheider, F.L., "Serial measurements of intra-oral air mercury: estimation of daily dose from dental amalgams," *J Dent Res,* 64(8) (August 1985): 1072–5.

Waalkes, M.P., Rehm, S., "Cadmium and prostate cancer," *J Toxicol Environ Health,* 43(3) (November 1994): 251–69.

Watts, D., "Tissue mineral analysis," *Clinical Chemistry and Nutrition Guidebook,* Vol. 1 (Eds. P. Yanick, Ph.D., and R. Jaffe, M.D.: T & H Publishing, 1988): 365–7.

White, K.P., et al., "Co-existence of chronic fatigue syndrome with fibromyalgia syndrome in the general population: a controlled study," *Scand J Rheumatol,* 29(1) (2000): 44–51.

Whitney, K.D., et al., "Developmental neurotoxicity of chlorpyrifos: cellular mechanisms." *Toxicol Appl Pharmacol,* 134(1) (September 1995): 53–63.

Wibberley, D.G., et al., "Lead levels in human placentae from normal and malformed births," *J Med Genet,* 14(5) (October 1977): 339–45.

Yang, R., "NTP technical report on the toxicity studies of a chemical mixture of 25 groundwater contaminants administered in drinking water to F344/N rats and B6C3F(1) mice," *Toxic Rep Ser.,* 35 (August 1993): 1–112.

Zabinski, Z., et al., "The activity of erythrocyte enzymes and basic indices of peripheral blood erythrocytes from workers chronically exposed to mercury vapours," *Toxicol Ind Health,* 16(2) (February 2000): 58–64.

Ziem, G., McTanney, J., "Profile of patients with chemical injury and sensitivity," *Environ Health Perspect,* 105 (S2) (March 1997): 417–36.

Ziff, S., Ziff, M.F., *Infertility and Birth Defects* (Orlando: Bio-Probe, Inc., 1987).

Chapter 11

Berson, E.L., "Nutrition and retinal degenerations," *Int Ophthalmol Clin,* 40(4) (Fall 2000): 93–111.

Blasiak, J., et al., "Protective action of vitamin C against DNA damage induced by selenium-cisplatin conjugate," *Acta Biochim Pol,* 48(1) (2001): 233–40.

Buttery, L.D., et al., "Differentiation of osteoblasts and *in vitro* bone formation from murine embryonic stem cells," *Tissue Eng,* 7(1) (February 2001): 89–99.

Carr, A., et al., "Does vitamin C act as a pro-oxidant under physiological conditions?" *FASEB J,* 13(9) (June 1999): 1007–24.

Chen, C.Y., et al., "Effects of nickel chloride on human platelets: enhancement of lipid peroxidation, inhibition of aggregation and interaction with ascorbic acid," *J Toxicol Environ Health A,* 62(6) (March 2001): 431–8.

Chithra, V., et al., "Hypolipidemic effect of coriander seeds (Coriandrum sativum): mechanism of action," *Plant Foods Hum Nutr,* 51(2) (1997): 167–72.

Chitra, V., et al., "Coriandrum sativum changes the levels of lipid peroxides and activity of antioxidant enzymes in experimental animals," *Indian J Biochem Biophys,* 36(1) (February 1999): 59–61.

Clemetson, C.A., "The key role of histamine in the development of atherosclerosis and coronary heart disease," *Med Hypotheses,* 52(1) (January 1999): 1–8.

Das, S., "Vitamin E in the genesis and prevention of cancer: a review," *Acta Oncol,*33(6) (1994): 615–19.

De la Fuente, M., et al., "Immune function in aged women is improved by ingestion of vitamins C and E," *Can J Physiol Pharmacol,* 76(4) (April 1998): 373–80.

Evans, W.J., "Vitamin E, vitamin C, and exercise," *Am J Clin Nutr,* 72(Suppl. 2) (August 2000): 647S–52S.

Ferslew, K.E., et al., "Pharmacokinetics and bioavailability of the RRR and all racemic stereoisomers of alpha-tocopherol in humans after single oral administration," *J Clin Pharmacol,* 33(1) (January 1993): 84–88.

Gao, F., Yao, C.L., Gao, E., et al., "Enhancement of glutathione cardioprotection by ascorbic acid in myocardial reperfusion injury," *J Pharmacol Exp Ther,* 301(2) (May 2002): 543–50.

Golan, R., *Optimal Wellness,* (New York: Ballantine Books, 1995): 157.

Head, K.A., "Ascorbic acid in the prevention and treatment of cancer," *Altern Med Rev,* 3(3) (June 1998): 174–86.

Heinemann, T., Kullak-Ublick, G.A., et al., "Mechanisms of action of plant sterols on inhibition of cholesterol absorption. Comparison of sitosterol and sitostanol," *Eur J Clin Pharmacol,* 40(Suppl 1) (1991): S59–63.

Kromhout, D., "Diet and cardiovascular diseases," *J Nutr Health Aging,* 5(3) (2001): 144–9.

Lee, C.Y., et al., "Vitamin E supplementation improves cell-mediated immunity and oxidative stress of Asian men and women," *J Nutr,* 130(12) (December 2000): 2932–7.

Miettinen, T.A, "Regulation of serum cholesterol by cholesterol absorption," *Agents Actions Suppl,* 26 (1988): 53–65.

Nardi, E.A., et al., "High-dose reduced glutathione in the therapy of alcoholic hepatopathy," *Clin Ter,* 136(1) (15 January 1991): 47–51.

Patra, R.C., et al., "Antioxidant effects of alpha tocopherol, ascorbic acid and L-methionine on lead induced oxidative stress to the liver, kidney and brain in rats," *Toxicology,* 162(2) (May 2001): 81–8.

Perticone, F., et al., "Obesity and body fat distribution induce endothelial dysfunction by oxidative stress: protective effect of vitamin C," *Diabetes,* 50(1) (January 2001): 159–65.

Pollak, O.J., "Effect of plant sterols on serum lipids and atherosclerosis," *Pharmacol Ther,* 31(3) (1985): 177–208.

Poo, J.L., Rosas-Romero, R., Montemayor, A.C., et al., "Diagnostic value of the copper/zinc ratio in hepatocellular carcinoma: a case control study," *J Gastroenterol,* 38(1) (January 2003): 45–51.

Qureshi, A.A., et al., "Tocotrienols: novel hypocholesterolemic agents with antioxidant properties," *Vitamin E in Health and Disease,* L. Packer & J. Fuchs, eds. New York: Marcel Dekker, 1993: 247–267.

Shenkin, A., "Trace elements: contribution to the efficacy of nutritional support," *Nestle Nutr Workshop Ser Clin Perform Programme,* 7:133–45 (2002): discussion 145–9.

Sundaram, V., et al., "Both hypothyroidism and hyperthyroidism enhance low-density lipoprotein oxidation," *J Clin Endocrinol Metal,* 82(10) (Oct 1997): 3421–4.

Vojdani, A., et al., "New evidence for antioxidant properties of vitamin C," *Cancer Detect Prev,* 24(6) (2000): 508–23.

Yin, L., et al., "Alterations of extracellular matrix induced by tobacco smoke extract," *Arch Dermatol Res,* 292(4) (April 2000): 188–94.

Zorn, N.E., et al., "A relationship between vitamin B_{12}, folic acid, ascorbic acid, and mercury uptake and methylation," *Life Sci,* 47(2) (1990): 167–73.

Chapter 12

Anderson, J.W., Smith, B.M., Gustafson, N.J., "Health benefits and practical aspects of high-fiber diets," *Am J Clin Nutr,* 59(5 Suppl) (May 1994): 1242S–1247S.

Ascherio, A.N., Willett, W.C., "Health effects of trans fatty acids," *Am J Clin Nutr,* 66(4s) (October 1997): 1006–1010s.

Baer, F.E., et al., "Variation in mineral composition of vegetables," *Soil Sci Soc Am,* 13 (1948): 380–84.

Bruinsma, N., Hutchison, J.M., Van Den Bogaard, A.E., et al., "Influence of population density on antibiotic resistance," *J Antimicrob Chemother,* 51(2) (February 2003): 385–90.

Buckley, J.D., et al., "Occupational exposures of parents of children with acute nonlymphocytic leukemia: a report from the Children's Cancer Study Group," *Cancer Res,* 49(14) (15 July 1989): 4030–7.

Chang, H.Y., Sharma, V.K., Howden, C.W., et al., "Knowledge, attitudes, and practice styles of North American Pediatric Gastroenterologists: helicobacter pylori infection," *J Pediatr Gastroenterol Nutr,* 36(2) (February 2003): 235–40.

Chiu, B.C., et al., "Diet and risk of non-Hodgkins lymphoma in older women," *JAMA,* 275(17) (1 May 1996): 1315–21.

Dayan, A.D., "Allergy to antimicrobial residues in food: assessment of the risk to man," *Vet Microbiol,* 35(3–4) (June 1993): 213–26.

Elbasha, E.H., "Deadweight loss of bacterial resistance due to overtreatment," *Health Econ,* 12(2) (February 2003): 125–38.

Fagan, J., "GM food labeling," *Nat Biotechnol,* 17(9) (September 1999): 836.

Fagan, J.B., "Assessing the safety and nutritional quality of genetically engineered foods," (online: www.natural-law.ca/genetic/geindex.html): 1–20.

Fidanza, A., "Therapeutic action of pantothenic acid," *Int J Vitam Nutr Res Suppl,* 24 (1983): 53–67.

Gaesser, G., "Roads to wellness may not be so narrow," *National Wellness Association,* (Online: www.nationalwellness.org/nwa, 1999).

Golan, R., *Optimal Wellness* (New York: Ballantine Books, 1995).

Gregory, K.E., Ford, J.J., "Effects of late castration, zeranol and breed group on growth, feed efficiency and carcass characteristics of late maturing bovine males," *J Anim Sci,* 56(4) (April 1983): 771–80.

Kohlmeier, L., et al., "Adipose tissue trans fatty acids and breast cancer in the European Community Multicenter Study on antioxidants, myocardial infarction, and breast cancer," *Cancer Epidemiol Biomarkers Prev,* 6(9) (September 1997): 705–10.

Kroes, R., Muller, D., Lambe, J., et al., "Assessment of intake from the diet," *Food Chem Toxicol,* 40(2–3) (February–March 2002): 327–85.

Kromhout, D., "Fatty acids, antioxidants, and coronary heart disease from an epidemiological perspective," *Lipids,* 34(S) (1999): 27–31s.

LeMarchand, L., Donlon, T., Seifried, A., et al., "Red meat intake, CYP2E1 genetic polymorphisms, and colorectal cancer risk," *Cancer Epidemiol Biomarkers Prev,* 11(10 pt 1) (October 2002): 1019–24.

Maliakal, P.P., Coville, P.F., Wanwimolruk, S., "Decreased hepatic drug metabolising enzyme activity in rats with nitrosamine-induced tumours," *Drug Metabol Drug Interact,* 19(1) (2002): 13–27.

McCann, S.E., et al., "Risk of human ovarian cancer is related to dietary intake of selected nutrients, phytochemicals, and food groups," *J Nutr.,* 133:1937–1942, June 2003.

Miller, J., Boswell, F.C., "Mineral composition of liver and kidney of rats fed corn, sorghum, and soybean grain grown with sewage sludges and NPK fertilizers," *J Agric Food Chem,* 24(5) (September–October 1976): 935–8.

National Research Council, *Toxicity Testing* (Washington: National Academy Press, 1984).

National Resource Defense Council, *Pesticide Fact Sheets: Highest Risk Pesticides,* (online: www.nrdc.org).

National Resource Defense Council, *The Food Quality Protection Act of 1996,* (online: www.nrdc.org).

Pao, E.M., Mickle, S.J., "Problem nutrients in the United States," *Food Technology* 35(1981): 58–62.

Partsch, C.J., Sippell, W.G., "Pathogenesis and epidemiology of precocious puberty: effects of exogenous oestrogens," *Hum Reprod Update,* 7(3) (May 2001–2002): 292–302.

Patterson, B.H., et al., "Fruit and vegetables in the American diet: data from the NHANES II Survey," *Am J Public Health,* 80(12) (1990): 1443–49.

Posner, B.M., et al., "Healthy People 2000: the rationale and efficacy of preventative nutrition in heart disease: The Framingham Offspring-Spouse Study," *Arch Intern Med,* 153 (13) (12 July 1993): 1549–56.

Raison-Peyron, N., Messaad, D., Bousquet, J., et al., "Anaphylaxis to beef in penicillin-allergic patient," *Allergy,* 56(8) (August 2001): 796–7.

Riboli, E., et al., "Dietary fiber in food and protection against colorectal cancer in the European prospective investigation into cancer and nutrition (EPIC): an observational study," *Lancet* 361 (2003): 1496–501.

Rogan, W.J., et al., "Polychlorinated biphenyls (PCBs) and dichlorodiphenyl dichloroethene (DDE) in human milk: effects on growth, morbidity, and duration of lactation," *Am J Public Health,* 77(10) (October 1987): 1294–7.

Rosenthal, M.S., *The Thyroid Sourcebook* (Los Angeles: Lowell House, 1996).

Sampson, M.J., et al., "Direct evidence of increased free-radical damage during acute hyperglycemia in type II diabetes," *Diabetes Care,* 25(3) (2002): 537–41.

Sears, B., *The Zone* (New York: Harper Collins, 1995).

Smith, B., "Organic foods vs. supermarket foods: element levels," *J Appl Nutr,* 45(1) (1993): 35–39.

Stevens, J., Juhaeri Ahn, K., Houston, D., et al., "Dietary fiber intake and glycemic index and incidence of diabetes in African-American and white adults: the ARIC study," *Diabetes Care,* 25(10) (October 2002): 1715–21.

Surgeon General's Report on Nutrition and Health, *DHHS,* Publication No. 88–50211.

Tepper, D., "Frontiers in congestive heart failure–lifetime risk for developing congestive heart failure: the Framingham Heart Study," *Congest Heart Fail,* 9(1) (January–February 2003): 51–2.

Thompson, D., et al., "Lifetime health and economic consequences of obesity," *Arch Intern Med,* 159(18) (11 October 1999): 2177–83.

Wilson, P.W., "Established risk factors and coronary artery disease: the Framingham Study," *Am J Hypertens,* 7(7 pt 2) (1994): 7s–12s.

Zand, J., et al., *Smart Medicine for Healthier Living,* (Garden City Park, NY: Avery Publishing, 1999).

Zima, T., "Free radicals in the pathogenesis of selected diseases," *Cas Lek Cesk,* 134(10) (17 May 1995): 291–5.

Zock, P.L., et al., "Dietary trans fatty acids: a risk factor for coronary heart disease," *Ned Tijdschr Geneeskd,* 142(30) (25 July 1998): 1701–4.

Chapter 13

Anderson, J.V., Palombo, R.D., Earl, R., "Position of the American Dietetic Association: the role of nutrition in health promotion and disease prevention programs," *J Am Diet Assoc,* 98(2) (February 1998): 205–8.

Boyd, J.N., et al., "Modification by beet and cabbage diets of aflatoxin B1 induced rat plasma alpha-fetoprotein elevation, hepatic tumorigenesis, and mutagenicity of urine," *Food Chen Toxicol,* 20 (1982): 47.

Chen, I., et al., "Aryl hydrocarbon receptor-mediated antiestrogenic and antitumorigenic activity of diindolylmethane," *Carcinogenesis,* 19 (1998): 1631–1639.

Feskanich, D., Willet, W., Colditz, G., "Calcium, vitamin D, milk consumption and hip fractures: a prospective study in postmenopausal women," *Am J Clin Nutr,* 77(2) (2003):504–511.

McDanell, R., et al., "Differential induction of mixed-function oxidase (MFO) activity in rat liver and intestine by diets containing processed cabbage: correlation with cabbage levels of glucosinolates and glucosinolate hydrolysis products," *Food Chem. Toxicicol,* 25 (1987): 363–368.

Press Release,"Report on the meeting of the American College of Sports Medicine where Cris Slentz lead author reported on the results of this yet unpublished study," *Reuters* (May 28, 2003).

Wattenberg, L.W., Loub, W.D., "Inhibition of polycyclic aromatic hydrocarbon-induced neoplasia by naturally occurring indoles," *Cancer Research,* 38 (1978): 1410–1413.

Zeligs, M.A., "Diet and estrogen status: the cruciferous connection," *J of Medicinal Food,* 1 (2 November 1998): 67–82.

Chapter 14

Aayo-Yusuf, O.A., et al., "Fluoride concentration of bottled drinking waters," *SADJ,* 56(6) (June 2001): 273–6.

Akpata, E.S., "Occurrence and management of dental fluorosis," *Int Dent J,* 51(5) (October 2001): 325–33.

Bar-Or, O., et al., "Swimming and asthma: benefits and deleterious effects," *Sports Med,* 14(6) (February 1992): 397–405.

Batmanghelidj, F., "A new and natural method of treatment of peptic ulcer disease," *J Clin Gastroenterol,* 5(3) (June 1983): 203–5.

Batmanghelidj, F., "Pain: a need for paradigm change," *Anticancer Res,* 7(5B) (1987): 971–89.

Bove, F., et al., "Drinking water contaminants and adverse pregnancy outcomes: a review," *Environ Health Perspect,* 110 (Suppl 1) (Feb 2002): 61–74.

Cabral, D., et al., "Fungal spoilage of bottled mineral water," *Int J Food Microbiol,* 72(1–2) (January 2002): 73–6.

Cotruvo, J.A., "EPA policies to protect the health of consumers of drinking water in the United States," *Sci Total Environ,* 18 (April 1981): 345–56.

"Fluorine and fluorides," Environmental Health Criteria 36, IPCS International Programme on Chemical Safety, WHO, 1984. (The WHO guideline values for fluoride in drinking water were reevaluated in 1996, without change, and the issue is currently under further review.)

Gniadecka, M., et al., "Water and protein structure in photoaged and chronically aged skin," *J Invest Dermatol,* 111(6) (December 1998): 1129–33.

Gostin, L.O., et al., "Water quality laws and waterborne diseases: cryptosporidium and other emerging pathogens," *Am J Public Health,* 90(6) (June 2000): 847–53.

Gupta, S.K., et al., "Reversal of clinical and dental fluorosis," *Indian Pediatr,* 31(4) (April 1994): 439–43.

Gupta, S.K., et al., "Reversal of fluorosis in children," *Acta Paediatr Jpn,* 38(5) (October 1996): 513–9.

James, S.C., "Metals in municipal landfill leachate and their health effects," *Am J Public Health,* 67(5) (May 1992): 29–32.

Kwak, S.Y., et al., "Structure-motion-performance relationship of flux-enhanced reverse osmosis (RO) membranes composed of aromatic polyamide thin films," *Environ Sci Technol,* 35(21) (November 2001): 4334–40.

LeChevallier, M.W., et al., "Giardia and cryptosporidium spp. in filtered drinking water supplies," *Appl Environ Microbiol,* 57(9) (September 1991): 2617–21.

Leigh, P., et al., "Costs of occupational COPD and asthma," *Chest,* 121(1) (January 2002): 264–72.

Li, X.Z., et al., "Further formation of trihalomethanes in drinking water during heating," *Int J Environ Health Res,* 11(4) (November 2001): 343–8.

Littleton, J., "Paleopathology of skeletal fluorosis," *Am J Phys Anthropol,* 109(4) (August 1999): 465–83.

Marier, J.R., "Some current aspects of environmental fluoride," *Sci Total Environ,* 8(3) (November 1977): 253–65.

McCloy, R.F., "Water in the treatment of peptic ulcer disease," *J Clin Gastroenterol,* 6(1) (1984): 95–6.

National Resources Defense Council Report, "Bottled Water. Pure Drink or Pure Hype?" (March 1999).

Noguchi, N., et al., "Formation of active oxygen species and lipid peroxidation induced by hypochlorite," *Arch Biochem Biophys,* 397(2) (January 2002): 440–7.

Ohnishi, S., et al., "DNA damage induced by hypochlorite and hypobromite with reference to inflammation-associated carcinogenesis," *Cancer Lett,* 178(1) (April 2002): 37–42.

Potera, C., "The price of bottled water," *Environ Health Perspect,* 110(2) (February 2002): A76.

Silvers, W.S., "Exercise-induced allergies: the role of histamine release," *Ann Allergy,* 68(1) (January 1992): 58–63.

Watts, A., et al., "Tooth discolouration and staining: a review of the literature," *Br Dent J,* 190(6) (March 2001): 309–16.

Wilhelm, K.P., et al., "Skin aging: effect on transepidermal water loss, stratum corneum hydration, skin surface pH, and casual sebum content," *Arch Dermatol,* 127(12) (December 1991): 1806–9.

Chapter 15

Abdulrahman, M., et al., "Effects of smoking on serum levels of lipid peroxides and essential fat-soluble antioxidants," *Nutrition and Health,* 12(1997): 55–65.

Alcocer, L., et al., "A comparative study of policosanol versus acipimox in patients with type II hypercholesterolemia," *Int J Tissue React,* 21(3) (1999): 85–92.

Ambrosio, G., Tritto, I., "Reperfusion injury: experimental evidence and clinical implications," *Am J Heart,* 138(2 Pt 2) (August 1999): 69–75.

Antila, E., Westermark, T., "On the etiopathogenesis and therapy of Down syndrome," *Int J Dev Biol,* 33(1) (March 1989): 183–8.

Arbuzova, S.B., "The age-dependent incidence of Down's syndrome and the free-radical theory," *Tsitol Genet,* 30(5) (September–October 1996): 27–35.

Barilla, J., (ed.), *The Nutrition Superbook* (Keats Publishing, 1995).

Batista, J., et al., "Effect of policosanol on hyperlipidemia and coronary heart disease in middle-aged patients: a 14-month pilot study," *Int J Clin Pharmacol Ther,* 34(3) (March 1996): 134–7.

Bendich, A., Olsen, J.A., "Biological actions of carotenoids," *FASEB,* 3(8) (June1989): 1927–32.

Benov, L., "How superoxide radical damages the cell," *Protoplasma,* 217(1–3) (2001): 33–6.

Borcea, V., Nourooz-Zadeh, J., Wolff, S.P., et al., "Alpha-lipoic acid decreases oxidative stress even in patients with poor glycemic control and albuminuria," *Free Radic Biol Med,* 26(11–12) (June 1999): 1495–500.

Breen, A.P., Murphy, J.A., "Reaction of oxyl radicals with DNA," *Free Radical Biol Med,* 18(6) (1995): 1035–77.

Burke, W.J., Kristal, B.S., Yu, B.P., et al., "Norepinephrine transmitter metabolite generates free radicals and activates mitochondrial permeability transition: a mechanism for DOPEGAL-induced apoptosis," *Brain Res,* 787(2) (23 March 1998): 328–32.

Calabrese, E., "Influence of dietary vitamin E on susceptibility to ozone exposure," *Bull Environ Contam Toxicol,* 34 (1985): 417–22.

Canetti, M., et al., "A two-year study on the efficacy and tolerability of policosanol in patients with type II hyperlipoproteinaemia," *Int J Clin Pharmacol Res,* 15(4) (1995): 159–65.

Christmas, C., O'Connor, K.G., Harman, S.M., et al., "Growth hormone and sex steroid effects on bone metabolism and bone mineral density in healthy aged women and men," *J Gerontol A Biol Sci Med Sci,* 57(1) (January 2002): M12–8.

Clarkson, P.M., Thompson, H.S., "Antioxidants: What role do they play in physical activity and health?" *Am J Clin Nutr,* 72(2s) (August 2000): 637s–46s.

Cranton, E., Frackelton, J., "Free radical pathology in age related diseases," *Journal of Holistic Medicine,* 6(1) (1984).

Cranton, E.M., Frackelton, J.P., "Treatment of free radical pathology in chronic degenerative diseases with EDTA chelation therapy," *Journal of Holistic Medicine,* 6(1) (1984): 6–37.

Davi, G., Guagnano, M.T., Ciabattoni, G., et al., "Platelet activation in obese women: role of inflammation and oxidant stress," *JAMA,* 288(16) (October 2002): 2008–14.

de la Monte, S.M., Luong, T., Neely, T.R., et al., "Mitochondrial DNA damage as a mechanism of cell loss in Alzheimer's disease," *Lab Invest,* 80(8) (August 2000): 1323–35.

Devaraj, S., Xu, D.Y., Jailal, I., "C-reactive protein increases plasminogen activator inhibitor-1 expression and activity in human aortic endothelial cells: implications for the metabolic syndrome and atherothrombosis," *Circulation,* 28; 107(3) (January 2003): 398–404.

Dhar, H.L.,"Newer approaches in increasing life span," *Indian J Med Sci,* 53(9) (September 1999): 390–2.

Di Maschio, P., et al., "Carotenoids, tocopherols, and thiols as biological singlet molecular oxygen quenchers," *Biochem Soc Trans,* 18(6) (December 1990): 1054–6.

Engelsen, J., Nielsen, J.D., Hansen, K.W., "Effects of coenzyme Q10 and gingko biloba on warfarin dosage in stable, long-term warfarin-treated outpatients," Ugeskr Laeger, 165 (18) (2003): 1868–71.

Franceschi, S., Favero, A., La Vecchia, C., "Influence of food groups and food diversity on breast cancer risk in Italy," *Int J Cancer,* 63(1995): 785–9.

Frankish, H., "Why do COX-2 inhibitors increase risk of cardiovascular events?" *Lancet,* 359(9315) (April 2002): 1410.

Funfgels, E.W., (ed.), *Rokan, Ginkgo biloba. Recent Results in Pharmacology and Clinic* (Berlin: Springer–Verlag, 1988).

Goel, A., Boland, C.R., Chauhan, D.P., "Specific inhibition of cyclooxygenase-2 (COX-2) expression by dietary curcumin in HT-29 human colon cancer cells," *Cancer Lett,* 172(2) (30 October 2001): 111–8.

Golan, R., *Optimal Wellness* (Newark: Ballantine Books, 1995).

Hansen, L.A., Sigman, C.C., Andreola, F., et al., "Retinoids in chemoprevention and differentiation therapy," *Carcinogenesis,* 21(7) (July 2000): 1271–9.

Hinokio, Y., Suzuki, S., Hirai, M., et al., "Oxidative DNA damage in diabetes mellitus: its association with diabetic complications," *Diabetologia,* 42(8) (August 1999): 995–8.

Holt, R.I., Webb, E., Pentecost, C., et al., "Aging and physical fitness are more important than obesity in determining exercise-induced generation of GH," *J Clin Endocrinol Metab,* 86(12) (December 2001): 5715–20.

Jacob, S., et al., "Enhancement of glucose disposal in patients with Type 2 diabetes by alpha-lipoic acid," *Arzneimittelforschung,* 45(8) (August 1995): 872–74.

Janero, D.R., "Therapeutic potential of vitamin E in the pathogenesis of spontaneous atherosclerosis," *Free Radical Biol Med,* 11(1) (1991): 129–44.

Ji, L.L., "Antioxidants and oxidative stress in exercise," *Proc Soc Exp Biol Med,* 222(3) (December 1999): 283–92.

Kaneto, H., Kajimoto, Y., Miyagawa, J., et al., "Beneficial effects of antioxidants in diabetes: possible protection of the pancreatic beta-cells against glucose toxicity," *Diabetes,* 48(12) (December 1999): 2398–406.

Kelm, M.A., Nair, M.G., Strasburg, G.M., et al., "Antioxidant and cyclooxygenase inhibitory phenolic compounds from *Ocimum sanctum Linn,*" *Phytomedicine,* 7(1) (March 2000): 7–13.

Kilic, F., et al., "Modelling cortical cataractogenesis XX. *In vitro* effect of alpha-lipoic acid on glutathione concentrations in lens in model diabetic cataractogenesis," *Biochem Mol Biol Int,* 46(3) (October 1998): 585–95.

Linnane, A.W., "Mitochondria and aging: the universality of bioenergetic disease," *Aging* (Milano), 4(4) (December 1992): 267–71.

Liu, D., Huang, Y., et al., "Effect of selenium on human myocardial glutathione peroxidase gene expression," *Chin Med J* (Engl), 113(9) (2000): 771–5.

Liu, T., et al., "The isoprostanes: novel prostaglandin-like products of the free radical-catalyzed peroxidation of arachidonic acid," *J Biomed Sci,* 6(4) (July–August 1999): 226–35.

Low, P.A., et al., "The roles of oxidative stress and antioxidant treatment in experimental diabetic neuropathy." *Diabetes,* 46 (Suppl 2) (September 97): S38–42.

Manev, H., Uz, T., Sugaya, K., et al., "Putative role of neuronal 5-lipoxygenase in an aging brain," *FASEB J,* 14(10) (July 2000): 1464–9.

McGahan, L., "COX-2 inhibitors: a Role in Alzheimer's Disease?" Issues Emerg Health Technol, (10) (December 1999): 1–6.

Menendez, R., et al., "Oral administration of policosanol inhibits in vitro copper ion-induced rat lipoprotein peroxidation," *Physiol Behav,* 67(1) (1 August 1999): 1–7.

Mortensen, S.A., et al., "Dose-related decrease of serum coenzyme Q10 during treatment with HMG-CoA reductase inhibitors," *Mol Aspects Med,* 18 (Suppl) (1997): S137–44.

Nagamatsu, M., et al., "Lipoic acid improves nerve blood flow, reduces oxidative stress, and improves distal nerve conduction in experimental diabetic neuropathy," *Diabetes Care,* 18 (1995): 1160–1167.

Okuda, M., Li, K., et al., "Mitochondrial injury, oxidative stress, and antioxidant gene expression are induced by hepatitis C virus core protein," *Gastroenterology,* 122(2) (February 2002): 366–75.

Olsen, J.A., "Carotenoids in human health," *Arch Latinoam Nutr,* 49(3Suppl) (September 1999): 7s–11s.

Opara, E.C., Abdal-Rahman, E., Soliman, S., "Depletion of total antioxidant capacity in type 2 diabetes," *Metabolism,* 48(11) (November 1999): 1414–7.

Packer, L., "Antioxidant properties of lipoic acid and its therapeutic effects in prevention of diabetes complications and cataracts," *Ann N Y Acad Sci,* 738 (November 1994): 257–64.

Patrignani, P., "Oxidized lipids" *Ital Heart J,* 2(12) (2002): 873–7.

Pearson, T.A., Mensah, G.A., Alexander, R.W., et al., "Markers of inflammation and cardiovascular disease: application to clinical and public health practice: a statement for healthcare professionals from the centers for disease control and prevention and the American Heart Association," *Circulation,* 107(3) (January 2003): 499–511.

Pelton, R., *Mind Food and Smart Pills* (New York: Doubleday, 1989).

Plenz, G., Robenek, H., "Monocytes/macrophages in atherosclerosis," *Eur Cytokine Netw,* 9(4) (December 1998): 701–3.

Poirier, P., Eckel, R.H., "Obesity and cardiovascular disease," *Curr Atheroscler Rep,* 4(6) (November 2002): 448–53.

Pompeia, C., Freitas, J.J., Kim, J.S., et al., "Arachidonic acid cytotoxicity in leukocytes: implications of oxidative stress and eicosanoid synthesis," *Biol Cell,* 94(4–5) (September 2002): 251–65.

Pratico, D., Lee, V.M.Y., Trojanowski, J.Q., et al., "Increased F2-isoprostanes in Alzheimer's disease: evidence for enhanced lipid peroxidation *in vivo,*" *FASEB,* 12(15) (December 1998): 1777–83.

Pressman, A.H., *The GSH Phenomenon* (New York: St. Martin's Press, 1997).

Pryor, W.A., "Cancer and free radicals," *Basic Life Sci,* 39 (1986): 45–59.

Retz, W., Gsell, W., et al., "Free radicals in Alzheimer's disease," *J Neural Transm Suppl,* 54 (1998): 221–36.

Ridker, P.M., Buring, J.E., Cook, N.R., et al., "C-reactive protein, the metabolic syndrome, and risk of incident cardiovascular events: an 8-year follow-up of 14,719 initially healthy American women," *Circulation,*107(3) (January 2003): 391–7.

Rousseau, E.J., Davidson, A.J., Dunn, B., "Protection by beta-carotene and related compounds against oxygen-mediated cytotoxicity and genotoxicity implications for carcinogenesis and anticarcinogenesis," *Free Radic Biol Med,* 13(4) (October 1992): 407–33.

Scharffetter-Kochanek, K., et al., "Photoaging of the skin from phenotype to mechanisms," *Exp Gerontol,* 35(3) (May2000): 307–16.

Schwartz, J.L., *The Dual Roles of Nutrients as Growth,* Symposium: Prooxidant Effects of Antioxidant Vitamins (American Institute of Nutrition, 1996).

Sharma, H., *Freedom from Disease* (Toronto: Veda Publishing, 1993).

Sharma, O.P., Krishna Murti, C.R., "Ascorbic acid—a naturally occurring mediator of lipid peroxide formation in rat brain," *J Neurochem,* 27(1) (July 1976): 299–301.

Siems, W., Quast, S., Carluccio, F., et al., "Oxidative stress in chronic renal failure as a cardiovascular risk factor," *Clin Nephrol,* 58 (Suppl 1) (July 2003): S12–9.

Simopoulos, A.P., "Omega-3 Fatty acids in inflammation and autoimmune diseases," *J Am Coll Nutr,* 21(6) (December 2002): 495–505.

Smith, D.W., "Centenarians: human longevity outliers," *Gerontologist,* 37(2) (April 1997): 200–6.

Steinberg, D.L., et al., "Beyond cholesterol. Modifications of low-density lipoprotein that increase its atherogenicity," *New Engl J Med,* 320 (1989): 915–24.

"Summaries for patients: aspirin for the prevention of heart attacks in people without previous cardio-vascular events: recommendations from the United States Preventive Services Task Force," *Ann Intern Med,* 136(2) (January 2002): 155.

Uchiyama, T., Kamikawa, H., et al., "Anti-ulcer effect of extract from phellodendri cortex," *Yakugaku Zasshi,* 109(9) (September 1989): 672–6.

Visser, M., et al., "Elevated inflammation status in obesity: NHANES III (Abstract 685.3)," *FASEB Journal,* (March 1999): A925.

Weltman, A., Weltman, J.Y., Veldhuis, J.D., et al., "Body composition, physical exercise, growth hor-mone and obesity," *Eat Weight Disord,* 6(3 Suppl) (September 2001): 28–37.

West, I.C., "Radicals and oxidative stress in diabetes," *Diabet Med,* 17(3) (March 2000): 171–80.

Williams, M., Stewart, R., "Inflammation, atherosclerosis and predicting cardiovascular risk," *N Z Med J,* 115(1163) (October 2002): U196.

Witt, E.H., Reznick, A.Z., Viguie, C.A., et al., *Exercise, Oxidative Damage and Effects of Antioxidant Manipulation,* Symposium: Nutrition and Exercise, (American Institute of Nutrition, 1992).

Chapter 16

"A New Niacin. Vitamin with an HDL kick," *US News World Rep,* 130(15) (April 2001): 54.

Agus, M.S., et al., "Cardiovascular actions of magnesium," *Crit Care Clin,* 17(1) (January 2001): 175–86.

"Can taking magnesium supplements help keep my bones strong?" *Mayo Clin Health Lett,* 17(9) (Sep-tember 1999): 8.

"Lowering blood homocysteine with folic acid-based supplements: meta-analysis of randomised tri-als," *Indian Heart J,* 52(7 Suppl) (November–December 2000): S59–64.

"The 8 most important supplements for people on HAART." *STEP Perspect,* 99(2) (Summer 1999): 18.

Ahmad, N., et al., "Green tea constituent epigallocatechin-3-gallate and induction of apoptosis and cell cycle arrest in human carcinoma cells," *J Natl Cancer Inst,* 89(24) (17 December 1997): 1881–6.

Anderson, J.J., "Calcium requirements during adolescence to maximize bone health," *J Am Coll Nutr,* 20 (2 Suppl) (April 2001): 186S–191S.

Anderson, R.A., "Chromium, glucose intolerance and diabetes," *J Am Coll Nutr,* 17(6) (December 1998): 548–55.

Anderson, R.A., "Effects of chromium on body composition and weight loss," *Nutr Rev,* 56(9) (Sep-tember 1998): 266–70.

Anderson, R.A., "Trace elements and cardiovascular diseases," *Acta Pharmacol Toxicol (Copenh),* 59 (Suppl 7) (1986): 317–24.

Anderson, R.A., et al., "Potential antioxidant effects of zinc and chromium supplementation in people with type 2 diabetes mellitus," *J Am Coll Nutr,* 20(3) (June 2001): 212–8.

Arsenio, L., et al., "Effectiveness of long-term treatment with pantethine in patients with dyslipidemia," *Clin Ther,* 8(5) (1986): 537–45.

Augustine, G.J., "How does calcium trigger neurotransmitter release?" *Curr Opin Neurobiol,* 11(3) (June 2001): 320–6.

Badmaev, V., et al., "Vanadium: a review of its potential role in the fight against diabetes," *J Altern Complement Med,* 5(3) (June 1999): 273–91.

Bahijiri, S.M., et al., "The effects of inorganic chromium and brewer's yeast supplementation on glucose tolerance, serum lipids and drug dosage in individuals with type 2 diabetes," *Saudi Med J,* 21(9) (September 2000): 831–7.

Barceloux, D.G., "Molybdenum," *J Toxicol Clin Toxicol,* 37(2) (1999): 231–7.

Baxxano, L.A., et al., "Dietary potassium intake and risk of stroke in US men and women: National Health and Nutrition Examination Survey I epidemiologic follow-up study," *Stroke,* 32(7) (July 2001): 1473–80.

Benzie, I.F., Szeto, Y.T., "Total antioxidant capacity of teas by the ferric reducing: Antioxidant Power Assay," *J Agric Food Chem,* 47(2) (February 1999): 633–6.

Berg, J.W., et al., "Epideminology of gastrointestinal cancer," *Proc Natl Cancer Congr,* 7 (1973): 459–63.

Berson, E.L., "Nutrition and retinal degenerations," *Int Ophthalmol Clin,* 40(4) (Fall 2000): 93–111.

Bertolini, S., et al., "Lipoprotein changes induced by pantethine in hyperlipoproteinemic patients: adults and children," *Int J Clin Pharmacol Ther Toxicol,* 24(11) (1986): 630–37.

Bettendorff, L., et al., "Thiamine, thiamine phosphates, and their metabolizing enzymes in human brain," *J Neurochem,* 55(1) (January 1996): 250–8.

Bonjour, J.P., "Biotin in man's nutrition and therapy – a review," *Int J Vitam Nutr Res,* 47(2) (1977): 107–18.

Brawley, O.W., Barnes, S., Parnes, H., "The future of prostate cancer prevention," *Ann N Y PacAcad Sci,* 952 (December 2001): 145–52.

Brooks, J.D., Metter, E.J., Chan, D.W., et al., "Plasma selenium level before diagnosis and the risk of prostate cancer development," *J Urol,* 166(6) (December 2001): 2034–8.

Brouwer, I.A., et al., "Low-dose folic acid supplementation decreases plasma homocysteine concentrations: a randomised trial," *Indian Heart J,* 52(7 Suppl) (November–December 2000): S53–58.

Bushman, J.L., "Green tea and cancer in humans: a review of the literature," *Nutr Cancer,* 31(3) (1998): 151–9.

Cao, G., et al., "Hyperoxia induced changes in antioxidant capacity and the dietary effects of antioxidants," *J Appl Physiol,* 86(6) (June 1999): 1817–22.

Challier, B., et al., "Garlic, onion and cereal fibre as protective factors for breast cancer: a French case-control study," *Eur J Epidemiol,* 14(8) (December 1998): 737–47.

Chen, Y.C., Shen, S.C., Chen, L.G., et al., "Wogonin, baicalin, and baicalein inhibition of inducible nitric oxide synthase and cyclooxygenase-2 gene expressions induced by nitric oxide synthase inhibitors and lipopolysaccharide," *Biochem Pharmacol,* 61(11) (June 2001): 1417–27.

Cheng, T., et al., "Effects of multinutrient supplementation on antioxidant defense systems in healthy human beings," *J Nutr Biochem,* 12(7) (July 2001): 388–395.

Clark, L.C., et al., "Effects of selenium supplementation for cancer prevention in patients with carcinoma of the skin: a randomized controlled trial, Nutritional Prevention of Cancer Study Group," *JAMA,* 276(24) (December 1996): 1957–63.

Clarke, R., et al., "Vitamin supplements and cardiovascular risk: review of the randomized trials of homocysteine-lowering vitamin supplements," *Semin Thromb Hemost,* 26(3) (2000): 341–8.

Costello, A.J., "A randomized, controlled chemoprevention trial of selenium in familial prostate cancer: rationale, recruitment, and design issues," *Urology,* 57(4 Suppl 1) (April 2001): 182–4.

Cuellar, M.J., Giner, R.M., Recio, M.C., et al., "Topical anti-inflammatory activity of some Asian medicinal plants used in dermatological disorders," *Fitoterapia,* 72(3) (March 2001): 221–9.

Cunningham, J.J., "Micronutrients as nutriceutical interventions in diabetes mellitus," *J Am Coll Nutr,* 17(1) (February 1998): 7–10.

Curhan, G.C., et al., "A prospective study of dietary calcium and other nutrients and the risk of symptomatic kidney stones," *N Engl J Med,* 328(12) (March 1993): 833–38.

Cymet, T.C., et al., "Osteoporosis," *J Am Osteopath Assoc,* 100 (10 Suppl Pt 1) (October 2000): S9–15.

Das, S., "Vitamin E in the genesis and prevention of cancer: a review," *Acta Oncol,* 33(6) (1994): 615–19.

Davies, B.E., et al., "The epidemiology of dental caries in relation to environmental trace elements," *Experientia,* 43(1) (January 1987): 87–92.

Dent, C.E., et al., "Calcium metabolism in bone disease: effects of treatment with microcrystalline calcium hydroxyapatite compound and dihydrotachysterol," *J R Soc Med,* 73(11) (1980): 780–785.

Dierkes, J., et al., "Vitamin supplementation can markedly reduce the homocysteine elevation induced by fenofibrate," *Atherosclerosis,* 158(1) (September 2001): 161–4.

Dorant, E., et al., "Consumption of onions and a reduced risk of stomach carcinoma," *Gastroenterology,* 110(1) (January 1996): 12–20.

Dunn, J.T., "What's happening to our iodine?" *J Clin Endocrinol Metab,* 83(10) (October 1998): 3398–400.

el-Yazigi, et al., "Urinary excretion of chromium, copper, and manganese in diabetes mellitus and associated disorders," *Diabetes Res,* 18(3) (November 1991): 129–34.

Eriksson, J.G., et al., "The effect of coenzyme Q10 administration on metabolic control in patients with type 2 diabetes mellitus," *Biofactors,* 9(2–4) (1999): 315–8.

Evans, W.J., "Vitamin E, vitamin C, and exercise," *Am J Clin Nutr,* 72(2 Suppl) (August 2000): 647S–52S.

Ferslew, K.E., et al., "Pharmacokinetics and bioavailability of the RRR and all racemic stereoisomers of alpha-tocopherol in humans after single oral administration," *J Clin Pharmacol,* 33(1) (January 1993): 84–88.

Field, C.J., Johnson, I.R., Schley, P.D., "Nutrients and their role in host resistance to infection," *J Leukoc Biol,* 71(1) (January 2002): 16–32.

Freeland-Graves, J., "Manganese: an essential nutrient for humans," *Nutrition Today,* (November–December 1988): 13–19.

French, R.J., et al., "Role of vanadium in nutrition: metabolism, essentiality and dietary considerations," *Life Sci,* 52(4) (1993): 339–46.

Friso, S., et al., "Low circulating vitamin B(6) is associated with elevation of the inflammation marker C-reactive protein independently of plasma homocysteine levels," *Circulation,* 103(23) (June 2001): 2788–91.

Fryer, M.J., "Selenium and human health," *Lancet,* 356(9233) (September 2000): 943.

Gaby, A.R., "Natural treatments for osteoarthritis," *Altern Med Rev,* 4(5) (October 1999): 330–41.

Ghirlanda, G., et al., "Evidence of plasma CoQ10-lowering effect by HMG-CoA reductase inhibitors: a double-blind, placebo-controlled study," *J Clin Pharmacol,* 22(3) (March 1993): 226–29.

Giovannucci, E., Rimm, E.B., Liu, Y., et al., "A prospective study of tomato products, lycopene, and prostate cancer risk," *J Natl Cancer Inst,* 94(5) (March 2002): 391–8.

Giugliano, D., "Dietary antioxidants for cardiovascular prevention," *Nutr Metab Cardiovasc Dis,* 10(1) (February 2000): 38–44.

Godfrey, J.C., et al., "Zinc for treating the common cold: review of all clinical trials since 1984," *Altern Ther Health Med,* 2(6) (November 1996): 63–72.

Grant, K.E., et al., "Chromium and exercise training: effect on obese women," *Med Sci Sports Exerc,* 29(8) (August 1997): 992–8.

Greenberg, S., et al., "Co-enzyme Q10: a new drug for cardiovascular disease," *J Clin Pharmacol,* 30(7) (July 1990): 596–608.

Greenwald, P., et al., "Diet and cancer prevention," *Eur J Cancer,* 37(8) (May 2001): 948–65.

Grimble, R.F., "Effect of antioxidative vitamins on immune function with clinical applications," *Int J Vitam Nutr Res,* 67(5) (1997): 312–20.

Haggi, T.M., Anthony, D.D., Gupta, S., et al., "Prevention of collagen-induced arthritis in mice by a polyphenolic fraction from green tea," *Proc Natl Acad Sci U S A,* 96(8) (April 1999): 4524–9.

Hamilton, E., Whitney, E., Sizer, F., *Nutrition Concepts and Controversies* (St. Paul: West Publishing, 1991).

Harland, B.F., et al., "Is vanadium of human nutritional importance yet?" *J Am Diet Assoc,* 4(8) (August 1994): 891–4.

Helen, A., et al., "Antioxidant role of oils isolated from garlic (*Allium sativum Linn*) and onion (*Allium cepa Linn*) on nicotine-induced lipid peroxidation," *Vet Hum Toxicol,* 41(5) (October 1999): 316–9.

Herbert, V., "The role of vitamin B12 and folate in carcinogenesis," *Adv Exp Med Biol.* 206 (1986): 293–311.

Herrera, E., Barbas, C., "Vitamin E: action, metabolism and perspectives," *J Physiol Biochem,* 57(2) (March 2001): 43–56.

Hochman, L.G., et al., "Brittle nails: response to daily biotin supplementation," *Cutis,* 51(4) (April 1993): 303–05.

Huttunen, J.K., "Selenium and cardiovascular diseases–an update," *Biomed Environ Sci,* 10(2–3) (September 1997): 220–26.

Ilich, J.Z., et al., "Nutrition in bone health revisited: a story beyond calcium," *J Am Coll Nutr,* 19(6) (November–December 2000): 715–37.

Imai, K., et al., "Cross sectional study of effects of drinking green tea on cardiovascular and liver diseases," *BMJ,* 310(6981) (March 1995): 693–96.

Jacob, S., et al., "Enhancement of glucose disposal in patients with Type 2 diabetes by alpha-lipoic acid," *Arzneimittelforschung,* 45(8) (August 1995): 872–74.

Jhamb, D.K., et al., "Magnesium in cardiovascular therapy," *J Assoc Physicians India,* 43(3) (March 1995): 201–3.

Johnson, S., "The multifaceted and widespread pathology of magnesium deficiency," *Med Hypotheses,* 56(2) (February 2001): 163–70.

Jones, P.W., et al., "Analysis and chemical speciation of copper and zinc in wound fluid," *J Inorg Biochem,* 81(1–2) (July 2000): 1–10.

Kelly, G.S., "Insulin resistance: lifestyle and nutritional interventions," *Altern Med Rev,* 5(2) (April 2000): 109–32.

Kelm, M.A., Nair, M.G., Strasburg, G.M., et al., "Antioxidant and cyclooxygenase inhibitory phenolic compounds from *Ocimum sanctum Linn, Phytomedicine,* 7(1) (March 2000): 7–13.

Kidd, P.M., "An integrative lifestyle: nutritional strategy for lowering osteoporosis risk," *Townsend Letter for Doctors,* (May 1992): 400–405.

Kilic, F., et al., "Modelling cortical cataractogenesis: XX. *In vitro* effect of alpha-lipoic acid on glutathione concentrations in lens in model diabetic cataractogenesis," *Biochem Mol Biol Int,* 46(3) (October 1998): 585–95.

Kimura, K., "Role of essential trace elements in the disturbance of carbohydrate metabolism," *Nippon Rinsho,* 54(1) (January 1996): 79–84.

Kishi, T., et al., "Bioenergetics in clinical medicine: XI. Studies on coenzyme Q and diabetes mellitus," *J Med,* 7(3–4) (1976): 307–21.

Kishi, T., et al., "Bioenergetics in clinical medicine: XV. Inhibition of coenzyme Q10-enzymes by clincically used adrenergic blockers of beta-receptors," *Res Commun Chem Pathol Pharmacol,* 17(1) (May 1997): 157–64.

Klaunig, J.E., Xu, Y., Han, C., et al., "The effect of tea consumption on oxidative stress in smokers and nonsmokers," *Proc Soc Exp Biol Med,* 220(4) (April 1999): 249–54.

Klein, C.J., "Zinc supplementation," *J Am Diet Assoc,* 100(10) (October 2000): 1137–8.

Knopp, R.H., "Evaluating niacin in its various forms," *Am J Cardiol,* 86(12A) (December 2000): 51L–56L.

Kokkonen, J., et al., "Residual intestinal disease after milk allergy in infancy," *J Pediatr Gastroenterol Nutr,* 32(2) (February 2001): 156–61.

Kong, L.D., Cai, Y., Huang, W.W., et al., "Inhibition of xanthine oxidase by some Chinese medicinal plants used to treat gout," *J Ethnopharmacol,* 73(1–2) (November 2000): 199–207.

Koutsikos, D., et al., "Biotin for diabetic peripheral neuropathy," *Biomed Pharmacother,* 44(10) (1990): 511–14.

Koyanagi, T., et al., "Effect of riboflavin on the metabolism of polyunsaturated fatty acids in the body of rat," *Tohoku J Exp Med,* 86(1) (June 1965): 19–22.

Kratzer, F.H., Vobra, P., *Chelates in Nutrition,* (Boca Raton: CRC Press, 1986).

Kristal, A.R., et al., "Vitamin and mineral supplement use is associated with reduced risk of prostate cancer," *Cancer Epidemiol Biomarkers Prev,* 8)10) (October 1999): 887–92.

Kromhout, D., "Diet and cardiovascular diseases," *J Nutr Health Aging,* 5(3) (2001): 144–9.

Lachance P., Langseth, L., "The RDA concept: time for a change?" *Nutrition Reviews,* 22(8) (1994): 266–67.

Lacroix, B., et al., "Role of pantothenic and ascorbic acid in wound healing processes: *in vitro* study on fibroblasts," *Int J Vitam Nutr Res,* 58(4) (1988): 407–13.

Lakshimi, A.V., "Riboflavin metabolism—relevance to human nutrition," *Indian J Med Res,* 108 (November 1998): 182–90.

Lall, S.B., et al., "Role of nutrition in toxic injury," *Indian J Exp Biol,* 37(2) (February 1999): 109–16.

Lavie, C.J., et al., "Niacin in patients with diabetes mellitus and coronary artery disease," *Am J Cardiol,* 87(9) (May 2001): 1137–8.

Lee, C.Y., et al., "Vitamin E supplementation improves cell-mediated immunity and oxidative stress of Asian men and women," *J Nutr,* 130(12) (December 2000): 2932–7.

Lee, I.P., Kim, Y.H., Kang, M.H., et al., "Chemopreventive effect of green tea (*camellia sinensis*) against cigarette smoke-induced mutations (SCE) in humans," *J Cell Biochem,* 27 (Suppl) (1997): 68–75.

Lee, N.A., et al., "Beneficial effect of chromium supplementation on serum triglyceride levels in NIDDM," *Diabetes Care,* 17(12) (December 1994): 1449–52.

Lee, Y., Kim, H., Choi, H.S., et al., "Effects of water extract of 1:1 mixture of Phellodendron cortex and Aralia cortex on polyol pathway and oxidative damage in lenses of diabetic rats," *Phytother Res,* 13(7) (November 1999): 555–60.

Levenson, D.I., et al., "A review of calcium preparations," *Nutr Rev,* 52(7) (1994): 221–232.

Lewin, A., et al., "The effect of coenzyme Q10 on sperm motility and function," *Mol Aspects Med,* 18(Suppl) (1997): S213–9.

Liang, J.Y., et al., "Inhibitory effect of zinc on human prostatic carcinoma cell growth," *Prostate,* 40(3) (August 1999): 200–7.

Loomis, D., "Fatalities from prescription drugs, non-prescription drugs, and nutrients," *Townsend Letter for Doctors,* (April 1992).

Low, P.A., et al., "The roles of oxidative stress and antioxidant treatment in experimental diabetic neuropathy," *Diabetes,* 46 (Suppl 2) (September 1997): S38–42.

Maebashi, M., et al., "Therapeutic evaluation of the effect of biotin on hyperglycemia in patients with non-insulin dependent diabetes mellitus," *J Clin Biochem Nutr,* 14 (1983): 211–18.

Manore, M.M., "Effect of physical activity on thiamine, riboflavin, and vitamin B-6 requirements," *Am J Clin Nutr,* 72 (2 Suppl) (August 2000): 598S–606S.

Mares-Perlman, J.A., Millen, A.E., Ficek, T.L., et al., "The body of evidence to support a protective role for lutein and zeaxanthin in delaying chronic disease," *J Nutr,* 132(3) (March 2002): 518S–524S.

Massey, V., "The chemical and biological versatility of riboflavin," *Biochem Soc Trans,* 28(4) (2000): 283–96.

Matsuoka, H., Seo, Y., Wakasugi, H., Saito, T., Tomoda, H., "Lentinan potentiates immunity and prolongs the survival time of some patients," *Anticancer Res,* 17(4A) (July–August 1997): 2751–5.

McCarron, D.A., et al., "Are low intakes of calcium and potassium important causes of cardiovascular disease?" *Am J Hypertens,* 14(6 Pt 2) (June 2001): 206S–212S.

McKenney, J.M., et al., "Effect of niacin and atorvastatin on lipoprotein subclasses in patients with atherogenic dyslipidemia," *Am J Cardiol,* (August 2001): 270–4.

Miesel, R., et al., "Copper-dependent antioxidase defenses in inflammatory and autoimmune rheumatic diseases," *Inflammation,* 17(3) (June 1993): 283–94.

Mitamura, T., Sakamoto, S., Suzuki, S., et al., "Effects of lentinan of colorectal carcinogenesis in mice with ulcerative colitits," *Oncol Rep,* 7(3) (May–June 2000): 599–601.

Miura, S., et al., "Effects of various natural antioxidants on the Cu(2+)-mediated oxidative modification of low density lipoprotein," *Biol Pharm Bull,* 18(1) (January 1995): 1–4.

Moneret-Vautrin, D.A., "Cow's milk allergy," *Allerg Immunol* (Paris), 31(6) (June 1999): 201–10.

Morgan, S.L., "Calcium and vitamin D in osteoporosis," *Rheum Dis Clin North Am,* 27(1) (February 2001): 101–30.

Moskovitz, J., Yim, M.B., Chock, P.B., "Free radicals and disease," *Arch Biochem Biophys,* 397(2) (January 2002): 354–9.

Mukhtar, H., Ahmad, N., "Green tea in chemoprevention of cancer," *Toxicol Sci,* 52(2s) (December 1999): 111–7.

Naghii, M.R., et al., "The role of boron in nutrition and metabolism," *Prog Food Nutr Sci,* 17(4) (October–December 1993): 331–49.

Nakagawa, K., Ninomiya, M., Okubo, T., et al., "Tea catechin supplementation increases antioxidant capacity and prevents phospholipid hydroperoxidation in plasma of humans," *J Agric Food Chem,* 47(10) (October 1999): 3967–73.

Nakamura, R., et al., "Study of CoQ10-enzymes in gingiva from patients with periodontal disease and evidence for a deficiency of coenzyme Q10," *Proc Natl Acad Sci U S A,* 71(4) (April 1974): 1456–60.

Neve, J., "The nutritional importance and physiopathology of molybdenum in man," *J Pharm Belg,* 46(3) (May–June 1991): 189–96.

Newnham, R.E., "Essentiality of boron for healthy bones and joints," *Environ Health Perspect,* 102 (Suppl 7) (November 1994): 83–5.

Nicolini, G., et al., "Anti-apoptotic effect of trans-resveratrol on paclitaxel-induced apoptosis in the human neuroblastoma SH-SY5Y cell line," *Neurosci Lett,* 302(1) (April 2001): 41–4.

Nilsson, K., et al., "Improvement of cognitive functions after cobalamin/folate supplementation in elderly patients with dementia and elevated plasma homocysteine," *Int J Geriatr Psychiatry,* 16(6) (June 2001): 609–14.

Niromanesh, S., et al., "Supplementary calcium in prevention of pre-eclampsia," *Int J Gynaecol Obstet,* 74(1) (July 2001): 17–21.

Obertreis, B., et al., "Anti-inflammatory effect of urtica dioica folia extract in comparison to caffeic malic acid," *Arzneim-Forsch/Drug Res,* 46(1) (January 1996): 52–56.

Okada, A., et al., "Zinc in clinical surgery: a research review," *Jpn J Surg,* 20(6) (November 1990): 635–44.

Omu, A.E., et al., "Magnesium in human semen: possible role in premature ejaculation," *Arch Androl,* 46(1) (January–February 2001): 59–66.

Ooi, V.E., Lui, F., "Immunomodulation and anti-cancer activity of polysaccharide-protein complexes," *Current Med Chem,* 7(7) (July 2000): 15–29.

Packer, L., "Antioxidant properties of lipoic acid and its therapeutic effects in prevention of diabetes complications and cataracts," *Ann N Y Acad Sci,* 738 (November 1994): 257–64.

Packer, L., Weber, S.U., Rimbach, G., "Molecular aspects of alpha-tocotrienol antioxidant action and cell signaling," *J Nutr,* 131(2) (February 2001): 369S–73S.

Pande, I., et al., "Osteoporosis in men," *Baillieres Best Pract Res Clin Rheumatol,* 15(3) (July 2001): 415–27.

Paschka, A.G., et al., "Induction of apoptosis in prostate cancer cell lines by the green tea component (-)-epigallocatechin-3-gallate," *Cancer Lett,* 130(1–2) (August 1998): 1–7.

Patki, P.S., et al., "Efficacy of potassium and magnesium in essential hypertension: a double-blind, placebo controlled, crossover study," *BMJ,* 301(6751) (September 1990): 521–23.

Pineau, A., et al., "A study of chromium in human cataractous lenses and whole blood of diabetics, senile, and normal population," *Biol Trace Elem Res,* 32 (January–March 1992): 133–8.

Prasad, A., et al., "Modern adjunctive pharmacotherapy of myocardial infarction," *Expert Opin Pharmacother,* 1(3) (March 2000): 405–18.

Pruthi, S., Allison, T.G., Hensrud, D.D., "Vitamin E supplementation in the prevention of coronary heart disease," *Mayo Clin Proc,* 76(11) (November 2001): 1131–6.

Qureshi, A.A., et al., "Tocotrienols: novel hypocholesterolemic agents with antioxidant properties," *Vitamin E in Health and Disease,* L. Packer & J. Fuchs, eds. New York: Marcel Dekker, 1993: 247–267.

Rayman, M.P., "The importance of selenium to human health," *Lancet,* 356(9225) (July 2000): 233–41.

Riccardi, D., "Calcium ions as extracellular, first messengers," *Z Kardiol,* 89(Suppl 2) (2000): 9–14.

Ritsema, G.H., et al., "Potassium supplements prevent serious hypokalaemia in colon cleansing." *Clin Radiol,* 49(12) (December 1994): 874–76.

Robins, Wahlin, T.B., et al., "The influence of serum vitamin B12 and folate status on cognitive functioning in very old age," *Biol Psychol,* 56(3) (June 2001): 247–65.

Rock, E., et al., "The effect of copper supplementation on red blood cell oxidizability and plasma antioxidants in middle-aged healthy volunteers," *Free Radic Biol Med,* 28(3) (February 2000): 324–9.

Rumi, L.A., et al., "The effect of calcium citrate on bone density in the early and mid-postmenopausal period: a randomized placebo-controlled study," *Am J Ther,* 6(6) (November 1999): 303–11.

Sardesai, V.M., "Molybdenum: an essential trace element," *Nutr Clin Pract,* 8(6) (December 1993): 277–81.

Saurat, J.H., "Skin, sun, and vitamin A: from aging to cancer," *J Dermatol,* 28(11) (November 2001): 595–8.

Schaafsma, G., "Bioavailability of calcium and magnesium," *Eur J Clin Nutr,* 51 (Suppl 1) (January 1997): S13–6.

Scopacasa, F., et al., "Inhibition of bone resorption by divided-dose calcium supplementation in early postmenopausal women," *Calcif Tissue Int,* 67(6) (December 2000): 440–2.

Seaborn, C.D., et al., "Effect of molybdenum supplementation on N-nitroso-N-methylurea-induced mammary carcinogenesis and molybdenum excretion in rats," *Biol Trace Elem Res,* 39(2–3) (November–December 1993): 245–56.

Simon, H.B., "Patient-directed, nonprescription approaches to cardiovascular disease," *Arch Intern Med,* 154(20) (24 October 1994): 2283–96.

Skelton, W.P., 3rd, et al., "Thiamine deficiency neuropathy. It's still common today," *Postgrad Med*, 85(8) (July 1989): 301–06.

Southon, S., "Increased fruit and vegetable consumption: potential health benefits," *Nutr Metab Cardiovasc Dis*, 11(4 Suppl) (August 2001): 78–81.

Sprecher, D.L., "Raising high-density lipoprotein cholesterol with niacin and fibrates: a comparative review," *Am J Cardiol*, 86(12A) (December 2000): 46L–50L.

Stojanoic, S., et al., "Efficiency and mechanism of the antioxidant action of trans-resveratrol and its analogues in the radical liposome oxidation," *Arch Biochem Biophys*, 391(1) (July 2001): 79–89.

Stoner, G.D., et al., "Polyphenols as cancer chemopreventive agents," *J Cell Biochem*, 22 (Suppl) (1995): 169–80.

Sunesen, V.H., et al., "Lipophilic antioxidants and polyunsaturated fatty acids in lipoprotein classes: distribution and interaction," *Eur J Clin Nutr*, 55(2) (February 2001): 115–23.

Sung, H., Nah, J., Chun, S., et al., "*In vivo* antioxidant effect of green tea," *Eur J Clin Nutr*, 54(7) (July 2000): 527–9.

Tarasov, I., et al., "Adrenal cortex functional activity in pantothenate deficiency and the administration of the vitamin or its derivatives," *Vopr Pitan*, 4 (July–August 1985): 51–54.

Tauler, P., Aguilo, A., Fuentespina, E., et al., "Diet supplementation with vitamin E, vitamin C and beta-carotene cocktail enhances basal neutrophil antioxidant enzymes in athletes," *Pflugers Arch*, 443(5–6) (March 2002): 791–7.

Thompson, K.H., "Vanadium and diabetes," *Biofactors*, 10(1) (1999): 43–51.

Toba, Y., et al., "Dietary magnesium supplementation affects bone metabolism and dynamic strength of bone in ovariectomized rats," *J Nutr*, 130(2) (February 2000): 216–20.

Tran, M.T., et al., "Role of coenzyme Q10 in chronic heart failure, angina, and hypertension," *Pharmacotherapy*, 21(7) (July 2001): 797–806.

Uchiyama, T., Kamikawa, H., et al., "Anti-ulcer effect of extract from phellodendri cortex," *Yakugaku Zasshi*, 109(9) (September 1989): 672–6.

Uusi-Rasi, K., et al., "Maintenance of body weight, physical activity and calcium intake helps preserve bone mass in elderly women," *Osteoporos Int*, 12(5) (2001): 373–9.

van den Berg, H., "Bioavailability of pantothenic acid," *Eur J Clin Nutr*, 51 (Suppl 1) (January 1997): S62–3.

Vessby, J., Basu, S., Mohsen, R., et al., "Oxidative stress and antioxidant status in Type 1 diabetes mellitus," *J Intern Med*, 251(1) (January 2002): 69–76.

Volpe, S.L., et al., "The relationship between boron and magnesium status and bone mineral density in the human: a review," *Magnes Res*, 6(3) (September 1993); 6(3): 291–96.

Ward, C.M., "Folate-targeted non-viral DNA vectors for cancer gene therapy," *Curr Opin Mol Ther*, 2(2) (April 2000): 182–7.

Weisburger, J.H., "Tea and health: a historical perspective," *Cancer Lett*, 114(1–2) (March 1997): 315–17.

Whitney, E.N., Cataldo, C.B., Rolfes, S.R., *Understanding Normal and Clinical Nutrition* (St. Paul: West Publishing Co., 1991).

Wikram Anayake, T.W., "Iodised salt and hyperthyroidism," *Ceylon Med J*, 45(4) (December 2000): 173–4.

Wilkinson, T.J., et al., "The response to treatment of subclinical thiamine deficiency in the elderly," *Am J Clin Nutr*, 66(4) (October 1997): 925–8.

Windham, C.T., et al., "Consistency of nutrient consumption patterns in the United States," *J Am Diet Assoc*, 78(6) (June 1981): 587–95.

Wu, J.M., et al., "Mechanism of cardioprotection by resveratrol, a phenolic antioxidant present in red wine (review)," *Int J Mol Med,* 8(1) (July 2001): 3–17.

Yazawa, K., Fujimori, M., Amano, J., et al., "Bifiodobacterium longum as a delivery system for cancer gene therapy: selective localization and growth in hypoxic tumors," *Cancer Gene Ther,* 7(2) (February 2000): 269–74.

Yegin, A., et al., "Erythrocyte selenium-glutathione peroxidase activity is lower in patients with coronary atherosclerosis," *Jpn Heart J,* 38(6) (November 1997): 793–98.

Yokozawa, T., et al., "Influence of green tea and its three major components upon low-density lipoprotein oxidation," *Exp Toxicol Pathol,* 49(5) (December 1997): 329–35.

Yu, H., et al., "Anticariogenic effects of green tea," *Fukuoka Igaku Zasshi,* 83(4) (April 1992): 174–80.

Appendix 1—Nutrient Reference Guide

[1] Kahn, R.S., et al., "L-5-Hydroxytryptophan in the treatment of anxiety disorders," *J Affect Disord,* 8(2) (March–April 1985): 197–200.

[2] van Praag, H.M., et al., 5-Hydroxytryptophan in combination with clomipramine in therapy-resistant depression," *Psychopharmacology,* 38 (1974): 267–69.

[3] Cruso, I., et al., "Double-blind study of 5-Hydroxytryptophan versus placebo in the treatment of primary fibromyalgia syndrome," *J Int Med Res,* 18(3) (May–June 1990): 201–09.

[4] De Benedittis, G., et al., "Serotonin precursors in chronic primary headache. A double-blind crossover study with L-5-Hydroxytryptophan vs. placebo," *J Neurosurg Sci,* 29(3) (July–September 1985): 239–48.

[5] Titus, F., et al., "5-Hydroxytryptophan versus methysergide in the prophylaxis of migraine. randomized clinical trial," *Eur Neurol,* 25(5) (1986): 327–29.

[6] Cangiano, C., et al., "Eating behavior and adherence to dietary prescriptions in obese adult subjects treated with 5-Hydroxytryptophan," *Am J Clin Nutr,* 56(5) (November 1992): 863–67.

[7] den Boer, J.A., et al., "Behavioral, neuroendocrine, and biochemical effects of 5-Hydroxytryptophan administration in panic disorder," *Psychiatry Res,* 31(3) (March 1990): 267–78.

[8] Spagnoli, A., et al., "Long-term acetyl-L-carnitine treatment in Alzheimer's disease," *Neurology,* 41 (1991): 1726–32.

[9] Tempesta, E., et al., "L-acetylcarnitine in depressed elderly subjects. A cross-over study vs. placebo," *Drugs Exp Clin Res,* 13 (1987): 417–23.

[10] Lowitt, S., et al., "Acetyl-L-carnitine corrects the altered peripheral nerve function of experimental diabetes," *Metabolism,* 44(5) (May 1995): 677–80.

[11] Haas, E., *Staying Healthy with Nutrition* (Berkeley, CA: Celestial Arts, 1992) 284.

[12] Intentionally omitted.

[13] Lipski, E., "*Digestive Wellness* (New Canaan, CT: Keats Publishing, Inc., 1996) 201–02.

[14] Gibson, G.R., et al., "Regulatory effects of bifidobacteria on the growth of other colonic bacteria," *J Appl Bacteriol,* 77(4) (October 1994): 412–20.

[15] Hochman, L.G., et al., "Brittle nails: response to daily biotin supplementation," *Cutis,* 51(4) (April 1993): 303–05.

[16] Koutsikos, D., et al., "Oral glucose tolerance test after high-dose I. V. Biotin administration in normoglucemic hemodialysis patients," *Ren Fail,* 18(1) (January 1996): 131–37.

[17] Koutsikos, D., et al., "Biotin for diabetic peripheral neuropathy," *Biomed Pharmacother,* 44(10) (1990): 511–14.

[18] Johnson, A.R., et al., "Biotin and the sudden infant death syndrome," *Nature,* 285(5761) (May 15, 1980): 159–60.

[19] Shelley, W.B., et al., "Uncombable hair syndrome: observations on response to biotin and occurrence in siblings with ectodermal dysplasia," *J Am Acad Dermatol,* 13(1) (July 1985): 97–102.

[20] Pan, S.A., et al., "Histological maturity of healed duodenal ulcers and ulcer recurrence after treatment with colloidal bismuth subcitrate or cimetidine," *Gastroenterology,* 101(5) (November 1991): 1187–91.

[21] Braverman, E.R., *The Healing Nutrients Within* (New Canaan, CT: Keats Publishing, Inc., 1997) 335–36.

[22] Travers, R.L., et al., "Boron and arthritis: the results of a double-blind study," *J Nutr Med,* 1 (1990): 127–32.

[23] Nielsen, F.H., et al., "Effect of dietary boron on mineral, estrogen, and testosterone metabolism in postmenopausal women," *Fed Am Soc Exp Biol,* 1(15) (1987): 394–97.

[24] Newnham, R.E., "Arthritis or skeletal fluorosis and boron," *Int Clin Nutr Rev,* 11(2) (1991): 68–70.

[25] Ghidini, O., et al., "Evaluation of the therapeutic efficacy of L-carnitine in congestive heart failure," *Int J Clin Pharmacol Ther Toxicol,* 26(4) (April 1988): 217–20.

[26] Abdel-Azid, M.T., et al., "Effect of carnitine on blood lipid pattern in diabetic patients," *Nutr Rep Internat,* 29 (1984): 1071–79.

[27] Giamberardino, M.A., et al., "Effects of prolonged L-carnitine administration on delayed muscle pain and CK release after eccentric effort," *Int J Sports Med,* 17(5) (July 1996): 320–24.

[28] Costa, M., et al., "L-carnitine in idiopathic asthenozoospermia: a multicenter study. Italian study group on carnitine and male infertility," *Andrologia,* 26(3) (May–June 1994): 155–59.

[29] Pittler, M.H., et al., "Randomized, double-blind trial of chitosan for body weight reduction," *Eur J Clin Nutr,* 53(5) (May 1999): 379–81.

[30] Uebelhart, D., et al., "Effects of oral chondroitin sulfate on the progression of knee osteoarthritis: a pilot study," *Osteoarthritis Cartilage,* 6 (Suppl A) (May 1998): 39–46.

[31] Anderson, R.A., et al., "Elevated intakes of supplemental chromium improve glucose and insulin variables in individuals with type 2 diabetes," *Diabetes,* 46(11) (November 1997): 1786–91.

[32] Press, R.I., et al., "The effect of chromium picolinate on serum cholesterol and apolipoprotein fractions in human subjects," *West J Med,* 152(1) (January 1990): 41–45.

[33] Lee, N.A., et al., "Beneficial effect of chromium supplementation on serum triglyceride levels in NIDDM," *Diabetes Care,* 17(12) (December 1994): 1449–52.

[34] Anderson, R.A., et al., "Effects of supplemental chromium on patients with symptoms of reactive hypoglycemia," *Metabolism,* 36(4) (April 1987): 351–55.

[35] Anderson, R.A., "Effects of chromium on body composition and weight loss," *Nutr Rev,* 56(9) (September 1998): 266–70.

[36] Kamikawa, T., et al., "Effects of coenzyme Q10 on exercise tolerance in chronic stable angina pectoris," *Am J Cardiol,* 56(4) (August 1, 1985): 247–51.

[37] Sinatra, S.T., "Coenzyme Q10: a vital therapeutic nutrient for the heart with special application in congestive heart failure," *Conn Med,* 61(11) (November 1997): 707–11.

[38] Kishi, T., et al., at pp. 157–64.

[39] Langsjoen, P., et al., "Treatment of essential hypertension with coenzyme Q10," *Mol Aspects Med,* 15 (Suppl) (1994): S265–72.

[40] Oda, T., "Effect of coenzyme Q10 on stress-induced cardiac dysfunction in paediatric patients with mitral valve prolapse: a study by stress echocardiography," *Drugs Exp Clin Res,* 11(8) (1985): 557–76.

[41] Folkers, K., et al., "Two successful double-blind trials with coenzyme Q10 (Vitamin Q10) on muscular dystrophies and neurogenic atrophies," *Biochem Biophys Acta,* 1271(1) (May 24, 1995): 281–86.

[42] van Gaal, L., et al., "Explatory study of coenzyme Q10 in obesity," *Biomedical and Clinical Aspects*

of Coenzyme Q, vol 4, Folkers, K., and Yamamura, Y., (eds.) (Amsterdam: Elsevier Science Publications, 1984) 369–73.

[43] Hansen, I.L., et al., "Bioenergetics in clinical medicine. IX. Gingival and leucocytic deficiencies of coenzyme Q10 in patients with periodontal disease," *Res Commun Chem Pathol Pharmacol,* 14(4) (August 1976): 729–38.

[44] Chvapil, M., and Van Winkle, W., Jr., "Medical and surgical applications of collagen," *International Review of Connective Tissue Research,* 6 (1973): 36.

[45] Rump, J.A., et al., "Treatment of diarrhea in human immunodeficiency virus-infected patients with immunoglobulins from bovine colostrum," *Clin Investig,* 70(7) (July 1992): 588–94.

[46] Wilson, D.C., et al., "Immune system breakthrough: colostrum," *Journal of Longevity,* 4(2) (1998): 43–46.

[47] Bertotto, A., et al., "Soluble CD30 antigen in human colostrum," *Biol Neonate,* 71(2) (1997): 69–74.

[48] Palmer, E.L., et al., "Antiviral activity of colostrum and serum immunoglobulins A and G," *J Med Virol,* 5(2) (1980): 123–29.

[49] West, D.B., et al., "Effects of conjugated linoleic acid on body fat and energy metabolism in the mouse," *Am J Physiol,* 275(3) (Pt 2) (September 1998): R667–72.

[50] Greenhaff, P.L., "Creatine and its application as an erogenic aid," *Am J Sport Nutr,* 5 (1995): 94–101.

[51] Song, M.K., et al., "Effects of bovine prostate powder on zinc, glucose, and insulin metabolism in old patients with non-insulin-dependent diabetes mellitus," *Metabolism,* 47(1) (January 1998): 39–43.

[52] Belluzzi, A., et al., "Effect of an enteric-coated fish oil preparation on relapses in Crohn's disease," *N Engl J Med,* 334 (1996): 1557–60.

[53] McManus, R.M., et al., "A comparison of the effects of n-3 fatty acids from linseed oil and fish oil in well-controlled type 2 diabetes," *Diabetes Care,* 19(5) (May 1996): 463–67.

[54] Bjorneboe, A., et al., "Effect of n-3 fatty acid supplement to patients with atopic dermatitis," *J Intern Med Supp.* 225(731) (1989): 233–36.

[55] Morris, M.C., et al., "Does fish oil lower blood pressure? A meta-analysis of controlled trials," *Circulation,* 88(2) (August 1993): 523–33.

[56] Prichard, B.N., et al., "Fish oils and cardiovascular disease," *BMJ,* 310(6983) (April 1995): 819–20.

[57] Bittiner, S.B., et al., "A double-blind, randomized, placebo-controlled trial of fish oil in psoriasis," *Lancet,* 1(8582) (February 20,1988): 378–80.

[58] Kremer, J.M., "Clinical studies of omega-3 fatty acid supplementation in patients who have rheumatoid arthritis," *Rheum Dis Clin North Am,* 17(2) (May 1991): 391–402.

[59] Yen, S.S., et al., "Replacement of DHEA in aging men and women: potential remedial effects," *Ann N Y Acad Sci,* 774 (December 29, 1995): 128–42.

[60] Wolkowitz, O.M., et al., "Dehydroepiandrosterone (DHEA) treatment of depression," *Biol Psychiatry,* 41(3) (February 1, 1997): 311–18.

[61] Casson, P., et al., "Replacement of DHEA enhances T-lymphocyte insulin binding in postmenopausal women," *Fertil Steril,* 63(5) (1995): 1027–31.

[62] Van Vollenhoven, R.F., et al., "Studies of dehydroepiandrosterone (DHEA) as a therapeutic agent in systemic lupus erythematosus," *Ann Med Interne (Paris),* 147(4) (1996): 290–96.

[63] Belluzzi, A., et al., "Effect of an enteric-coated fish oil preparation on relapses in Crohn's disease," *N Engl J Med,* 334 (1996): 1557–60.

[64] McManus, R.M., et al., "A comparison of the effects of n-3 fatty acids from linseed oil and fish oil in well-controlled type 2 diabetes," *Diabetes Care,* 19(5) (May1996): 463–67.

[65] Bjorneboe, A., et al., "Effect of n-3 fatty acid supplement to patients with atopic dermatitis," *J Intern Med Supp,* 225(731) (1989): 233–36.

[66] Morris, M.C., et al., "Does fish oil lower blood pressure? A meta-analysis of controlled trials," *Circulation,* 88(2) (August 1993): 523–33.

[67] Prichard, B.N., et al., "Fish oils and cardiovascular disease," *BMJ,* 310(6983) (April.1, 1995): 819–20.

[68] Bittiner, S.B., et al., "A double-blind, randomized, placebo-controlled trial of fish oil in psoriasis," *Lancet,* 1(8582) (February 20, 1988): 378–80.

[69] Kremer, J.M., "Clinical studies of omega-3 fatty acid supplementation in patients who have rheumatoid arthritis," *Rheum Dis Clin North Am,* 17(2) (May 1991): 391–402.

[70] Sinclair, H.M., "Essential fatty acids in perspective," *Hum Nutr Clin Nutr,* 38 (July 1984): 245–60.

[71] Pujalte, J.M., et al., "Double-blind clinical evaluation of oral glucosamine sulfate in the basic treatment of osteoarthrosis," *Curr Med Res Opin,* 7(2) (1980): 110–14.

[72] Rogers, L.L., et al., "Voluntary alcohol consumption by rats following administration of glutamine," *J Biol Chem,* 220 (1) (1956): 321–23.

[73] Shive, W., et al., "Glutamine in treatment of peptic ulcer," *Texas State J Med,* 53 (1957): 840–43.

[74] Hammarqvist, F., et al., "Addition of glutamine to total parenteral nutrition after elective abdominal surgery spares free glutamine in muscle, counteracts the fall in muscle protein synthesis, and improves nitrogen balance," *Ann Surg,* 209(4) (April 1989): 455–61.

[75] Fujita, T., et al., "Efficacy of glutamine-enriched enteral nutrition in an experimental model of mucosal ulcerative colitis," *Br J Surg,* 82(6) (June 1995): 749–51.

[76] Altomare, E., et al., "Hepatic glutathione content in patients with alcoholic and non-alcoholic liver diseases," *Life Sci,* 43(12) (1988): 991–98.

[77] Spallholz, J.E., "Selenium and glutathione peroxidase: essential nutrient and antioxidant component of the immune system," *Adv Exp Med Biol,* 262 (1990): 145–58.

[78] Hirokawa, K., et al., "Changes in glutathione in gastric mucosa of gastric ulcer patients," *Res Commun Mol Pathol Pharmacol,* 88(2) (May 1995): 163–76.

[79] Nissen, S., Sharp, R., Ray, M., et al., "Effect of leucine metabolite beta-hydroxy-beta-methylbutyrate on muscle metabolism during resistive-exercise training," *J Appl Phys,* 81 (1996): 2095–104.

[80] Messina, M., et al., *The Simple Soybean and Your Health* (Garden City Park, NY: Avery Publishing Group, 1994) 75–76.

[81] Devi Saraswathy, K., et al., "Hypolipaemic activity of *phaseolus mungo* (blackgram) in rats fed a high-fat, high-cholesterol diet," *Atherosclerosis,* 15 (1972): 223–30.

[82] Katagiri, S., "Study on the anti-diarrhea effect-combined use of augmentin and lactic acid bacteria product of multiple resistance," *Basics and Clinics,* 20(17) (December 1986): 651–53.

[83] Schiffrin, E.J., et al., "Immune modulation of blood leukocytes in humans by lactic acid bacteria: criteria for strain selection," *Am J Clin Nutr,* 66(2) (August 1997): 515S–20S.

[84] Michielutti, F., et al., "Clinical assessment of a new oral bacterial treatment for children with acute diarrhea," *Minerva Med,* 87(11) (November 1996): 545–50.

[85] Anderson, J.W., et al., "Effect of fermented milk (yogurt) containing lactobacillus acidophilus L1 on serum cholesterol in hypercholesterolemic humans," *J Am Coll Nutr,* 18(1) (February 1999): 43–50.

[86] Kim, H.S., et al., "Lactobacillus acidophilus as a dietary adjunct for milk to aid lactose digestion in humans," *J Dairy Sci,* 66(5) (May 1983): 959–66.

[87] Elmer, G.W., et al., "Biotherapeutic agents. A neglected modality for the treatment and prevention of selected intestinal and vaginal infections," *JAMA,* 275(11) (March 20, 1996): 870–76.

[88] Haas, E., *Staying Healthy with Nutrition* (Berkeley, CA: Celestial Arts, 1992) 286.

[89] Nagamatsu, M., et al., "Lipoic acid improves nerve blood flow, reduces oxidative stress, and improves distal nerve conduction in experimental diabetic neuropathy," *Diabetes Care,* 18(8) (August 1995): 1160–67.

[90] Packer, L., et al., "Alpha-lipoic acid as a biological antioxidant," *Free Radic Biol Med,* 19(2) (August 1995): 227–50.

[91] Packer, L., et al., "Neuroprotection by the metabolic antioxidant alpha-lipoic acid," *Free Radic Biol Med,* 22(1–2) (1997): 359–78.

[92] Lyle, B.J., et al., "Antioxidant intake and risk of incident age-related nuclear cataracts in the Beaver Dam eye study," *Am J Epidemiol,* 149(9) (May 1, 1999): 801–09.

[93] Hammond, B.R., Jr., et al., "Dietary modification of human macular pigment density," *Invest Ophthalmol Vis Sci,* 38(9) (August 1997): 1795–801.

[94] Agarwal, S., et al., "Tomato lycopene and low density lipoprotein oxidation: a human dietary intervention study," *Lipids,* 33(10) (October 1998): 981–84.

[95] Giovannucci, E., "Tomatoes, tomato-based products, lycopene, and cancer: Review of the epidemiologic literature," *J Natl Cancer Inst,* 91(4) (February 17, 1999): 317–31.

[96] Mares-Perlman, J.A., et al., "Serum antioxidants and age-related macular degeneration in a population-based case-control study," *Arch Ophthalmol,* 113(12) (December 1995): 1518–23.

[97] Pauling, L., "Case report: Lysine/ascorbate-related amelioration of angina pectoris," *J Orthomolecular Med,* 6 (1991): 144–46.

[98] Griffith, R.S., et al., "Success of L-lysine therapy in frequently recurrent herpes simplex infection. Treatment and prophylaxis," *Dermatologica,* 175(4) (1987): 183–90.

[99] Civitelli, R., et al., "Dietary L-lysine and calcium metabolism in humans," *Nutrition* 8(6) (November–December 1992): 400–05.

[100] Abraham, G.E., et al., "Management of fibromyalgia: rationale for the use of magnesium and malic acid," *J Nutri Med,* 3 (1992): 49–50.

[101] Domingo, J.L., et al., "Citric, malic, and succinic acids as possible alternatives to deferoxamine in aluminum toxicity," *Clin Tox,* 26 (1, 2) (1988): 67–79.

[102] Zisapel, N., "The use of melatonin for the treatment of insomnia," *Biol Signals Recep,* 8(1–2) (January–April 1999): 84–89.

[103] Suhner, A., et al., "Comparative study to determine the optimal melatonin dosage form for the alleviation of jet lag," *Chronobiol Int,* 15(6) (November 1998): 655–66.

[104] Rosenbaum, J.F., et al., "An open-label pilot study of oral S-adenosyl-L-methionine in major depression: interim results," *Psychopharmacol Bull,* 24(1) (1988): 189–94.

[105] Jacob, S.W., et al., *The Miracle of MSM: The Natural Solution for Pain* (New York: G. P. Putnam's Sons, 1999) 57–58.

[106] Childs, S.J., "Dimethyl sulfone (DMSO2) in the treatment of interstitial cystitis," *Urol Clin North Am,* 21(1) (February 1994): 85–88.

[107] Morton, J.I., and Moore, R.D., "Lupus nephritis and deaths are diminished in B/W mice drinking 3% water solutions of dimethyl sulfoxide (DMSO) and dimethyl sulfone (DMSO$_2$)," *Journal of Leukocyte Biology,* 40(3) (1986): 322.

[108] Rizzo, R., "Calcium, sulfur and zinc distribution in normal and arthritic articular equine cartilage: a synchrotron radiation induced x-ray emission study," *Journal of Experimental Zoology,* 237(1) (September 1995): 82–86.

[109] Perry, H.E., et al., "Efficacy of oral versus intravenous N-acetylcysteine in acetaminophen overdose: results of an open-label, clinical trial," *J Pediatr,* 132(1) (January 1998): 149–52.

[110] Droge, W., "Cysteine and glutathione deficiency in AIDS patients: a rationale for the treatment with N-acetyl-cysteine," *Pharmacology,* 46(2) (1993): 61–65.

[111] Millman, M., et al., "Use of acetylcysteine in bronchial asthma-another look," *Ann Allergy,* 54(4) (April 1985): 294–96.

[112] Hansen, N.C., et al., "Orally administered N-acetylcysteine may improve general well-being in patients with mild chronic bronchitis," *Respir Med,* 88(7) (August 1994): 531–35.

[113] Swerdlow, R.H., "Is NADH effective in the treatment of Parkinson's disease?" *Drugs Aging* 13(4) (October 1998): 263–68.

[114] Forsyth, L.M., et al., "Therapeutic effects of oral NADH on the symptoms of patients with Chronic Fatigue Syndrome," *Ann Allergy Asthma Immunol,* 82(2) (February 1999): 185–91.

[115] Carson, C.C., "Potassium para-aminobenzoate for the treatment of Peyronie's disease: is it effective?" *Tech Urol,* 3(3) (Fall 1997): 135–39.

[116] Zarafonetis, C.J., et al., "Retrospective studies in scleroderma: effect of potassium para-aminobenzoate on survival," *J Clin Epidemiol,* 41(2) (1988): 193–205.

[117] Hughes, C.G., "Oral PABA and vitiligo," *J Am Acad Dermatol,* 9(5) (November 1983): 770.

[118] Mann, J., et al., "D-phenylalanine in endogenous depression," *Am J Psychiatry,* 137(12) (December 1980): 1611–12.

[119] Walsh, N.E., et al., "Analgesic effectiveness of D-phenylalanine in chronic pain patients," *Arch Phys Med Rehabil,* 67(7) (July 1986): 436–39.

[120] Camacho, F., et al., "Treatment of vitiligo with oral and topical phenylalanine: 6 years of experience," *Arch Dermatol,* 135(2) (February 1999): 216–17.

[121] Chwiecko, M., et al., "Inhibition of non-enzymatic lipid peroxidation by 'Essentiale' a drug enriched in phosphatidylcholine in ethanol-induced liver injury," *Drug Alcohol Depend,* 33(1) (June 1993): 87–93.

[122] Little, A., et al., "A double-blind, placebo controlled trial of high-dose lecithin in Alzheimer's disease," *J Neurol Neurosurg Psychiatry,* 48(8) (August 1985): 736–42.

[123] Jenkins, P.J., et al., "Use of polyunsaturated phosphatidylcholine in HBsAg negative chronic active hepatitis: results of prospective double-blind controlled trial," *Liver,* 2(2) (June 1982): 77–81.

[124] Engel, R.R., et al., "Double-blind cross-over study of phosphatidylserine vs. placebo in patients with early dementia of the Alzheimer type," *Eur Neuropsychopharmacol,* 2(2) (June 1992): 149–55.

[125] Maggioni, M., et al., "Effects of phosphatidylserine therapy in geriatric patients with depressive disorders," *Acta Psychiatr Scand,* 81(3) (March 1990): 265–70.

[126] Crook, T.H., et al., "Effects of phosphatidylserine in age-associated memory impairment," *Neurology,* 41(5) (May 1991): 644–49.

[127] Freeman, H., et al., "Therapeutic efficacy of delta-5–pregnenolone in rheumatoid arthritis," *J Am Med Assn,* 142(15) (1950): 1124–28.

[128] Pincus, G., et al., "Effects of administered pregnenolone on fatiguing psychomotor performance," *J Aviat Med,* 15 (1944): 98–115.

[129] Lee, J.R., et al., *What Your Doctor May Not Tell You About Menopause* (New York: Warner Books, Inc., 1996) 117–28.

[130] Martorano, J.T., et al., "Differentiating between natural progesterone and synthetic progestins: clinical implications for premenstrual syndrome and perimenopause management," *Compr Ther,* 24(6–7) (June–July 1998): 336–39.

[131] Chang, K.J., et al., "Influences of percutaneous administration of estradiol and progesterone on human breast epithelial cell cycle in vivo," *Fertil Steril,* 63(4) (April 1995): 785–91.

[132] Stanko, R.T., et al., "Enhancement of arm exercise endurance capacity with dihydroxyacetone and pyruvate," *J Apply Phys,* 68(1) (1990): 119–24.

[133] Stenko, R.T., et al., "Body composition, energy utilization, and nitrogen metabolism with a 4.25–MJ/d low-energy diet supplemented with pyruvate," *Am J Clin Nutr,* 56(4) (1992): 630–35.

[134] Bronner, C., Landry, Y., "Kinetics of the inhibitory effect of flavonoids on histamine secretion from mast cells," *Agents Actions,* 16 (1985): 147–51.

[135] Negre-Salvayre, A., et al., "Quercetin prevents the cytotoxicity of oxidized LDL on lymphoid cell lines," *Free Radic Biol Med,* 12(2) (1992): 101–06.

[136] Beyer-Mears, A., et al., "Diminished sugar cataractogenesis by quercetin," *Exp Eye Res,* 28(6) (June 1979): 709–16.

[137] Alarcon de la Lastra, C., et al., "Antiulcer and gastroprotective effects of quercetin: a gross and histologic study," *Pharmacology,* 48(1) (January 1994): 56–62.

[138] Loehrer, F.M., et al., "Low whole-blood S-adenosylmethionine and correlation between 5–methyltetrahydrofolate and homocysteine in coronary artery disease," *Arterioscler Thromb Vasc Biol,* 16(6) (June 1996): 727–33.

[139] Kagan, B.L., et al., "Oral S-adenosylmethionine in depression: a randomized, double-blind, placebo-controlled trial," *Am J Psychiatry,* 147(5) (May 1990): 591–95.

[140] Jacobsen, S., et al., "Oral S-adenosylmethionine in primary fibromyalgia. Double-blind clinical evaluation," *Scand J Rheumatol,* 20(4) (1991): 294–302.

[141] Sitaram, B.R., et al., "Nyctohemeral rhythm in the levels of S-adenosylmethionine in the rat pineal gland and its relationship to melatonin biosynthesis," *J Neurochem,* 65(4) (October 1995): 1887–94.

[142] Miglio, F., et al., "Double-blind studies of the therapeutic action of S-adenosylmethionine (SAMe) in oral administration, in liver cirrhosis and other chronic hepatitides," *Minerva Med,* 66(33) (May 2, 1975): 1595–99.

[143] Polli, E., et al., "Pharmacological and clinical aspects of S-adenosylmethionine (SAMe) in primary degenerative arthropathy," *Minerva Med,* 66(83) (December 5, 1975): 4443–59.

[144] di Padova, C., "S-adenosylmethionine in the treatment of osteoarthritis. Review of the clinical studies," *Am J Med,* 83(5A) (November 20, 1987): 60–65.

[145] Prudden, J.F., "The treatment of human cancer with agents prepared from bovine cartilage," *J Biol Response Mod,* 4(6) (December 1985): 551–84.

[146] Lane, I.W., et al., *Sharks Don't Get Cancer* (Garden City Park, New York: Avery Publishing Group, 1992) 110–18.

[147] Lane, I.W., et al., *Sharks Don't Get Cancer* (Garden City Park, New York: Avery Publishing Group, 1992) 107–10.

[148] Azuma, J., et al., "Therapy of congestive heart failure with orally administered taurine," *Clin Ther,* 5(4) (1983): 398–408.

[149] Franconi, F., et al., "Plasma and platelet taurine are reduced in subjects with insulin-dependent diabetes mellitus: effects of taurine supplementation," *Am J Clin Nutr,* 61(5) (May 1995): 1115–19.

[150] Fukuyama, Y., et al., "Therapeutic trial by taurine for intractable childhood epilepsies," *Brain Dev,* 4(1) (1982): 63–69.

[151] Fujita, T., et al., "Effects of increased adrenomedullary activity and taurine in young patients with borderline hypertension," *Circulation,* 75(3) (March 1987): 525–32.

[152] Kosmala, K., et al., "Pharmacological properties of the extract of thymus gland (Thymomodulin-TFX) and its effect on reproduction," *Acta Pol Pharm,* 50(6) (1993): 447–52.

[153] Haas, E., *Staying Healthy with Nutrition* (Berkeley, CA: Celestial Arts, 1992) 285.

[154] Meyer, J.S., et al., "Neurotransmitter precursor amino acids in the treatment of multi-infarct dementia and Alzheimer's disease," *J Am Ger Soc,* 7(1977): 289–98.

[155] Gelenberg, A.J., et al., "Tyrosine for the treatment of depression," *Nutr Health,* 3(3) (1984): 163–73.

[156] Rohr, F.J., et al., "Tyrosine supplementation in the treatment of maternal phenylketonuria," *Am J Clin Nutr,* 67(3) (March 1998): 473–76.

[157] Blum, K., et al., "Effects of catecholamine synthesis inhibition on ethanol-induced withdrawal symptoms in mice," *Br J Pharmacol,* 51(1) (May 1974): 109–11.

[158] Badmaev, V., et al., "Vanadium: a review of its potential role in the fight against diabetes," *J Altern Complement Med,* 5(3) (June 1999): 273–91.

[159] Boden, F., et al., "Effects of vanadyl sulfate on carbohydrate and lipid metabolism in patients with non-insulin-dependent diabetes mellitus," *Metabolism,* 45(9) (September 1996): 1130–35.

[160] Brignall, M.S., "Prevention and treatment of cancer with indole-3–carbinol," *Altern Med Rev,* 6(6) (December 2001): 580–9.

[161] Staub, E.E., et al., "Fate of indole-3–carbinol in cultured human breast tumor cells," *Chem Res Toxicol,* 15(2) (February 2002): 101–9.

Appendix 2—Herbal Reference Guide

[1] Ghoneum, M, et al., NK Immunomodulatory function in 27 cancer patients by MGN-3, a modified arabinoxylane from rice bran, *87th Annual Meeting of the American Association for Cancer Research,* (April 20–24, 1996), Washington, DC.

[2] Ghoneum, M., "Anti-HIV activity in vitro of MGN-3, an activated arabinoxylane from rice bran," *Biochem Biophys Res Commun,* 243(1) (February 1998): 25–9.

[3] Ghoneum, M., et al., "Effect of MGN-3 on human natural killer cell activity and interferon-γ synthesis in vitro," *FASEB JOURNAL,* (June 1996): 26.

[4] Kirchhoff, R., et al., "Increase in choleresis by means of artichoke extract," *Pytomedicine,* 1 (1994): 107–115.

[5] Khadzhai, I., et al., "Effect of artichoke extracts on the liver," *Farmakol Toksikol,* 34(6) (November 1971): 685–687.

[6] Maros, T., et al., "Effect of cynara scolymus-extracts on the regeneration of rat liver. 2," *Arzneimittelforschung,* 18(7) (July 1968): 884–886.

[7] Kirchhoff, R., et al., "Increase in choleresis by means of artichoke extract," *Pytomedicine,* 1 (1994): 107–115.

[8] DeSmet, P., et al., *Adverse Effects of Herbal Drugs 2* (Berlin, Springer-Verlag, 1993), 45.

[9] Grandhi, A., et al., "A comparative pharmacological investigation of ashwagandha and ginseng," *J Ethnopharmaco,* 44(3) (December 1994): 131–35.

[10] Ziauddin, M., et al., "Studies on the immunomodulatory effects of ashwagandha," *J Ethnopharmacol,* 50(2) (February 1996): 69–76.

[11] Kuttan, G., "Use of withania somnifera dunal as an adjuvant during radiation therapy," *Indian J Exp Biol,* 34(9) (September 1996): 854–56.

[12] Devi, P.U., et al., "Withaferin A: a new radiosensitizer from the Indian medicinal plant withania somnifera," *Int J Radiat Biol,* 69(2) (February 1996): 193–97.

[13] McGuffin, M., et al., *Botanical Safety Handbook* (Boca Raton, FL: CRC Press, 1997) 124.

[14] Chang, H., et al., *Pharmacology and Application of Chinese Materia Medica* (Singapore: Chinese University of Hong Kong, World Scientific, 1987) 4.

[15] Zhao, K.S., et al., "Enhancement of the immune response in mice by astragalus membranaceus extracts," *Immunopharmacology,* 20(3) (1990): 225–33.

[16] Geng, C.S., et al., "Advances in immuno-pharmacological studies on astragalus membranaceus," *Chung Hsi I Chieh Ho Tsa Chih,* 6(1) (1986): 62–64.

[17] Griga, I.V., "Effect of a summary preparation of astragalus cicer on the blood pressure of rats with renal hypertension and on the oxygen consumption by the tissues," *Farm Zh,* 6 (1977): 64–66.

[18] Kidd, P.M., pp. 144–61.

[19] Morazonni, P., et al., "Vaccinium myrtillus," *Fitoterapia,* vol. LXVII, no. 1 (1996): 3–29.

[20] Bottecchia, D., et al., "Vaccinium myrtillus," *Fitoterapia,* 48 (1977): 3–8.

[21] Morazzoni, P., et al., "Vaccinium myrtillus anthocyanosides pharmacokinetics in rats," *Arzneim-Forsch/Drug Res,* 41(2) (1991): 128–31.

[22] Leatherdale, B.A., et al., "Improvement in glucose tolerance due to momordica charantia (Karela)," *Br Med J,* (Clin Res Ed) 282(6279) (June 1981): 1823–1824.

[23] Welihinda, J., et al., "Effect of momordica charantia on the glucose tolerance in maturity onset diabetes," *J Ethnopharmacol,* 17(3) (September 1986): 277–282.

[24] Lee-Huang, S., et al., at pp. 151–156.

[25] Sarkar, S., et al., "Demonstration of the hypoglycemic action of momordica charantia in a validated animal model of diabetes," *Pharmacol Res,* 33(1) (January 1996): 1–4.

[26] Jarry, H., et al., "The endocrine effects of constituents of cimicifuga racemosa. 2. *In vitro* binding of constituents to estrogen receptors," *Planta Med,* 4 (August 1985): 316–19.

[27] Lieberman, S., "A review of the effectiveness of cimicifuga racemosa (black cohosh) for the symptoms of menopause," *J Womens Health,* 7(5) (June 1998): 525–529.

[28] Shibata, M., et al., "Pharmacological studies on the Chinese crude drug 'Shoma' III. Central depressant and antispasmodic actions of cimicifuga rhizoma, cimicifuga simplex wormsk," *Yakugaku Zasshi,* 100(11) (November 1980): 1143–50.

[29] Duker, E.M., et al., "Effects of extracts from cimicifuga racemose on gonadotropin release in menopausal women and ovariectomized rats," *Planta Med,* 57(5) (October 1991): 420–24.

[30] Duker, E.M., et al., "Effects of extracts from cimicifuga racemosa on gonadotropin release in menopausal women and ovariectomized rats," *Planta Med,* 57(5) (October 1991): 420–24.

[31] Taussig, S.I., "The mechanism of the physiological action in bromelain," *Med Hypoth,* 6 (1980): 99–104.

[32] Heinicke, R., et al., "Effect of bromelain (anase) on human platelet aggregation," *Experientia,* 28 (1972): 844–45.

[33] Petticrew, M., et al., "Systematic review of the effectiveness of laxatives in the elderly," *Health Technol Assess,* 1(13) (1997): 1–52.

[34] Bradley, P.R., ed., *British Herbal Compendium, vol. 1,* (Bournemouth: British Herbal Medicine Association, 1992) 52–54.

[35] Wagner, H., et al., "The alkaloids of uncaria tomentosa and their phagocytosis-stimulating action," *Planta Med,* 5 (1995): 419–23.

[36] Aquino, R., et al., "Plant metabolites. Structure and in vitro antiviral activity of quinovic acid glycosides from uncaria tomentosa and guettarda platypoda. *J Nat Prod,* 52(4) (1989): 679–85.

[37] Senatore, A., et al., "Phytochemical and biological study of uncaria tomentosa," *Boll Soc Ital Biol Sper,* 65(6) (1989): 517–20.

[38] Aquino, R., et al., "Plant metabolites. New compounds and anti-inflammatory activity of uncaria tomentosa," *J Nat Prod,* 54(2) (1981): 453–59.

[39] Aquino, R., et al., "New polyhydroxylated triterpenes from uncaria tomentosa," *J Nat Prod,* 53(3) (1990): 559–64.

[40] Aquino, R., et al., "New polyhydroxylated triterpenes from uncaria tomentosa," *J Nat Prod,* 53(3) (1990): 559–64.

[41] Haginiwa, J., et al., "Studies of plants containing indole alkaloids. 2. On the alkaloids of uncaria rhynchophylla miq," *Yakugaku Zasshi,* 93(4) (1973): 448–52.

[42] Newall, C.A., et al., *Herbal Medicines: A Guide for Health Care Professionals* (London: The Pharmaceutical Press, 1996) 28–30.

[43] Nagy, J.I., et al., "Fluoride-resistant acid phosphatase-containing neurones in dorsal root ganglia are separate from those containing substance P or somatostatin," *Neuroscience,* 7(1) (January 1982): 89–97.

[44] Magnusson, B.M., "Effects of topical application of capsaicin to human skin: a comparison of effects evaluated by visual assessment, sensation registration, skin blood flow and cutaneous impedance measurements," *Acta Derm Venereol,* 76(2) (March 1996): 129–132.

[45] Rains, C., et al., "Topical capsaicin. A review of its pharmacological properties and therapeutic potential in post-herpetic neuralgia, diabetic neuropathy and osteoarthritis," *Drugs Aging,* 7(4) (October 1995): 317–328.

[46] Newall, C.A., et al., *Herbal Medicines: A Guide for Health Care Professionals* (London: The Pharmaceutical Press, 1996) 60–61.

[47] Newall, C.A., et al., *Herbal Medicines: A Guide for Health Care Professionals* (London: The Pharmaceutical Press, 1996) 69–71.

[48] Snow, J.M., "Vitex agnus-castus L. (Verbenaceae)," *Protocol Journal of Botanical Medicine,* 1(4) (1996): 20–23.

[49] Amann, W., "Premenstrual water retention. Favorable effect of agnus castus (agnolyt) on premenstrual water retention," *ZFA* (Stuttgart), 55(1) (1979): 48–51.

[50] Milewicz, A., et al., "Vitex agnus castus extract in the treatment of luteal phase defects due to latent hyperprolactinemia. Results of a randomized placebo-controlled double-blind study. *Arzneim Forsch/Drug Res,* 43(7) (1993): 752–56.

[51] Sliutz, G., et al., "Agnus castus extracts inhibit prolactin secretion of rat pituitary cells," *Hormone and Metabolic Research,* 25 (1993): 253–55.

[52] Newall, C.A., et al., *Herbal Medicines: A Guide for Health Care Professionals* (London: The Pharmaceutical Press, 1996) 19–20.

[53] Baumann, G., et al., "Cardiovascular effects of forskolin (HL 362) in patients with idiopathic congestive cardiomyopathy - a comparative study with dobutamine and sodium nitroprusside. *Cardiovasc Pharmacol,* 16(1) (1990): 93–100.

[54] Kreutner, R.W., "Bronchodilator and antiallergy activity of forskolin," *European Journal of Pharmacology,* 111 (1985): 1–8.

[55] Ammon, H.P., et al., "Forskolin: from an Ayurvedic remedy to a modern agent," *Planta Medica,* 51 (1985): 473–77.

[56] Lindner, E., et al., "Positive inotropic and blood pressure lowering activity of a diterpene derivative isolated from coleus forskohli: forskolin," *Arzneim-Forsch/Drug Res,* 28 (1978): 284–89.

[57] Christenson, J.T., et al., "The effect of forskolin on blood flow, platelet metabolism, aggregation and ATP release," *Vasa,* 24(1) (1995): 56–61.

[58] Zhu, J., et al., "CordyMax Cs-4: A scientific product review," *Pharmanex Phytoscience Review Series,* 1997.

[59] Lei, J., et al., "Pharmacological study on cordyceps sinensis (Berk.) sacc. and ze-e cordyceps," *Chung Kuo Chung Yao Tsa Chih,* 17(6) (June 1992): 364–66.

[60] Bao, T.T., et al., "Pharmacological actions of cordyceps sinensis," *Chung Hsi I Chieh Ho Tsa Chih,* 8(6) (June 1988): 352–54.

[61] Sun, Y.H., "Cordyceps sinensis and cultured mycelia," *Chung Yao Tung Pao,* 10(12) (December 1985): 3–5.

[62] Chen, Y.P., "Studies on immunological actions of cordyceps sinensis. I. Effect on cellular immunity," *Chung Yao Tung Pao,* 8(5) (September 1983): 33–35.

[63] Xu, R.H., et al., "Effects of cordyceps sinensis on natural killer cell activity and colony formation of B16 melanoma," *Chinese Medical Journal,* 105 (1992): 97–101.

[64] Wan, F., et al., "Sex hormone-like effects of JinShiuBao capsule: pharmacology and clinical studies," *Chinese Traditional Patent Medicine,* 9 (1988): 29–31.

[65] Zhou, L.T., et al., "Short-term curative effect of cultured cordyceps sinensis mycelia in chronic hepatitis B," *China Journal of Chinese Materia Medica,* 115 (1990): 53–55.

[66] Hammerschmidt, D.E., "Szechwan purpura," *New England Journal of Medicine,* 302 (1980): 1191–1193.

[67] Xu, W.Z., et al., "Effects of cordyceps mycelia on monoamine oxidase and immunity," *Shanghai Journal of Traditional Chinese Medicine,* 1 (1988): 48–49.

[68] Newall, C.A., et al., at pp. 96–97.

[69] Racz-Kotilla, E., Racz, G., and Solomon, A., "The action of taraxacum officinale extracts on body weight and diuresis of laboratory animals," *Planta Med,* 26(1974): 212–17.

[70] McGuffin, M., et al., *Botanical Safety Handbook* (Boca Raton: CRC Press, 1997) 114.

[71] Bauer, R., "Echinacea drugs-effects and active ingredients," *Z Arztl Fortbild* (Jena), 90(2) (1996): 111–15.

[72] Luettig, B., et al., "Macrophage activation by the polysaccharide arabinogalactan isolated from plant cell cultures of echinacea purpurea," *Journal of the American Cancer Institute,* 81(9) (1989): 669–75.

[73] Bradley, P.R., ed., *British Herbal Compendium,* vol. 1 (Bournemouth: British Herbal Medicine Association, 1992) 81–83.

[74] Murray, M.T., "Echinacea: pharmacology and clinical applications," *American Journal of Natural Medicine,* 2 (1995): 18–24.

[75] Li Wan Po, A., "Evening primrose oil," *Pharm J,* 246 (1991): 670–76.

[76] Khoo, S.K., et al., "Evening primrose oil and treatment of premenstrual syndrome," *Med J Aust,* 153(4) (1990): 189–92.

[77] Miller, L.G., "Herbal medicinals: selected clinical considerations focusing on known or potential drug-herb interactions," *Arch Intern Med,* 158(20) (November 1998): 2200–11.

[78] De La Cruz, J.P., et al., "Effect of evening primrose oil on platelet aggregation in rabbits fed an atherogenic diet," *Thromb Res,* 87(1) (July 1997): 1414–19.

[79] Miller, L.G., "Herbal medicinals: selected clinical considerations focusing on known or potential drug-herb interactions," *Arch Intern Med,* 158(20) (November 1998): 2200–11.

[80] Johnson, E.S., et al., "Efficacy of feverfew as prophylactic treatment of migraine," *British Medical Journal,* 291 (1985): 569–73.

[81] Newall, C.A., et al., *Herbal Medicines: A Guide for Health Care Professionals* (London: The Pharmaceutical Press, 1996) 119–21.

[82] Makheja, A.N., et al., "A platelet phospholipase inhibitor from the medicinal herb feverfew (tanacetum parthenium)," *Prostaglandins Leukot Med,* 8(6) (June 1982): 653–60.

[83] Agarwal, K.C., "Therapeutic actions of garlic constituents," *Med Res Rev,* 16(1) (1996): 111–24.

[84] Steiner, M., et al., "A double-blind crossover study in moderately hypercholesterolemic men that compared the effect of aged garlic extract and placebo administration on blood lipids," *Am J Clin Nutr,* 64(6) (1996): 866–70.

[85] Bordia, A., et al., "Effect of garlic (allium sativum) on blood lipids, blood sugar, fibrinogen and fibrinolytic activity in patients with coronary artery disease," *Prostaglandins Leukot Essent Fatty Acids,* 58(4) (April 1998): 257–63.

[86] Adetumbi, M., et al., "Allium sativum (garlic)-a natural antibiotic," *Med Hypoth,* 12 (1983): 227–37.

[87] Pai, S.T., et al., "Antifungal effects of allium sativum (garlic) extract against the aspergillus species involved in otomycosis," *Lett Appl Microbiol,* 20(1) (1995): 14–18.

[88] Le Bars, P.L., et al., "A placebo-controlled, double-blind, randomized trial of an extract of ginkgo biloba for dementia, North American EGb Study Group," *JAMA,* 278(16) (October 1997): 1327–32.

[89] Kleijnen, J., et al., "Ginkgo biloba," *Lancet,* 340(8828) (1992): 1136–39.

[90] Odawara, M., et al., "Ginkgo biloba," *Neurology,* 48(3) (March 1997): 789–90.

[91] Skogh, M., "Extracts of ginkgo biloba and bleeding or haemorrhage," *Lancet,* 352(9134) (October 1998): 1145–46.

[92] Vale, S., "Subarachnoid haemorrhage associated with ginkgo biloba," *Lancet,* 352(9121) (July 1998): 36.

[93] Grontved, A., et al., "Ginger root against seasickness. A controlled trial on the open sea," *Acta Otolaryngol* (Stockh), 105(1–2) (1998): 45–9.

[94] Bone, M.E., et al., "Ginger root-A new antiemetic. The effect of ginger root on postoperative nausea and vomiting after major gynaecological surgery," *Anaesthesia,* 45(8) (1990): 669–71.

[95] Chong, S.K., et al., "Ginseng-Is there a use in clinical medicine?" *Postgrad Med J,* 64(757) (November 1988): 841–46.

[96] Kim, J.Y., et al., "Panax ginseng as a potential immunomodulator: studies in mice," *Immunopharmacol Immunotoxicol,* 12(2) (1990): 257–76.

[97] Siegel, R.K., "Ginseng and high blood pressure," *JAMA,* 243(1) (January 1980): 32.

[98] Teng, C.M., et al., "Antiplatelet actions of panaxynol and ginsenosides isolated from ginseng," *Biochim Biophys Acta,* 990(3) (March 1989): 315–20.

[99] Janetzky, K., et al., "Probable interaction between warfarin and ginseng," *Am J Health Syst Pharm,* 54(6) (March 1997): 692–93.

[100] Jones, B.D., et al., "Interaction of ginseng with phenelzine," *J Clin Psychopharmacol,* 7(3) (June 1987): 201–02.

[101] Dukes, M.N., "Ginseng and mastalgia," *Br Med J,* 1(6127) (June 1978): 1621.

[102] Hopkins, M.P., et al., "Ginseng face cream and unexplained vaginal bleeding," *Am J Obstet Gynecol,* 59(5) (November 1988): 1121–22.

[103] Brekhman, I.I., et al., "Eleutherococcus-a means of increasing the nonspecific resistance of the organism," *Izv Akad Nauk SSSR* [Biol], 5 (1965): 762–65.

[104] Brekhman, I.I., et al., "Effect of eleutherococcus on alarm-phase of stress," *Life Sci,* 8(3) (1969): 113–21.

[105] Hikino, H., et al., "Isolation and hypoglycemic activity of eleutherans A, B, C, D, E, F and G: glycans of eleutherococcus senticosus roots," *J Nat Prod,* 49(2) (1986): 293–97.

[106] McRae, S., "Elevated serum digoxin levels in a patient taking digoxin and Siberian ginseng," *CMAJ,* 155(3) (August 1996): 293–95.

[107] Medon, P.J., et al., "Effects of eleutherococcus senticosus extracts on hexobarbital metabolism in vivo and in vitro," *J Ethnopharmacol,* 10(2) (April 1984): 235–41.

[108] Newall, C.A., et al., *Herbal Medicines: A Guide for Health Care Professionals* (London, England; The Pharmaceutical Press, 1996) 151–52.

[109] Sabir, M., et al., "Study of some pharmacological actions of berberine," *Indian J Physiol Pharmacol,* 15(3) (1971): 111–32.

[110] Maffei Facino, R., et al., "Regeneration of endogenous antioxidants, ascorbic acid, alpha tocopherol, by the oligomeric procyanide fraction of vitus vinifera L:ESR study. *Boll Chim Farm,* 136(4) (1997): 340–44.

[111] Jonadet, M., et al., "Anthocyanosides extracted from vitis vinifera, vaccinium myrtillus and pinus maritimus. I. Elastase-inhibiting activities in vitro. II. Compared angioprotective activities in vivo," *J Pharm Belg,* 38(1) (1983): 41–46.

[112] Frankel, E.N., et al., "Inhibition of oxidation of human low-density lipoprotein by phenolic substances in red wine," *Lancet,* 341(8843) (1993): 454–57.

[113] Yokozawa, T., et al., "Influence of green tea and its three major components upon low-density lipoprotein oxidation," *Exp Toxicol Pathol,* 49(5) (December 1997): 329–35.

[114] Stoner, G.D., et al., "Polyphenols as cancer chemopreventive agents," *J Cell Biochem*, (Suppl 22) (1995): 169–80.

[115] Mitscher, L.A., et al., "Chemoprotection: a review of the potential therapeutic antioxidant properties of green tea (camellia sinensis) and certain of its constituents," *Med Res Rev*, 17(4) (July 1997): 327–65.

[116] Yang, T.T., et al., "Hypocholesterolemic effects of Chinese tea," *Pharmacol Res*, 35(6) (June 1997): 505–12.

[117] Sagesaka-Mitane, Y., et al., "Platelet aggregation inhibitors in hot water extract of green tea," *Chem Pharm Bull* (Tokyo), 38(3) (March 1990): 790–93.

[118] Snow, J., "Camellia sinensis (L.) Kuntze (Theaceae)," *Protocol Journal of Botanical Medicine*, Autumn (1995): 47–51.

[119] Singh, R.B., et al., "Hypolipidemic and antioxidant effects of commiphora mukul as an adjunct to dietary therapy in patients with hypercholesterolemia," *Cardiovasc Drugs Ther*, 8(4) (1994): 659–664.

[120] Nityanand, S., et al., Clinical trials with gugulipid. A new hypolipidaemic agent," *J Assoc Physicians India*, 37(5) (1989): 323–328.

[121] Agarwal, R.C., et al., "Clinical trial of gugulipid-a new hypolipidemic agent of plant origin in primary hyperlipidemia," *Indian J Med Res*, 84 (1986): 626–634.

[122] Satyavati, G.V., et al., "Guggulipid: a promising hypolipidemic agent from gum guggul (commiphora wightii)," *Econ Med Plant Res*, 5 (1991): 48–82.

[123] Dalvi, S.S., et al., "Effects of gugulipid on bioavailability of diltiazem and propranolol," *J Assoc Physicians India*, 42(6) (1994): 454–55.

[124] Baskaran, K., et al., "Antidiabetic effect of a leaf extract from gymnema sylvestre in non-insulin-dependent diabetes mellitus patients," *J Ethnopharmacol*, 30(3) (October 1990): 295–300.

[125] Schussler, M., et al., "Myocardial effects of flavonoids from crataegus species," *Arzneimittelforschung*, 45(8) (August 1995): 842–45.

[126] Weihmayr, T., et al., "Therapeutic effectiveness of crataegus," *Fortschr Med*, 114(1–2) (January 1996): 27–29.

[127] McGuffin, M., et al., *Botanical Safety Handbook* (Boca Raton: CRC Press, 1997) 37.

[128] Singh, S., "Mechanism of action of anti-inflammatory effect of fixed oil of *ocimum basilicum linn*," *Indian J Exp Biol*, 37(3) (March 1999): 248–52.

[129] Kelm, M.A., et al., "Antioxidant and cyclooxygenase inhibitory phenolic compounds from *ocimum sanctum linn*," *Phytomedicine*, 7(1) (March 2000): 7–13.

[130] Sembulingam, K., et al., "Effect of *ocimum sanctum linn* on noise-induced changes in plasma corticosterone level," *Indian J Physiol Pharmacol*, 41(2) (1997): 139–43.

[131] Wohlfart, R., et al., "Detection of sedative-hypnotic active ingredients in hops. Degradation of bitter acids to 2-methyl-3-buten-2-ol, a hop constituent with sedative-hypnotic activity," *Arch Pharm* (Weinheim), 316(2) (1983): 132–7.

[132] Hansel, R., et al., "Sedative-hypnotic compounds in the exhalation of hops, II," *Z Naturforsch* [C], 35(11–12) (December 1980): 1096–7.

[133] Lee, K.M., et al., "Effects of humulus lupulus extract on the central nervous system in mice," *Planta Medica*, 59 (Suppl.) (1993): A691.

[134] Pittler, M.H., et al., "Horse-chestnut seed extract for chronic venous insufficiency. A criteria-based systematic review," *Arch Dermatol*, 134(11) (November 1998): 1356–60.

[135] Simini, B., "Horse-chestnut seed extract for chronic venous insufficiency," *Lancet*, 347(9009) (April 1996): 1182–83.

[136] Skogh, M., "Extracts of ginkgo biloba and bleeding or haemorrhage," *Lancet*, 352(9134) (October 1998): 1145–46.

[137] Vale, S., "Subarachnoid haemorrhage associated with ginkgo biloba," *Lancet,* 352(9121) (July 1998): 36.

[138] Urbaniuk, K.G., et al., "The anticoagulant action of horse chestnut and eskuzan," *Klin Med (Mosk),* 45(2) (February 1967): 129–33.

[139] Tiktinskii, O.L., et al., "Therapeutic action of java tea and field horsetail in uric acid diathesis," *Urol Nefrol* (Mosk), (1) (1993): 47–50.

[140] Meyer, P., "Thiaminase activities and thiamine content of pteridium aquilinum, equisetum ramo-sissimum, malva parviflora, pennisetum clandestinum and medicago sativa," *Onderstepoort J Vet Res,* 56(2) (June 1989): 145–46.

[141] Intentionally deleted.

[142] Intentionally deleted.

[143] Singh, Y.N., "Kava: an overview," *J Ethnopharmacol,* 37(1) (1992): 13–45.

[144] Davies, L.P., "Kava pyrones and resin: studies on $GABA_A$, $GABA_B$ and benzodiazepine binding sites in rodent brain," *Pharmacol Toxicol,* 71(2) (1992): 120–26.

[145–147] Intentionally omitted.

[148] Jamieson, D.D., et al., "Positive interaction of ethanol and kava resin in mice," *Clin Exp Pharmacol Physiol,* 17(7) (July 1990): 509–14.

[149] Herberg, K.W., "Effect of kava-special extract WS 1490 combined with ethyl alcohol on safety-relevant performance parameters," *Blutalkohol,* 30(2) (March 1993): 96–105.

[150] Schelosky, L., et al., "Kava and dopamine antagonism," *J Neurol Neurosurg Psychiatry,* 58(5) (May 1995): 639–40.

[151] Davis, E.A., et al., "Medicinal uses of licorice through the millennia: the good and plenty of it," *Mol Cell Endocrinol,* 78(1–2) (June 1991): 1–6.

[152] Newall, C.A., et al., *Herbal Medicines: A Guide for Health Care Professionals* (London, England: The Pharmaceutical Press, 1996): 183–86.

[153] Dehpour, A.R., et al., "The protective effect of liquorice components and their derivatives against gastric ulcer induced by aspirin in rats," *J Pharm Pharmacol* 46(2) (February 1994): 148–49.

[154] Balakrishnan, V., et al., "Deglycyrrhizinated liquorice in the treatment of chronic duodenal ulcer," *J Assoc Physicians India,* 26(9) (September 1978): 811–4.

[155] de Klerk, G.J., et al., "Hypokalaemia and hypertension associated with use of liquorice flavoured chewing gum," *BMJ,* 314(7082) (March 1997): 731–32.

[156] de Klerk, G.J., et al., "Hypokalaemia and hypertension associated with use of liquorice flavoured chewing gum," *BMJ,* 314(7082) (March 1997): 731–32.

[157] Stormer, F.C., et al., "Glycyrrhizic acid in liquorice-evaluation of health hazard," *Food Chem Toxicol,* 31(4) (April 1993): 303–12.

[158] Carrescia, O., et al., "Silymarin in the prevention of hepatic damage by psychopharmacologic drugs. Experimental premises and clinical evaluations," *Clin Ter,* 95(2) (1980): 157–64.

[159] Flora, K., et al., "Milk thistle (silybum marianum) for the therapy of liver disease," *Am J Gastroenterol,* 93(2) (1998): 139–43.

[160] Kropacova, K., et al., "Protective and therapeutic effect of silymarin on the development of latent liver damage," *Radiats Biol Radioecol,* 38(3) (May 1998): 411–15.

[161] Morazzoni, P., et al., "Silybum marianum," *Fitoterapia,* 66 (1995): 3–42.

[162] Vogel, G., et al., "Protection by silibinin against amanita phalloides intoxication in beagles," *Toxicol Appl Pharm,* 73 (1984): 355–62.

[163] Desplaces, A., et al., "The effects of silymarin on experimental phalloidine poisoning," *Arzneim-Forsch/Drug Res,* 25 (1975): 89–96.

[164] Gonzalez, M., et al., "Hypoglycemic activity of olive leaf," *Planta Med,* 58(6) (December 1992): 513–5.

[165] Fehri, B., et al., "Hypotension, hypoglycemia and hypouricemia recorded after repeated administration of aqueous leaf extract of olea europaea L," *J Pharm Belg,* 49(2) (March–April 1994): 101–8.

[166] Wolfman, C., et al., "Possible anxiolytic effects of chrysin, a central benzodiazepine receptor ligand isolated from passiflora coerulea," *Pharmacol Biochem Behav,* 47(1) (January 1994): 1–4.

[167] Spreoni, E., et al., at pp. 488–491.

[168] Aoyagi, N., et al., "Studies on passiflora incarnata dry extract, isolation of maltol and pharmacological action of maltol and ethyl maltol," *Chem Pharm Bull* (Tokyo), 22(5) (May 1974): 1008–13.

[169] Jong, S.C., et al., "Medicinal benefits of the mushroom ganoderma," *Adv Appl Microbiol,* 37 (1992): 101–34.

[170] Tao, J., et al., "Experimental and clinical studies on inhibitory effect of ganoderma lucidum on platelet aggregation," *J Tongii Med Unive,* 10(4) (1990): 240–43.

[171] Sufka, K.J., Roach, J.T., Chambliss, W.G., Jr., et al., "Anxiolytic properties of botanical extracts in the chick social separation-stress procedure," *Psychopharmacology* (Berl), 53(2) (2000): 219–24.

[172] Rege, N.N., et al., "Adaptogenic properties of six rasayana herbs used in Ayurvedic medicine," *Phytother Res,* 13(4) (June 1999): 275–91.

[173] Lishmanov, Iu.B., et al., "Contribution of the opioid system to realization of inotropic effects of rhodiola rosea extracts in ischemic and reperfusion heart damage in vitro," *Eksp Klin Farmakol,* 60(3) (May–June 1997): 34–36.

[174] Al-Sereiti, M.R., et al., "Pharmacology of rosemary (rosmarinus officinalis linn.) and its therapeutic potentials," *Indian J Exp Biol,* 37(2) (February 1999): 124–30.

[175] Kelm, M.A., et al., "Antioxidant and cyclooxygenase inhibitory phenolic compounds from ocimum sanctum linn," *Phytomedicine,* 7(1) (March 2000): 7–13.

[176] Plosker, G.L., et al., "Serenoa repens (permixon). A review of its pharmacology and therapeutic efficacy in benign prostatic hyperplasia," *Drugs Aging,* 9(5) (196): 379–95.

[177] Strauch, G., et al., "Comparison of finasteride (proscar) and serenoa repens (permixon) in the inhibition of 5-alpha reductase in healthy male volunteers," *European Urology,* 26 (1994): 247–52.

[178] Braeckman, J., "The extract of serenoa repens in the treatment of benign prostatic hyperplasia: a multicenter open study," *Curr Ther Res,* 55(7) (1994): 76–84.

[179] Yamada, S., et al., "Preventive effect of gomisin A, a lignan component of shizandra fruits, on acetaminophen-induced hepatotoxicity in rats," *Biochem Pharmacol,* 46(6) (September 1993): 1081–85.

[180] Liu, G.T., "Pharmacological actions and clinical use of fructus schizandrae," *Chin Med J* (Engl), 102(10) (October 1989): 740–49.

[181] Lin, T.J., "Antioxidation mechanism of schizandrin and tanshinonatic acid A and their effects on the protection of cardiotoxic action of adriamycin," *Sheng Li Ko Hsueh Chin Chan,* 22(4) (October 1991): 342–45.

[182] Liu, G.T., "Pharmacological actions and clinical use of fructus schizandrae," *Chin Med J* (Engl), 102(10) (October 1989): 740–49.

[183] Newall, C.A., et al., *Herbal Medicines: A Guide for Health Care Professionals* (London: The Pharmaceutical Press, 1996) 243–244.

[184] Bradley, P.R., ed., *British Herbal Compendium, vol. 1* (Bournemouth: British herbal Medicine Association, 1992) 52–54.

[185] Wang, G.L., et al., "The immunomodulatory effect of lentinan," *Yao Hsueh Hsueh Pao,* 31(2) (1996): 86–90.

[186] Tochikura, T.S., et al., "Antiviral agents with activity against human retroviruses," *J Acquir Immune Defic Syndr,* 2(5) (1989): 441–47.

[187] Chihara, G., et al., "Fractionation and purification of the polysaccharides with marked antitumor activity, especially lentinan, from lentinus edodes (berk.) Sing. (An edible mushroom)," *Cancer Res,* 30(11) (November 1970): 2776–81.

[188] Murkies, A.L., et al., "Dietary flour supplementation decreases post-menopausal hot flushes: effect of soy and wheat," *Maturitas,* 21 (1995): 189.

[189] Cott, J.M., et al., "Is St. John's wort (hypericum perforatum) an effective antidepressant?" *J Nerv Ment Dis,* 186(8) (August 1998): 500–01.

[190] Hippius, H., "St John's wort (hypericum perforatum)—an herbal antidepressant," *Curr Med Res Opin,* 14(3) (1998): 171–84.

[191] Volz, H.P., "Controlled clinical trials of hypericum extracts in depressed patients-an overview," *Pharmacopsychiatry,* 30 (Suppl 2) (1997): 72–76.

[192] Miller, A.L., "St. John's wort (hypericum perforatum): clinical effects on depression and other conditions," *Altern Med Rev,* 3(1) (February 1998): 18–26.

[193] Chatterjee, S.S., et al., "Hyperforin as a possible antidepressant component of hypericum extracts," *Life Sci,* 63(6) (1998): 499–510.

[194] Bennett, D.A., Jr, et al., "Neuropharmacology of St. John's wort," *Ann Pharmacother,* 32(11) (November 1998): 1201–08.

[195] Nebel, A., et al., "Potential metabolic interaction between St. John's wort and theophylline," *Ann Pharmacother,* 33(4) (April 1999): 502.

[196] Johne, A., et al., "Pharmacokinetic interaction of digoxin with an herbal extract from St John's wort (hypericum perforatum)," *Clin Pharmacol Ther,* 66(4) (October 1999): 338–45.

[197] Piscitelli, S.C., et al., "Indinavir concentrations and St. John's wort," *Lancet,* 355 (9203) (February 2000): 547–48.

[198] Rey, J.M., et al., "Hypericum perforatum (St John's wort) in depression: pest or blessing?" *Med J Aust,* 169(11–12) (December 1998): 583–86.

[199] Rey, J.M., et al., "Hypericum perforatum (St John's wort) in depression: pest or blessing?" *Med J Aust,* 169(11–12) (December 1998): 583–86.

[200] Piscitelli, S.C., et al., "Indinavir concentrations and St. John's wort," *Lancet,* 355 (9203) (February 2000): 547–48

[201] Brockmoller, J., et al., "Hypericin and pseudohypericin: pharmacokinetics and effects of photosensitivity in humans," *Pharmacopsychiatry,* 30 (Suppl 2) (1990): 94–101.

[202] Brockmoller, J., et al., "Hypericin and pseudohypericin: pharmacokinetics and effects on photosensitivity in humans," *Pharmacopsychiatry,* 30 (Suppl 2) (September 1997): 94–101.

[203] Carson, C.F., et al., "Efficacy and safety of tea tree oil as a topical antimicrobial agent," *J Hosp Infect,* 40(3) (November 1998): 175–8.

[204] Concha, J.M., et al., "Antifungal activity of melaleuca alternifolia (tea-tree) oil against various pathogenic organisms,"*J Am Podiatr Med Assoc,* 88(10) (October 1998): 489–92.

[205] Rubel, D.M., et al., "Tea tree oil allergy: what is the offending agent? Report of three cases of tea tree oil allergy and review of the literature," *Australas J Dermatol,* 39(4) (November 1998): 244–47.

[206] Ammon, H.P., et al., "Mechanism of anti-inflammatory actions of curcumin and boswellic acids," *J Ethnopharmacol,* 38 (1993): 113.

[207] Ammon, H.P., et al., "Pharmacology of curcuma longa," *Planta Med,* 57(1) (February 1991): 1–7.

[208] Srivastava, K.C., et al., "Curcumin, a major component of food spice turmeric (curcuma longa) inhibits aggregation and alters eicosanoid metabolism in human blood platelets," *Prostaglandins Leukot Essent Fatty Acids,* 52(4) (April 1995): 223–27.

[209] Snow, J.M., "Curcuma Longa L. (Zingiberaceae)," *Protocol Journal of Botanical Medicine,* 1(2) (Autumn 1995): 43–46.

210 Houghton, P.J., "The biological activity of valerian and related plants," *J Ethnopharmacol* 22(2) (1988): 121–42.

211 Balderer, G., et al., "Effect of valerian on human sleep,"*Psychopharmacology,* 87 (1985): 406–09.

212 "Valerianae radix," *German Commission E Monograph,* May 15, 1985, Bundesanzeiger, no. 90.

213 Hendriks, H., et al., "Central nervous depressant activity of valerenic acid in the mouse," *Planta Med,* (1) (February 1985): 28–31.

Index